Handbook of
RENAL
THERAPEUTICS

Handbook of
RENAL
THERAPEUTICS

Edited by
Manuel Martínez-Maldonado

Veterans Administration Hospital
and University of Puerto Rico School of Medicine
San Juan, Puerto Rico

PLENUM MEDICAL BOOK COMPANY
New York and London

Library of Congress Cataloging in Publication Data

Main entry under title:

Handbook of renal therapeutics:

  Includes bibliographical references and index.
  1. Kidneys—Diseases—Treatment—Handbooks, manuals, etc. I. Martínez-
Maldonado, Manuel.
RC903.H36 1983   616.6′106   82-24516
ISBN 0-306-41096-6

Notice: The indications and dosages of all drugs in this book are essentially those recommended in the medical literature. They are also those utilized by the general medical community. The usages recommended by the Food and Drug Administration (FDA) should be obtained from the package insert of each drug. In the *Handbook* the indications and uses of some drugs do not always conform to the FDA recommendations. The readers and users of the *Handbook* are urged to consult references on drug dosage and uses to keep abreast of revised recommendations or changes regarding new or old drugs.

©1983 Plenum Publishing Corporation
233 Spring Street, New York, N.Y. 10013

Plenum Medical Book Company is an imprint of Plenum Publishing Corporation

Printed in the United States of America

To Nivia, Manuel, David, Ricardo, and Pablo

Contributors

GERALD B. APPEL, M.D., Medical Director, Hemodialysis Unit, Columbia Presbyterian Medical Center and Departments of Pharmacology and Medicine, Divisions of Nephrology and Infectious Diseases, College of Physicians and Surgeons, Columbia University, New York, New York 10032

THOMAS R. BECK, M.D., Assistant Professor, Department of Medicine, Temple University Health Sciences Center, Philadelphia, Pennsylvania 19140

D. CRAIG BRATER, M.D., Assistant Professor, Departments of Pharmacology and Internal Medicine, Southwestern Medical School at the University of Texas Health Science Center at Dallas, Dallas, Texas 75235

JACK W. COBURN, M.D., Director, Research and Training Program in Nephrology, Veterans Administration Wadsworth Medical Center; and Professor, Department of Medicine, UCLA School of Medicine, Los Angeles, California 90024

CECIL H. COGGINS, M.D., Associate Professor, Department of Medicine, Harvard Medical School; and Associate Physician, Renal Unit, Massachusetts General Hospital, Boston, Massachusetts 02114

ALLAN J. COLLINS, M.D., Assistant Professor, Department of Medicine, University of Minnesota Medical School; and Director, Renal Intensive Care Unit, Regional Kidney Disease Program, Hennepin County Medical Center, Minneapolis, Minnesota 55415

RALPH A. DeFRONZO, M.D., Associate Professor, Department of Internal Medicine, Renal Division, Yale University School of Medicine, New Haven, Connecticut 06510

GARABED EKNOYAN, M.D., Professor, Department of Medicine, Renal Section, Baylor College of Medicine, Houston, Texas 77030

THOMAS F. FERRIS, M.D., Professor and Chairman, Department of Internal Medicine, University of Minnesota, Minneapolis, Minnesota 55455

LINDA L. FRANCISCO, M.D., Assistant Professor, Department of Internal Medicine, University of Minnesota, Minneapolis, Minnesota 55455

ALFREDO GARCÍA, M.D., Clinical Instructor, Medical Service, Veterans Administration Hospital, San Juan, Puerto Rico 00936; and Department of Internal Medicine, University of Puerto Rico School of Medicine, San Juan, Puerto Rico 00931.

HANS J. GLOOR, M.D., Fellow, Division of Nephrology, Department of Medicine, University of Missouri Health Sciences Center; and Harry S. Truman Memorial Veterans Hospital, Columbia, Missouri 65211; present address: Kantonsspital Schaffhausen, Geissberg, Switzerland

EDWARD R. JONES, M.D., Assistant Professor, Departments of Medicine and Physiology, Temple University Health Sciences Center, Philadelphia, Pennsylvania 19140

CARL M. KJELLSTRAND, M.D., Professor, Departments of Medicine and Surgery, University of Minnesota Medical School; and Department of Medicine, Regional Kidney Disease Program, Hennepin County Medical Center, Minneapolis, Minnesota 55415

JAMES P. KNOCHEL, M.D., Chief, Medical Service, Veterans Administration Medical Center, Dallas, Texas 75216; and Professor and Vice-Chairman, Department of Internal Medicine, Southwestern Medical School at the University of Texas Health Science Center at Dallas, Dallas, Texas 75235

MANUEL MARTÍNEZ-MALDONADO, M.D., Chief, Medical Service, Veterans Administration Hospital, San Juan, Puerto Rico 00936; and Departments of Internal Medicine and Physiology, University of Puerto Rico School of Medicine, San Juan, Puerto Rico 00931

EDWIN MEJÍAS, M.D., Chief, Rheumatology Section, Assistant Professor, Department of Internal Medicine, Veterans Administration Hospital, San Juan, Puerto Rico 00936

WILLIAM E. MITCH, M.D., Associate Professor, Department of Medicine, Harvard Medical School; and Brigham and Women's Hospital, Boston, Massachusetts 02115

ROBERT G. NARINS, M.D., Chief, Renal Division, Professor, Department of Medicine, Temple University Health Sciences Center, Philadelphia, Pennsylvania 19140

HAROLD C. NEU, M.D., Chief, Division Infectious Diseases, Columbia Presbyterian Medical Center; and Departments of Pharmacology and Medicine, Divisions of Nephrology and Infectious Diseases, College of Physicians and Surgeons, Columbia University, New York, New York 10032

KARL D. NOLPH, M.D., Director, Division of Nephrology, and Professor, Department of Medicine, University of Missouri Health Sciences Center; and Harry S. Truman Memorial Veterans Hospital, Columbia, Missouri 65211

CHARLES Y. C. PAK, M.D., Professor, Department of Internal Medicine, Section of Mineral Metabolism, Southwestern Medical School at the University of Texas Health Science Center at Dallas, Dallas, Texas 75235

CESAR E. PRU, M.D., Medical Associate, Nephrology and Renal Transplant Unit, University Hospital, Caracas, Venezuela

C. VENKATA S. RAM, M.D., Assistant Professor, Department of Internal Medicine, Southwestern Medical School at the University of Texas Health Science Center at Dallas, Dallas, Texas 75235; and St. Paul Hospital, Dallas, Texas 75235

K. VENKATESWARA RAO, M.D., Assistant Professor, Department of Medicine, University of Minnesota Medical School; and Department of Nephrology, Regional Kidney Disease Program, Hennepin County Medical Center, Minneapolis, Minnesota 55415

EDUARDO SLATOPOLSKY, M.D., Professor, Department of Medicine, Washington University School of Medicine; Attending Physician, Renal Division, Barnes Hospital; and Director, Chromalloy American Kidney Center, St. Louis, Missouri 63110

MARY C. STOM, M.D., Assistant Professor, Department of Medicine, Temple University Health Sciences Center, Philadelphia, Pennsylvania 19140

SAMUEL O. THIER, M.D., Sterling Professor and Chairman, Department of Internal Medicine, Yale University School of Medicine, New Haven, Connecticut 06510

Preface

This book started out as a "Manual." The idea was to offer straightforward instruction on how to handle patients in whom renal function is altered by intrinsic as well as systemic or extrarenal disease. While we have attempted to provide simple approaches to most conditions, we have gone beyond that and offer here more detailed description of pathophysiology, diagnosis and therapy. Thus, the "Manual" has become a *Handbook*. In so doing we hope we have widened the audience for which the book may be useful. As it now stands, we envision that students, house staff, nephrology trainees, nephrologists, primary-care physicians, and nurses of specialized units, interested in kidney-related disturbances and in alterations of the composition of the extracellular fluid, will benefit from reading the *Handbook*.

While providing a rational background for the treatments outlined, each author has attempted to narrate the reasons why such therapy is utilized. Frequently, the information is provided in tables and figures to which ready reference can be made. The flow-chart approach has also been utilized to illustrate pathophysiological sequence or steps in therapy. In most instances, the discussion of pathophysiology has been limited to what is widely accepted rather than treading into anything controversial, unless the nature of the problem or the nature of our knowledge is ambiguous.

The chapters are grouped by types of disturbances and by clinical conditions to make it easy to find information which can be applied to actual patients. The treatment of each condition has been highlighted for practical purposes.

The authors have had extensive experience in the fields which they cover. This experience comes, not only from practical knowledge, but also from their contributions to clinical investigation in each area.

Their approach to each subject has been to make information as readily accessible as possible. In this way, the *Handbook* can be consulted for bedside use with speed and efficiency.

I would like to thank the contributors and Anna Carmen Rivera, my outstanding secretary, for making this *Handbook* possible.

Manuel Martínez-Maldonado

San Juan, Puerto Rico

Contents

Chapter 13. Management of Hypertension: Management of Essential and Secondary Hypertension 263
C. Venkata S. Ram

Chapter 14. Management of Hypertension: Hypertensive Emergencies 301
C. Venkata S. Ram

Chapter 17. Diagnosis and Therapy of Nephrolithiasis 375
Charles Y. C. Pak

Chapter 18. Bone and Mineral Disturbances in Renal Insufficiency 397
Eduardo Slatopolsky and Jack W. Coburn

Chapter 19. Therapy of the Acute Renal Failure Syndrome 425
Garabed Eknoyan

Fluid and Electrolyte Disturbances
Hypo- and Hypernatremia

RALPH A. DeFRONZO and SAMUEL O. THIER

I. NORMAL PHYSIOLOGY OF URINARY DILUTION

The treatment of hyponatremia (serum sodium concentration less than 135 mEq/liter) is critically dependent on establishing the correct diagnosis. Fortunately, both the diagnosis and approach to therapy rest firmly on physiological principles. The presence of low serum sodium concentration indicates an excess of water relative to sodium and can occur in the face of increased, normal, or decreased total body sodium content. To maintain a normal serum sodium concentration, it is necessary for the kidney to excrete an amount of free water that is equal to the free water intake (minus insensible losses, about 400 ml/day). Therefore, to understand the pathophysiology of hyponatremia, it is important to review briefly free water generation by the kidney.

Normal urinary dilution depends on three factors (Fig. 1): (1) adequate delivery of solute to the distal diluting sites (ascending loop of Henle and early distal tubule); (2) functional intactness of the distal diluting sites so that sodium, along with chloride, can be removed at a point where the tubule is impermeable to water, thereby generating free water; and (3) suppression of antidiuretic hormone (ADH) so that any free water generated by the distal diluting sites will not be reabsorbed by the collecting duct.

Adequate sodium delivery to the distal nephron is in turn also dependent on three factors (Fig. 1, sites 1A, 1B, 1C): (1) adequate renal plasma flow;

RALPH A. DeFRONZO and SAMUEL O. THIER • Department of Internal Medicine, Renal Division, Yale University School of Medicine, New Haven, Connecticut 06510.

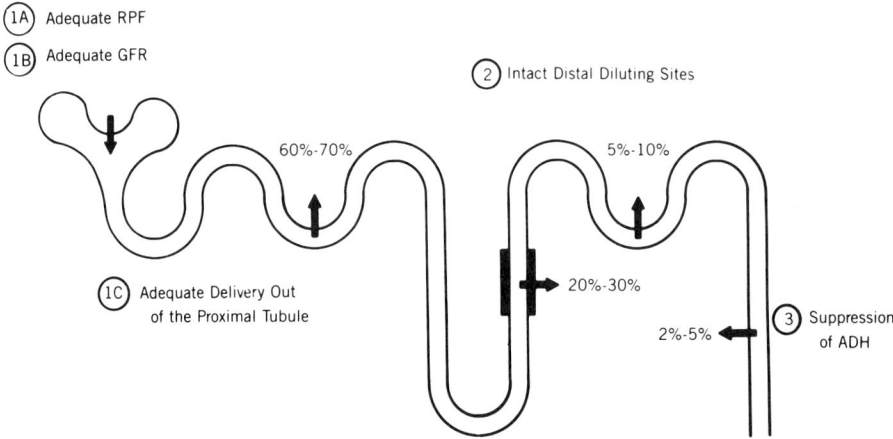

Figure 1. Free water generation. To excrete a water load normally (1A,B,C,), there must be adequate delivery of salt and water to the thick ascending limb of Henle and early distal tubule; (2) these distal diluting sites must be functionally intact so that sodium can be removed without water; and (3) there must be suppression of antidiuretic hormone (ADH) so that free water generated at distal diluting sites is not reabsorbed by collecting duct. Arrows indicate relative amounts of sodium that are reabsorbed in proximal tubule, loop of Henle, distal tubule, and collecting duct; RPF, renal plasma flow; GFR, glomerular filtration rate.

(2) adequate glomerular filtration rate (GFR); and (3) adequate delivery of sodium and chloride out of the proximal tubule. A decrease in renal plasma flow (RPF) (Fig. 1, site 1A) may occur when the intravascular volume is either acutely or chronically reduced. This will cause a decrease in GFR (Fig. 1, site 1B) and stimulate proximal tubular sodium reabsorption (Fig. 1, site 1C). Solute and fluid delivery to the distal diluting sites will thus be reduced, and free water generation will be impaired. In edematous states (congestive heart failure, nephrosis, cirrhosis), the kidney acts as though it is being hypoperfused even though total body and extracellular sodium content is absolutely increased. The result is a decrease in the "effective plasma volume," leading to a decrease in "effective renal plasma flow," a fall in GFR, and an enhancement in proximal tubular sodium and water reabsorption. The decrease in "effective circulating plasma volume" and "effective renal plasma flow" may result from low cardiac output (congestive heart failure), peripheral and splanchnic venous pooling (cirrhosis, nephrosis, congestive heart failure), or hypoalbuminemia (cirrhosis and nephorsis). Increased sympathetic nervous system activity and intrarenal redistribution of GRF or RPF may also contribute to increased proximal tubular salt and water reabsorption. It should be emphasized that sodium reabsorption in the proximal tubule is isotonic, and enhanced solute reabsorption at this site cannot cause hyponatremia. It is the decrease in solute delivery to the distal diluting sites and resultant impairment in free water generation that leads to hyponatremia.

Even if RPF and GFR are adequate and excessive amounts of salt and water are not reabsorbed by the proximal tubule, the distal diluting sites must be functionally intact so that sodium can be removed, leaving free water behind (Fig. 1, site 2). Thus, any chronic renal disease (particularly interstitial nephritis) that injures the tubular epithelial cells of this thick ascending limb of Henle's loop or early distal tubule may cause an impairment in sodium reabsorption, urinary sodium wasting, and diminished free water generation. Similarly, loop diuretics (furosemide, ethacrynic acid) or diuretics (such as thiazides) that act on the distal tubule will also impair urinary dilution and may lead to hyponatremia.

Finally, even if salt and water delivery to the distal diluting sites is adequate, and even if these sites are functionally intact, the free water that is generated must still escape reabsorption in the collecting duct (Fig. 1, site 3). For this to happen, ADH must be suppressed, and there must be an absence of substances that possess ADH-like activity.

II. ETIOLOGY OF HYPONATREMIA

With this brief review of renal physiology in mind, one can begin logically to approach the work-up of the patient with hyponatremia. However, the clinician must be cognizant of certain factitious causes of a low serum sodium concentration.

A. Factitious Hyponatremia

Both hyperproteinemia and hyperlipidemia may cause a factitiously low serum sodium concentration by a volume-displacing effect. The clinical laboratory reports the sodium content per unit volume of plasma, not plasma water. Therefore, if a significant percentage of plasma is comprised of macromolecules or lipid, a falsely low sodium concentration will be reported. A clue to this diagnosis is provided by the plasma osmolality which is normal. This type of hyponatremia occurs in patients with marked hyperlipidemia and severe hyperproteinemia ($> 12–15$ g/dl). Since these patients are not truly hyponatremic, no therapy is needed to correct the sodium concentration.

B. Redistribution of Water

The presence of a nonsodium solute that is poorly diffusable across cell membranes will cause an osmotic gradient that favors water movement from the intracellular to the extracellular compartment, resulting in hyponatremia. This type of hyponatremia is most commonly observed with hyperglycemia. Each 100 mg/dl rise in plasma glucose above the fasting level will decrease the serum sodium concentration by about 1.6 mEq/liter. Treatment of this type of hyponatremia should be directed at lowering the plasma glucose concentration with insulin. The result will be that water will move into the intracellular space, and the sodium concentration will return to normal.

Once factitious causes of hyponatremia and abnormal water distribution have been excluded, the rational approach to the patient with hyponatremia involves only an accurate assessment of the total body sodium content and determination of the urinary osmolality and urine sodium concentration (Table 1). Serum urea nitrogen and creatinine measurements are also helpful. In most patients, a careful physical examination will establish whether the total body salt and water content is increased, decreased, or close to normal. In occasional patients, it may be difficult to determine clinically whether the total body salt and water content is slightly increased versus normal or slightly decreased versus normal. Fortunately, this clinical distinction is not critical, since the urine osmolality and sodium concentrations will help to separate these cases. To establish the etiology of the hyponatremia, it is necessary only to differentiate clinically those patients with obviously increased from those with obviously decreased total body salt and water content.

C. Hyponatremia with Increased Total Body Salt and Water Content

Hyponatremia with an increase in total body salt and water content may occur in three common clinical situations: cirrhosis, nephrosis, and congestive heart failure. Common to each of these conditions is a decrease in the "effective" circulating plasma volume so that the kidney responds as though it were being hypoperfused. In patients with cirrhosis and nephrosis, an actual decrease in plasma volume may be present because of a decrease in colloid osmotic pressure. In congestive heart failure, extracellular fluid volume is absolutely increased, but the "effective" circulating volume is dimished because of the decreased cardiac output and/or redistribution of renal blood flow.

Thus, in all three conditions, the kidney responds as though being hypoperfused, and proximal tubular sodium reabsorption is enhanced. Consequently, the urine sodium concentration will be low—usually less than 10 to 15 mEq/liter—and the urine osmolality will be high—usually more than 350 to 400 mOsm/kg (Table I). The high urine osmolality results from a combination of high circulating plasma vasopressin levels and a decreased urine flow which permits a greater passive back diffusion of water out of the distal tubule and collecting duct. With increasing severity of cirrhosis, nephrosis, or heart failure, the urine becomes isotonic with plasma. This is an ominous sign and indicates a marked reduction in RPF and GFR with intense proximal

Table I. Pathophysiological Approach to the Diagnosis of Hyponatremia

	Urine sodium concentration	Urine osmolality	BUN	Treatment
Increased extracellular fluid (cirrhosis, nephrosis, congestive heart failure)	↓	↑ → Isotonic	Normal → increased	Sodium and water restriction
Decreased extracellular fluid Nonrenal loss (gastrointestinal, skin)	↓	↑ → Isotonic	Normal → increased	Isotonic sodium chloride
Renal loss (diuretics, renal disease, Addison's disease)	↑	Isotonic	Normal → increased	Isotonic sodium chloride
Normal extracellular fluid SIADH[a]	↑	↑	Decreased	Water restriction
"Reset osmostat"	Variable	Variable	Normal	Treat underlying disease

[a]SIADH indicates syndrome of inappropriate antidiuretic hormone secretion.

tubular reabsorption of salt and water, resulting in decreased sodium delivery to the loop of Henle and dissipation of the normal medullary osmotic gradient. Early in the course of these clinical conditions, the serum urea nitrogen concentration will be normal, but with increasing renal hypoperfusion, it will rise disproportionately to the increase in serum creatinine concentration.

D. Hyponatremia with Decreased Total Body Salt and Water Content

Hyponatremia with a decrease in total body salt and water content may occur with both nonrenal and renal losses of sodium. Sodium may be lost from the gastrointestinal tract (diarrhea, vomiting) and skin (burns, rarely with sweating) or by third-space fluid acumulation (pancreatitis, peritonitis, burns, traumatized muscle, etc.; Table I). All of these situations are characterized by a decrease in the ECF volume with resultant renal hypoperfusion and decreased GFR. These alterations stimulate proximal tubular sodium reabosorption and decrease sodium delivery to the distal diluting sites. The volume stimulus to ADH release further impairs free water generation. Occasionally, moderate to severe dietary sodium restrictions may be associated with sufficient negative sodium balance and volume contraction to cause hyponatremia if free water intake is excessive.

It is important to remember that patients with extrarenal routes of sodium loss have normal, functioning kidneys, and sodium and water reabsorption will be maximally stimulated in an attempt to reexpand the extracellular fluid volume. Volume depletion will also provide a stimulus for ADH secretion. Consequently, urine sodium concentration will be low ($<$5–10 mEq/liter) and urine osmolality will be high ($>$400 mOsm/kg). Initially, the serum urea nitrogen (SUN) and creatinine concentrations will be normal. With time and continued renal hypoperfusion, however, the SUN will rise disproportionately to the increase in serum creatinine. It should be noted from Table I that the only overlap in the approach to hyponatremia occurs between the volume-contracted individual who has lost salt and water via extrarenal routes and the previously discussed patients with excess total body sodium and water content (i.e., cirrhosis, nephrosis, congestive heart failure). However, these two groups are easily separated on physical examination by evidence of extracellular volume contraction in the former and ECF volume expansion in the latter. With the exception of these two groups, which can be easily distinguished on clinical examination, the urine sodium concentration and urine osmolality will differentiate all other causes of hyponatremia.

Excessive renal loss of sodium may also be associated with hyponatremia and a decrease in total body salt and water content (Table I). This occurs in three clinical situations: (1) diuretic effects, (2) chronic renal disease, usually of the interstitial variety, and (3) Addison's disease.

Hyponatremia with a decrease in total body salt and water content may also result from excessive renal sodium losses (Table I). Diuretics impair urinary dilution and free water generation via two mechanisms: (1) furosemide, ethacrynic acid, and thiazides inhibit sodium chloride reabsorption at the distal diluting sites (Fig. 1, site 2); and (2) all diuretics cause negative sodium balance, leading to ECF volume contraction and renal hypoperfusion. The latter effect results in enhanced proximal sodium reabsorption and diminished solute delivery to the distal diluting sites.

Chronic renal disease, particularly of the interstitial variety, may also be associated with renal sodium wasting and hyponatremia. Damage of the tubular epithelial cells of the loop of Henle and distal tubule as well as disruption of the normal interstitial architecture by scarring and inflammation leads to impaired sodium reabsorption and free water clearance. Hyponatremia may develop despite GFRs (>20–30 liter/day) that would not be expected to cause an impairment in water excretion *per se*.

The third cause of hyponatremia with excessive renal sodium losses and ECF volume depletion is mineralocorticoid deficiency. This is common in Addison's disease but infrequently may be observed with selective aldosterone deficiency. The defect in urinary dilution results from the negative sodium balance and decreased RPF and GFR which limit salt and water delivery to the distal diluting sites. Additionally, both volume contraction and glucocorticoid lack increase ADH secretion. When hyponatremia is associated with excessive renal sodium losses, the urine sodium concentration will be high (>20–30 mEq/liter), and the urine osmolality will be nearly isotonic to plasma since the kidney cannot generate a concentrated medullary interstitium. If the volume contraction is particularly severe and orthostatic signs are present, the urine may become slightly concentrated (300–450 mOsm/kg). The serum urea nitrogen will usually be elevated, either because of intrinsic renal disease or prerenal azotemia resulting from volume contraction. From Table I, it can be seen that the urine osmolality and sodium concentration in this group show no overlap with any of the other causes of hyponatremia.

E. Hyponatremia and "Normal" Total Body Salt and Water Content

The presence of hyponatremia in an individual who clinically appears to be euvolemic occurs in two situations: (1) the syndrome of inappropriate antidiuretic hormone secretion (SIADH) and (2) a resetting of the osmostat. In patients with SIADH, the urine osmolality and sodium concentration are inappropriately elevated despite the presence of hypoatremia and hypoosmolality. It is important that renal and adrenal disorders be excluded in order to establish the diagnosis of SIADH. This syndrome may be observed with (1) excessive production of ADH or an ADH-like substances by a wide variety of tumors; (2) excessive hypothalamic–pituitary release of ADH from

(a) a spectrum of pulmonary diseases including tuberculosis, pneumonia, lung abscess, fungal infections; (b) literally any CNS disorder; (c) endocrinopathies—glucocorticoid deficiency and myxedema; (d) drugs—opiates, barbiturates, chlorpropamide, tolbutamide, nicotine, clofibrate, tricyclic antidepressants, vincristine, thiazide diuretics, β-adrenergic agents (isoproterenol); (3) exogenous ADH administration; (4) potentiation of ADH action or a direct renal ADH-like effect (chlorpropamide, cyclophosphamide, or oxytocin).

The primary pathophysiological disturbance responsible for the hyponatremia is an excess of circulating ADH or ADH-like activity. This causes enhanced water reabsorption by the collecting duct (Fig. 1, step 3) and resultant expansion of the ECF volume. However, clinical evidence of hypervolemia is not evident, since only one-third of the retained water remains in the extracellular space, two thirds moving intracellularly. Nevertheless, the modest ECF volume expansion is sufficient to enhance RPF and GFR, to inhibit proximal sodium reabsorption, and to decrease aldosterone secretion and distal tubular sodium reabsorption as well. All of these factors contribute to an enhancement in sodium excretion in excess of dietary intake. Furthermore, whatever free water is generated by sodium removal at the distal diluting sites will be reabsorbed in the collecting duct under the influence of excess ADH. Precisely how concentrated the urine is depends on the balance between the plasma hypotonicity (which will tend to inhibit ADH secretion) and the nonosmotic stimulus for ADH release. In most patients with SIADH, the urine osmolality will exceed the plasma osmolality (Table I). This need not always be the case, however. In some patients the urine osmolality will be less than the plasma tonicity, but it will never be maximally dilute (<100 mOsm/kg). A urine osmolality significantly above this (i.e., >150 mOsm/kg) in the face of plasma hypotonicity signifies a defect in urinary diluting ability even though the urine may be hypotonic to plasma (Table I).

The serum urea nitrogen in SIADH is often low (<8–10 mg/dl) because of the high GFR and urine flow. Hyponatremia with a truly normal ECF volume may also be observed in patients with chronic debilitating diseases (Table I) such as tuberculosis, malnutrition, and cancer. These patients have a resetting of the osmostat. They behave as normal individuals, appropriately diluting or concentrating the urine when plasma osmolality (and plasma sodium concentration) deviates from its reset level.

F. Acute Water Intoxication

The previous discussion has focused on the causes of chronic hyponatremia. However, hyponatremia may also develop acutely in patients following ingestion of excessive amounts of water. This is most commonly seen in advanced renal failure (GFR less than 5 to 10 ml/min), where the marked reduction in GFR becomes the rate-limiting factor in excretion of the water load. Occasionally, patients with normal GFR (psychogenic polydipsia) may ingest enough water (more than 15 to 20 liters/day) to overcome the kidneys' ability to excrete the water load.

III. TREATMENT OF HYPONATREMIA

From Table I it can be seen that two simple laboratory determinations (urine osmolality and urine sodium concentration) in conjunction with a careful clinical examination to assess the patient's extracellular volume status will suffice to categorize the causes of hyponatremia. Furthermore, this simple box diagram approach provides the necessary framework for a rational approach to therapy.

A. Duration of Hyponatremia

The development of acute hyponatremia, as defined by a drop in serum sodium concentration from normal to less than 128 mEq/liter within 24–36 hr, usually leads to stupor, coma, or seizures and therefore should be considered a medical emergency. Such acute hyponatremia is associated with a high mortality rate, in excess of 40–50% in some series. When the development of hyponatremia is more chronic, occurring over several days to several weeks, it is common to see patients with serum sodium concentrations in the low 120 mEq/liter range who manifest no symptoms at all. However, the morbidity and mortality in such individuals is still significant, and CNS symptoms may develop acutely without any premonitory changes. Therefore, even if the hyponatremia is known to be chronic, therapy should be initiated in anyone with a serum sodium concentration less than 125 mEq/liter, and more aggressive treatment should be employed if the sodium concentration is ≤120 mEq/liter. It is important to remember that in individual patients with chronic hyponatremia, the signs and symptoms may not correlate well with the serum sodium concentration. This is in contrast to acute hyponatremia in which serum sodium concentrations less than 125 mEq/liter are usually associated with significant disturbances in CNS function.

B. Hyponatremia and Diminished Extracellular Fluid Volume

In the patient with hyponatremia and contraction of the extracellular fluid volume, the mainstay of treatment is isotonic soldium chloride. In this situation, morbidity and mortality are most closely related to the consequences of hypovolemia and tissue hypoperfusion (acute renal failure, stroke, myocardial infarction, etc.). It should be remembered that isotonic saline has a sodium concentration of 155 mEq/liter, and this will automatically be hypernatric to the patient's plasma. How fast normal saline is administered will be determined by the patient's blood pressure and overall clinical condition. The goal of therapy is to restore blood pressure and tissue perfusion to normal. Correction of the hyponatremia will follow normally. As the extracellular fluid volume is expanded, both renal plasma flow and GFR will increase, and the stimulus for sodium reabsorption in the proximal tubule will be diminished. This will enhance delivery of sodium to the distal diluting sites and lead to an increase in free water generation. Since the volume stimulus to ADH secretion is removed, the free water generated by the loop of Henle and early distal tubule will escape reabsorption in the collecting duct, thereby correcting the hyponatremia.

C. Assessment of Extracellular Fluid Volume and Sodium Deficit

Initial assessment of the extracellular volume deficit can be made as follows: if less than 5% of the ECFV is lost, no clinical findings will be present; with losses amounting to 5–10% of the ECFV (1.5–2 liters for a 70-kg man), an orthostatic increase in pulse will be present; if ECFV loss is 15–20% (3–4 liters for a 70-kg man), an orthostatic drop in blood pressure will occur. This evaluation provides only a rough estimate of the patient's volume status and should not be used as a substitute for close monitoring of the patient's vital signs and frequent clinical examinations. In addition to isotonic saline, volume expanders such as colloid may also be used to improve renal hemodynamics and increase distal sodium delivery. In some situations, the anion accompanying sodium may need to be altered, depending on the patient's acid–base status. If neurological symptoms (stupor, seizures, coma, muscle cramps, myoclonus) are present, and they are believed to be related to the hyponatremia, then more aggressive therapy with hypertonic saline is indicated to rapidly restore the plasma tonicity and sodium concentration towards normal.

One can make a rough estimate of the total body sodium deficit by assuming a distribution space equal to that for total body water. If one wishes to restore the plasma sodium concentration completely to normal, then the total sodium requirement is (140 mEq/liter − patients Na concn.) × (body weight × 0.60). Normally, however, only enough sodium is given to increase the sodium concentration to ~125–130 mEq/liter, a level that is usually sufficient to reverse any clinical symptoms of hyponatremia. The major complication associated with rapid correction of hyponatremia is circulatory overload. This risk can be reduced (but not eliminated) by using either 3% (513 mM) or 5% (855 mM) NaCl. Half of the calculated sodium deficit should be given over the first 8 hr and the remaining half over the subsequent 8–16 hr. The patient's fluid and sodium balance, sodium concentration, and mental status should be evaluated at frequent intervals during therapy.

D. Hyponatremia and Expanded Extracellular Fluid Volume

In patients with hyponatremia and expanded ECF volume (cirrhosis, nephorsis, congestive heart failure), both salt and water are present in excess, but the latter is disproportionately increased. Since total body sodium content is increased, moderate to severe sodium restriction is indicated. The degree of sodium restriction will be dependent on the patient's clinical status and urinary sodium excretion. To achieve negative sodium balance, the dietary intake must be reduced below the urinary excretion. For correction of the hyponatremia, water restriction is the mainstay of therapy. Again, the degree of water restriction will vary according to the severity of the hyponatremia.

Since the underlying pathophysiological disturbance in all of these conditions (cirrhosis, nephrosis, congestive heart failure) is a decrease in the "effective" circulating plasma volume therapy should be aimed at increasing renal perfusion and increasing sodium delivery to the distal diluting sites. In the person with congestive heart failure, an attempt should be made to increase cardiac output. This is best accomplished with digitalization and diuretics. Those agents that act in the proximal tubule (i.e., acetazolamide) are the most efficacious, but the development of a metabolic acidosis inhibits their effectiveness. Although the loop diuretics, furosemide and ethacrynic acid, have a theoretical disadvantage in that they directly inhibit free water generation, the improvement in cardiac and renal hemodynamics offsets this inhibitory effect on sodium reabsorption. The net result is an increase in sodium delivery to the distal diluting sites and the excretion of a dilute urine. It is also possible that these potent diuretics have a site of action in the proximal tubule as well. Diuretics (thiazides) that act in the distal tubule are not helpful in the treatment of hyponatremia associated with congestive heart failure. In fact, they may actually make the hyponatremia worse by inhibiting free water generation in the early distal tubule.

In the hyponatremic patient with refractory congestive heart failure who requires hospitalization, low-dose intravenous dopamine therapy (2–5 μg/kg·min) is particularly efficacious. Not only does it increase cardiac output, but it specifically causes renal vasodilation and markedly increases renal sodium excretion. A similar pharmacological approach can be employed in hyponatremic patients with cirrhosis and nephrosis. In addition, volume expanders (such as colloid or mannitol), which are contraindicated in congestive heart failure, have been shown to be particularly useful in improving renal hemodynamics and increasing distal sodium delivery in patients with cirrhosis and nephrosis.

E. Inappropriate ADH Secretion

In all patients with SIADH, the cornerstones of therapy are water restriction and removal of the cause of ADH secretion (i.e., drug, tumor, infection, etc.). The degree of water restriction should be sufficient to cause a net negative water balance of 0.5–1.0 liters per day. This will lead to a gradual reduction of the ECF volume and a concomitant decrease in RPF and GFR. As the intravascular volume declines, proximal tubular sodium reabsorption will be enhanced, and stimulation of aldosterone will increase distal tubular sodium reabsorption. The net result will be a marked decrease in urinary sodium excretion. Since the source of excessive ADH secretion has not been removed, the urine will remain concentrated, and there will be no increase in free water excretion. However, if water intake is sufficiently restricted, net negative water balance will still be achieved.

If the hyponatremia is particularly severe (<115–120 mEq/liter), or evidence of neuromuscular irritability is present, then more aggressive therapy is indicated. In the past, such patients have been treated with hypertonic saline as described earlier. However, many of these patients are elderly and have compromised cardiac function, making volume overload a serious consideration. Furthermore, treatment with hypertonic saline alone often results in only a transient rise in the serum sodium concentration, since the ECF volume is already expanded, and the administered sodium is rapidly excreted. More recently, the use of a potent loop diuretic with meticulous replacement of urinary sodium losses with 3% sodium chloride has been shown to be an efficacious and rapid means of correcting the low serum sodium concentration. Ideally, urinary sodium losses should be replaced on an hourly basis to avoid hypotension. If facilities are not readily available to measure urinary sodium excretion, it is wise to replace all urinary losses quantitatively with normal saline. Since the urine composition following furosemide or ethacrynic acid approximates half-normal saline, for each liter of urine excreted, 500 cc of free water will be generated.

In patients with SIADH in whom the source of the excessive vasopressin secretion cannot be removed, chronic water restriction is often poorly tolerated. In such individuals, demeclocycline (600–1200 mg/day) will induce a state of nephrogenic diabetes insipidus, and even though circulating ADH will remain elevated, its effect on the collecting duct will be inhibited. However, several recent reports have documented nephrotoxicity and sodium wasting, particularly in patients with impaired hepatic function. Although earlier reports suggested that lithium might be effective in treating chronic SIADH, its effectiveness is quite unpredictable, and its use is accompanied by a high incidence of side effects. Lastly, in patients with SIADH secondary to glucocorticoid or thyroid hormone deficiency, specific hormonal replacement will rapidly reverse the diluting defect and correct the hyponatremia.

F. Hypokalemia-Associated Hyponatremia

In patients with moderate to severe potassium deficiency, hyponatremia will often be present. Potassium is the major intracellular cation. If intracellular potassium stores become depleted, sodium ions will move into cells in an attempt to maintain cell volume. Such shifts may decrease the serum sodium concentration by as much as 10–15 mEq/liter without any significant total body sodium deficits. Adequate potassium replacement will cause a dramatic correction of the hyponatremia.

IV. CLINICAL DISORDERS OF HYPERNATREMIA

The pathophysiological approach to the hypernatremic patient is simplified by the realization that an elevated serum sodium concentration usually results from one of three primary disturbances: sodium gain, water loss, or water loss in excess of sodium loss.

A. Sodium Gain

Hypernatremia resulting from sodium gain is much more common in children than adults. Accidental addition of large sodium loads as the result of errors in preparation of formula may overwhelm the young child's ability to excrete sodium and lead to hypernatremia. In adults, excessive administration of sodium bicarbonate during a cardiac arrest or to a patient with severe metabolic acidemia often results in hypernatremia. It is unusual to observe other than transient hypernatremia in adults with normal renal function despite the infusion of large sodium loads. However, with patients with severe metabolic acidosis or in those who have experienced a cardiac arrest, a marked reduction in RPF and GFR is often present, and the administered sodium cannot be excreted. Salt-water drowning may be associated with hypernatremia in both adults and children, since large quantities of sodium are rapidly absorbed from the alveolar surface at a time when renal function is impaired. Malfunction of hemodialysis or peritoneal dialysis proportioning systems have also been reported as a cause of hypernatremia. Other therapeutic measures associated with hypernatremia are the administration of isotonic sodium sulfate (200 mEq of sodium and 100 mEq of sulfate) for the treatment of hypercalcemia and the use of hypertonic NaCl for therapeutic abortions.

B. Water Loss

Pure water loss may occur (1) via nonrenal routes or (2) via the kidney (diabetes insipidus).

In the elderly patient exposed to a hot climate, excessive sweating added to respiratory water loss may lead to a vicious cycle. A debilitated person loses water, becoming dehydrated and hypernatremic. The dehydration, in turn, causes further weakness, and the hypernatremia may depress the sensorium to a point where thirst is no longer appreciated. Lack of water intake with continued skin and respiratory losses results in severe hypertonicity and eventually CNS changes including seizures and coma.

Excessive renal water losses may result from either central diabetes insipidus (deficiency of arginine vasopressin, ADH) or from the inability of the kidney to respond to ADH (nephrogenic diabetes insipidus). Clinically, diabetes insipidus is manifested by polyuria and polydipsia. The urine is dilute despite serum hypertonicity.

To establish the diagnosis of diabetes insipidus, one must exclude other conditions in which polyuria may be the presenting feature. The first step is to define the water and solute content of the urine. If solute comprises a major portion of the urinary composition, then the excessive water loss may be the consequence of an osmotic diuresis, and a primary defect in renal water conservation need not be invoked. The urine of patients undergoing a solute diuresis will be isotonic with plasma. If significant volume contraction is present, the urine may become slightly concentrated. Water loss resulting from an osmotic diuresis is commonly encountered in patients with diabetes mellitus and chronic interstitial renal diseases in which impaired glucose and sodium reabsorption, respectively, obligate the excretion of excessive amounts of water. In these situations, therapy should be directed at the underlying disease process.

In a pure water diuresis, the urine osmolality is quite low (<150–200 mOsm/kg) in contrast to the near isotonic urine elaborated during an osmotic diuresis, and pathological amounts of glucose, sodium, and urea are not present. Such a water diuresis may be the result of excessive water intake, as occurs in subjects with psychogenic polydipsia, or may be caused by an alteration in the renal handling of water *per se*. The latter may be secondary to inadequate secretion of arginine vasopressin by the posterior pituitary or the inability of the renal tubule to respond normally to secreted ADH.

The diagnosis of diabetes insipidus is best established by comparing the urine and plasma osmolalities after 16 to 24 hr of fluid deprivation (or 3–5% loss of body weight) and after the administration of exogenous vasopressin (Table II). In patients with psychogenic polydipsia, random plasma osmolality will usually be reduced (<280 mOsm/kg), and after dehydration, the urine/plasma osmolality ratio will significantly exceed 1 and frequently 2. In contrast, the patient with complete central or nephrogenic diabetes insipidus will often have a high random plasma osmolality (>295 mOsm/kg), and the urine/plasma osmolality ratio will fail to exceed 1 during fluid deprivation. If exogenous vasopressin is administered after the period of fluid deprivation, the subject with psychogenic polydipsia will manifest little additional increase in urine osmolality (<50 mOsm/kg), whereas the person with central diabetes insipidus will demonstrate a significant rise (>100 mOsm/kg). The patient with nephrogenic diabetes insipidus will respond neither to fluid deprivation nor to exogenous vasopressin. It should be emphasized that although the diagnosis of complete central diabetes insipidus is excluded by

Table II. Evaluation of Polyuric States Based on the Response of Urine Osmolality to Fluid Deprivation and Arginine Vasopressin Administration

	Central diabetes insipidus	Psychogenic polydipsia	Nephrogenic diabetes insipidus
Plasma osmolality (mOsm/kg)	>295	<280	>290
Urine/plasma osmolality after fluid restriction	<1	>1	<1
Increase in U_{Osm} after vasopressin	>100	<100	<50

the ability to elaborate a concentrated urine, a partial defect in vasopressin release may still exist. Patients with incomplete central diabetes insipidus can concentrate their urine above the plasma osmolality, but they are unable to elaborate a maximally concentrated urine (i.e., 1000–1200 mOsm/kg). The diagnosis of partial diabetes insipidus may be difficult to establish in some subjects, and a closely monitored therapeutic trial with vasopressin may be indicated.

Once the diagnosis of central diabetes insipidus has been established, a careful search should be made for potentially remediable causes. Although the majority of cases of central diabetes insipidus will be idiopathic or secondary to trauma, approximately 25% will be caused by surgically correctable lesions such as pituitary tumors or craniopharyngiomas or granulomatous processes that are amenable to specific medical therapy.

C. Water Loss in Excess of Sodium Loss

This is the most dangerous type of hypernatremia because it is usually associated with significant depletion of the extracellular fluid volume. In children, water loss in excess of sodium most commonly occurs with gastroenteritis and copious diarrhea. In adults, hypertonic dehydration resulting from water loss in excess of sodium usually is observed in association with an osmotic diuresis. The most common clinical situation in which this occurs is hyperglycemic hyperosmotic nonketotic coma (HHNK), but it may also be observed during mannitol infusion or following relief of urinary tract obstruction.

In HHNK, relative insulin deficiency leads to hyperglycemia and, when the rise in plasma glucose concentration exceeds the renal threshold for glucose reabsorption (180–200 mg/dl), an osmotic diuresis ensues. The solute content of the urine is equal to about half-normal saline. The urinary losses can, therefore, be conceptualized as containing equal volumes of isotonic saline and free water. The loss of isotonic saline results in contraction of the ECF volume, and the loss of free water causes hypernatremia. The decrease in intravascular volume leads to organ system hypoperfusion and may result in myocardial infarction, stroke, acute tubular necrosis, etc. To the extent that the glomerular filtration rate falls, renal glucose losses will diminish, and the hyperglycemia will be made worse. In turn, both the hyperglycemia and the hypernatremia will contribute to the increase in plasma tonicity, which in turn will cause cellular dehydration and CNS dysfunction. The effect of changes in brain water and electrolyte composition on cerebral function will be discussed subsequently.

The osmotic effects of mannitol and urea on renal electrolyte and water excretion are similar to those previously described for hyperglycemia with attendant glucosuria. Since mannitol, like glucose, is excluded from cells, it will also result in intracellular dehydration. In contrast, urea, which is freely diffusible, will not obligate any movement of water out of cells as long as sufficient time has elapsed (36–48 hr) for urea to equilibrate with the intracellular fluid compartment.

D. Reset Osmostat

Sustained hypernatremia may also occur in patients whose osmostat is reset at a higher than normal level. Such patients will concentrate and dilute the urine perfectly normally, but they do so at a plasma osmolality and sodium concentration that are higher than in the normal individual. The importance of recognizing this syndrome is that no therapy need be instituted. Occasionally, these patients have been found to have small hypothalamic tumors encroaching on the area of the supraoptic and paraventricular nuclei.

V. CLINICAL MANIFESTATIONS OF HYPERNATREMIA

Avoidance of major swelling or contraction in response to changes in extracellular fluid osmolality is an inherent property of most cells, and this is particularly critical for the brain with its fixed attachments within a rigid chamber. When the serum sodium concentration (and serum osmolality) increases acutely, there is a net movement of water from the intracellular to the extracellular space. As brain cells lose volume, traction is placed on the delicate bridging cerebral veins, and this may result in their rupture. Within 4–6 hr after brain cells begin to lose water, there is an influx of sodium, chloride, and potassium into cerebral tissues, and the resultant increase in intracellular tonicity tends to oppose further water loss. Following 2–3 days of persistent hypernatremia, intracellular brain water content returns to normal. Total brain osmolality is elevated at this time, but the increase in brain cell sodium, chloride, and potassium content can only account for about 40% of the increase in brain osmolality. Of the remaining 60%, a small percentage can be accounted for by amino acids, but the majority remains unexplained and has been termed "idiogenic osmoles." The importance of recognizing the appearance of these so-called idiogenic osmoles is that they are slow to disappear following correction of the hypernatremia with hypotonic fluid. Thus, if free water replacement is too rapid, brain cells may swell, resulting in cerebral edema.

Clinically, the changes in intracellular brain composition are reflected by restlessness and irritability followed by lethargy, stupor, and eventually coma. Neuromuscular irritability and seizures are commonly observed. The reported mortality of acute hypernatremia in adults is high, ranging from 40 to 60%. However, this is in large part related to the severity of the patient's underlying medical problems. In children, acute hypernatremia is associated with a lower mortality (20–40%), but approximately half of the survivors have some type of residual neurological deficit. Since, in children, hypernatremia is usually associated with reversible medical illnesses, the high morbidity and mortality suggest that hypernatremia per se is responsible for the poor prognosis. When the hypernatremia develops more chronically, the outcome is more favorable. In recent years, a better understanding of the pathophysiological consequences of hypernatremia have lead to a more rational approach to therapy and a considerable improvement in morbidity and mortality.

VI. TREATMENT OF HYPERNATREMIA

There are few data on which to base therapeutic recommendations. Because of the high morbidity and mortality associated with hypernatremia, therapeutic intervention is clearly indicated. However, how much free water should be given and how quickly remains controversial. As discussed earlier, since there is an increase in idiogenic brain osmoles, which are slow to disappear, too vigorous hydration may result in a rapid influx of water into brain cells and the development of cerebral edema. A reasonable therapeutic regimen should attempt to correct one-third of the water deficit over the first 12 hr and the remaining two-thirds over the subsequent 36 hr. If seizures or coma develop during the course of therapy and are believed to result from cerebral edema, water replacement should be stopped and mannitol administered to reverse the presumed increase in CSF pressure.

A. Treatment of Hypernatremia Resulting from Sodium Gain

If the patient is asymptomatic and has intact renal function, no specific therapy is indicated. The kidneys will eventually excrete the excess sodium, and the hypernatremia will spontaneously correct itself. If symptoms are present, however, free water must be given. It is important to remember that these patients have a marked increase in total body sodium content and that excesive water administration may lead to circulatory overload. Therefore, only the minimum amount of water necessary to reverse the neurological manifestations should be given. Eventually, the kidney will excrete the excess sodium, and this will restore the serum sodium concentration to normal. If kidney function is impaired, as is often the case following cardiac arrest and in many of the other syndromes associated with hypernatremia and excess sodium administration, then the only way to remove the excess sodium from the body is by either hemodialysis or peritoneal dialysis.

B. Treatment of Hypernatremia Resulting from Pure Water Loss

When excessive water losses are incurred via nonrenal routes, simple water replacement will suffice to correct the hypernatremia. Water deficits should be calculated using a space of water distribution that is equal to 60% of body weight. Assuming a body weight of 70 kg and a starting sodium concentration of 180 mEq/liter, the amount of water required to restore the serum sodium concentration to 140 mEq/liter can be calculated from the following equation:

$$(180 \text{ mEq/liter}) \ (42 \text{ liters}) = (140 \text{ mEq/liter}) \ (X)$$

where $X = 54$ liters and represents the total amount of water in the body after correction of the hyponatremia. The different, $54 - 42 = 12$ liters, is the total amount of water needed to lower the sodium concentration from 180 to 140 mEq/liter. One-third of this or 4 liters should be given over the first 12 hr.

In the patients whose water loss is renal in origin, the approach to therapy is quite different. The inital water deficit should be replaced as described in the preceding paragraph. Subsequent therapy, however, is dependent on establishing whether the patient has central or nephrogenic diabetes insipidus.

1. Central Diabetes Insipidus

Although several newer nonhormonal modalities have been advocated in the treatment of central diabetes insipidus, the mainstay of therapy still remains some form of vasopressin.

a. Vasopressin (Pitressin®) Tannate in Oil

This dosage form (supplied as 1-ml ampules containing 5 units per ml) is a long-acting preparation that may be administered subcutaneously or intramuscularly. After the usual dose of 2–5 units, antidiuresis ensues within 2 to 4 hr and affords relief of symptoms for up to 24 to 48 hr. When the ampule is examined, a brown precipitate will be noticed on the bottom. This is the hormone. Before injection, the ampule must be shaken thoroughly and warmed under tap water to insure the proper suspension of hormone in an emulsion. Failure to achieve such suspension is the most common cause of treatment failure. To prevent excessive water retention and dilutional hyponatremia, each dose of vasopressin (Pitressin®) should be repeated only after symptoms recur.

Local and systemic allergic reactions are uncommon. If they occur, desensitization can be achieved by starting with a dose of 0.01 ml per day and increasing in a stepwise fashion. Since vasopressin causes contraction of smooth muscle, abdominal cramps may occur in some patients. Hypertension and coronary insufficiency are unusual with the recommended doses, but patients with known coronary artery disease should be observed closely when therapy is started. Acquired refractoriness secondary to the development of antibodies is unusual.

b. Aqueous Vasopressin (Pitressin®)

This preparation is a water-soluble pituitary extract containing a variable mixture of arginine and lysine vasopressin. Each vial contains 20 units dissolved in 1 ml of diluent. Although useful for diagnostic purposes and in the management of the unconscious patient, it has almost no place in the treatment of uncomplicated diabetes insipidus. The usual dose is 5 to 10 units administered subcutaneously or intramuscularly. Onset of action is within 30 min, and the effect lasts 4–6 hr. Intravenous use is investigational, and when it is so administered, the dose is 1–5 milliunits per min. The onset of action is immediate and lasts 30–60 min. Adverse reactions are similar to those of vasopressin (Pitressin®) tannate in oil.

c. Synthetic Lysine Vasopressin (Diapid®)

This drug comes as a nonirritating saline solution (50 units per ml) which is sprayed deep into the nasal passages from a plastic squeeze bottle, one to two sprays in each nostril. Onset of action is within 30 min. It is administered every 4–6 hr with an additional dose just before bedtime. Its major limitation is its short duration of action, but it may be employed as a useful adjunct during travel or at bedtime. This lysine vasopressin spray has almost completely replaced the use of posterior pituitary snuff or powder which is quite irritating to the nasal mucosa.

d. DDAVP (1-Desamino-8-d-arginine Vasopressin)

This is a new synthetic vasopressin analogue with increased antidiuretic and decreased pressor activity. It can be administered as a nasal spray (5–20 μg per inhalation) and has the advantage of long duration, 10–20 hr. Recent studies in Europe and in this country have documented its efficacy in the treatment of central diabetes insipidus with minimal side effects. Because this preparation is effective, long lasting, largely free of side effects, and does not require an injection, it has rapidly gained popularity over vasopressin tannate in oil as the mainstay of therapy in patients with central diabetes insipidus.

e. Nonhormonal Drugs

Chlorpropamide, clofibrate, and thiazides, alone or in combination, have proved useful in reducing polyuria in patients with central diabetes insipidus. The mechanisms of action of these drugs are described below. When employed in combination with dietary restriction of protein and salt, urine volume may be reduced by as much as one-third to one-half. Such dietary restriction is useful, because for any degree of limitation of urine-concentrating ability, urine volume will depend on the solute load to be excreted. These nonhormonal measures are most effective in patients with incomplete diabetes insipidus and may obviate the need for vasopressin treatment in such patients. This form of therapy should be considered whenever significant sensitivity to vasopressin exists or when vasopressin must be given too frequently to be practical.

Chlorpropamide (Diabinese®) is an oral sulfonylurea hypoglycemic agent capable of reducing polyuria to an acceptable level in as many as one-half of the patients with vasopressin-sensitive diabetes insipidus. (This use of chlorpropamide is not listed in the manufacturer's official directive and must be considered experimental.) When chlorpropamide is administered in a single dose of 250–500 mg/day, the onset of antidiuresis begins within 1–2 hr and reaches peak effectiveness in 1–2 days. Urine flow may decrease to one-half to one-third of the predrug level, and this is associated with a significant rise in urine osmolality. The magnitude of the response is proportional to the amount of chlorpropamide, but doses in excess of 500–750 mg/day are often associated with an increased incidence of side effects, the most troublesome of which is hypoglycemia. This is particularly likely to occur in people with associated anterior pituitary insufficiency. The patient should be warned of hypoglycemic symptoms, which may be alleviated by small between-meal and bedtime feedings.

The drug, which is ineffective in patients with nephrogenic diabetes insipidus and in patients with complete central diabetes insipidus, probably acts by potentiating the effect of low circulating levels of arginine vasopressin on the distal nephron. Some evidence also has been accumulated to suggest that it stimulates pituitary release of residual ADH. Chlorpropamide may be tried in patients with central diabetes insipidus but would be expected to be most beneficial to those in whom the diabetes insipidus is incomplete. The starting dose is 250 mg/day, and this can be increased by 250 mg every 3–4 days up to a maximum dose of 750 mg/day. In many patients, chlorpropamide alone may be sufficient to control symptoms. If a partial response is observed, the addition of thiazides will often be effective in achieving adequate antidiuresis.

The thiazide diuretics have long been known to be effective in reducing urine flow in patients with both central and nephrogenic diabetes insipidus. Recent studies have also demonstrated that other diuretics, as well as rigid sodium restriction, are equally effective in producing antidiuresis and that the antidiuretic effect of these diuretics can be prevented by concomitant salt administration. These results imply that the efficacy of the thiazides as well as other diuretics is related to the induction of negative salt balance. The resultant decrease in extracellular fluid volume and the accompanying fall in glomerular filtration rate serve to enhance fluid reabsorption in the proximal nephron. Since the mechanism of action of the thiazides differs from that of chlorpropamide, the action of the two drugs is additive. Conventional doses of chlorothiazide (500–1000 mg/day) or hydrochlorothiazide (50–100 mg/day) are effective, and side effects other than hypokalemia and hyperuricemia are unusual. (This use of chlorothiazide or hydrochlorothiazide is not listed in the manufacturer's official directive and therefore should be considered experimental.)

f. Clofibrate (Atromid-S®)

Clofibrate is an oral hypolipidemic agent that, when administered in conventional doses of 1–2 g/day, is capable of reducing urine flow in patients with central but not nephrogenic diabetes insipidus. (This use of clofibrate is not listed in the manufacturer's official directive and therefore should be considered experimental.) Its mechanism of action is similar to that of chlorpropamide, but its antidiuretic potency is somewhat less. As its duration of action is short (6–8 hr), it must be administered in divided doses every 6 hr. A variety of side effects have been reported with this agent, but the most common are gastrointestinal symptoms, myositis, and abnormalities of liver function. The drug has an additive effect with the thiazides but has little additional antidiuretic effect when employed with chlorpropamide. Compared with clorpropamide, its only advantage is its freedom from hypoglycemic reactions.

2. Nephrogenic Diabetes Insipidus

Nephrogenic diabetes insipidus may be caused by a variety of treatable lesions (ingestion of lithium and tetracycline derivatives, hypercalcemia, hypokalemia, obstructive uropathy, amyloidosis, and sickle cell disease) which should be carefully excluded before therapy is initiated. Since these patients are refractory to the action of vasopressin and agents such as chlorpropamide and clofibrate, which work by potentiating the effect of circulating ADH, therapy is limited to the thiazides and dietary solute restriction as previously discussed. Although several recent studies have suggested that indomethacin may be useful in treating patients with nephrogenic diabetes insipidus, such reports should be considered preliminary and experimental at the present time.

a. Treatment of Hypertonic Dehydration (HHNK)

The treatment of the hypertonic patient with volume contraction requires close attention to the consequences of both volume depletion and plasma hypertonicity with its concomitant intracellular dehydration. The most serious medical complications usually result from organ (brain, heart, kidney) hypoperfusion. Therefore, the first step in therapy should be directed at reexpanding the intravascular volume and restoring blood pressure and organ perfusion to normal. Isotonic saline should be infused as rapidly as possible to stabilize the cardiovascular system. Once the intravascular volume has been repleted, correction of the water deficit should be undertaken with hypotonic fluid replacement. As discussed earlier, approximately one-third of the water deficit should be administered over the first 12 hr and the remaining two-thirds over the subsequent 24–36 hr. If fluid replacement is too rapid, cerebral edema may result.

It should be noted that even though patients with HHNK will have an elevated plasma osmolality, the serum sodium concentration may be high, normal, or low. This will depend on the balance between two pathophysiological disturbances: (1) the relatively greater loss of water than sodium by the kidney which will tend to increase the serum sodium concentration and (2) plasma hypertonicity which will extract water from the intracellular space and dilute down the serum sodium concentration. Therefore, in calculating the free water replacement in patients with hypertonic dehydration, one should use the plasma osmolality and not the sodium concentration. If an individual weighs 70 kg and has a plasma osmolality of 400 mOsm/kg, then the water deficit would be calculated from the following equation:

$$(400 \text{ mOsm/kg}) (70 \text{ kg} \times 0.60) = (300 \text{ mOsm/kg}) (x)$$

where $x = 56$ liters and represents the total amount of water in the body after correction of the hypertonicity. The difference, $56 - 42$ liters, is the total amount of water needed to lower the plasma tonicity from 400 to 300 mOsm/kg.

In the treatment of HHNK, several other important considerations must be kept in mind. When the patient is first seen, the blood pressure and intravascular volume may be marginally maintained. If insulin is administered before sodium deficits are corrected, the fall in plasma glucose concentration will be associated with a shift of water from the ECF to ICF volume, and this may lead to disastrous hypotension and tissue hypoperfusion. Insulin therapy will also stimulate cellular potassium uptake. Since the osmotic diuresis has already caused a marked decrease in total body potassium stores, profound hypokalemia may be precipitated by insulin therapy. A normal or low serum potassium concentration in these individuals is an indication for aggressive potassium replacement (see Section vl.B.1). In patients with hypertonic dehydration secondary to mannitol and urea osmotic diuresis, sodium and water deficits should be replaced as described previously. Urine sodium and water excretion should be followed closely, and any subsequent losses should be replaced quantitatively until the mannitol or urea has been excreted and the osmotic diuresis has ended.

SUGGESTED READINGS

Brenner BM, Stein JH (eds): *Sodium and Water Homeostasis.* New York, Churchill Livingstone, 1978.

DeFronzo RA, Thier SO: Pathophysiologic approach to hyponatremia. *Arch Intern Med* 140:897–902, 1980.

Hays RM, Levine SD: Pathophysiology of water metabolism, in Brenner BM, Rector FC (eds): *The Kidney.* Philadelphia, WB Saunders, 1981, pp 777–840.

Schrier R: Water metabolism (symposium). *Kidney Int* 10:1–132, 1976.

Fluid and Electrolyte Disturbances
Hypo- and Hyperkalemia

RALPH A. DeFRONZO and SAMUEL O. THIER

I. POTASSIUM DISTRIBUTION

The total amount of potassium in a healthy adult is approximately 50 mEq/kg body weight or about 3500 mEq for a 70-kg man. The vast majority of potassium is intracellular (Fig. 1), primarily in muscle, and is present at a concentration of about 150 mEq/liter. Only 2% of total body potassium is located in the extracellular fluid, normally at a concentration of 3.5–5.0 mEq/liter. The large difference in plasma potassium concentration across the cell membrane is critical for normal cell function since it is the primary determinant of the resting membrane potential. Small changes in the intracellular/extracellular potassium ratio can lead to severe disturbances in neuromuscular function, particularly of the heart. A change (gain or loss) in the amount of extracellular potassium equal to only 1% of the total body potassium content (35 mEq) can cause a 50% increase (or decrease) in the plasma potassium concentration. Such a change might result from redistribution of potassium between the intracellular and extracellular fluid compartments or from net gain or loss of potassium from the body. Thus, it is important that (1) the total amount of potassium within the body and (2) the distribution of potassium between intracellular and extracellular fluid compartments be closely regulated.

In healthy man potassium can only enter the body by ingestion. Approximately 100 mEq of potassium is ingested per day, and essentially all of this

RALPH A. DeFRONZO and SAMUEL O. THIER • Department of Internal Medicine, Renal Division, Yale University School of Medicine, New Haven, Connecticut 06510.

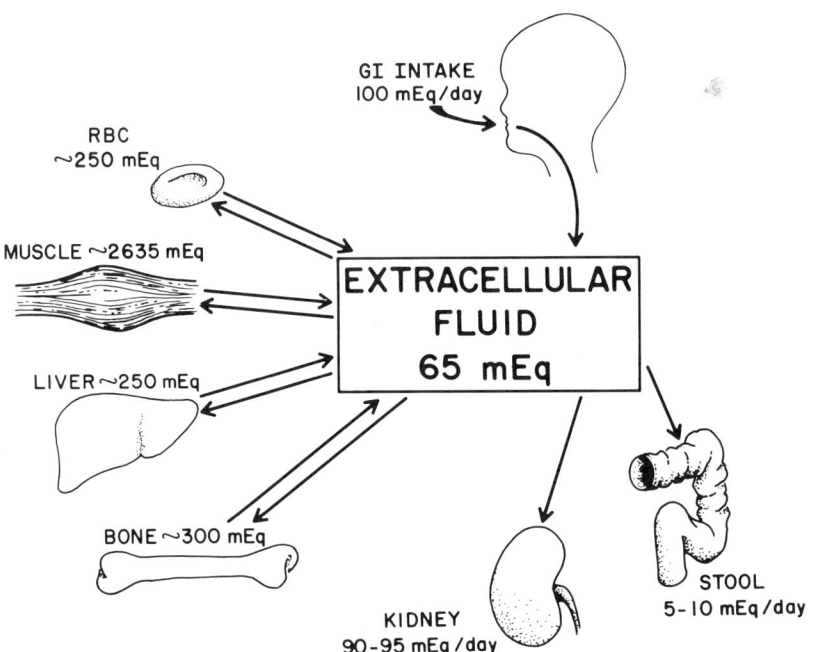

Figure 1. Internal and external potassium balance in man. See text for a more detailed discussion.

is absorbed from the stomach and upper gastrointestinal tract (Fig. 1). Approximately 10 mEq of potassium per day is excreted in stool. Although the epithelial cells of the colon are capable of potassium secretion, under physiological conditions the kidney is the major organ responsible for the maintenance of chronic potassium balance. In contrast, acute potassium homeostasis is primarily regulated by extrarenal tissues. During the first 4–6 hr following both oral and intravenous potassium administration, only half of the potassium load appears in the urine. If all of the infused or ingested potassium that was not excreted were retained in the extracellular fluid compartment, the increase in plasma potassium concentration would produce life-threatening hyperkalemia. Hyperkalemia does not occur, however, since nearly 80% of the retained potassium load is translocated into cells.

II. RENAL REGULATION OF POTASSIUM EXCRETION

Micropuncture studies indicate that the majority of the potassium excreted in the urine is derived from secretion in the distal nephron (distal tubule and collecting duct). Of the 600–700 mEq of potassium filtered by the glomerulus each day, less than 10% remains by the early distal tubule. The percent reabsorbed is quite constant despite a variety of maneuvers known to either increase or decrease the amount of potassium excreted in the urine. Approximately 60–70% of the filtered potassium load is reabsorbed by the accessible portion of the proximal convoluted tubule, and an additional 20–30% is reabsorbed by the time the fluid reaches the first accessible segment of the distal tubule. The mid to late distal convoluted tubule represents the first major site of potassium secretion. Both the cortical and medullary collecting tubule are capable of secreting potassium, but their precise contribution to overall potassium homeostasis is presently unknown.

A schematic representation of the mechanism of distal tubular potassium secretion is shown in Fig. 2. This diagram takes into account data gathered from micropuncture, microperfusion, and other techniques, and the reader is referred to several recent excellent reviews for a more detailed discussion. The salient features of this model are the following. (1) The lumen is electronegatively charged by approximately 50 mV compared to the pericapillary surface. (2) There is an active pump located in the pericapillary membrane which pumps potassium into the cell against a large concentration gradient. Once within the cell, the potassium may either back diffuse into the capillary blood or enter the tubular lumen. However, the electrical gradient (lumen negative) favors the net secretion of potassium into the tubular fluid. (3) Potassium transport by the active pump is coupled in some loose fashion to sodium transport, and the integrity of the pump is influenced by the enzyme sodium–potassium ATPase. (4) The pump system is regulated by aldosterone. Aldosterone deficiency is associated with a marked impairment in potassium secretion, whereas aldosterone excess enhances distal potassium secretion. (5) The activity of the pump is exquisitely sensitive to small changes in the potassium concentration in the pericapillary

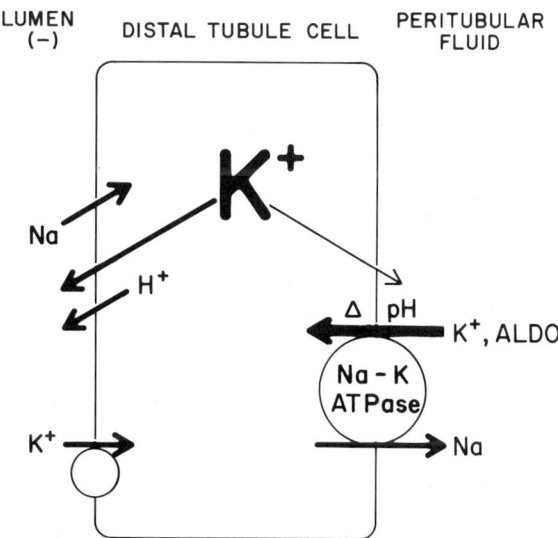

Figure 2. Schematic representation of potassium secretion by an individual distal tubular cell. See text for a more detailed discussion.

blood, with hyperkalemia providing a potent stimulus to enhance potassium secretion. (6) Both an increase in sodium delivery and an increase in urine flow, independent of sodium delivery, stimulate potassium secretion. (7) The activity of the pump is strongly influenced by changes in acid–base status, with acidemia inhibiting and alkalemia stimulating potassium secretion acutely. (8) A potassium reabsorptive mechanism also must exist in the distal tubule, since urinary potassium excretion may approach zero despite delivery of 5–10% of the filtered load to the early distal tubule. The cells responsible for potassium reabsorption need not be the same as those responsible for potassium excretion.

III. EXTRARENAL POTASSIUM HOMEOSTASIS

As discussed in the preceding section, the maintenance of chronic potassium balance is primarily regulated by the kidney. However, acute potassium tolerance is in large part dependent on extrarenal tissues. During the first 4–6 hr following the administration of an oral or intravenous potassium load, only half of the potassium appears in the urine. If all of the administered load that is not excreted were retained within the extracellular space, dangerous hyperkalemia would result. This does not happen, however, since nearly 80% of the retained potassium is translocated into cells. In recent years, much progress has been made in defining those factors that contribute to the regulation of extrarenal potassium homeostasis. Three hormones—insulin, aldosterone, and epinephrine—have all been shown to be important in extrarenal potassium metabolism.

If basal insulin secretion is inhibited with somatostatin, fasting plasma insulin levels decline by 50% and the serum potassium concentration rises by 0.4–0.5 mEq/liter. More importantly, if potassium is infused at a time when insulin secretion has been inhibited, a marked deterioration in potassium tolerance is observed. The protective effect of insulin has been shown to be related to its ability to stimulate potassium uptake by muscle and liver cells.

Epinephrine or, more specifically, agents that act via the β_2-adrenergic receptor also exert a stimulatory effect on potassium uptake by muscle and liver cells. As with insulin, the simple maintenance of basal epinephrine levels is necessary for normal potassium homeostasis. Although physiological increments in plasma potassium concentration appear to have no stimulatory effect on catecholamine secretion, if potassium is administered at a time when the β_2-adrenergic receptor has been blocked, marked hyperkalemia will ensue. β_1-Adrenergic agonists and antagonists do not appear to exert any effect on potassium metabolism. Aldosterone also plays an important regulatory role in extrarenal potassium homeostasis both by stimulating colonic potassium secretion and enhancing cellular potassium uptake by nonrenal, nongastrointestinal tissues.

Defects in insulin, epinephrine, and aldosterone secretion have all been associated with clinically significant hyperkalemia and are discussed in Sections IV.F and IV.H. In addition to these hormones, metabolic acidemia and plasma hypertonicity are also known to affect overall potassium tolerance adversely by inhibiting net potassium uptake by extrarenal tissues. It should also be pointed out that factors in addition to those described above must be important in extrarenal potassium metabolism. Even when insulin, epinephrine, and aldosterone secretion are blocked and blood pH and serum tonicity are controlled, approximately half of the retained potassium is still taken up by cells. Whether this regulation represents the intrinsic ability of extrarenal tissues to respond to a rise in serum potassium concentration or is mediated by other yet unidentified mechanisms is not yet established.

IV. CLINICAL DISORDERS OF HYPERKALEMIA

The pathophysiology of clinical disorders complicated by an impairment in renal potassium secretion and consequent hyperkalemia follows directly from the model described above (Table I). Thus, decreased renal potassium excretion and the potential for hyperkalemia can result from: inadequate sodium delivery to the distal nephron; decreased distal tubular urine flow; a defect in the renin–angiotensin–aldosterone axis; a primary renal tubular secretory defect; inhibition of distal potassium secretion by acidemia, drug, or toxin; or the presence of renal disease, usually of the interstitial variety, that directly affects the integrity of the potassium secretory cells located in the distal nephron. In addition, nonrenal disturbances resulting in an abnormal distribution of potassium between intracellular and extracellular environment can result in hyperkalemia.

A. Factitious Hyperkalemia

Before embarking on an extensive investigation of etiology and before instituting therapy, one should be certain that the patient is truly hyperkalemic. Laboratory error and factitious causes of hyperkalemia (Table I) should be excluded. Erythrocytes, leukocytes, and platelets are all high in potassium content. If there is an abnormality in the red blood cell membrane, or if the white blood cell ($>$50,000–100,000/mm^3) or platelet ($>$10^6/mm^3) counts are extremely high, significant amounts of potassium may be released from cells during the clotting process, and this may result in a falsely elevated potassium level. This can easily be checked by comparing the potassium measurements on simultaneously drawn serum and plasma samples. They should agree within 0.2–0.3 mEq/liter. A difference of greater than 0.2–0.3 mEq/liter suggests pseudohyperkalemia. Most importantly, since the serum potassium

Table I. Etiology of Hyperkalemia

Factitious
    Laboratory error
    Pseudohyperkalemia: *in vitro* hemolysis, thrombocytosis, leukocytosis
Acidemia (acute)
Increased potassium input into ECF compartment
    Exogenous: diet, salt substitutes, low-sodium diet, medications
    Endogenous: hemolysis, GI bleeding, catabolic states, crush injury
Inadequate distal delivery of sodium and decreased distal tubular flow
Renal failure
    Acute
    Chronic: GFR < 15–20 ml/min
Impaired renin–aldosterone axis
    Addison's disease
    Enzyme deficiency
    Primary hypoaldosteronism
    Primary hyporeninism
    Angiotensin deficiency or insensitivity
    Other (heparin, β-adrenergic blockers, prostaglandin synthesis inhibitors,
       captopril)
Primary renal tubular potassium secretory defect
    Sickle cell disease
    Systemic lupus erythematosus
    Post renal transplantation (? rejection)
    Obstructive uropathy
    Amyloidosis
    Congenital (children with short stature)
    Familial
Inhibition of tubular potassium secretion
    Spironolactone
    Triamterene
    Amiloride
    Digitalis
Abnormal potassium distribution
    Acidemia
    Insulin deficiency
    Hypertonicity (hyperglycemia)
    Aldosterone deficiency
    β-Adrenergic blockers
    Exercise
    Periodic paralysis
    Tissue damage
    Succinylcholine
    Digitalis
    Arginine hydrochloride

level *in vivo* is normal, electrocardiographic manifestations of hyperkalemia will be absent. An EKG should be performed in every patient with laboratory evidence of hyperkalemia.

B. Acidemia

Acidemia may cause hyperkalemia via two mechanisms: (1) acutely, acidemia exerts a direct inhibitory effect on distal tubular secretion of potassium; this effect lasts only a few hours and wanes as the acidemia becomes more chronic; and (2) as the extracellular hydrogen ion concentration increases, there is a shift of potassium from the intracellular to the extracellular space as hydrogen ions move into cells to be buffered. Although it is commonly stated that for every 0.1-unit increase in blood pH, the potassium concentration will increase by 0.6 mEq/liter, the literature indicates considerable variation, with 0.1-unit changes in blood pH being associated with rises in plasma potassium concentration ranging from 0.3 to 1.3 mEq/liter. Recent studies have indicated that this relationship is quite complex and can be influenced by multiple factors.

Respiratory acidemia causes little increase (0.1–0.3 mEq/liter) in the plasma potassium concentration, whereas metabolic acidemia results in a more pronounced rise in the potassium level, 0.5–1.3 mEq/ liter per 0.1 unit. The anion accompanying the increase in hydrogen ion influences the increase in plasma potassium concentration. Hydrochloric acid causes marked hyperkalemia, whereas organic acids (lactic acid and β-hydroxybutyric acid) cause a much smaller rise in plasma potassium. Changes in plasma bicarbonate concentration *per se*, independent of changes in blood pH, also influence the potassium concentration. When acid is infused to lower the bicarbonate concentration but the blood pH is maintained constant by simultaneous reduction of the P_{CO_2}, the plasma potassium concentration still rises substantially. Lastly, the duration of metabolic acidemia and, presumably, the extent of intracellular buffering also affect the plasma potassium concentration. Immediately following an acid load, the serum bicarbonate concentration and blood pH demonstrate their greatest decline, yet little change in plasma potassium concentration occurs. With time, as more of the hydrogen ions move into cells to be buffered, plasma bicarbonate and blood pH levels return to normal, and plasma potassium concentration rises to its highest level.

C. Increased Potassium Intake or Release from Cells

Increased intake of potassium or potassium release from cells may result in a transient rise in plasma potassium concentration. Sustained hyperkalemia, however, is unusual unless an underlying defect in renal potassium excretion also exists. During intravenous potassium chloride infusion, the plasma potassium concentration may rise into the 5–5.4 mEq/liter range initially, but it returns to normal within 24–36 hr even though the infusion is sustained. This results from a combination of enhanced renal potassium excretion and increased cellular uptake of potassium. The persistence of hyperkalemia even in the face of an increased potassium load should suggest the presence of an underlying defect in the potassium homeostatic system.

D. Inadequate Distal Delivery of Sodium and Fluid

Diminished sodium delivery to the distal sites of potassium secretion is commonly cited as a cause of hyperkalemia. However, this situation is unusual unless urinary sodium excretion is markedly reduced, i.e., less than 5–10 mEq/day. The reason for this is that the majority of potassium secretion occurs in the distal tubule, and sodium delivery to this segment is rarely rate limiting even when dietary sodium intake is markedly reduced. Furthermore, recent studies suggest that flow, rather than sodium delivery, is the primary determinant of potassium secretion; clinically, however, the two almost always go hand in hand. The most common situation in which decreased distal sodium delivery results in hyperkalemia is acute pulmonary edema, particularly in an individual with underlying chronic renal disease. The acute reduction in renal plasma flow and glomerular filtration rate markedly enhances proximal tubular salt and water reabsorption, thereby limiting the delivery of sodium and fluid to distal sites of potassium secretion.

E. Renal Failure

Acute oligo- to anuric renal failure is almost universally accompanied by hyperkalemia. The reasons for this are: (1) glomerular filtration rate is often reduced to less than 10 ml/min, and such a severe reduction may of itself become rate limiting for potassium excretion; (2) distal sodium delivery and urine flow are markedly decreased; (3) the most common cause of acute renal failure is acute tubular necrosis which results in widespread damage to the distal tubule and collecting duct cells, the sites primarily responsible for potassium secretion; (4) because of the acuteness of the renal failure, there is insufficient time for the normal renal and extrarenal adaptive mechanisms to develop; and (5) these factors are often coupled with increased tissue catabolism or frank tissue breakdown, releasing cellular potassium and adding to the likelihood of developing hyperkalemia.

In contrast, it is unusual to observe significant hyperkalemia in the patient with chronic renal failure unless the glomerular filtration rate is reduced to less than 15–20 ml/min. With progressive reduction in nephron mass, there is a marked adaptive increase in the ability of the remaining tubules to secrete potassium.

F. Impaired Renin–Aldosterone Axis

1. Addison's Disease

Both aldosterone and, to a lesser extent, glucocorticoids are known to have important kaliuretic effects in man (Fig. 3). Both hormones also stimulate potassium secretion by the colonic epithelium. Therefore, it is not surprising that patients with Addison's disease (combined mineralocorticoid and glucocorticoid deficiency resulting from destruction of the adrenal gland) are predisposed to hyperkalemia. In contrast, patients with pituitary disease and ACTH deficiency, in whom aldosterone production is relatively well maintained, rarely develop hyperkalemia. This clinical observation indicates that of the two hormones, aldosterone plays a quantitatively

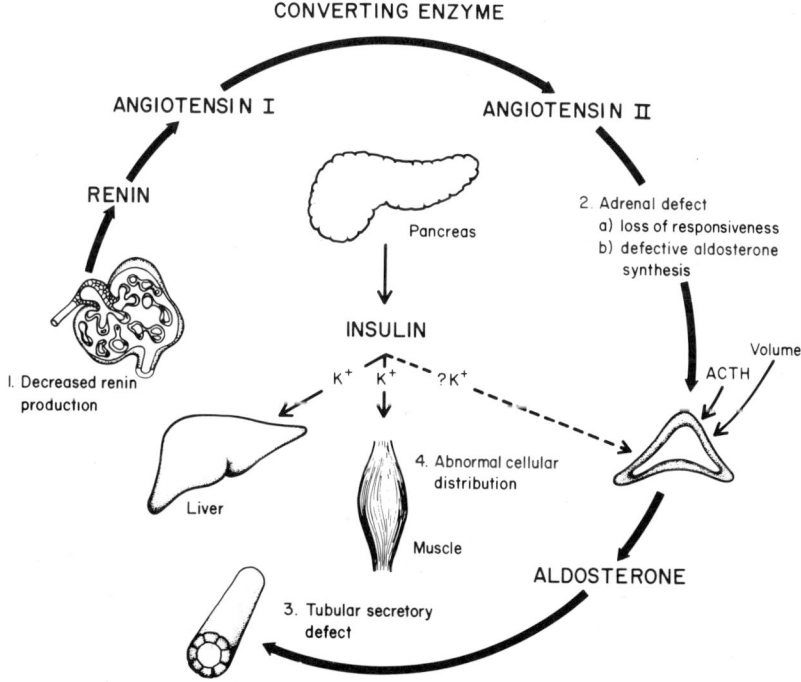

Figure 3. Schematic representation of potential hormonal, renal, and extrarenal defects resulting in hyperkalemia. Hyperkalemia may result as a consequence of the following: (1) decreased renin production; (2) decreased aldosterone production despite normal renin secretion (adrenal defect); (3) a renal tubular secretory defect; (4) an abnormal distribution of potassium between intracellular and extracellular fluid compartments.

more important role than glucocorticoids in the defense of body potassium homeostasis.

Aldosterone stimulates potassium secretion by the distal tubule and collecting duct, and, conversely, aldosterone deficiency is associated with a decrease in distal tubular fluid potassium concentration. In addition to their well-known kaliuretic action, mineralocorticoids are also known to enhance potassium uptake by extrarenal tissues. However, despite these important effects on both renal and extrarenal potassium metabolism, moderate to severe hyperkalemia (5.5–6 mEq/liter) is uncommon in adult subjects with mineralocorticoid lack and normal renal function who are not volume contracted. As long as the dietary intake of sodium chloride is sufficient to maintain the intravascular volume and to insure an adequate delivery of fluid and sodium to the distal sites of potassium secretion, the Addisonian patient will be able to excrete sufficient potassium to maintain normal potassium balance.

2. Enzyme Defects

Aldosterone deficiency can be associated with a variety of enzymatic defects, of which the most common is the 21-hydroxylase deficiency. This results in a combined deficiency of both mineralocorticoid and glucocorticoid function with the clinical presentation as renal salt wasting, hyperkalemia, virilization, and failure to thrive. Such individuals almost always present in childhood, and only rarely, when a partial enzymatic defect is present, do they escape undiagnosed into adulthood. The final two steps in the biosynthesis of aldosterone involve mixed-function oxidation reactions in which corticosterone is converted to 18-hydroxycorticosterone and then to aldosterone. Defects in both of these enzymatic reactions have been described. Because these enzymes are not necessary for cortisol biosynthesis, evidence of glucocorticoid insufficiency and virilization are not part of the clinical presentation.

3. Hyporeninemic Hypoaldosteronism

At present, this is the most common cause of hypoaldosteronism. The clinical presentation is quite typical. Most patients are old, and this may be an important underlying substrate since both renin and aldosterone secretion are known to descrease with advancing age. The majority of patients are asymptomatic and are diagnosed on routine laboratory screening or during evaluation for some other unassociated illness. Only 25% of patients present with symptoms referrable to the hyperkalemia, i.e., muscle weakness and cardiac arrhythmias. A hyperchloremic metabolic acidosis is present in over half the cases. Salt wasting is distinctly uncommon. Most of these patients have a partial defect in aldosterone secretion, and the plasma aldosterone concentration, although reduced, is adequate to maintain normal sodium balance unless the dietary sodium intake is markedly restricted. However, although the low circulating aldosterone concentrations are sufficient to maintain normal sodium balance, they are clearly insufficient to prevent the development of hyperkalemia. Baseline cortisol levels and the cortisol response to ACTH have been normal in all reported patients.

The majority of patients have some degree of chronic renal insufficiency. The two most frequently encountered types of renal disease are diabetic glomerulosclerosis and a variety of interstitial renal diseases (i.e., gouty nephropathy, nephrolithiasis, analgesic nephropathy, obstructive uropathy, and sickle cell disease). The syndrome has occasionally been described in patients with glomerulonephritis.

Baseline plasma aldosterone concentrations are low or low normal, and following volume contraction, a subnormal increase has been observed in all reported cases. In the great majority of patients with selective hypoaldosteronism, the low circulating plasma aldosterone levels can be explained, in large part, by the hyporeninemia. However, several lines of evidence suggest that, at least in a significant minority of patients, in addition to hyporeninemia a primary adrenal defect may contribute to the hypoaldosteronism. First, baseline and/or stimulated renin levels have been reported to be normal in about 20% of patients. Second, the aldosterone response to intravenous angiotensin II and ACTH is frequently abnormal. Since both angiotensin II and ACTH directly stimulate aldosterone release by the zona glomerulosa, one would anticipate a normal response if adrenal gland function were intact. A variety of pathogenetic mechanisms have been suggested to explain the hyporeninemia and hypoaldosteronism. The reader is referred to several excellent recent reviews.

4. Other Causes of an Impairment in the Renin–Aldosterone Axis

A variety of drugs produce a state of functional hypoaldosteronism. The β-adrenergic blocking agents, by inhibiting renin secretion and impairing potassium uptake by extrarenal tissues, can lead to hyperkalemia. Captopril, an antihypertensive agent that works by inhibiting the conversion of angiotensin I to angiotensin II, has also been reported to cause hyperkalemia. Prostaglandin inhibitors such as indomethacin have also been associated with hyperkalemia and hyporeninemic hypoaldosteronism.

G. Renal Tubular Secretory Defect

An increasing number of patients are being described in whom hyperkalemia is associated with normal or high circulating levels of renin and aldosterone and who fail to respond to large doses of mineralocorticoid replacement. Such patients are characterized by a defect in the renal tubular secretion of potassium (Fig. 3). This primary renal tubular secretory defect has been described in patients with sickle cell disease, systemic lupus erythematosus, renal transplantation, obstructive uropathy, and amyloidosis.

Several diuretics (spironolactone, triamterene, amiloride) can result in hyperkalemia by inhibiting renal tubular potassium secretion.

H. Abnormal Potassium Distribution

As discussed in Section I, only about 2% of the body's potassium stores is located in the extracellular fluid compartment. The remaining 98% is located within cells. Thus, anything that causes even the slightest imbalance of potassium between the intracellular and extracellular space can result in profound hyperkalemia. Metabolic acidemia is one of the most common clinical situations in which a shift of potassium from the intracellular to extracellular space can result in signficiant hyperkalemia.

Insulin plays a very important role in maintaining the normal distribution of potassium between intracellular and extracellular compartments. When fasting insulin levels are decreased by 50%, a predictable rise in plasma potassium concentration of 0.4–0.5 mEq/liter occurs. More importantly, if an exogenous potassium load is administered at a time when insulin secretion has been blocked, a marked deterioration in potassium tolerance ensues. Insulin has been shown to exert its protective effect on potassium metabolism by enhancing hepatic and muscle cell uptake of potassium. Lack of insulin is one of the major factors that predispose the insulin-dependent diabetic to hyperkalemia. Hyperglycemia, particularly in diabetics who lack adequate aldosterone (see below), is often associated with a rise in the plasma potassium concentration. The increase in blood glucose induces a shift of water and potassium from the intracellular to the extracellular space. Normally, the efflux of potassium from cells is opposed by the action of insulin and aldosterone to enhance cellular uptake of potassium. With a deficiency of both of these hormones, clinically significant hyperkalemia may develop.

Two other hormones, aldosterone and epinephrine, also have important extrarenal mechanisms of actions. Although the primary effect of aldosterone is to enhance potassium excretion by the kidney, it also has an important extrarenal mechanism of action, and impaired uptake of potassium by nonrenal tissues likely contributes to the hyperkalemia observed in selective hypoaldosteronism. Epinephrine enhances potassium uptake by extrarenal tissues, an effect mediated via the β_2-adrenergic receptor. In contrast, β-adrenergic blockers such as propranolol inhibit epinephrine-mediated stimulation of potassium uptake by extrarenal tissues and result in a deterioration of potassium tolerance.

V. TREATMENT OF HYPERKALEMIA

Treatment of the patient with hyperkalemia is dependent on two factors: (1) the severity of the hyperkalemia and (2) definition of the etiology.

Whether or not aggressive therapy should be instituted is dictated by both the degree of hyperkalemia and the presence of cardiac or neuromuscular manifestations. Obviously, if a specific cause for the increase in serum potassium concentration can be identified, this should be eliminated. Regardless of etiology, however, there will be certain patients in whom acute correction of the hyperkalemia is indicated. In order to appreciate who should be treated aggressively, the clinician must be familiar with the clinical manifestations of hyperkalemia.

A. Clinical Manifestations

All of the important clinical manifestations of hyperkalemia are related to alterations in the electrical excitability of the cell membrane. A detailed description of the precise electrophysiological events that govern excitation and conduction of the electrical impulse are beyond the scope of the present chapter. Briefly, in the basal state, the transmembrane electrical potential difference is about -80 mV, with the cell interior negative. This resting potential is primarily determined by the high concentration difference of potassium ions between the intracellular ($\sim$150 mEq/liter) and extracellular (3.5–5.0 mEq/liter) fluid volumes. This high intracellular/extracellular potassium (K_i/K_e) ratio (35–40:1) is maintained by active extrusion of sodium from the cell interior in exchange for potassium. When the serum potassium concentration rises, the ratio of K_i/K_e falls, and the resting potential becomes less negative; i.e., it moves closer to the threshold for excitation. The electrophysiological consequences resulting from this alteration are complex, but the end result is a decrease in conduction velocity and an increase in the rate of repolarization.

1. Cardiac Toxicity

The heart is particularly vulnerable to increases in the serum potassium concentration. The earliest EKG change suggesting hyperkalemia is a symmetrical increase in the amplitude or tenting of the T waves, best seen in the precordial leads and occasionally associated with some ST depression. These changes result from an increase in the rate of repolarization of the action potential. Such changes usually become apparent with serum potassium levels of 5.5–6.0 mEq/liter. As the serum potassium concentration rises further (6.0–7.0 mEq/liter), slowed conduction through the His–Purkinje system and ventricular muscle is reflected by a lengthening of the PR interval and widening of the QRS complex. With potassium concentrations of 7.0–7.5 mEq/liter, conduction by atrial muscle becomes impaired as reflected by progressive flattening of the P wave; there is continued widening of the QRS complex and a further delay in A–V conduction. At potassium concentrations in excess of 8 mEq/liter, atrial conduction ceases, and the P waves disappear. As the QRS complex widens further, it merges with the T wave to produce a sine-wave pattern that is frequently misdiagnosed as ventricular tachycardia. If these ominous changes go unrecognized, and appropriate therapy is not instituted, ventricular fibrillation or asystole will follow shortly. In addition to the classical sequence of events outlined above, virtually any arrhythmia or conduction disturbance may be seen in hyperkalemic patients. Various forms of fasicular and A–V nodal block are particularly common.

It is important to recognize that many factors can alter the effects of hyperkalemia on the heart. If the hyperkalemia develops more slowly (i.e., as occurs in chronic renal failure), cardiac manifestations may be minimal or even absent despite serum concentrations of 7.0–7.5 mEq/liter. In contrast, certain metabolic derangements such as hyponatremia, hypocalcemia, and acidemia will potentiate the effects of hyperkalemia, and severe cardiotoxicity may be observed with serum potassium concentrations of only 6.0–6.5 mEq/liter. Lastly, it should be emphasized that cardiac toxicity may develop without any premonitory changes in the electrocardiogram. Thus, a perfectly normal EKG may degenerate directly to ventricular tachycardia. Regardless of the EKG, therapeutic intervention should be initiated when the serum potassium concentration has risen acutely to 6.0 mEq/liter.

2. Neuromuscular Manifestations

The first symptoms include paresthesias and weakness in the arms and legs. These are followed by a symmetrical flaccid paralysis which ascends toward the trunk and may involve the muscles of respiration, leading to hypoxemia and carbon dioxide retention.

B. Acute Treatment of Hyperkalemia

If the serum potassium concentration has risen acutely to levels in excess of 6.0 mEq/liter, or if EKG changes of hyperkalemia are present regardless of the degree of hyperkalemia, treatment should be initiated. Therapy can be divided into four general categories (Table II): measures designed (1) to oppose directly the effects of hyperkalemia on the cell membrane; (2) to enhance the transfer of potassium from extracellular to intracellular fluid compartments; (3) to remove potassium from the body; and (4) to reverse specifically the cause of the hyperkalemia.

1. Direct Antagonism of Membrane Effects

a. Calcium

The infusion of calcium will immediately antagonize the effects of hyperkalemia on the heart, even in normocalcemic patients. Although calcium does not alter the resting membrane potential, it causes an increase in

Table II. Acute Therapy of Hyperkalemia

	Mechanism	Dose	Onset	Duration of hypokalemic effect
Calcium gluconate (10%)	Membrane antagonism	10–20 ml IV	1–3 min	30–60 min
Sodium bicarbonate	Membrane antagonism and redistribution	50–100 mEq IV	5–10 min	~2 hr
Sodium chloride (3%)	Membrane antagonism	50–100 mEq IV	5–10 min	~2 hr
Insulin plus glucose	Redistribution	20 units of regular insulin with 50 g of glucose IV over 1 hr	30 min	4–6 hr
Cation exchange resin (Kayexalate)	Excretion	20–50 g PO or per rectum with sorbitol	1–2 hr	4–6 hr
Peritoneal or hemodialysis	Excretion	—	Within minutes after starting	Until dialysis is completed
Diuretics	Excretion		With start of diuresis	Until diuresis ends
Furosemide		40 mg IV		
Ethacrynic acid		50 mg IV		

the threshold potential at which excitation occurs. This restoration of the normal difference between the resting and threshold potentials reverses the depolarization blockade seen with hyperkalemia. The increase in calcium ion concentration also increases the number of sodium channels within the cell membrane, resulting in faster conduction. The infusion of a 10- to 20-ml bolus of a 10% solution of calcium gluconate will have an immediate onset (1–3 min) of action that will last for approximately 30–60 min. If no effect is seen within 5–10 min, the dose can be repeated. Failure to respond to the second dose makes it unlikely that further doses will be of benefit. If an initial response is observed, but the beneficial effect wanes, repeated doses can be given as the electrocardiographic changes of hyperkalemia begin to reappear. When calcium is administered, it is always preferable to have continuous EKG monitoring.

In patients with renal failure, the serum phosphate concentration is often elevated. The administration of calcium under such circumstances runs the risk of elevating the calcium phosphate in tissues. If a life-threatening arrhythmia is present, however, its treatment must take precedence, and calcium should be administered even though its full effect may be partially offset by its binding with phosphate.

A note of caution should be inserted concerning the administration of calcium to patients who are taking digitalis. Hypercalcemia will potentiate the toxic effects of digitalis on the heart. Therefore, if calcium must be given to patients taking digitalis, it should be added to 100 ml of dextrose 5% in water and infused slowly over 20–30 min to allow a more even distribution throughout the extracellular space. Since hypocalcemia will potentiate all of the toxic effects of hyperkalemia on neuromuscular function, restoration of the serum calcium concentration to normal in these individuals will have a particularly dramatic effect in reversing the manifestations of cardiac toxicity.

b. Sodium

Changes in serum sodium concentration (either hyper- or hyponatremia) have little or no effect on the heart in the absence of other electrolyte or acid–base disturbances. In the presence of hyperkalemia, the number of sodium channels (which are responsible for the conduction of electrical impulse once the threshold potential has been reached) is diminished, and the decrease in conduction velocity is amplified. Administration of hypertonic saline (50–100 mEq of NaCl) to such a hyponatremic individual may have the dramatic effect of reversing the deleterious effects of hyperkalemia on the heart. The action of hypertonic saline is less predictable in the patient with a normal serum sodium concentration.

Although hypertonic NaCl has been shown to be effective in reversing the cardiac effects of hyperkalemia, sodium bicarbonate has largely replaced its use because hyperkalemia is frequently associated with acidemia.

2. Redistribution of Potassium from Extracellular to Intracellular Space

a. Sodium Bicarbonate

Even in the absence of acidemia, an increase in serum bicarbonate concentration and blood pH will cause a shift of potassium into cells and increase the K_i/K_e ratio. The increase in blood pH will have the additional effect of acutely stimulating potassium secretion by the distal tubule. In addition, if the renal threshold (Tm_{HCO_3}) is exceeded, the excess bicarbonate along with sodium will be delivered to the distal tubules and further augment potassium secretion. Sodium bicarbonate can be administered intravenously as a 50-mEq bolus given over 5–10 min. The onset of action in correcting hyperkalemia is 5–10 min, and the duration is approximately 2 hr. If no effect is observed within 10–15 min, an additional 50 mEq can be infused. The major contraindication to $NaHCO_3$ is volume overload. It should also be remembered that alkalemia may precipitate tetany or seizures in a patient with preexisting hypocalcemia. If neurological symptoms develop, intravenous calcium chloride should be administered in a dose to increase the plasma ionized calcium concentration by approximately 1 mg/dl.

b. Insulin–Glucose

Infusion of insulin has long been known to stimulate potassium uptake by cells, particularly in muscle. This is the result of a direct depolarizing effect of insulin on the cell membrane and is independent of glucose transport. Glucose is administered solely for the purpose of preventing hypoglycemia. A 10-unit dose of insulin is usually administered with 50 g of glucose over 1 hr. This is most easily accomplished by adding the insulin to 500 ml of a 10% glucose solution. The onset of action in correcting hyperkalemia is approximately 30 min, and the effect may last for 4–6 hr. One can expect a 0.5–1.2 mEq/liter decrease in the plasma potassium concentration within 1–2 hr. The dose of insulin–glucose can be repeated as frequently as needed. The major side effect is hypoglycemia. This can be avoided by infusing the insulin with glucose as previously described.

3. Removal of Potassium by the Body

None of the therapeutic maneuvers discussed so far will result in a net removal of potassium from the body. Thus, they serve solely as temporizing measures until more definitive therapy can be instituted to decrease the total body potassium content.

a. Increased Renal Excretion

Unfortunately, hyperkalemia is most frequently encountered in the setting of renal failure, and little can be done to enhance renal potassium excretion. However, in the patient with relatively intact kidney function, measures that enhance urine flow and sodium delivery to the distal tubular sites of potassium secretion will markedly enhance renal potassium excretion. Diuretics acting proximal to the potassium secretory sites such as furosemide (40–80 mg IV) and ethacrynic acid (50–100 mg IV) have proven effective in this regard.

b. Cation-Exchange Resins

Cation-exchange resins such as Na polystyrene sulfonate (Kayexalate®) will reduce the plasma potassium concentration by exchanging sodium for potassium within the gastrointestinal tract. Each gram of resin removes 0.5–1 mEq of potassium in exchange for 2–3 mEq of sodium. Significant amounts of calcium and magnesium may also be removed. The usual dose of Kayexalate® is 25 g given orally or as a retention enema. Since Kayexalate® is constipating, it should be given with sorbitol to induce diarrhea: 15 ml of 70% sorbitol is given every 30 min to induce diarrhea, which can usually be sustained by administering the same dose of sorbitol every 6–8 hr. If the patient is unable to tolerate oral administration, 50 g of Kayexalate® with 50 g of sorbitol can be added to 200 ml of 10% dextrose in water and given per rectum with an inflatable rectal catheter. Retention for 30–60 min is needed for the best therapeutic results. Enemas can be repeated 4–6 times per day as necessary. It usually takes 1–2 hr to see the onset of Kayexalate® action. On average, 50 g of Kayexalate® will lower the serum potassium concentration by 0.5–1.0 mEq/liter over the 4–6 hr period following its administration. The serum potassium concentration should be checked after each enema to guide further therapy. It is noteworthy that in the original studies examining the efficacy of Kayexalate®, the administration of oral sorbitol alone was almost as effective as the combination of sorbitol plus Kayexalate®. The major side effects are nausea and vomiting with oral administration. In patients with underlying cardiac disease, the increased sodium load may precipitate congestive heart failure.

c. Dialysis

Both peritoneal dialysis and hemodialysis are effective means of removing potassium from the body. If acute reduction of the serum potassium concentration is desired, hemodialysis is preferred. Using standard dialysis coils (with no addition of potassium to the dialysate), if an individual starts with a plasma potassium concentration of 7 mEq/liter, one will remove approximately 40 mEq of potassium during the first hour of dialysis. The plasma potassium concentration will begin to fall within minutes after the start of dialysis, and the hypokalemic effect will last for as long as the dialysis is continued. The major disadvantage of hemodialysis is the time required to prepare the equipment and insert the catheter. Peritoneal dialysis is also an effective way to remove potassium from the body, but its potassium-lowering effect is much slower than that of hemodialysis or resins. If the standard 2-liter exchanges are employed, and if each exchange takes 1 hr, approximately 5 mEq of potassium per hour will be removed. This will have little acute impact on either hyperkalemia or total body potassium content, but over 36–48 hr, approximately 180–240 mEq of potassium will be removed, and this will have a pronounced potassium-lowering effect.

C. Treatment of Chronic Hyperkalemia

Once the acute effects of hyperkalemia on cardiovascular and neuro-muscular function have been reversed, the specific etiology of the hyperkalemia should be sought (Table I) and more specific therapy instituted to prevent recurrence of hyperkalemia. If a reversible cause for the hyperkalemia cannot be identified, then more general therapeutic interventions should be initiated.

1. Dietary Management

All patients with chronic hyperkalemia should be placed on a diet containing less than 60 mEq of potassium per day. If the hyperkalemia is particularly severe and/or associated with signs of cardiac toxicity, dietary potassium should be reduced to less than 40 mEq/day. Some foodstuffs particularly rich in potassium are shown in Table 3. Sources of increased potassium input (both exogenous and endogenous) should be sought and eliminated. A low-sodium diet is by definition a high-potassium diet, since the dietician usually replaces sodium-rich foods with those high in potassium content. Low-sodium foods have sodium removed with exchange for potassium. Salt substitutes, which contain 10–13 mEq of potassium per gram, are another source of increased potassium intake. Endogenous input of potassium may be more difficult to recognize. Rhabdomyolysis, burns, crush injuries, and chemotherapy are obvious causes. Chronic hemolysis and gastrointestinal bleeding may be less obvious.

2. Acidemia

Metabolic acidemia should be corrected. Recent studies have shown that a decrease in the serum bicarbonate concentration, independent of a decrease in blood pH, will also cause a shift of potassium from the intracellular to extracellular fluid compartment. Correction of a low serum bicarbonate concentration is best accomplished with sodium bicarbonate, using a bicarbonate distribution space equal to 40% of body weight. For example, if a person weighs 70 kg, to raise his serum bicarbonate concentration from 15 to 25 mEq/liter will require:

Bicarbonate replacement (mEq) = (70 kg) (0.60) (25 − 15 mEq/liter)

Table III. Potassium Content of Some Commonly Eaten Foods[a]

	K per serving[b]			K per serving[b]	
	mg	mEq		mg	mEq
Vegetables			Fruits and fruit juice		
Chick peas, raw	1594	41	Raisins, whole fresh	1106	28
Butternut squash, boiled, mashed	835	21	Prunes, dried, cooked	695	18
Pea beans, cooked	790	20	Avocado, fresh, 1/2 medium	684	17
Potato, baked, 1 medium	782	20	Cantaloupe, 1/2 medium	682	17
Acorn squash, baked, 1/2 medium	749	19	Apricots, canned	605	15
Lima beans, cooked	717	18	Prune juice, canned	602	15
Red kidney beans, cooked	629	16	Pumpkin, canned	588	15
Blackeye peas, cooked	625	16	Rhubarb, cooked	548	14
Parsnips, diced, cooked	587	15	Orange juice, canned or fresh	496	13
Spinach, cooked	583	15	Orange juice, frozen	476	12
Tomato juice, canned	552	14	Orange and grapefruit juice, canned	454	12
Vegetable juice cocktail, canned	535	14	Banana, medium	440	11
Tomatoes, canned	523	13	Melon balls, frozen	432	11
Lentils, cooked	498	13	Nectarine, 1 medium	406	10
Winter squash, frozen, cooked	497	13	Grapefruit juice, canned	400	10
Beet greens, cooked	481	12	Pomegranate, 1 medium	399	10
Broccoli, cooked, 1 medium stalk	481	12	Apricot nectar	379	10
Swiss chard, cooked	465	12	Plums, canned	368	9

Food			Food		
Brussels sprouts, cooked	423	11	Apricot halves, dried, 10 medium	343	9
Succotash, frozen, cooked	418	11	Peaches, canned	334	9
Sweet potato, canned	400	10	Papaya, cubed	328	8
Beets, sliced, cooked	354	9	Mango, sliced	312	8
Mixed vegetables, frozen, cooked	348	9	Apricots, fresh, 3	301	8
Collards, cooked	339	9	Raspberries, red, canned	277	7
Sauerkraut, canned	329	9	Raspberries, black, fresh	267	7
Green peas, cooked	314	8	Orange, 1 medium	263	7
Mustard greens, frozen, cooked	308	8	Raspberries, red, frozen	250	6
Okra, cooked	303	8	Raspberries, red, raw	207	5
Tomato, raw, 1 medium	300	8			
Turnips, cubed, cooked	291	7	Some other sources		
Rutabagas, cooked	284	7			
			Peanuts, 2 oz.	382	10
Meat, poultry, fish (3-oz. serving)			Milk, 1 cup	351	9
Flounder	498	13	Cashews, 2 oz.	264	7
Halibut	447	11	Walnuts, 2 oz.	260	7
Chicken	273–351	7–9	Peanut butter, 2 tablespoons	200	5
Beef	225–282	6–7			
Lamb	241–273	6–7			

[a] Potassium values are from Nutritive Value of American Food—Handbook No. 456, USDA, Washington.
[b] Serving size is 1 cup unless otherwise indicated.

or 420 mEq. The major complication of bicarbonate therapy is volume over-load. If this is a concern, sodium bicarbonate should be administered slowly and cautiously and with a diuretic to promote sodium excretion. Alternative-ly, calcium carbonate can be substituted. One gram of calcium carbonate contains 10 mEq of bicarbonate.

3. Avoidance of Drugs That Predispose to Hyperkalemia

A large number of drugs are known to predispose to hyperkalemia. Some inhibit the renin–angiotensin–aldosterone axis (β-adrenergic blockers, i.e., propranolol; prostaglandin inhibitors, i.e., indomethacin; captopril), whereas others directly block potassium secretion by the distal tubule (spiro-nolactone, triamterene, amiloride). Most recently, intravenous glucose (hyperglycemia) and β-adrenergic blocking agents have also been shown to enhance the movement of potassium from the intracellular to the extracellu-lar fluid compartment, with resultant hyperkalemia.

4. Volume Expansion

Since both a decrease in distal sodium delivery and a decrease in distal tubular urine flow are known to inhibit potassium secretion, care should be taken to maintain adequacy of the intravascular volume at all times.

5. Specific Therapeutic Interventions

In the patient with documented aldosterone deficiency and hyperkale-mia, the treatment of choice is fluorocortisone acetate (Florinef®). The normal replacement dose is 0.1 mg per day orally. However, many of these individuals have underlying renal disease and are refractory to the mineralo-corticoid effect. Consequently, larger doses, 0.3–0.5 mg/day, may be neces-sary to correct the hyperkalemia. Unfortunately, significant sodium retention often accompanies the use of such large doses of Florinef®, and this may require the concomitant use of diuretic therapy.

Patients with a renal tubular secretory defect are more difficult to treat. Furosemide or the combination of acetazolamide with sodium bicarbonate have been tried, but these agents often prove unsuccessful. Recently, thiazide diuretics have been shown to enhance renal potassium excretion even though the more potent loop diuretics have failed. The mechanism of the effect of thiazides in patients with a renal secretory defect has not yet been worked out.

VI. HYPOKALEMIA: ESTIMATION OF POTASSIUM DEFICIT

Hypokalemia is defined by a serum potassium concentration less than 3.5 mEq/liter. As with hyperkalemia, treatment of the patient with hypokalemia is dependent on (1) definition of the etiology and (2) the severity of the hypokalemia.

In the absence of cellular shifts of potassium (as may occur with alkalemia, insulin, epinephrine), a serum potassium concentration between 2.5 and 3.5 mEq/liter signifies approximately a 10% reduction (200–400 mEq) in total body potassium content. Such deficits are not usually associated with any clinical manifestations and usually can be corrected more slowly with oral potassium replacement. Serum potassium concentrations less than 2.5 mEq/liter imply a 15–20% or greater decrease in total body potassium stores (400–700 mEq) and may need to be replaced more aggressively depending on the presence or absence of clinical manifestations. When the serum potassium level drops to less than 1.8–2.0 mEq/liter, it becomes difficult to estimate the true potassium deficit because the relationship between serum potassium concentration and total body potassium content becomes less linear. With serum potassium levels less than 2.0 mEq/liter, small additional decreases may be associated with huge deficits in total body potassium. The treatment of hypokalemia is potassium replacement, usually in the form of KCl. How rapidly potassium is replaced and whether the potassium is given intravenously or orally will depend both on the absolute serum potassium concentration and its clinical manifestations.

VII. CLINICAL MANIFESTATIONS

When the plasma potassium concentration falls as a result of potassium loss from the body, potassium moves out of cells in an attempt to replenish the extracellular stores. The intracellular loss of potassium is in large part replaced by sodium, so cell volume changes little. Even though the intracellular potassium concentration decreases, there is a proportionately greater decline in the extracellular potassium concentration, and the K_i/K_e actually increases. When extracellular potassium concentration falls as the result of potassium shifts from the extracellular to the intracellular space, obviously the K_i/K_e ratio must increase. The rise in K_i/K_e, as well as the absolute decline in intracellular potassium content, is responsible for the clinical manifestations of hypokalemia.

A. Cardiac Toxicity

Electrocardiographic changes of hypokalemia are unusual with serum potassium levels above 3.0 mEq/liter unless the potassium has fallen very rapidly. Progressively more severe hypokalemia is manifested by flattening of the T wave, ST depression, and the emergence of U waves. If the hypokalemia is particularly severe, prolongation of the PR and QRS intervals may be observed. If the serum potassium falls below 2.0–2.5 mEq/liter, significant AV conduction problems and potentially lethal ventricular arrhythmias may occur. Any evidence of ventricular irritability is an indication for aggressive therapy. Premature atrial contractions and supraventricular tachycardias may also be seen in hypokalemic patients. Particular attention should be directed to patients on digitalis in whom hypokalemia is known to potentiate digitalis toxic rhythms.

B. Neuromuscular Manifestations

The increase in K_i/K_e causes the resting cellular potential to become more negative and widens the gap between it and the threshold potential. This causes a decrease in excitability and a delay in impulse conduction and muscle contraction. The earliest clinical manifestation is weakness of the limb muscles which later extends to involve the trunk and respiratory muscles. Smooth muscle dysfunction is manifested by gastric distension, ileus, and urinary retention. In the presence of hypokalemia, the normal increase in muscle blood flow that normally accompanies exercise may be blunted, and this may precipitate rhabdomyolysis.

C. Renal–Metabolic

If hypokalemia is prolonged and severe (<2.5–3.0 mEq/liter), a vasopressin-resistant defect in urine-concentrating ability may develop and lead to polyuria and polydipsia. Mild to moderate azotemia (SUN < 40–50 mg/dl) may also occur. Hypokalemia is also associated with development of metabolic alkalosis. As the plasma potassium concentration falls, potassium moves out of cells to replenish the extracellular stores. This shift occurs in exchange for H^+ and Na^+ and leads to a metabolic alkalosis. The low serum potassium concentration also enhances proximal tubular bicarbonate reabsorption, contributing to the maintenance of the metabolic alkalosis. Glucose intolerance is also common in hypokalemic states and has been shown to result from an impairment in insulin secretion.

VIII. ETIOLOGY AND SPECIFIC THERAPY OF HYPOKALEMIA

The cause of the hypokalemia (Table IV) should be carefully sought and corrected if possible. In the absence of total-body potassium deficits, hypokalemia can result from a shift of potassium into cells. This is most commonly observed following insulin administration or during metabolic alkalemia (Table IV). Before potassium is administered in such instances, the insulin dose should be adjusted or the alkalemia corrected. Dietary deficiency of potassium is unusual and can be easily excluded by history. In patients with nonrenal potassium losses, the urinary excretion of potassium will be low (<10 mEq/liter). Excessive skin losses of potassium are usually obvious.

Table IV. Etiology of Hypokalemia

Redistribution

   Alkalemia
   Insulin excess
   Catecholamine excess
   Periodic paralysis

Dietary deficiency

Nonrenal losses ($U_kV < 10$ mEq/day)

   Gastrointestinal

      Diarrhea (and cathartics)
      Villous adenoma
      Watery diarrhea syndrome
      Fistulae (and other GI drainage)

   Skin

      Sweat
      Burns

Renal losses ($U_kV > 20$–30 mEq/day)

   Normotensive

      Diuretics
      Vomiting (loss is largely renal)
      Renal tubular dysfunction (RTA, Fanconi syndrome)
      Barter's syndrome
      Welt's syndrome[a]
      Hypomagnesemia
      Amphotericin B
      Potassium-losing nephritis

   Hypertensive

      Elevated plasma renin, high aldosterone
         Renovascular hypertension
         Malignant hypertension
         Renin-secreting tumor

      Low renin, high aldosterone
         Adrenal adenoma
         Adrenal hyperplasia

      Low renin, low aldosterone
         Exogenous mineralocorticoid excess
         Licorice ingestion
         Pseudoaldosteronism (Liddle's syndrome)
         Congenital adrenal hyperplasia (17- and 11-hydroxylase deficiency)

      Low renin, variable aldosterone
         Cushing's syndrome
         ACTH excess

[a] Welt's syndrome is characterized by hypokalemia, hypomagnesemia, elevated serum but normal aldosterone levels, and normotension. The hypokalemia is unresponsive to magnesium replacement but corrects with either aldactone or triamterene.

Gastrointestinal losses may be less obvious, particularly in the patient with self-induced vomiting or cathartic abuse. The low urinary potassium concentration will be helpful in establishing the diagnosis. If a tumor (villous adenoma) is found to be responsible for the excessive potassium losses, it should be removed surgically if possible.

The physiological framework for evaluating excessive renal potassium wasting is shown in Table IV. Division of patients into normotensive and hypertensive categories and further subdivision of the hypertensive group are based on the plasma renin and aldosterone levels.

A. Diuretics

Of the renal causes of hypokalemia in the normotensive patient, diuretics are far and away the most common. Any diuretic that inhibits sodium reabsorption in the more proximal parts of the nephron will enhance urine flow and sodium delivery to the more distal sites of potassium secretion. Both enhanced tubular flow and sodium delivery, even in the absence of volume contraction and secondary hyperaldosteronism, will increase renal potassium excretion. It is unusual, however, for diuretics alone to cause a serious deficit in total body potassium stores. In fact, several recent studies have suggested that the risk of developing significant hyperkalemia with the routine administration of potassium supplements in patients taking diuretics is at least as great as (if not greater than) the incidence of significant hypokalemia (<3.0 mEq/liter), which has been reported to be about 5%. It seems wise, therefore, to measure the serum potassium concentration after institution of diuretic therapy and to start potassium supplementation only in those individuals who demonstrate persistent hypokalemia (<3.0 mEq/liter). There are two exceptions to this rule. The first is the patient who is taking digitalis. Since hypokalemia is known to potentiate digitalis toxicity, these individuals should either be instructed in a high-potassium diet or receive oral potassium supplementation. The second is those patients with secondary hypoaldosteronism (i.e., cirrhosis, nephrosis) who initially present with hypokalemia. Obviously, it is important to follow the serum potassium concentration in these latter two groups very closely. The use of combination diuretics (i.e., a thiazide plus spironolactone or triamterene) is not routinely recommended when initiating therapy.

B. Other Forms of Renal Losses

In the hypertensive patient with excessive renal potassium losses, a careful evaluation of the renin–angiotensin–aldosterone axis should be carried out (Table IV). In many cases, either definitive surgical (renovascular hypertension, renin secreting tumor, adrenal adenoma, Cushing's syndrome, ACTH secreting tumor, etc.) or medical (dexamethasone-suppressible adrenal hyperplasia, congenital adrenal hyperplasia, renovascular hypertension, etc.) therapy will correct the excessive renal potassium losses. In some instances, neither surgical nor medical therapy will be practical. Since potassium losses may be particularly severe in such instances, hypokalemia may prove refractory to therapy. If oral potassium replacement leads to gastrointestinal symptoms, spironolactone can be added to the regimen. Great caution should be taken to monitor the serum potassium concentration closely in such individuals.

IX. GENERAL TREATMENT OF HYPOKALEMIA

Except when severe hypokalemia is associated with disturbances in cardiac conduction, arrhythmias, neuromuscular weakness, or paralysis, treatment of a low serum potassium concentration is not an emergency. It should be emphasized that during the replenishment of total body deficits, potassium must first move through the extracellular space, and therapy always has with it the risk of hyperkalemia. Whenever possible, potassium replacement should be given orally. The best guide to the adequacy of potassium replacement is sequential serum potassium measurements. Although changes in total body potassium content are roughly reflected by changes in the serum potassium concentration, there is considerable variation from one individual to another.

A. Oral Potassium Replacement

Since many patients find oral potassium supplements irritating to their gastrointestinal tract, it is wise to start replacement therapy with foods that are rich in potassium (Table III). Such dietary supplementation, if well planned, can provide an extra 40–60 mEq per day of potassium. If oral potassium supplementation is necessary, a variety of preparations are available. Some of the more commonly employed preparations are listed in Table V. In general, the drug of choice is 10% potassium chloride. This is best administered in a liquid form and is better tolerated if dissolved in juice and taken with meals. Potassium chloride may also be administered in a wax matrix (Slow-K®) from which it is slowly absorbed in the stomach and small bowel. Many patients who cannot tolerate liquid KCl will experience no gastrointestinal side effects with Slow-K®. In rare instances, ulceration of the gastrointestinal tract has been reported with Slow-K®.

In general, KCl is the preferred salt and is the required salt in the hypokalemic patient with an accompanying metabolic alkalosis and volume depletion. Unless contraction of the intravascular volume is corrected, the metabolic alkalosis will prove refractory to therapy and will oppose correc-

Table V. Potassium and Chloride Content in Some of the More Commonly Employed Potassium Supplements

Preparation	Ingredient	K+ (mEq)	Cl− (mEq)	Per volume
Liquids				
Kaochlor® 10%	KCl	20	20	15 ml
Kaochlor S-F® 10% (sugar free)	KCl	20	20	15 ml
Kaon Elixir®	K gluconate	20		15 ml
Kaon-Cl® 20%	KCl	40	40	15 ml
Kay Ciel Elixir®	KCl	20	20	15 ml
Klorvess® 10%	KCl	20	20	15 ml
Kolyum®	KCl	20	3.34	15 ml
Potassium Chloride®				
Oral solution 5%	KCl	10	10	15 ml
Sugar free 10%	KCl	20	20	15 ml
Potassium Triplex®	K acetate, K bicarbonate, K citrate	15		5 ml
Rum-K®	KCl	20	20	10 ml
Tablets				
Kaon-Cl Tabs® (slow release, wax matrix)	KCl	6.67	6.67	
Slow-K® (slow release, wax matrix)	KCl	8	8	
Kaochlor-Eff®	KCl, K citrate, K bicarbonate, betaine HCl	20	20	
Kaon®	K gluconate	5		
KEFF®	KCl, betaine HCl, K bicarbonate, K carbonate	20	20	
Klorvess Effervescent®	K bicarbonate, L-lysine monohydrochloride	20	20	
K-Lyte®	K bicarbonate, K citrate	25		
PfiKlor-F Effervescent®	KCl, K bicarbonate, L-lysine monohydrochloride	20	20	
Powder				
Kato®	KCl	20	20	
Kay Ciel Solodose®	KCl	20	20	
K-Lor®	KCl	20	20	
K-Lyte/Cl®	KCl	25	25	
Kolyum®	KCl, K gluconate	20	3.34	
PfiKlor® for oral solution	KCl	20	20	
Potassium Chloride® (sugar free)	KCl	20	20	

tion of the hypokalemia. With volume expansion, the elevated Tm for bicarbonate in the proximal tubule will return to normal. Consequently, chloride will be preferentially reabsorbed, and the retained bicarbonate will be excreted in the urine. As the extracellular fluid volume is restored to normal, plasma aldosterone levels will decline, and potassium secretion by the distal tubule will fall. Alkalosis *per se* also aggravates the hypokalemia by directly stimulating renal potassium secretion and causing a shift of potassium into cells. With return of the serum bicarbonate concentration and blood pH to normal, these adverse effects on potassium homeostasis are reversed.

In two clinical situations (diarrhea, renal tubular acidosis), hypokalemia is associated with metabolic acidosis. In these conditions, potassium should be replaced as potassium bicarbonate or its equivalent (potassium gluconate, citrate, or acetate). If these alkalinizing potassium salts are not available, KCl can be given. Correction of the hypokalemia should always be initiated before or concomitantly with correction of the acidosis, since the rise in pH and bicarbonate concentration will be associated with a shift of potassium into cells.

In the nonemergency situation, correction of the hypokalemia can be carried out over several days to avoid gastrointestinal upset and the risk of hyperkalemia. Ultimately, however, replacement of potassium stores can only be gauged by monitoring the serum potassium concentration. When the serum potassium concentration rises to 3.5 mEq/liter, the rate of replacement should be cut back and the clinical situation reassessed.

B. Intravenous Potassium Replacement

Potassium can be administered intravenously as the chloride or bicarbonate salt depending on the accompanying acid–base disturbance (see previous discussion). Evidence of cardiac or neuromuscular dysfunction, the presence of severe hypokalemia (<2.0–2.5 mEq/liter), and the inability to administer potassium orally (i.e., post surgery, vomiting, etc.) are indications for intravenous potassium. Most texts state that no more than 40 mEq of potassium chloride should be added to each liter of IV fluid and that this should not be administered in less than 60 min; this is a safe approach. If one infuses 0.75 mEq/kg of body weight (or 30 mEq/m^2 of surface area for obese persons) during 1 to 2 hr, the rise in plasma potassium concentration will be 1 to 1.5 mEq/liter. Thus, even if the base-line plasma potassium concentration is only slightly reduced (i.e., 3.0 mEq/liter), the plasma potassium level will increase to only 4.0–4.5 mEq/liter. Although this might lead to EKG changes (i.e., tented T waves), it would be unlikely to cause a life-threatening arrhythmia. Furthermore, when potassium is given to patients with more profound hypokalemia (i.e., <2.0–2.5 mEq/liter) and total-body potassium deficits in the 15–20% range, a greater percentage of the administered potassium will enter cells, and the absolute rise in plasma potassium concentration will be less than the 1 to 1.5 mEq/liter seen in normokalemic patients or in patients with only mild hypokalemia. Thus, 0.75 mEq/kg of body weight administered over 1 to 2 hr is a safe means of replacing potassium IV.

If hypokalemia is severe (less than or equal to 2.0 mEq/liter) and associated with cardiac arrhythmias such as premature ventricular contractions or ventricular tachycardia, potassium replacement must be more aggressive, and as much as 80 to 100 mEq may have to be infused during 1 hr to suppress the ventricular irritability. With these high doses, the factor limiting the rate of potassium infusion will be local pain, which can be overcome by using two peripheral IVs containing 40 to 50 mEq/liter infused during 1 hr. Since most hypokalemic patients will have concomitant volume contraction or be euvolemic, the large volume load should not present a problem. If, however, volume overload is a consideration, a high concentration of potassium can be infused through a larger vein with higher blood flow, e.g., the femoral vein. The infusion of high concentrations of potassium chloride via a subclavian, jugular, or right atrial catheter should be avoided, since local potassium concentrations achieved in the heart may be high enough to cause serious cardiac disturbances. Any time that emergency intravenous potassium therapy is indicated, it is advisable to employ continuous electrocardiographic monitoring and to check the serum potassium concentration every 2–4 hr.

Urine output should be monitored closely. Administration of potassium to patients who are oliguric or who have chronic renal insufficiency is potentially hazardous, since the kidneys are the major route of potassium excretion. Lastly, when potassium is infused intravenously, glucose-containing solutions should be avoided, since hyperglycemia will stimulate insulin secretion which in turn will drive potassium into cells.

C. Antagonists of Potassium Secretion

In some patients with excessive renal potassium loss, the use of spironolactone and triamterene may prove efficacious. The former works by inhibiting aldosterone-mediated potassium secretion, whereas the latter blocks aldosterone-independent potassium secretion. The usual dose of spironolactone is 25–50 mg every 6 hr. Triamterene is given as 100 mg every 8–12 hr. Except in very unusual circumstances, where urinary potassium losses are marked and refractory to therapy, the combined use of potassium supplements and aldactone (or triamterene) is contraindicated. Severe hyperkalemia is commonly observed when potassium is administered to patients whose ability to excrete potassium is impaired. Amiloride, a new diuretic agent, has also been shown to lead to hyperkalemia. This drug, which inhibits potassium secretion by the distal tubule, should not be used in patients with preexisting hyperkalemia and should be used cautiously in patients with significant renal impairment and diabetes mellitus.

SUGGESTED READINGS

Bia MJ, DeFronzo RA: Extrarenal potassium homeostasis. A review. *Am J Physiol* 240:F257–F268, 1981.

Brenner BM, Stein JH (eds): *Acid–Base and Potassium Homeostasis.* New York, Churchill Livingstone, 1978.

Cohen JJ, Gennari FJ, Harrington JJ: Disorders of potassium balance, in Brenner BM, Rector FC (eds): *The Kidney.* Philadelphia, W B Saunders, 1981, pp 908–939.

DeFronzo RA: Hyperkalemia and hyporeninemic hypoaldosteronism. *Kidney Int* 17:118–134, 1980.

Giebisch G, Malnic G, Berliner RW: Renal transport and control of potassium excretion, in Brenner BM, Rector FC (eds): *The Kidney.* Philadelphia, W B Saunders, 1981, pp 408–439.

3

Fluid and Electrolyte Disturbances
Hypo- and Hypercalcemia

MANUEL MARTÍNEZ-MALDONADO and ALFREDO GARCÍA

I. PHYSIOLOGICAL ROLE OF CALCIUM

A. Physicochemical Aspects

Calcium is the third most abundant ion in the body; it represents about 2% of the body weight. Calcium constitutes about 21% of wet weight of adult bone which in turn is 10–15% of the body weight. The distribution of calcium in the body tissue is summarized in Tables I and II.

Normal calcium requirements are approximately 9 mg/kg or 500–600 mg/day. This may vary with age. In aging adults over 60 years old, the requirement is higher because of a decline in intestinal calcium absorption, a rise in bone resorption, and loss of calcium in the urine.

Calcium exists in plasma in different forms. Total plasma calcium may be calculated as follows:

$$\text{Total plasma calcium} = \text{Ionized calcium} + \text{Complexed calcium} + \text{CaAlb} + \text{CaGlob} \qquad (1)$$

where Ca Alb is calcium bound to albumin, and Ca Glob is calcium bound to globulin.

MANUEL MARTINEZ-MALDONADO and ALFREDO GARCÍA ● Medical Service, Veterans Administration Hospital, San Juan, Puerto Rico 00936; and Departments of Internal Medicine and Physiology, University of Puerto Rico School of Medicine, San Juan, Puerto Rico 00931.

Table I. Distribution of Calcium in a 70-kg Adult Man[a]

Organ	Ca Content	Percent of total
Skeleton	1300 g	99
Teeth	7 g	0.6
Soft tissues	7 g	0.6
Plasma	350 mg	0.03
Extravascular fluid	700 mg	0.06
Total (approximately)	1315 g	100

[a] Average values.

With respect to blood calcium distribution, approximately 50% of Ca is diffusable, and 50% is bound to plasma protein. This does not change much even when subjects have renal failure (Table III).

Calcium binding strength is as follows:

$$\beta\text{-globulin} > \alpha_2\text{-globulin} > \gamma\text{-globulin} > \text{albumin}$$

Since albumin is the most abundant protein in plasma, 90% of calcium is bound to albumin. Hypoalbuminemia leads to reduction in total serum calcium (0.7 to 1 mg/dl for every 1 g/dl decrease when serum albumin falls from 4 g/dl). Abnormal increases in plasma protein such as those seen in multiple myeloma and other gammapathies will increase the total plasma calcium concentration.

Of the diffusable calcium, 90% is in the ionized (ultrafiltrable) form, and the other 10% is bound to citrate, phosphate, and bicarbonate molecules. Reduction in blood pH to the acid range will favor a change from bound calcium to the ionized fraction. Details of the effect of the ionized versus the complexed calcium fraction on the cellular membrane have not been clearly defined.

Significant reductions in ionized calcium can occur during massive blood transfusions in which large amounts of citrate are present. Reduction

Table II. Approximate Calcium Content of Cells in Some Tissues of Man[a]

High-Ca tissues	Calcium (mmol/kg wet wt.)	Low-Ca tissues	Calcium (mmol/kg wet wt.)
Platelets	5–15	Skeletal muscle	1.3
Cartilage	7–10	Liver	1.6
Smooth muscle	8	Heart	1.9
Placenta	6	Brain	2.1
Lungs	6	Spleen	2.0

[a] Adapted from Nordin BEC (ed): *Calcium, Phosphate and Magnesium Metabolism. Clinical Physiology and Diagnostic Procedures.* Churchill Livingstone, Edinburgh, London, New York, 1976, p 231. Bone, of course, is very high in calcium. It is clear that tissue destruction is an unlikely cause of alterations in serum calcium. Exceptions would be circumstances in which soft tissue or organ calcification has occurred as a result of serum calcium-phosphate product alteration (particularly skeletal muscle).

Table III. Concentration and Physicochemical State of Calcium in Blood of Normal Subjects (N), Patients with Chronic Renal Disease (CRD), and Patients on Long-Term Hemodialysis[a]

	Total	Diffusible	Ionized	Complexed
Normal	10.4[b]	6.3 (60 ± 5)[c]	5.8 (54 ± 5)	0.8 (6 ± 4)
CRD	10.0	5.8 (62 ± 6)	4.9 (51 ± 7)	1.20 (12 ± 7)
Hemodialysis	10.0	5.6 (58 ± 5)	4.8 (48 ± 5)	1.10 (11 ± 4)

[a] Values in mg/100 ml serum water. Total calcium is the sum of protein-bound calcium (not shown) and diffusible calcium. Diffusible calcium the sum of the ionized and complexed fractions. Since total calcium is expressed as concentration in serum water, it will be 6–10% higher than the mean of plasma calcium concentration. It is to be noted that ionized calcium is essentially unchanged in CRD and hemodialysis patients as compared to normals. Modified and adapted from Coburn et al: *Arch Intern Med* 124:302–311, 1969.
[b] Mean values.
[c] Values in parentheses indicate mean percentage of total serum calcium (±1 SD) of each fraction.

of ionized calcium in this manner leads to symptoms of hypocalcemia. Since citrate also induces alkalosis, increased protein binding of ionized calcium may contribute to the problem.

B. Functions in the Body

Essential steps in the maintenance of body functions are controlled by calcium. Calcium ion continuously recycles between the intracellular and the extracellular space. Because of its wide effects, alterations in its concentration bring about profound effects in general body function. In all cells, calcium is necessary for membrane stability and for control of Na^+ and K^+ transport. In glandular tissue, it is necessary for microtubule formation and secretory functions. In bone, it serves as a depot for rapid utilization and at the same time strengthens structure.

Some of the most important effects of calcium are on neural and muscular integrity. A summary of these effects follows.

1. Nerve Conduction

Calcium ions are necessary for nervous excitation and neuromuscular transmission since they regulate nerve cell permeability to sodium and potassium. Changes in the permeability of all membranes result from the release of Ca^{2+} ions during the propagation of the action potential.

Reductions in the concentration of calcium ion in the extracellular fluid will leave sodium gates (which regulate the entry of Na^+ ions into the membrane) open. This will make the membrane leaky to Na^+ ions so that the membrane remains continuously depolarized or fires repetitively. This probably results from the binding of calcium to the protein lining the sodium channels, creating an electrical field in or near the channel which blocks the entry of sodium ions.

The release of acetylcholine from the vesicles beneath the presynaptic membrane requires the presence of Ca^{2+} ions in the extracellular fluid.

2. Effect on Muscle

Calcium is a central regulator of contraction in skeletal, smooth, and cardiac muscle. It is important in regulating the steady-state permeability of the muscle membrane and in changing its ability to generate an action potential. The binding of calcium to cell surface sites determines the level of depolarization needed to initiate contraction. In addition, the intensity of contraction is determined by the intracellular concentration of ionized calcium. Finally, the duration of the contraction is controlled by the rate of removal of the calcium by the sarcoplasmic reticulum.

a. Skeletal Muscle

Reduction in extracellular Ca^{2+} concentration causes a rapid fall in the excitation potential in skeletal muscle and a fall in the electrical resistance of the membrane. An elevation increases cellular polarization and electrical resistance.

A change in sodium permeability dominates the depolarization mechanism, and there is a net movement of calcium into the cell. A small elevation of the intracellular calcium ion concentration will bind to troponin, and then will fall until it reaches a value close to its resting level as muscle tension reaches its peak. Depolarization appears to release calcium from intracellular stores, and activation proceeds as the contractile proteins bind the released calcium. Relaxation of muscle tension occurs as the calcium is returned to its intracellular store. The main store of intracellular calcium is the lateral cisterna of the sarcoplasmic reticulum. Relaxation is an active process requiring ATP. Calcium must react with contractile proteins and activate a calcium-dependent adenosinetriphosphatase to cause interaction of myosin and actin.

b. Cardiac Muscle

The relationship between contractility and extracellular calcium in cardiac muscle is different from that in skeletal muscle. In the first place, tension in response to electrical stimulation of the heart varies according to the ratio $[Ca^{2+}]/[Na^+]^2$ in the extracellular fluid. A rise in calcium in the extracellular fluid initiates a lasting contraction in skeletal muscle, whereas short contractions are initiated in heart muscle. These findings suggest that intracellular fluid calcium plays a more important role in excitation–contraction coupling in heart muscle than in skeletal muscle.

The effects of calcium ion on the heart are almost exactly opposite to those of potassium. Hypercalcemia causes spastic contraction and increases the heart rate. It also increases conduction through the cardiac muscle and through the AV node and, by increasing the intensity of the action potential, increases contraction. This is probably the result of the ability of calcium ions to excite the contractile process.

c. Smooth Muscle

In contrast to nerve fibers and skeletal muscle, the first phase of the action potential of smooth muscle includes the rapid movement of a large quantity of sodium ions in addition to calcium ions. The beginning of depolarization is believed to be caused by the influx of Ca^{2+} ions and not Na^+. The actual contractile process in both skeletal and smooth muscle is initiated by Ca^{2+}. However, the sarcoplasmic reticulum in smooth muscle is poorly developed as compared to skeletal muscle, and calcium must diffuse passively into the cell. In some types of smooth muscle, most of the ions causing contraction enter the fiber at the time of the action potential generation. Calcium pumps in smooth muscle remove intracellular calcium back to the extracellular fluid, stopping the interaction of contractile proteins. Nevertheless, removal of calcium is slower, so contraction lasts longer than in skeletal muscle.

C. Calcium Homeostasis

1. Gastrointestinal

a. Dietary

Calcium intake is approximately 15 mg/kg per day on a normal diet. Digestive juice calcium adds 3 mg/kg per day to this. The total net reabsorption is approximately 25–30% of the dietary intake. Using these values, a net absorption of 4–5 mg/kg per day would take place, all of which will appear in the urine if the patient is in calcium balance.

b. Absorption

Calcium absorption is mostly active and occurs predominantly in the duodenum. The jejunum, ileum, and colon have a much lower ability to transport calcium actively. This difference seems to depend on the effect of $1,25(OH)_2D_3$ on the various segments of the intestine. Calcium must be ionized to be transported, and the active process is saturable and requires aerobic conditions. It is carrier mediated and is independent of phosphorus. In addition, at concentrations higher than 13 mg/dl, a diffusion process seems to predominate in the net movement of calcium ions from lumen to blood.

A calcium binding protein (CaBP) that participates in calcium absorption has been found. This protein shows a high correlation between its concentration in the different segments of the intestine and the capacity for each segment to carry out calcium reabsorption. The activity and concentration of the protein is modulated by $1,25(OH)_2D_3$. It is not completely clear whether CaBP is the direct mediator of the vitamin D-induced calcium absorption or if it is just an initial step of a complex transferring system or a modulator of luminal permeability.

c. Factors That Influence Calcium Absorption

The effect of parathyroid hormone on gastrointestinal calcium reabsorption is controversial, and its action may be mediated through $1,25(OH)_2D_3$. Calcitonin has no consistent effect. On the other hand, chronic administration of corticosteroids in man reduces intestinal calcium absorption. Thyroid hormone also decreases intestinal calcium, whereas human growth hormone increases it. A relationship between sodium and calcium absorption has not been shown in humans. Increased intake of protein or amino acids as well as of carbohydrates and sugars (lactose, xylose, and sorbitol) increases calcium absorption.

2. Renal Handling

a. Filtration

About 60% of all calcium is filtered at the glomerulus. Only that portion in plasma that is ultrafilterable will appear in the glomerular filtrate. Conditions that increase diffusible calcium or the GFR will increase filtered load.

$$\text{Filtered load} = \text{Plasma diffusible fraction} \times \text{GFR} \qquad (2)$$

where GFR is the creatinine clearance in ml/min or, if available, the clearance of inulin or another marker of glomerular filtration. One may also estimate filtered load of calcium by multiplying total serum calcium by 0.65 (see Table III) and by the creatinine clearance.

b. Reabsorption

Calcium is reabsorbed actively by the nephron. This occurs in the proximal tubule, the thick ascending limb of Henle's loop, and the distal convolution. It is important to point out that little if any calcium is reabsorbed in the cortical ascending thick limb (so-called cortical diluting segment). This fact is important in understanding why inhibition of this site by some pharmacological agents (thiazide diuretics) does not appreciably increase urine calcium excretion, whereas agents working in the thick medullary limb such as furosemide and ethacrynic acid augment calcium excretion.

c. Secretion

No evidence has been advanced to indicate that calcium is secreted by the renal tubules.

d. Maximal Reabsorptive Capacity

No evidence exists to indicate a maximum reabsorptive capacity for calcium in man (Tm_{Ca}). Neither has a Tm been shown in experimental animals.

3. Factors That Influence Renal Handling of Calcium

a. Parathyroid Hormone

Parathyroid hormone acts directly on the kidney to increase the tubular reabsorption of calcium. Because PTH also increases the filtered load by raising serum calcium, the calcium-retaining effects of PTH may be obscured. Similarly, in the absence of PTH, there is a tendency for calcium excretion to rise, which in turn is offset by the fall in filtered load. The action of PTH is mediated through the cyclic AMP–adenylate cyclase system.

b. Vitamin D

Parathyroid hormone requires vitamin D and its metabolites for its normal action on the gastrointestinal tract and on bone, but conclusive evidence of this interaction in the kidney is lacking.

c. Calcitonin

Calcitonin acts on the kidney of man by decreasing tubular reabsorption of calcium, phosphate, sodium, potassium, and magnesium. Although CT appears to have an effect through adenylate cyclase in the kidney, unlike PTH, it does not increase the urinary excretion of cyclic AMP.

d. Growth Hormone

Growth hormone increases calcium excretion. Possibly the increase results from raised serum calcium secondary to enhanced intestinal absorption.

e. Thyroid Hormone

Thyroid hormone may lead to hypercalcemia when its secretion is above normal as in primary hyperthyroidism. This effect is principally mediated by enhanced bone resorption which tends to cause hypercalcemia. Moreover, hypercalciuria results which is secondary to increased filtered load and diminished tubular reabsorption of calcium.

f. Corticosteroids

In general chronic administration of all glucocorticoids (prednisolone, 6-methylprednisolone, and cortisone) increases the urine excretion of calcium. This seems to be the result of inhibition of tubular reabsorption of calcium. Mineralocorticoids tend to reduce calcium reabsorption by the kidney. The effect of mineralocorticoids in causing enhanced calcium excretion in the face of sodium retention is mediated by expansion of the extracellular fluid and inhibition of tubular reabsorption of calcium.

g. Gonadal Hormones

Estrogenic hormones reduce urine calcium excretion; this seems to be the result of a fall in filtered load of calcium.

h. Prostaglandins

Prostaglandins increase calcium excretion, most likely as a result of increased filtered load but perhaps also by direct inhibitory effect on tubular calcium reabsorption.

The factors that influence the urinary excretion of calcium (and magnesium) are summarized in Table IV.

Table IV. Factors That Alter Urinary Excretion of Calcium and Magnesium

	Urine calcium	Urine magnesium
Expansion of ECF	↑	↑
Changes in renal hemodynamics		
Renal vasodilation	↑	↑
↑ GFR	No Δ	No Δ
Diuretics		
Osmotic	↑	↑
Chronic thiazide therapy	↓	Slight ↑
Furosemide and ethacrynic acid	↑	↑
Cardiac glycosides	↑	↑
Alcohol ingestion	↑	↑
Changes in plasma composition		
Hypercalcemia	↑	↑
Hypermagnesemia	↑	↑
Phosphate depletion	↑	↑
Phosphate loading	↓	No Δ
Acidosis	↑	↑
High salt intake	↑	↑
Endocrine factors		
PTH	↓	↓
Vitamin D		
Acute	↓	?
Chronic	↑	?
Growth hormone	↑	↑
Thyroid hormone	↑	↑
Mineralocorticoid		
Acute administration	No Δ	No Δ
Chronic administration	↑	↑

II. HYPOCALCEMIA

Hypocalcemia is a common electrolyte disturbance. Because of the frequency with which it is associated with hypoalbuminemia, for the proper clinical assessment of patients it is essential to measure albumin. Total serum calcium will fall by 0.7 to 1.0 mg/dl for every decrement in serum albumin of 1 g/dl from 4 g/dl. Ionized calcium remains unchanged in hypoalbuminemia, and, thus, patients are asymptomatic.

A. Causes and Mechanisms

The causes and mechanisms of hypocalcemia are listed in Table V.

Table V. Causes and Mechanisms of Hypocalcemia

Causes	Mechanisms
Endocrine	
Hypoparathyroidism	
Idiopathic	Autoimmunity; absence of parathyroid hormone. Decreased calcium absorption from the intestine.
Acquired	Infarct of parathyroid adenoma. Metastasis to parathyroid glands.
Surgical; postthyroidectomy	Removal of parathyroid gland during thyroidectomy (necessary or inadvertent). Ligation of parathyroid artery. Hungry-bone phenomenon (increased skeletal uptake of calcium). Parathyroid hormone deficiency; chronic renal failure; hypomagnesemia.
Familial (sex-linked recessive, autosomal recessive)	
Associated with multiple endocrinopathies	
Associated with iron storage disease	Hemosiderin deposits in parathyroid glands.
Pseudohypoparathyroidism	
Type I	Renal and skeletal resistance to PTH. Skeletal and renal binding of PTH, but failure of calcium and transport systems to respond to the cyclic AMP generated.
Hyperparathyroidism	
Adult and children (secondary)	Chronic renal failure as result of hypercalcemia with hyperphosphatemia leading to hypocalcemia.
Infants of hyperparathyroid mothers	Hypercalcemia of mother inhibits infant's PTH secretion.
Hypovitaminosis D and resistance to vitamin D	Low gastrointestinal calcium absorption.
Hyperaldosteronism (primary)	Increased calcium excretion secondary to expansion of extracellular fluid volume. Diminished PTH sensitivity secondary to hypomagnesemia.

(continued)

Table V. Causes and Mechanisms of Hypocalcemia (*Continued*)

Causes	Mechanisms
Renal disorders	
Acute renal failure	Hyperphosphatemia decreases calcium. Deficiency of $1,25(OH)_2D_3$ and skeletal resistance to PTH.
Chronic renal failure	Decreased $1,25(OH)_2$. Decrease in calcium absorption by gut. Skeletal resistance to PTH. Hyperphosphatemia complexes calcium.
Renal tubular acidosis	Loss of calcium in urine. Loss of magnesium in urine.
Respiratory alkalosis	Increased calcium bound to albumin; decreased ionized calcium.
Gastrointestinal disturbances	
Malabsorption syndrome	Malabsorption of vitamin D. Malabsorption of calcium. Hypomagnesemia. Saponification of calcium salts in the gut. Loss of albumin in feces.
Pancreatitis (acute)	Extraskeletal sequestration of calcium (saponification of calcium salts in the pancreas). Hypomagnesemia. Skeletal resistance to PTH. Hyperglucagonemia stimulates calcitonin secretion which blunts PTH action on bone.
Acute and chronic alcoholism	Hypomagnesemia. Decreased $1,25(OH)_2D_3$. Phosphate depletion leading to hypercalciuria. Malabsorption of calcium. Hypoalbuminemia.
Hypomagnesemia	Skeletal resistance to PTH. Increased calcium influx into bone. Decreased parathyroid secretion.
Hypermagnesemia	Decreased PTH secretion (experimentally).
Major surgical procedures	Increased serum phosphate (trauma). Lactate accumulation during hypotension. Reduced by citrate administered in transfusions (calcium–citrate complex).
Gentamycin	Renal wastage of magnesium.
Neoplasms	Increased activity of skeleton for calcium. Production of hypocalcemic agent.
Mithramycin	Inhibits bone resorption. Interferes with PTH action.
Phosphate infusion	Increases complexed calcium. Inhibits $1,25(OH)_2D_3$ production.
Edetic acid (EDTA)	Complexes calcium.
Radioactive iodine treatment for hyperthyroidism	Radiation damage to parathyroid glands; functional hypoparathyroidism.

B. Consequences

1. General

Most of the symptoms are a reflection of altered neuromuscular irritability resulting from a decreased concentration of ionized calcium. Tetany and convulsions represent the most serious complication. Latent tetany can be elicited by tapping the facial nerve and producing a contraction of the facial muscles (Chvostek's sign) or by application of a tourniquet or blood pressure cuff leading to carpopedal spasm (Trousseau's sign). This test is performed by raising cuff pressure to above systolic blood pressure levels for 3 min but has the weakness that it is negative in 34% of patients with latent tetany and is positive in 4% of the normal population.

2. Central Nervous System

Hypocalcemia can lead to a variety of emotional disturbances including irritability, emotional lability, depression, impairment of memory, confusion, delusions, and hallucinations.

3. Neurological

Epileptiform seizures are not uncommon in hypocalcemia, especially in hypoparathyroidism. Grand mal seizures are usual, but Jacksonian seizures have been described. Tendon reflexes tend to increase in hypocalcemia but may disappear if hypocalcemia is profound.

4. Cardiovascular

The EKG is usually normal except for prolongation of the QT interval, but low-voltage and T-wave abnormalities have been reported.

5. Ectodermal Lesions

Abnormalities of the skin, hair, nails, teeth, and ocular lens are frequently found if hypocalcemia is longstanding. Eczema and psoriasis may be worsened by hypocalcemia. The skin will become coarse, dry, and scaly. This and patchy scalp hair, scanty eyelashes and eyebrows, and absence of axillary and pubic hair are frequent. Bilateral cataracts involving the anterior and posterior subcapsular areas of the cortical portion of the lens may be seen after 1 year of hypocalcemia.

6. Gastrointestinal

Severe diarrhea with B_6 and fat malabsorption may present occasionally. Constipation and abdominal pain have been reported.

III. HYPERCALCEMIA

Multiple causes of hypercalcemia exist, but basically there are two sources of elevated serum calcium. First, excessive external administration, as seen in patients who receive toxic doses of parenteral calcium or patients with an increased intestinal absorption as occurs in sarcoidosis, vitamin D intoxication, and tuberculosis.

Second, an endogenous source such as increased bone resorption may be brought about by an increase in osteoclastic activity. This is usually seen in conditions with excessive circulating parathyroid hormone or when an osteoclast-stimulating factor is produced by tumoral cells (e.g., lympho-proliferative disorders).

Causes of hypercalcemia and their mechanisms are described in Table VI, and the consequences of hypercalcemia are summarized in Table VII.

Table VI. Causes and Mechanisms of Hypercalcemia

Causes	Mechanisms
Primary hyperparathyroidism	Bone: Cyclic AMP-mediated increased resorption; increased number and activity of osteoclasts; osteoprogenitor cells proliferate, deep osteocytes mobilize calcium from perilacunar bone, surface osteocytes regulate calcium flux and so maintain a steady-state level of plasma calcium. Renal: Increased distal renal calcium reabsorption. Gut: Increased calcium reabsorption mediated by $1,25(OH)_2D_3$; other possible factors include pro-PTH, prostaglandins, osteoclast-activating factor.
Carcinomatosis (pseudohyperparathyroidism)	Osteoclast-activating factor, a substance secreted by lymphocytic cells and activated by antigens or phytomitogen around metastases. Prostaglandin E_2 increases PTH-mediated bone resorption. PTH-like substances secreted by tumors. Vitamin D metabolites produced by neoplastic tissue.
Absorptive hypercalcemia	$\uparrow 1,25(OH)_2D_3$ increases intestinal absorption. Frequently accompanied by renal tubular acidosis and nephrocalcinosis.
Vitamin D intoxication	Increases Ca absorption from intestine by increasing synthesis of Ca-binding protein and Ca-dependent ATPase in intestinal mucosa. Recent investigations suggest that this is mediated by 25(OH)D and not $1,25(OH)_2D_3$. The diagnosis can be established by measuring 25(OH)D. Also causes bone resorption.

(continued)

Table VI. Causes and Mechanisms of Hypercalcemia (*Continued*)

Causes	Mechanisms
Sarcoidosis, tuberculosis	Impaired regulation of production of and/or response to $1,25(OH)_2D_3$.
Estrogen therapy	↑ Sensitivity to $1,25(OH)_2D_3$.
Diuretics (thiazides)	↓ Urinary Ca^{2+}. Intravascular volume depletion. Potentiate the peripheral effect of PTH on skeletal system.
Adrenal insufficiency	Intravascular volume depletion. ↑ Plasma protein (ionized Ca^{2+} is normal).
Vitamin A intoxication	↑ Bone resorption.
Hyperthyroidism	Thyroxine inhibits phosphodiesterase which increases skeletal cyclic AMP and increases bone resorption.
Acute renal failure (particularly in presence of muscle damage)	Release of calcium from soft tissue in which it has been complexed with inorganic and organic anions.
Milk alkali syndrome	Increases intake of milk and alkali. Calcium carbonate absorption from intestine is enhanced. Calcium inhibits PTH secretion which enhances renal phosphate reabsorption. Metastatic calcification occurs from increased calcium–phosphate product. Continued calcium carbonate intake worsens picture as does immobilization.
Paget's disease	Increased bone turnover and bone resorption. Immobilization may cause hypercalcemia.
Immobilization	↑ Bone resorption, particularly in the presence of increased bone turnover.
Primary hypercalcemia	Stimulation of adenylate cyclase in bone; ↑ bone resorption mediated by cyclic AMP. ↑ Number and activity of osteosclasts.

Table VII. Consequences of Hypercalcemia

System affected	Mechanism
Central nervous system Memory impairment, acute psychosis, and bizarre behavior	Although mechanism is not clear, increased free Ca^{2+} in CNS fluid may decrease conduction in nerve terminals. Synaptosomal ATPase may be inhibited. Intracerebral dehydration may also play a role.

(*Continued*)

Table VII. Consequences of Hypercalcemia (*Continued*)

System affected	Mechanism
Cardiovascular	
Cardiac effects	Shortening of PR and ST intervals occurs.
Blood vessels	Vasoconstriction leading to hypertension seen in acute and chronic hypercalcemia.
Pulmonary	Thick secretions and inhibitory effects on motion of bronchial cilia. Pulmonary calcification.
Gastrointestinal	Constipation resulting from diminished motility and dehydration. Paralytic ileus caused by the effect of the ion on smooth muscle and nerve conduction. Anorexia and vomiting, altered gastrointestinal motility, and gastric emptying because of effect of calcium on smooth muscle. Duodenal ulcer from increased acid secretion by direct effect on parietal cells and gastrin secretion.
Hematological	Bone marrow fibrosis and anemia in cases of primary hyperparathyroidism.
Musculoskeletal	Arthralgias and arthritis in cases of PTH-mediated bone resorption. In neoplasia as a result of metastases, OAF, or prostaglandins.
Ocular	Calcification of conjuctival tissue and corneal area as a result of alkanization secondary to exposures to low-P_{CO_2} ambient air. Impaired vision. Gritty eyes from the presence of calcium deposits.
Renal	Diminished GFR per nephron as a result of a reduction in ultrafiltration coefficient and reduced plasma flow. Renal salt and water losses leading to volume contraction; ↑ bicarbonate reabsorption and hypokalemia. Polyuria resulting from inhibition of ADH effects in collecting ducts. Sodium wastage as a result of inhibition of tubular reabsorption in ascending limb of Henle's loop. Azotemia and hyperuricemia as a result of volume contraction. Interstitial nephritis from deposition of calcium and uric acid in the parenchyma. Chronic renal failure as a result of interstitial nephritis and an increase in intravascular resistance or low GFR. Acute renal failure from alterations in renal hemodynamics and interstitial reactions.

IV. TREATMENT OF HYPO- AND HYPERCALCEMIA

A. Hypocalcemia

1. Acute

The symptoms of acute tetany can be corrected or alleviated by the intravenous injection of 10 to 20 ml of 10% calcium gluconate (see Table VIII). The infusion rate should not exceed 2 ml/min. If the patient has been receiving digitalis, it should be recalled that calcium sensitizes the myocardium to the glycoside. The EKG should be monitored.

In severe cases, an intravenous drip of calcium gluconate may be necessary (see Table VIII).

The oral administration of calcium salts should be instituted as quickly as possible. During this period, phosphate intake should be restricted since it will retard calcium absorption. When indicated, pharmacological doses of vitamin D should also be administered, particularly if hypocalcemia persists for longer than 14 days or if the hypocalcemia is known to be long standing.

When the cause of hypocalcemia is not clear, serum magnesium should be measured. If the concentration is less than 1.0 mg/dl, intravenous treatment should be given (see Chapter 4). We also administer $MgSO_4$ intramuscularly if Mg^{2+} values are just slightly below normal. When large doses of magnesium are to be given, they should be administered with 1% procaine, since magnesium is a very painful medication (see Chapter 4 for dose).

2. Chronic

The oral administration of calcium and vitamin D should be considered when deficiency of the vitamin and/or markedly depressed parathyroid function are present. Calcium should be provided in the range of 2 to 4 g per day (see Table VIII for the amounts of elemental calcium provided by the various compounds). If the response to oral calcium loads is not adequate and serum calcium is still below normal, a vitamin D preparation should be added to the regimen. The doses and characteristics of various preparations of vitamin D (or analogues) are shown in Table IX. In subjects with surgical hypoparathyroidism, the use of a thiazide and a low-salt diet may permit reduction of the amount of vitamin D and calcium administered.

Some conditions, such as decreased intake and drugs (see Table X), may lead to reduced availability of vitamin D. If hypocalcemia supervenes during their use, supplementation with 500 to 10,000 units of vitamin D per day is indicated. (There are 40,000 units per milligram of ergocalciferol.)

B. Hypercalcemia

Hypercalcemia is a frequent electrolyte disturbance which may result in dehydration, azotemia, stupor, and coma, and unless it is rapidly recognized

Table VIII. Calcium Preparations for Clinical Use

	Doses	Indications	Mechanisms	Complications
Calcium carbonate[a]	1–2 g three times daily (260 mg elemental calcium per 650-mg tablet).	Mild hypocalcemia Osteomalacia Osteoporosis Renal osteodystrophy	Converted in stomach to soluble calcium salt by HCl. Therefore, ineffective in patients with achloridia.	Hypercalcemia after long-term therapy, particularly if vitamin D given concomitantly.
Calcium chloride	5 to 10 ml of 10% (360 mg per 10-ml ampule) solution given slowly IV (rarely given orally because of irritation of GI tract).	Severe hypocalcemia	Increase ionized calcium rapidly.	Irritant to vein and subcutaneous tissue if extravasated. Hypercalcemia during long-term therapy, particularly if given with vitamin D therapy.
Calcium gluceptate	5 to 10 ml IV solution (220 mg/ml or 80 mg/ml of calcium in 5-ml container). In newborn infants, 0.5 ml after every 100 ml in exchange transfusion; 2 to 5 mg IM in gluteal region.	Severe hypocalcemia Exchange transfusion	Increases ionized Ca^{2+}.	Transient tingling and metallic taste after IV infusion. Can enhance digitalis effect in the heart, precipitating arrhythmia.

Calcium gluconate	20 ml of 10% solution (one 10-ml ampule contains 90 mg of elemental calcium) injected slowly followed by slow infusion of 30–40 ml of 10% solution in 500 ml or 1 liter of 5% glucose or 0.9% NaCl over a 4-hr period. Children should receive 500 mg/kg of body weight daily in divided doses. For adults, 15 g daily in divided doses. Tablets have 90 mg elemental calcium per gram.	Severe hypocalcemia, IV In mild hypocalcemia, oral	Same as above.	Same as above.
Calcium lactate	Adults 1.5 to 3.0 g three times daily with meals. Children 500 mg/kg of body weight PO in divided doses (60 mg elemental calcium per 300-mg tablet).	Mild hypocalcemia and maintenance therapy	Same as above.	Same as above.

ᵃCalcium should not be mixed with any solution containing bicarbonate because of the possibility of precipitation.

Table IX. Dose Requirements of Vitamin D and Metabolites[a]

	Vitamin D$_2$ (ergocalciferol)	DHT (dihydrotachysterol)	25(OH)D (calcifeidol)	1,25(OH)$_2$D$_3$ (calcitrol)
Hypoparathyroidism daily dose (μg)	750–3000	250–1000	50–200	0.5–2.0
Time required to achieve normocalcemia (weeks)	4–8	1–2	2–4	0.5–1
Maximal effect (weeks)	4–10	2–4	4–20	0.5–1
Persistence of effect after cessation (weeks)	6–18	1–3	4–12	0.5–1

[a] Earliest times for maximal effects are not certain. Adapted from Agus ZS, Goldfarb S, Wasserstein A: In Brenner BM, Rector FC Jr (eds): *The Kidney*, ed 2. Philadelphia, W B Saunders, 1980.

Table X. Disturbances in Vitamin D Metabolism

Decreased production
  Liver disease; 25(OH)D ↓
  Renal disease, hereditary; 1,25(OH)$_2$D$_3$ ↓
Increased metabolism; 25(OH)D ↓
  Phenobarbital
  Phenytoin
  Alcohol
  Glutethimide
Decreased intake; malnutrition
Decreased absorption; malabsorption
Increased loss of 25(OH)D
  Nephrotic syndrome
  Disturbance of enterohepatic circulation

and treated, it is accompanied by a high mortality. As already described, hypercalcemia has varied etiologies, but the clinical consequences of hypercalcemia are the same regardless of its origin.

The principal aim of the therapy is to reduce the serum calcium concentration to normal levels. The management should be directed at recognition and definite treatment of the underlying disease and at instituting treatment that will increase the renal excretion of calcium and/or diminish bone resorption.

Adequate hydration and volume reexpansion should be the first step. One to 2 liters of 0.9% normal saline solution must be given hourly. Forced diuresis must be induced when necessary, and at all times precise records of fluid and electrolyte balance must be kept. Central venous pressure should be monitored as well. It is to be understood that forced diuresis is an acute palliative measure and that concomitant permanent control of the cause of the hypercalcemia must also be attempted.

The following are the most useful courses of therapy.

1. Forced Diuresis with Furosemide (Lasix®)

a. Mechanisms of Action

Furosemide inhibits tubular sodium chloride and calcium reabsorption.

b. Method

Induce forced diuresis with saline as described above. Administer furosemide, 80 to 100 mg IV every 1 to 2 hr, until an adequate response is obtained. Concomitant replacement of water, sodium, potassium (60 mEq/hr), and magnesium (15 mg/hr) is essential. If calcium is below 15 mg/dl, smaller doses of furosemide (20–80 mg IV) can be given every 2 to 4 hr together with saline infusion.

In children, give 25 mg every 4 hr with serum calcium below 15 mg/dl and 60 mg with serum calcium over 15 mg/dl.

c. Complications

Furosemide may cause severe volume depletion, hyper- or hyponatremia, hypomagnesemia, and hypokalemia.

2. Mithramycin (Mithracin®)

a. Mechanisms of Action

Mithramycin has a direct toxic effect on osteoclasts in bone and thus decreases bone turnover.

b. Method

Administer 25 μg/kg of body weight by direct intravenous injection or, preferably, added to 5% dextrose and infused over a period of 4 to 8 hr. Failure of serum calcium to fall in 12–24 hr is an indication to continue the same dose for 2 to 4 days. If hypercalcemia is not controlled, additional courses could be given at weekly intervals. When calcium levels fall, the effects of mithramycin will last for 3 to 7 days.

c. Complications

Mithramycin may cause anorexia, nausea and vomiting, severe thrombocytopenia which may progress to severe bleeding, and hepato- and nephrotoxicity.

3. Salmon Calcitonin (Calcimar®)

a. Mechanisms of Action

Calcitonin reduces bone resorption and is therefore particularly effective in Paget's disease.

b. Method

Administer 100 to 400 MRC units once or twice daily (4 units/kg of body weight intravenously followed by 4 units/kg subcutaneously at 12–14 hr). Prednisone succinate, 20 to 100 mg/day IV or IM, may be added for severe hypercalcemia.

c. Complications

For hypercalcemia the results are erratic, and the effect may be lost after several weeks of use, although occasionally addition of oral phosphate will restore responsiveness. Not all patients (20–25%) with acute hypercalcemia respond. Nausea, vomiting, diarrhea, facial flushing, malaise, and soreness and inflammation at the site of injection may occur. Patients may develop secondary hyperparathyroidism or the appearance of cellular resistance with long-term administration. Patients may form antibodies to the salmon hormone.

4. Steroids

a. Mechanisms of Action

Steroids can inhibit intestinal absorption of calcium by antagonizing vitamin D and its metabolites. They have their best effect in vitamin D intoxication and sarcoidosis but are also effective in malignancies such as breast carcinoma and multiple myeloma. In these conditions, they also have tumoricidal effects and inhibit bone resorption.

b. Method

Administer hydrocortisone, 5 mg/kg per day, for 2–3 days and then reduce to a maintenance level. Prednisone in a dose of 40–80 mg/day can be given until the serum calcium level is satisfactorily controlled. Dosage can then be decreased until normal serum calcium can be maintained. Steroids may be combined with oral phosphate in long-term treatment.

c. Complications

Steroids can induce a cushingoid syndrome, infections, peptic ulcer disease, hyperkalemia, and glucose intolerance.

Table XI. Oral Phosphate Preparations

Preparation	Content/tablet
K-Phos Original® (sodium free)	Phosphorus 114 mg; K 114 mg
K-Phos Neutral®	Phosphorus 250 mg; K 45 mg; sodium 298 mg
K-Phos Alkaline®	Phosphorus 250 mg; K 90 mg; sodium 319 mg
K-Phos MF®	Phosphorus 126 mg; K 45 mg; sodium 67 mg
K-Phos No. 2®	Phosphorus 250 mg; K 88 mg; sodium 134 mg
Neutra-Phos®	Each capsule or 75 ml of solution after reconstitution contains phosphorus 250 mg; sodium 7.125 mEq; potassium 7.125 mEq
Neutra-Phos K®	Each capsule or 75 ml of solution after reconstitution contains phosphorus 250 mg; potassium 14.25 mEq; sodium-free

5. Phosphate Salts

a. Mechanisms of Action

Phosphate salts (Table XI) bring about movement of calcium into cells, decrease bone resorption, increase bone formation, and reduce calcium resorption as a result of diminished synthesis of $1,25(OH)_2D_3$.

b. Method

Administer 2 to 4 g orally daily in divided doses. The dose should be adjusted downward after remission to maintain the serum calcium concentration. Intravenously, 1.5 g can be infused over a period of 6 to 8 hr. The dose may be repeated daily, but no more than two infusions are required.

c. Complications

Intravenous administration is effective but dangerous. We do not recommend it. Hypocalcemia, hypertension, myocardial infarction, tetany, acute renal failure, and death have occurred. Ectopic calcification may also occur.

Oral administration is safer, but serum calcium, phosphate, and renal function must be monitored closely. Oral phosphates should not be given to a patient with impaired renal function.

Nausea, vomiting, and diarrhea may occur after oral administration. Concomitant use of antacids with aluminum or magnesium should be avoided because they bind phosphate and diminish absorption.

6. Dialysis

In an occasional patient hemodialysis or peritoneal dialysis may be used (particularly if oliguria is present).

The average clearances of calcium are shown in Table XII.

Clearly, dialytic procedures should be reserved for a few patients, since only low calcium bath dialysis is clearly better than forced diuresis.

Table XII. Calcium Clearances Produced by Dialysis

Procedure	Clearance
Forced saline diuresis with furosemide	
Average clearance	82 mg/hr
Maximum clearance	150 mg/hr
Peritoneal dialysis	
Average clearance	60 mg/hr
Maximum clearance	124 mg/hr
Hemodialysis	
Using 0–3 mEq/liter dialysis concentrate	
Maximum clearance	680 mg/hr
Using 4 mEq/liter dialysis concentrate	
Maximum clearance	163 mg/hr

Some cases treated with hemodialysis have exhibited a rebound of hypercalcemia. These patients had parathyroid adenomas. Hemodialysis has aided in preparing patients for surgery; it also has an important use in some patients with multiple myeloma in whom renal failure and congestive heart failure prevent the use of saline and furosemide.

Low-Ca^{2+} hemodialysis increases patient survival and decreases morbidity and is, thus, an effective adjunct to the therapy of hypercalcemic crisis that does not respond to other forms of therapy.

Note in proof: Dichloromethylene diphosphonate, a potent inhibitor of osteoclast-mediated bone resorption, can lower serum calcium in patients with hypercalcemia as a result of primary hyperparathyroidism, parathyroid carcinoma, malignancy, multiple myeloma, and Paget's disease. It may be given orally (1600 mg daily for as long as 12 weeks) or intravenously (over 2 hr, 2.5 mg/kg on Day 1 and 5 mg/kg for 2–7 days) without significant side effects.(From Shane et al: *Ann Int Med* 95:23–27, 1981; Shane et al: *Am J Med* 72:939–944, 1982.)

SUGGESTED READINGS

Agus ZS, Goldfarb S, Wasserstein A: Disorders of calcium and phosphate, in Brenner BM, Rector FC Jr (eds): *The Kidney*, ed 2. Philadelphia, WB Saunders, 1981, pp 940–1022.

Bell N: Hypercalcemic and hypocalcemic disorders: Diagnosis and treatment. *Nephron* 23:147–151, 1979.

Benabe J, Martínez-Maldonado M: Hypercalcemic nephropathy. *Arch Intern Med* 138:777–779, 1978.

Besarab A, Caro JF: Mechanisms of hypercalcemia in malignancy. *Cancer* 41:2276–2285, 1978.

Dennis VW, Stead WW, Myers JL. Renal handling of phosphate and calcium. *Annu Rev Physiol* 41:257–271, 1979.

Kleeman CR (ed): Divalent ion metabolism and osteodystrophy in chronic renal failure. *Arch Intern Med* 124:261–683, 1969.

Muggia F, Heinemann HO: Hypercalcemia associated with neoplastic disease. *Ann Intern Med* 73:281–290, 1970.

Nysynowitz ML, Frame B, Kolb FO: The spectrum of the hypoparathyroid states. *Medicine* 55:105, 1976.

Norman AW: Vitamin D metabolism and calcium absorption. *Am J Med* 67:989–998, 1979.

Schweitzer VG, Thompson NW, Harness JK, Nishiyama RH: Management of severe hypercalcemia caused by primary hyperparathyroidism. *Arch Surg* 113:373–381, 1979.

Suki WN, Yium JJ, Von Minden M, Saller-Hebert C, Eknoyan G, Martínez-Maldonado M: Acute treatment of hypercalcemia with furosemide. *N Engl J Med* 283:836–840, 1970.

4

Fluid and Electrolyte Disturbances
Hypo- and Hypermagnesemia

MANUEL MARTÍNEZ-MALDONADO and
ALFREDO GARCÍA

I. PHYSIOLOGICAL ROLE OF MAGNESIUM

A. Physicochemical Aspects

Magnesium is the fourth most abundant cation in the body. The body of the adult human contains 2000 mEq of Mg; 50% is in the skeleton, and the remainder is in soft tissues. Almost 90% is intracellular and is distributed among bone, muscles, and blood cells. Of this, 60% is in the bone, and the other 30% is distributed in muscle and blood cells. The usual RBC magnesium concentration is 4.60 ± 0.34 mEq/liter. Most of this is acquired during hematopoiesis. Fluctuations of serum Mg will not affect total RBC pool content. The usual plasma concentration of magnesium is 1.5 to 2.0 mEq/liter of which 65–75% is diffusable, and the rest is bound to protein (mostly albumin). The concentration of magnesium in various cells and tissues is shown in Table 1.

Fluctuations in the intracellular level of Mg^{2+} occur following K^+ ion fluxes. When the cell loses potassium, magnesium is also lost. The exact mechanism and the reason for this finding are not known.

MANUEL MARTÍNEZ-MALDONADO and ALFREDO GARCÍA • Veterans Administration Hospital, San Juan, Puerto Rico 00936; and Departments of Internal Medicine and Physiology, University of Puerto Rico School of Medicine, San Juan, Puerto Rico 00931.

Table I. Normal Values of Magnesium[a]

Total serum	1.56 ± 0.08 mEq/liter
Ultrafiltrable	1.15 ± 0.05 mEq/liter
Erythrocyte	4.60 ± 0.34 mEq/liter
Muscle	75.6 ± 8.6 mEq/kg FFDS[b]
Cortical bone	352 ± 20 mEq/kg ash

[a] Adapted from Alfrey AC et al: *J Lab Clin Med* 84:153, 1974. Values are mean $\pm$ SE.
[b] Fat-free dry solids.

B. Functions in the Body

The following are some of the intracellular functions of magnesium in metabolism:

1. Necessary for hydrolysis and transfer of phosphate groups including phosphatases and adenosine triphosphate.
2. Cofactor for oxidative phosphorylation.
3. Stabilization of DNA and RNA.
4. Necessary for structural integrity of ribosomes.
5. Contributes to the binding of messenger RNA to ribosomes.
6. Needed in the amino acid activating system.
7. Possesses curariform activity presumably by interference with the release of acetylcholine from motor nerve terminals.

In animals, magnesium is essential for all enzymatic reactions requiring ATP including oxidative phosphorylation and as a cofactor in enzymatic protein metabolism. This is necessary for maintenance of cellular integrity and intact membrane potentials.

C. Magnesium Homeostasis

1. Gastrointestinal

a. Dietary Influence

The usual occidental diet contains 4.0 mg/kg per day of magnesium. Studies done by Stanbury and King show that the percentage of Mg absorbed in a diet of less than 2 mg/kg per day is around 75–80%, but when the dietary intake increases above 2 mg/kg per day, the absorption stabilizes at 35–40% of the ingested Mg.

b. Absorption

Most of the absorption occurs in the small intestine, particularly in the ileum. Diseases involving this area may be associated with severe magnesium deficiency. The colon also absorbs Mg but to a lesser extent than the small intestine. In conditions with severe diarrhea, large fecal losses of magnesium occur. Since the mechanism of gut absorption is an active process, particularly large losses will occur if the diarrhea is of the secretory type.

c. Excretion

It is important to recall that gastrointestinal secretions contain magnesium, so that up to 30–40 mg/day can be lost in stool. Considerable losses of the ion continue to occur in a man fed a low-Mg diet in the presence of diarrhea, or in a patient placed on nasogastric suction (0.5 mg/kg per day).

d. Factors That Influence the Absorption of Magnesium

Proteins have been found to stimulate absorption of magnesium. Carbohydrates also stimulate absorption, apparently through the enhancement of sodium and water reabsorption in the ileum. Vitamin D also stimulates absorption directly, independent of calcium or phosphate, but the mechanism is not clearly elucidated. Other modulators of Mg^{2+} absorption are $Na,^+$ which increases absorption, and phosphate which decreases net absorption.

2. Renal Handling

a. Filtration

Approximately 1800 mg of Mg is filtered at the glomerulus daily. Of this, 95% is reabsorbed. The absorption is through an active process exibiting tubular maximum characteristics and via a passive diffusion process throughout the entire nephron. Patients placed on low-magnesium diets are able to decrease magnesium excretion to less than 1 mEq/day.

b. Reabsorption

The major site of reabsorption is the thick ascending limb of Henle (50–70%), and 15–20% is reabsorbed in the proximal tubule. Both processes are known to be active. The mechanism of reabsorption in the distal tubule is not clear. A maximal reabsorptive capacity for magnesium probably exists in man as it does in the dog. The values for Tm obtained in the dog are about 140 mg/min per kg body weight. The splay (deviation from an idealized linear relationship between filtered load and reabsorption) is great, and the Tm can only be demonstrated when the filtered load is twice the Tm value. The Tm value is significantly reduced by (1) volume expansion and (2) calcium infusion.

Studies done in rats have demonstrated a recycling of magnesium in the loop of Henle: magnesium is added to the tubular fluid in the descending limb and reabsorbed in the ascending limb. During hypermagnesemia, the percentage of magnesium filtered increases, and the reabsorption also increases until the Tm for Mg^{2+} is reached.

c. Factors That Influence Magnesium Excretion

1. Extracellular fluid volume expansion (EFVE): Despite a significant reduction in the filtered load, there is a depression of tubular reabsorption of Mg^{2+} brought by EFVE. This has been demonstrated by micropuncture techniques to occur in the proximal tubule.
2. Renal vasodilation with bradykinin and acetylcholine causes an increased excretion as a result of a decrease in tubular resorption. The close relationship between Na^+ clearance and Mg^{2+} clearance after vasodilatation is similar to that seen after saline infusion (EFVE).
3. Osmotic diuresis: Mannitol, glucose, and urea inhibit tubular reabsorption of Mg^{2+} because of a decrease in the concentration of Mg^{2+} in tubular fluid secondary to the inhibition of water reabsorption.
4. Diuretics: Furosemide and ethacrynic acid reduce ascending limb reabsorption of magnesium. Thiazides cause a transient loss during the first days, but later the excretion returns to base line. This is in contrast to the hypocalciuria which occurs with chronic thiazide administration. Acetazolamide produces no change in Mg reabsorption. This suggests that Mg^{2+} reabsorption is not linked to Na^+–H^+ exchange.
5. The effects of PTH on magnesium are similar to those on calcium: the hormone increases tubular reabsorption of magnesium. Most clinical conditions do not permit a clear-cut separation of the actions of calcium from those of PTH on magnesium reabsorption. Nevertheless, high plasma calcium is almost always associated with low magnesium and decreased tubular reabsorption of magnesium.
6. The effects of calcitonin (CT) on urinary magnesium are highly variable. In man, acute infusion of CT causes an increase or no change in magnesium excretion.
7. Urinary magnesium is high in hyperthyroidism and low in hypothyroidism. The hypermagnesemia seems to be a consequence of a direct effect of thyroid hormone to decrease the tubular reabsorption of magnesium.
8. Adrenal steroids: Acute mineralocorticoid therapy has no effect on magnesium excretion, whereas chronic therapy decreases reabsorption (most likely through volume expansion).
9. Other drugs such as cardiac glycosides cause a decrease in reabsorption. Similar effects are induced by gentamicin and cis-platinum, drugs that may result in a reversible defect in renal Mg^{2+} conservation. Alcohol is also known to cause a decrease in magnesium reabsorption. The mechanism is not completely clear.
10. Starvation: During periods of starvation, the urinary excretion of magnesium increases. This is believed to result from an impairment

Table II. Plasma Magnesium (mM) in Normal Subjects and Uremic Individuals[a]

	Total	Protein bound	Complexed	Free or ionized
Normal	1.0	0.375	0.125	0.5
Uremics				
Type I	0.7	0.37	0.13	0.2
Type II	1.1	0.32	0.10	0.68
Type III	1.4	0.39	0.19	0.82

[a] Mean values are given. The types have been selected arbitrarily based on values of total and free or ionized magnesium. From Coburn et al: *Arch Intern Med* 124:302–311, 1969.

of tubular reabsorption as a result of metabolic acidosis secondary to ketone body accumulation.

11. Early in renal disease, there is a reduction in absorption manifested as a decrease in serum Mg levels. As azotemia and renal function deteriorate, hypermagnesemia usually occurs (see Table II). The levels of magnesium vary, however, among uremic individuals.

D. Interaction with Other Ions

Interactions between Mg^{2+} and other ions have been documented. Of, these, one of the most important is the inhibitory effect of calcium on the absorption of magnesium in the gastrointestinal tract. The exact mechanism is not known. Calcium is also known to inhibit magnesium reabsorption in the renal tubule. A shift of concentration from intracellular to extracellular depots follows hypokalemia.

II. HYPOMAGNESEMIA

A. Causes

Table III summarizes the major causes of hypomognesemia.

1. Diuretics

Loop diuretics can increase urinary excretion up to 50% over control values.

2. Excessive Lactation

High fluid loss of approximately 2400 ml/day can cause severe losses. A case of tetany secondary to magnesium losses from lactation has been reported.

Table III. Causes of Hypomagnesemia

Dietary deficiency
   Very severe dietary restriction
      Starvation
      Protein–calorie (malnutrition)
   Hyperalimentation

Gastrointestinal
   Prolonged gastric suction
   Malabsorption
      Tropical sprue
      Celiac disease
      Regional enteritis
      Biliary cirrhosis
   Excessive use of laxatives
   Fistulae (GI)
   Massive rejection of small intestine

Renal
   Prolonged osmotic diuresis
      Glucosuria
      Mannitol administration
      Alcohol diuresis
   Postobstructive diuresis (urea)
   Diuretics therapy
      Furosemide
      Ethacrinic acid
      Thiazides
   Saline diuresis
      Hypotonic saline
      Isotonic saline
      Hypertonic saline
   Renal tubular acidosis
      Fanconi syndrome
      Distal RTA

Endocrine
   Insulin administration
      (diabetic ketoacidosis)
   Hyperparathyroidism
      Decreased tubular reabsorption
   Hyperaldosteronism
      Decreased renal tubular reabsorption
      Decreased GI reabsorption
   Hyperthyroidism

Drugs
   Antibiotics
      Gentamycin
      Amphotericin B (?)
      Outdated tetracycline
   Antineoplastic drugs
      Cis-platinum

Pancreatitis

3. Endocrine Disorders

a. Inappropriate ADH

The syndrome of inappropriate ADH secretion increases renal losses of Mg^{2+} in addition to the effect of hemodilution of its plasma concentration.

b. Thyrotoxicosis

Thyrotoxicosis is associated with hypomagnesemia and negative Mg^{2+} balance. This is caused by diminished intestinal absorption; the mechanism is not known.

c. Hyperparathyroidism

Marked increases in urinary Mg^{2+} excretion are found in patients with parathyroid tumors or hyperplasia.

d. Primary Aldosteronism

Studies in the rat have demonstrated that aldosterone causes a dose-related increase in excretion of Mg^{2+} in feces and urine. Patients with primary aldosteronism are frequently hypomagnesemic. This is reversed by spironolactone.

e. Diabetes Mellitus

A loss of 0.9 mEq/kg over a period of 3.5 days of insulin deprivation has been measured in insulin-dependent patients. Up to 23 mEq is lost in the urine during the initial fluid and insulin therapy of diabetic coma.

4. Alcohol

Alcohol inhibits the renal tubular reabsorption of magnesium.

5. Renal Diseases

Renal diseases in which a tubular defect is present can lead to hypomagnesemia. These include spontaneous and drug-induced distal renal tubular acidosis and tubulointerstitial disease. The nephropathies produced by cis-platinum and gentamycin are particularly prone to induce hypomagnesemia.

6. Vitamin D

Vitamin D in pharmacological doses leads to hypomagnesemia, although physiological doses increase absorption.

7. Gastrointestinal Disorders

1. Malabsorption syndrome, tropical and nontropical sprue, extensive bowel resection, and bowel and biliary fistulas all lead to Mg^{2+} losses. When steatorrhea is present, large amounts of Mg soaps are lost. Prolonged nasogastric suction with administration of Mg-free parenteral fluids are a common cause of hypomagnesemia. Gastric fluid contains approximately 1 mEq of Mg^{2+} per liter.
2. Prolonged diarrhea.
3. Protein–calorie malnutrition.
4. Pancreatitis with precipitation of magnesium soaps.
5. High oral Ca^{2+} loads which compete for the transport system.

B. Consequences of Hypomagnesemia

1. Central Nervous System

Irritability, ataxia, vertigo, and seizures result from outburst of synaptic transmission.

2. Cardiovascular

Cardiac arrhythmias, prolonged P–R and Q–T intervals, and prolonged, broad T waves are usual. These changes are similar to those seen in hypokalemia. Depression of ST segment and inversion of T waves in precordial leads are also common. Increased susceptibility to digoxim intoxication has been noted.

3. Pulmonary

No significant disturbances of lung function have been associated with hypomagnesemia.

4. Renal

There is diminished PTH response which leads to increased urinary Ca^{2+} losses.

5. Musculoskeletal

Tetany can occur in magnesium deficiency; this is potentiated by concomitant hypokalemia which frequently coexists with hypomagnesemia.

6. Gastrointestinal

Paralytic ileus or vomiting can occur secondary to hypotonic smooth muscle tone. Dysphagia has been associated with Mg deficiency. This is completely reversible after repletion. An increase in neuronal excitability and neuromuscular transmission has been suggested as a cause of muscle spasms.

7. Hematological

Magnesium deficiency can result in anemia through shortened RBC survival and spherocytosis associated with a striking reticulocytosis. Increased destruction of erythocytes in the spleen leads to intravascular hemolysis. The exact mechanism of hemolysis is unclear.

III. HYPERMAGNESEMIA

A. Causes

1. Excessive Intake

a. Oral

Patients receiving oral magnesium for peptic ulcer disease therapy frequently develop hypermagnesemia, particularly if renal disease is present. Magnesium is excreted mainly by the kidney; thus, diseases that reduce glomerular filtration rate will also affect magnesium excretion. As GFR decreases below 30 ml/min, hypermagnesemia develops.

b. Parenteral

The parenteral administration of magnesium in patients with toxemia of pregnancy can result in severe neurological depression as a result of magnesium excess. Optimal blood levels for control are from 3–6 mEq/liter. In some patients, symptoms of Mg toxicity may start at 4 mEq/liter. Adequate monitoring of the patient's clinical status is best followed by assessment of deep tendon reflexes and frequent serum Mg determinations. Another possible complication of parenteral therapy with magnesium in eclamptic females is intoxication of the newborn because of transplacental passage of the ion.

c. Enemas

Several cases have been reported of patients in whom cleansing enemas containing high magnesium concentration have lead to toxicity.

d. Miscellaneous

A case has been reported of hypermagnesemia following irrigation of the renal pelvis (as conservative management for urolithiasis) with a solution of magnesium oxide at 0.30%. The patient developed respiratory arrest as a manifestation of the hypermagnesemia that ensued.

B. Consequences

Degrees of hypermagnesemia producing various effects are summarized in Fig. 1.

1. Central Nervous System

Block of central synaptic transmission by decreased impulse transmission across neural junctions may occur. General somnolence, drowsiness, and anesthesia occur when plasma concentration is 4–7 mEq/liter. Diminished deep tendon reflexes, encephalopathy, ataxia, dysarthria, dilated pupils, and even coma may occur.

2. Cardiovascular

As Mg levels increase, conduction and cardiac contractility decrease. When Mg levels reach 14 to 25 mEq/liter, cardiac standstill in diastole is

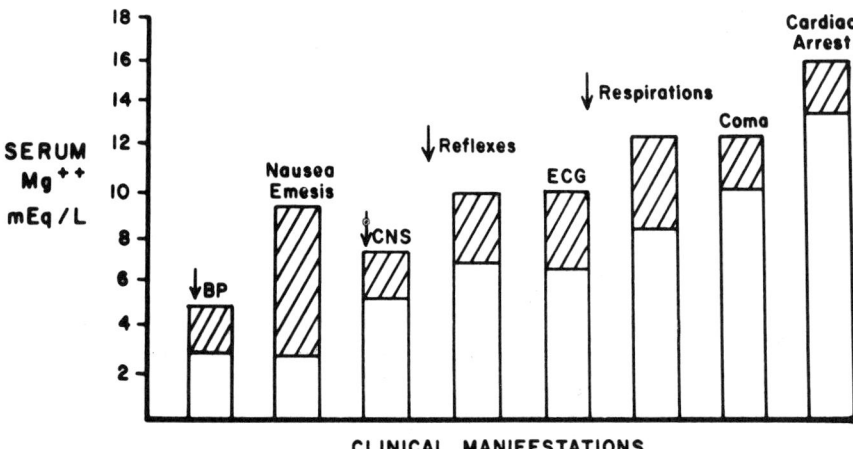

Figure 1. The signs and symptoms of hypermagnesemia begin to arise when serum values exceed 3 mEq/liter. In this graph, the clear portion of the bar represents values at which the given manifestation is usually not present, whereas the hatched areas are the range at which toxic phenomena may start to occur. Above these concentrations, clinical manifestations of toxicity are commonly present. (Reproduced with permission from Ferdinandus and Whang, Clinical Fluid and Electrolyte Management II, Veterans Administration Department of Medicine and Surgery, pp 130–138, 1978.)

observed. An increase in the P–R interval and intraventricular conduction defects with increased QRS and Q–T interval occur at plasma Mg concentrations of 6–10 mEq/liter. Moderate hypermagnesemia (3–5 mEq/liter) may result in bradycardia and hypotension.

3. Pulmonary

Respiratory paralysis occurs when Mg^{2+} levels reach 12 mEq/liter. Weakness of respiratory muscles leading to apnea or respiratory failure can occur soon after deep tendon reflexes are lost.

4. Renal

Inhibition of passive sodium entry in the proximal renal tubule may lead to natriuresis.

5. Musculoskeletal

Decreased deep tendon reflexes may be present when Mg^{2+} levels approach 7 mEq/liter. Hypermagnesemia increases the threshold of axonal excitation and decreases impulse transmission across neural junctions. The first signs of intoxication are decreased or absent deep tendon reflexes which are usually seen at values of 4 mEq/liter or higher.

6. Gastrointestinal

Hypermagnesemia may inhibit jejunal sodium and water transport, but the mechanism is unknown. Diminished peristalsis secondary to neuromuscular effects leads to nausea and vomiting.

7. Hematological

Hypermagnesemia may cause impairment of clotting mechanisms and may play a role in uremic bleeding disorders.

IV. TREATMENT OF HYPO- AND HYPERMAGNESEMIA

A. Treatment of Magnesium Excess

1. Discontinue Mg-containing medications.
2. If possible, correct renal insufficiency if present.
3. Calcium will transiently reverse the symptoms. The usual dose is 10 ml of 10% of calcium gluconate or calcium chloride administered intravenously which may be repeated as necessary. In the meanwhile,

other permanent measures such as peritoneal dialysis or hemodialysis, which rapidly and effectively lower the plasma Mg^{2+} concentration, should be started.

B. Treatment of Magnesium Deficiency

Magnesium administration is indicated whenever symptoms of deficiency are documented. These may fluctuate from tetany or seizures to resistant hypocalcemia without any other manifestation except the concomitant hypomagnesemia.

Replacement should be started with oral supplements of magnesium salts whenever the patient can tolerate them. Prior to magnesium replacement, renal function should be assessed (measure BUN and creatinine). If renal function is impaired, daily assessment of serum magnesium concentration must be done to avoid intoxication.

At least 1 mEq/kg of body weight should be given parenterally the first day. During the next 2 to 5 days, this should be reduced to 0.5 mEq/kg followed by 0.2 mEq/kg per day if parenteral fluid therapy is to continue. An effective regimen of replacement is 2 g of $MgSO_4 \cdot 7H_2O$ (8.12 mEq Mg^{2+}) every 4–6 hr during the first 24 hr followed by 1 g every 4–6 hr for the next 5 days. This can be given intramuscularly as a 50% solution. Procaine (1%) should be added to reduce the pain of the injection.

Intravenous replacement (infusion) is well tolerated and less painful than intramuscular injections. The first day, 5 g (42 mEq) in each of 2 liters of saline should be given for a total of 84 mEq. This is followed by a total of 6 g (50 mEq) distributed equally in the fluids given the next 2 to 5 days. A dose of 4 g a day of $MgSO_4$ (32 mEq) will maintain adequate serum concentrations. A 5-day regimen should be given to patients manifesting hypocalcemia secondary to magnesium deficiency. In patients unable to eat, there is a continuous loss of approximately 8 mEq/day which should be replaced daily. The rate of intravenous injection should not exceed 1.5 ml/min of 10% solution.

When losses are continuous because of steatorrhea, oral supplementation is essential. A solution of 4.0 g magnesium chloride ($MgCl_2 \cdot 6H_2O$) and 6.0 g magnesium citrate ($MgC_6H_5O_7 \cdot 5H_2O$) in 100 ml of water will provide 0.8 mEq/ml of magnesium.

Other oral preparations exist, but one must keep in mind that magnesium salts can produce diarrhea, and this becomes a limiting factor in their use.

1. Liquid milk of magnesia, one teaspoonful four times a day as tolerated.
2. Magnesium hydroxide tablets (milk of magnesia), one 300-mg tablet four times a day as tolerated; may be increased to two tablets four times a day if tolerated.

3. Magnesium acetate (9.35 mEq/g) as 10% solution: 10 ml in water four times a day as tolerated.

SUGGESTED READINGS

Ferdinandus J, Whang R: Hypermagnesemia, in: Clinical Fluid and Electrolyte Management II. Veterans Administration Department of Medicine and Surgery, 1978, pp 140–144.

Flink EB: Hypomagnesemia and magnesium depletion, in: Clinical Fluid and Electrolyte Management II. Veterans Administration Department of Medicine and Surgery, 1978, pp 130–138.

Massry SG: Magnesium homeostasis and its clinical pathophysiology. *Res and Staff Physician* (June) 105–109, 1981.

Massry SG, Seeling MS: Hypo- and hypermagnesemia. *Clin Nephrol* 7:147–153, 1977.

Mordes JP, Wacker WE: Excess magnesium. *Pharmacol Rev* 29:273–300, 1978.

Rude RK, Singer FR: Magnesium deficiency and excess. *Annu Rev Med* 32:245–259, 1981.

Wacker WEC, Parisi AE: Magnesium metabolism. *N Engl J Med* 278:658–661, 712–717, 1968.

5

Fluid and Electrolyte Disturbances
Treatment of Hypophosphatemia and Phosphate Depletion

JAMES P. KNOCHEL

I. HYPOPHOSPHATEMIA

Phosphate is a highly reactive ion involved in many chemical reactions. It is readily taken up from extracellular fluid into cells and incorporated into numerous organic compounds. Because of this lability, modest depression of serum phosphate to values between 2.0 and 2.5 mg/dl is common (Table I). In most instances, hypophosphatemia of itself is no more than an interesting transient finding. Little difficulty appears to result from moderate hypophosphatemia *per se*. However, moderate hypophosphatemia is an important finding, since it may reflect such disorders as vitamin D deficiency, hyperparathyroidism, or a reabsorptive defect of the renal tubule.

In contrast to moderate hypophosphatemia, when phosphate concentrations fall below 1.0 mg/dl and remain at that level for 2 or more days, serious consequences may occur. The conditions associated with severe hypophosphatemia, herein defined as a serum phosphorus less than 1 mg/dl, are shown in Table II.

JAMES P. KNOCHEL • Medical Service, Veterans Administration Medical Center, Dallas, Texas 75216; and Department of Internal Medicine, Southwestern Medical School at the University of Texas Health Science Center at Dallas, Dallas, Texas 75235.

Table I. Causes of Moderate Hypophosphatemia

Hemodialysis	Volume expanion
Hyperparathyroidism	Aldosteronism (licorice)
Starvation	Saline infusion
Administration of:	Hypokalemia
Glucose	Hypomagnesemia
Fructose	Gram-negative bacteremia
Glycerol	Administration of:
Lactate	Insulin
$NaHCO_3$	Gastrin
Osteomalacia	Glucagon
Renal tubular defects	Epinephrine
Pregnancy	Corticosteroids
Malabsorption	Diuretic therapy
Vitamin D deficiency	Androgen therapy
Acute gout	Recovery from hypothermia
Salicylate poisoning	

A. Relationship to Alcohol

The most common cause of severe hypophosphatemia is chronic alcoholism and alcohol withdrawal. Hypophosphatemia is especially common in hospitalized alcoholics. In such patients, serum phosphorus may be normal initially but decline to extremely low values over a period of 1–3 days. With the onset of hypophosphatemia, phosphorus in the urine virtually disappears. This presumably indicates cellular uptake of inorganic phosphate as administered nutrients are metabolized. As will be discussed later, such severe hypophosphatemia could also be the result of acute respiratory alkalosis. Nearly all severe alcoholics display respiratory alkalosis during withdrawal.

Measurement of skeletal muscle composition in severe alcoholics shows that phosphorus deficiency almost always exists. The cause of phosphorus deficiency in these patients is not completely understood. Although one could certainly implicate deficient intake, this cannot always be demonstrated. Experimentally, chronic alcoholic intoxication causes a substantial reduction of total muscle phosphorus despite a nutritious diet and an abundant intake of phosphorus.

B. Role of Antacid

Ingestion of phosphorus-binding antacids such as aluminum hydroxide or aluminum carbonate may cause phosphorus depletion and hypophosphatemia. Experimental studies by Lotz and Bartter showed clearly that human volunteers fed a low-phosphorus diet and large quantities of phosphorus-binding antacids developed severe hypophosphatemia and phosphorus de-

Table II. Causes of Severe Hypophosphatemia

Chronic alcoholism and alcoholic withdrawal
Pharmacological phosphate binding
Severe thermal burns
Recovery from diabetic ketoacidosis
Hyperalimentation
Nutritional recovery syndrome
Respiratory alkalosis
Renal transplantation

ficiency. In most clinical circumstances, ingestion of antacids does not cause phosphorus deficiency unless dietary intake of phosphorus is severely restricted.

C. Burns

Severe hypophosphatemia has been noted in patients suffering extensive thermal burns. It usually appears during the first few days after the burn. In such patients, phosphorus excretion is markedly depressed, and respiratory alkalosis is the rule.

D. Role of Nutrients

Administration of calories from any nutrient source to patients who have lost weight may result in severe hypophosphatemia. Their shrunken cells must be capable of an anabolic response. Hypophosphatemia occurs as a result of synthesis of protoplasm with inadequate quantities of phosphorus. Until this problem was recognized, hypophosphatemia occurred commonly in patients being treated by hyperalimentation. It usually became most prominent between the fifth and tenth days of treatment.

E. Diabetes Mellitus

In uncontrolled diabetes mellitus with prolonged heavy glycosuria, phosphorus is excreted excessively into the urine as a result of osmotic diuresis. In addition, metabolic acidosis decomposes phosphorylated compounds in cells, elevates serum phosphorus concentration, and thereby intensifies phosphaturia.

Diabetic ketoacidosis of mild to moderate intensity and of only a few days' duration does not usually cause an important degree of phosphorus deficiency. Such cases present with hyperphosphatemia as a rule, and with administration of fluids and insulin, serum phosphorus falls rapidly to values ranging between 1 and 3 mg/dl. During this time, urinary phosphorus becomes almost immeasurably low, reflecting cellular uptake.

F. Nutritional Recovery Syndrome

The nutritional recovery syndrome represents a constellation of findings observed during refeeding of patients with severe protein calorie malnutrition or starvation. In contrast to hyperalimentation, hypophosphatemia may occur during administration of calories in normally required quantities. Most observations on this syndrome were made on prisoners of war at the end of World War II. Refeeding, especially when overzealous and with simple carbohydrates, was sometimes followed by peripheral edema, ascites, and hydrothorax. Sudden death was common. Administration of brewer's yeast did not consistently prevent these complications. However, refeeding with skim milk was apparently associated with less morbidity. Unfortunately, measurements of chemical composition of the blood or urine from those patients were not possible.

This syndrome can be reproduced in experimental animals and is commonly seen during overzealous feeding of patients who have lost marked quantities of weight as result of food fadism or anorexia nervosa. Based on clinical description, such patients closely resemble the prisoners after World War II. In addition to hypophosphatemia provoked by nutrients, most of these patients show other serious disturbances such as hypokalemia, hypomagnesemia, and severe glucose intolerance. The observation that feeding with small quantities of skim milk rather than pure carbohydrates caused less morbidity is very likely ascribable to the reduced calories and phosphorus and potassium content of skim milk.

G. Acid–Base Alteration

Respiratory alkalosis can cause severe hypophosphatemia. Mostellar and Tuttle studied normal subjects and showed that serum phosphorus concentration may fall below 0.5 mg/dl after voluntary hyperventilation. Respiratory alkalosis is probably one of the most common causes of severe hypophosphatemia in hospitalized patients. Hyperventilation may apparently accompany metabolic encephalopathy associated with alcoholic withdrawal or simply may be the result of fear and pain. Respiratory alkalosis can be especially prominent in patients with sepsis and bacteremia.

The mechanism of hypophosphatemia under such conditions is quite clear. Reduction of carbon dioxide in blood is associated with an equally rapid reduction of carbon dioxide in the cell. The associated elevation of intracellular pH activates phosphofructokinase which in turn accelerates phosphorylation of glucose. Thereby, phosphate ions are rapidly taken up from serum, and hypophosphatemia results. Simultaneously, phosphorus virtually disappears from the urine.

On the other hand, if an equal degree of alkalosis is induced by infusing sodium bicarbonate, serum phosphorus concentration falls only slightly, and excretion of phosphorus in the urine increases. The increase of phosphorus excretion occurs by two mechanisms. First, there occurs slight expansion of extracellular fluid volume as a result of bicarbonate infusion, and this reduces reabsorption of phosphorus in the proximal tubule. Secondly, because of plasma volume expansion and a slight reduction of serum calcium concentration, parathyroid hormone levels increase during bicarbonate infusion and serve to decrease tubular reabsorption of phosphate.

Severe hypophosphatemia has also been noted in some patients who have undergone renal transplantation. Such patients apparently have a renal tubular reabsorptive defect which permits excessive phosphate loss into the urine. This has often occurred in the setting of corticosteroid therapy and administration of phosphate-binding antacids, both of which could conceivably favor development of hypophosphatemia.

II. THE CONSEQUENCES OF ACUTE HYPOPHOSPHATEMIA

Current evidence suggests that there are at least eight definite harmful consequences of severe hypophosphatemia. These are illustrated in Table III. That other tissues, organs, or physiological functions are affected would appear likely.

A. Rhabdomyolysis

Rhabdomyolysis, or acute necrosis of skeletal muscle, is one of the most common and reproducible consequences of phosphorus deficiency and severe hypophosphatemia. In the majority of cases, it is recognized by the appearance of abnormal elevations of muscle enzymes in serum, such as

Table III. Consequences of Severe Hypophosphatemia

Rhabdomyolysis
Red cell dysfunction and hemolysis
Myocardial dysfunction
Leukocyte dysfunction
Platelet dysfunction
Central nervous system dysfunction
Metabolic acidosis
Osteomalacia

creatine phosphokinase or aldolase. When severe, it may be associated with overt physical findings of muscle necrosis including profound weakness, pain, stiffness, tenderness, and edema of involved muscles and sometimes the appearance of myoglobin in the urine. In most cases of hypophosphatemia, rhabdomyolysis is clinically mild or asymptomatic and reflected only by elevated muscle enzymes. This has most commonly occurred in chronic alcoholics. It has also been seen in patients who become hypophosphatemic as a result of hyperalimentation.

Although slight to moderate elevations of enzyme activity are common, frank rhabdomyolysis is rarely observed during recovery from diabetic keto-acidosis. Measurements of muscle composition in chronic alcoholics have invariably shown severe deficiency of phosphorus. In the latter group, phosphorus deficiency occurs in association with other disturbances including magnesium deficiency and, in some but certainly not all cases, a moderately low content of potassium. Tissue content of sodium, chloride, water, and calcium are nearly always substantially elevated in such patients. To my knowledge, there have been no reports of rhabdomyolysis with severe hypophosphatemia as a result of respiratory alkalosis if body stores of phosphorus are normal. Experimental studies on dogs support this observation. On the other hand, a reversible electrochemical defect of skeletal muscle cells appears after feeding of a diet containing all essential nutrients except phosphorus. This defect is reversible on repletion with phosphorus. However, if an animal with preexisting phosphorus deficiency is subjected to hyperalimentation without phosphorus, hypophosphatemia is promptly induced, and severe rhabdomyolysis supervenes. Ongoing studies in our laboratory show that dogs fed intoxicating doses of ethanol each day eventually show depletion of skeletal muscle phosphorus despite an adequate phosphorus intake.

B. The Red Cell in Hypophosphatemia

The most important biochemical abnormalities of erythrocytes associated with phosphorus deficiency and severe hypophosphatemia include a decline of 2,3-diphosphoglycerate (2,3-DPG) and a decline of adenosine triphosphate (ATP). As will be described in more detail later, red cell inorganic phosphate is thought to be in diffusion equilibrium with plasma phosphorus. Consequently, both 2,3-DPG and ATP may become reduced in the presence of severe phosphorus deficiency and hypophosphatemia.

An important interaction occurs between hemoglobin and 2,3-DPG that promotes release of oxygen. This has been quantitated by means of the index, P_{50}, which is the value for oxygen tension of mixed venous blood at 37°C, pH 7.4, at which hemoglobin is 50% saturated (Fig. 1).

Low levels of 2,3-DPG may depress P_{50} values or shift the oxyhemoglobin saturation curve to the left so that release of oxygen to peripheral tissues is diminished. Thus, acute hypophosphatemia, when associated with a seri-

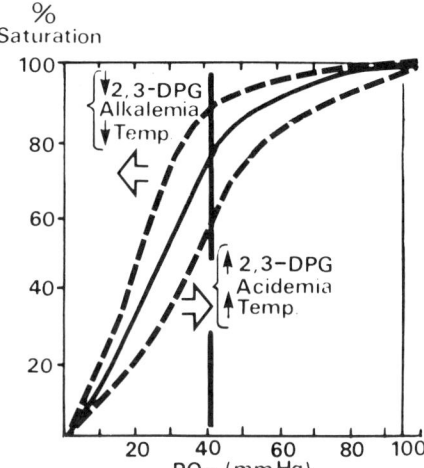

Figure 1. The oxyhemoglobin dissociation curve and factors that affect it. Decreased 2,3-DPG concentrations, alkalemia, and a decreased temperature will shift the curve to the left, resulting in an increased affinity of hemoglobin for oxygen with possible tissue hypoxia. Increased 2,3-DPG, acidemia, and temperature will produce an opposite effect.

ous decline of 2,3-DPG, may limit oxygen release at the cellular level and thereby cause anoxia. Respiratory alkalosis displaces the oxyhemoglobin dissociation curve to the left and consequently would aggravate the effects of an abnormally low red cell 2,3-DPG content. Metabolic acidosis displaces the curve to the right, and consequently, the P_{50} may be normal in the presence of diabetic ketoacidosis even though red cell 2,3-DPG may be low. The problem in diabetic ketoacidosis becomes apparent after 12–20 hr as acidosis is corrected and the curve shifts to the left. Speculation has been placed on this cause of hypoxia as an explanation for those rare patients who either awaken and return to a comatose state or those who fail to awaken at all despite correction of hyperglycemia and acidosis. I should like to emphasize that this issue is unsettled.

The interaction of hemoglobin with 2,3-DPG occurs at the same molecular site of hemoglobin glycosylation in patients with persistent hyperglycemia. It seems possible, therefore, that a potentiation of impaired oxygen delivery could occur in the phosphorus-deficient, hypophosphatemic, and persistently hyperglycemic patient with diabetes mellitus. An additional potentiating factor in diabetes could be the presence of metabolic acidosis. This would favor decomposition of 2,3-DPG independently of hyperglycemia or phosphorus deficiency.

Structural defects of the red cell in phosphorus deficiency and hypophosphatemia include increased ridigity (implying resistance to the normal deformity required to negotiate the microcirculation) and, in rare instances, hemolytic anemia. Hemolysis has also been described in patients with chronic uremic acidosis whose serum phosphorus has been profoundly depressed by excessive ingestion of phosphate-binding antacids. Hemolysis is actually a rare complication of severe hypophosphatemia. When it has occurred, ATP content has invariably been less than 15% of normal. Hemolysis is usually provoked by an unusual stress on the metabolic requirements of the red cell such as severe metabolic acidosis.

C. Myocardial Dysfunction

If phosphorus deficiency and hypophosphatemia were sufficiently severe to reduce red cell content of 2,3-DPG, one might predict that release of oxygen to tissues would diminish as a result of shifting the oxyhemoglobin dissociation curve to the left, and in response, the resting cardiac output would necessarily rise. One might further speculate that if a high resting cardiac output occurred by this means, such a condition, especially in the severe alcoholic, might lead one to suspect underlying vitamin deficiency and beri-beri heart disease. However, data are not available to verify such a speculation.

Fuller has examined the effects of pure phosphorus deficiency on myocardial performance in dogs. These animals were gavage-fed a diet that was normal in all respects except that it contained only trace quantities of phosphorus. Transducers were implanted surgically for measurement of ascending aortic root blood velocity and left ventricular pressure. The dogs were studied while awake. Their serum phosphorus values had fallen from 5.1 to 0.9 mg/dl, and their muscle phosphorus values had fallen from 28 to 22.6 mmol/100 g FFDW. When phosphorus deficiency existed, stroke volume, peak blood flow velocity, maximum ascending aortic blood flow acceleration, and maximum left ventricular rate of change of pressure (dP/dt) had decreased significantly. Restoration of phosphorus to the diet corrected all of these abnormalities. Although dogs may not have the same relationship between 2,3-DPG in red cells and oxyhemoglobin dissociation as man, it was clear that experimental phosphorus deficiency and hypophosphatemia resulted in a hypodynamic effect on the heart rather than the speculated high-output state.

Somewhat similar observations have been made on critically ill patients whose average serum phosphorus concentration was 0.97 mg/dl (range 0.7–1.4 mg/dl). After infusion of 1000 mg of elemental phosphorus in 60 cc of fluid volume, cardiac output did not change significantly, but calculated stroke work rose. This occurred independently of Starling effects and was attributed to an improvement in myocardial contractility.

Perhaps the most important clinical observations to date on hypophosphatemia were made on three patients with severe congestive cardiomyopathy and florid heart failure. The first was an alcoholic whose serum phosphorus was 0.4 mg/dl; the second was a 42-year-old man who had ingested large quantities of aluminum hydroxide gel for several months and whose serum phosphorus was 0.6 mg/dl; and the third was a patient whose serum phosphorus was 0.3 mg/dl who also had consumed aluminum hydroxide gel. All patients recovered completely from their congestive cardiomyopathy following restoration of serum phosphorus to normal. Of importance, only the first patient received digitalis and diuretics; the second and third patients did not. These observations suggest that correction of hypophosphatemia itself reversed cardiomyopathy.

Although severe hyphosphatemia occurs commonly in a wide variety of circumstances, recognition of congestive cardiomyopathy or overtly impaired ventricular function in hypophosphatemia is highly unusual. The reason for this may be explained by preliminary experimental studies from two different laboratories.

The effects of hyperalimentation-induced hypophosphatemia have been examined in dogs whose weight had been reduced by caloric restriction. Despite an appreciable fall of skeletal muscle phosphorus content during hyperalimentation, myocardial content of inorganic phosphate, ATP, ADP, and total phosphorus remained within normal limits. These findings existed in the face of serum phosphorus concentrations of less than 1 mg/dl. They suggest that the heart, being vital to life, has protective mechanisms that maintain vital energy substrates at the expense of skeletal muscle.

In rats maintained on a phosphorus-free diet and phosphate-binding antacids for 7 weeks, serum and skeletal muscle phosphorus were depressed significantly, but cardiac muscle phosphorus levels were normal. Preliminary studies suggest that the clinical appearance of hypophosphatemic cardiomyopathy was usually preceded by an event that caused sudden release of residual myocardial phosphorus into the bloodstream.

In dogs, it has been shown that following a 10-min occlusion of the midportion of the left anterior descending coronary artery, myocardial contractility was significantly decreased in phosphorus-depleted but not in normal dogs with the same duration of coronary occlusion. Such findings might mean that although total phosphorus, inorganic phosphorus, and perhaps even the adenylic acid pool (ATP and related metabolites) remain normal in hearts of phosphorus-deficient dogs, the metabolic state and potential contractility of the myocardium is extremely tenuous and fails with insults that would not ordinarily affect muscle performance.

It seems clear that increased attention should be paid to the effects of phosphorus deficiency on the heart. Although frank congestive cardiomyopathy under such conditions appears to be rare, it nevertheless appears to be one of the rare types of congestive cardiomyopathy that is curable.

D. Leukocyte Function during Hypophosphatemia

A serious complication of intravenous hyperalimentation therapy is systemic infection by bacterial and fungal organisms. Hypophosphatemic dogs show severe depression of chemotactic, phagocytic, and bactericidal activity of granulocytes. These abnormalities are reversed on correction of hypophosphatemia. Similar observations have been made on a patient who became hypophosphatemic during hyperalimentation.

Respiratory alkalosis and hypophosphatemia may occur in association with gram-negative bacteremia. Guinea pigs infected with *Salmonella* organisms became hypophosphatemic before death. When given phosphate, mortality was significantly reduced, and the number of organisms found in their tissues was smaller.

Apparently, hypophosphatemia impairs granulocytic function by impairing ATP synthesis. ATP provides energy for contractions of microfilaments, which in turn regulate the mechanical properties of leukocytes, viz., pseudopod and vacuole formation.

E. Platelet Function during Hypophosphatemia

Seven abnormalities of platelet function and structure have been observed in hypophosphatemic dogs: (1) thrombocytopenia, (2) increase in platelet diameter, suggesting shortened platelet survival, (3) megakaryocytosis of the marrow, (4) a five- to tenfold acceleration of the rate of labeled platelet disappearance from blood, (5) impairment of clot retraction, (6) a 44% reduction in platelet ATP content, and (7) hemorrhage into the gut and skin. These abnormalities are circumvented if phosphorus supplements are provided. Whether or not similar changes occur in man is unknown.

F. Effects of Hypophosphatemia on the Central Nervous System

Some patients with severe hypophosphatemia display symptoms compatible with a metabolic encephalopathy. In sequence, they show irritability, apprehension, weakness, numbness, paresthesias, dysarthria, confusion, obtundation, convulsive seizures, and coma. This clinical syndrome has been observed in patients without other apparent causes for encephalopathy who have been treated with IV hyperalimentation and also in patients with withdrawal from chronic alcoholism. In contrast to delerium tremens, hallucinations have not been observed. Obviously, both conditions may coexist.

The relationship between hypophosphatemia and the decline of red cell 2,3-DPG becomes especially important in tissues in which oxygen is necessary for energy production. This could have an important role in the brain where oxidation of glucose through the Krebs cycle is necessary for synthesis of ATP. In one report, three of the eight patients who became hypophosphatemic during hyperalimentation developed paresthesias, mental obtundation, and hyperventilation. Those whose P_{50} values were abnormally low showed diffuse slowing of their electroencephalograms. These changes disappeared when the hypophosphatemia was corrected. Perhaps the best evidence that hypophosphatemia plays a role in this encephalopathy has been the observation that it does not occur in patients receiving hyperalimentation with adequate phosphorus.

G. Metabolic Acidosis

Substantial clinical and experimental evidence is now available indicating that severe metabolic acidosis may occur in the presence of phosphorus deficiency and severe hypophosphatemia. When phosphorus is removed from the diet or its absorption is prevented by binding with antacids, bone minerals are promptly mobilized. This apparently occurs even before the advent of hypophosphatemia and suggests operation of an unidentified hormone. Phosphorus deficiency in a child or in an adult who has a disease process causing rapid turnover of bone may cause hypercalcemia. Independently of hypercalcemia, phosphorus deficiency nearly always causes hypercalciuria. Phosphorus deficiency thus induced is seldom associated with metabolic acidosis. However, as hypophosphatemia becomes more severe, phosphate ions virtually disappear from the urine, thereby eliminating the capacity to excrete metabolic hydrogen as titratable acid.

The bulk of metabolic acid is excreted by exchange of H^+ from the cell with Na^+ from the renal tubular lumen. In this process, Na_2HPO_4 is normally converted to NaH_2PO_4, and the hydrogen ions are measurable as titratable acid. If phosphate is absent from the urine, metabolic acid can be excreted by the reaction $NH_3 + H \rightarrow NH_4^+$. Ordinarily, a decline of intracellular pH would augment production of NH_3. However, in phosphorus deficiency, it has been proposed that intracellular pH rises, thereby decreasing NH_3 production. A rise of intracellular pH in phosphorus deficiency has been reported in liver and muscle. Whether similar changes occur in the kidney cell have not been determined.

Nevertheless, abundant evidence shows that phosphorus deficiency reduces ammonia excretion and thus supports the theory that intracellular pH of the renal cell rises. Thus, the decrease in ammonia production and unavailability of buffer phosphate in the urine essentially prevent excretion of metabolic acids. Therefore, the question arises as to why individuals who cannot excrete titratable acid or form ammonium in adequate quantity do not regularly develop profound metabolic acidosis. The explanation lies in the fact that during mobilization of bone mineral, there also occurs mobilization of carbonate which is an important component of bone apatite (Fig. 2). Sufficient carbonate is mobilized from bone to titrate metabolic acid. In fact, in animal studies it has been found that carbonate mobilization may overshoot and result in slight metabolic alkalosis.

However, should some event occur that prevents mobilization of bone mineral, metabolic acidosis of severe proportion can occur. This has been described in children with severe lactase deficiency and protein–calorie malnutrition during refeeding without adequate phosphorus. Addition of phosphorus to their dietary mixture resulted in marked increments of acid excretion into the urine and correction of metabolic acidosis. Experimentally, bone mobilization resulting from phosphorus deficiency also prevents metabolic acidosis. However, metabolic acidosis rapidly supervenes if

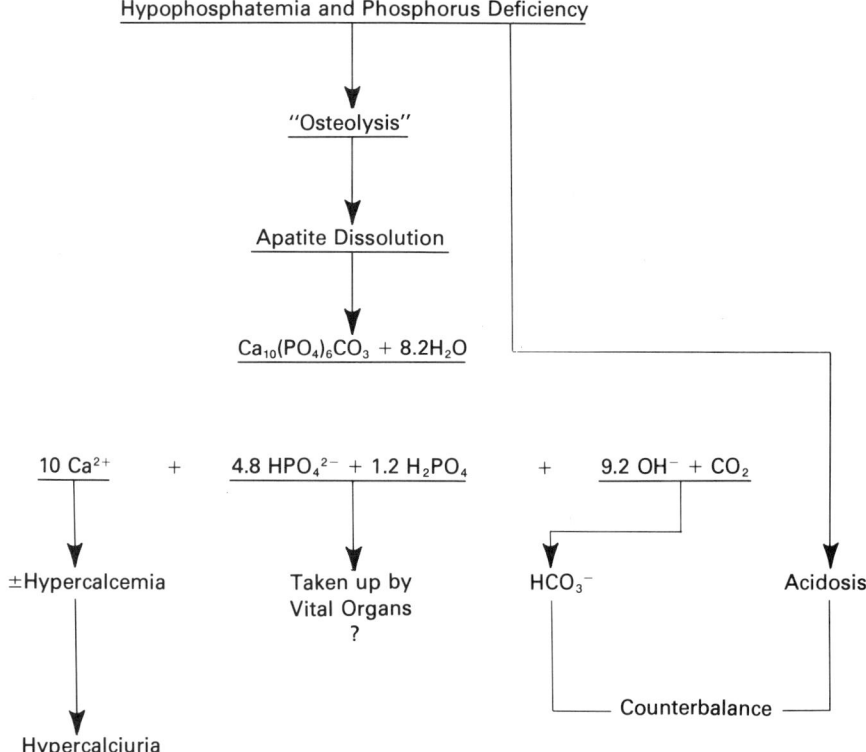

Figure 2. Deprivation of phosphorus stimulates dissolution of the skeleton in an apparent attempt to maintain a normal serum phosphorus concentration. Apatite breaks down to calcium, phosphate, carbonate, and water. Hypercalcemia occurs in children or in adults in any state in which increased bone turnover prevails. Hypercalciuria is a regular feature. Although urine phosphate is sufficiently depressed to prevent acid excretion as titratable acidity, carbonate ions mobilized from apatite titrate metabolic acids sufficiently to prevent metabolic acidosis. If this process is long standing, classical osteomalacia may result.

agents are administered that interrupt mobilization of bone mineral such as diphosphonate or colchicine. Although the possibility might be considered that the mild state of hyperchloremic metabolic acidosis that regularly occurs during recovery from diabetic ketoacidosis might be the result of phosphorus deficiency and hypophosphatemia, there is no evidence to support this notion.

Besides the aforementioned metabolic interplay of bone mineral mobilization and altered excretion of acid by the kidney, there also may occur a depression of bicarbonate reabsorption in the proximal tubule. The potential clinical importance of proximal tubular bicarbonate wasting in phosphorus depletion has not been established.

H. Osteomalacia

Mobilization of bone mineral during phosphorus deficiency and hypophosphatemia, when present for a sufficiently long period of time, may result in frank osteomalacia. A patient has been described who ingested a diet deficient in phosphorus and consumed large quantities of phosphate-binding antacids for a prolonged time. Dietary deprivation of phosphorus and ingestion of phosphate-binding antacids have been associated with hypercalciuria. When serum phosphorus levels approached 1 mg/dl or less, patients complained of weakness and bone pain and were thought to show all findings consistent with osteomalacia. Their symptoms were relieved promptly on restoration of phosphorus to their diets and elimination of phosphate-binding antacids. Hypercalciuria appears to be a feature of phosphorus deficiency in women more than in men.

I. Unproved Consequences of Hypophosphatemia

Since adequate supplies of inorganic phosphate are critical for repletion of ATP stores in every cell, it seems conceivable that any tissue or organ may become damaged in the presence of severe hypophosphatemia. Descriptions of muscular paralysis independent of rhabdomyolysis have appeared. Unfortunately, the patients in one report were also acutely hypokalemic. Thus, the role of hypophosphatemia was unclear.

Hepatocellular dysfunction was first suggested in studies of a 51-year-old woman with alcoholic cirrhosis whose serum phosphorus had fallen to 0.5 mg/dl in the wake of respiratory alkalosis. Her bilirubin rose appreciably and she became comatose. Over the following few days, serum phosphorus became normal, and her neurological findings cleared. We have also observed this sequence of events in hospitalized alcoholics and therefore question the possibility that spontaneous correction of hypophosphatemia by release of phosphorus from injured skeletal muscle may inadvertently be life saving in such patients.

Severe hypophosphatemia may alter the redox state of cytosol and conceivably be responsible for lactic acidosis or β-hydroxybutyric ketoacidosis. Unfortunately, studies have not been conducted to determine if pancreatitis or even intestinal function could be impaired by hypophosphatemia.

In hypophosphatemia and phosphorus deficiency, critical determinants of cellular injury appear to be the prevailing concentrations of inorganic phosphate and adenine nucleotides in the cytosol. In particular, if the concentration of cytosolic ATP falls to a critically low level, cellular dysfunction or disintegration may follow. Studies by a number of investigators have shown that the supply of inorganic phosphate in the cytosol is critical for resynthesis of ATP from ADP.

J. Mechanism of Cellular Injury in Hypophosphatemia

Unquestionably, combined phosphorus deficiency and severe hypophosphatemia can result in widespread cellular damage. On the other hand, whether hypophosphatemia independently of phosphorus deficiency can induce cellular damage or dysfunction is unclear. One study published only in abstract form showed that experimental animals given *Salmonella* organisms intravenously become hypophosphatemic as the result of respiratory alkalosis. When sufficient phosphate to prevent hypophosphatemia was given along with the same dose of bacteria, the LD_{50} was significantly reduced. Similarly, unpublished observations on patients with severe thermal burns suggest that prevention of severe hypophosphatemia reduces the incidence and morbidity from burn wound sepsis and bacteremia.

Energy requirements to maintain cellular function and integrity may undergo rapid fluctuation, and these variable demands must be integrated and transmitted to mitochondria where energy is produced. At any given instant, the mitochondrial respiratory rate must respond to these minute-to-minute changes in cellular demands. This cellular energy state is reflected by several substrate concentration ratios. For example, the lactate/pyruvate ratio indicates the cytosolic redox state, whereas that of mitochondria is reflected by the ratio of β-hydroxbutyrate to acetoacetate. However, the overall energy state of the cell is perhaps best represented by the phosphorylation potential. This is defined as the ratio of cytosolic ATP to the product of cytosolic ADP and inorganic phosphate:

$$\text{Phosphorylation potential} = [\text{ATP}]/([\text{ADP}] \times [\text{Pi}])$$

Any metabolic alteration that increases the value of the phosphorylation potential slows mitochondrial respiration. In contrast, if the phosphorylation potential decreases, mitochondrial respiration accelerates. Thus, a reduction of cytosolic inorganic phosphate increases the potential and slows mitochondrial respiration. By this mechanism, ATP falls and reduces the ATP/ADP ratio, thereby normalizing the phosphorylation potential.

Besides affecting the mitochondrial respiratory rate, intracellular inorganic phosphate concentration is also an important regulator of the overall adenine nucleotide pool size. Thus, ADP, AMP, and ATP are in equilibrium through the myokinase reaction:

$$2 \text{ ADP} \rightleftharpoons \text{AMP} + \text{ATP}$$

A major degradation pathway for the adenylate pool is the irreversible deamination of AMP to IMP catalyzed by the enzyme AMP deaminase. This reaction is strongly inhibited by a normal concentration of intracellular phosphate. Thus, a marked reduction in intracellular phosphate disinhibits AMP deaminase, resulting in AMP degradation which is, in turn, reflected throughout the adenylate pool.

A good example of this phenomenon is the response to intravenous fructose. Fructose is metabolized by three tissues, intestinal mucosa, liver, and renal cortex. Its phosphorylation by these tissues is facilitated by fructokinase. Formation of fructose phosphate is unregulated, meaning that increasing concentrations of fructose phosphate in the cytosol do not inhibit further uptake of fructose. The cytosolic concentration of inorganic phosphate is thereby sharply lowered, AMP-deaminase is disinhibited, and the adenylate pool is reduced. In patients with hereditary fructose intolerance, the product of AMP deamination, inosine, and its product, uric acid, appear in the urine in increased quantities following administration of fructose. This reaction is illustrated as follows:

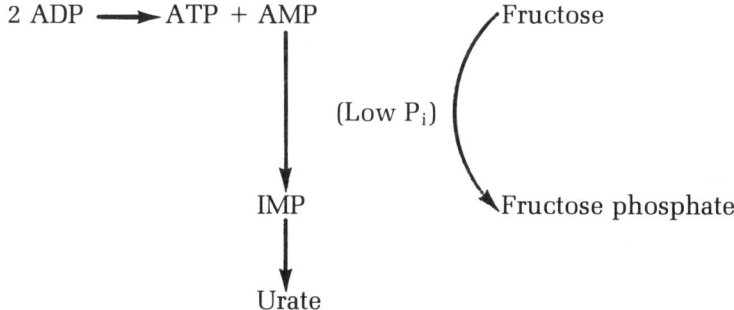

This sequence of events occurs very rapidly and has been associated with functional and structural disturbances in the liver and kidney. Administration of inorganic phosphorus provides partial protection against these harmful effects.

With the foregoing in mind, it becomes apparent that a sustained, severe reduction of inorganic phosphate concentration in the cell with reduce the cytosolic concentration of ATP. This can potentially result in a critical deficiency of ATP for energy-requiring reactions. Although information is not complete, certain tissues appear to be more susceptible to hypophosphatemia than others. For example, intracellular concentration of inorganic phosphate in the red cell is dependent on diffusion down a chemical gradient from plasma. Thus, hypophosphatemia leads to a reduction of cellular inorganic phosphate, and this in turn reduces the cell's capacity to produce ATP. This process would apparently be quite independent of the reduced 2,3-DPG which in turn would alter the cell's capacity to release oxygen. If an additional metabolic stress is superimposed such as severe acidosis, hemolysis may occur. Hemolysis has been observed only when ATP concentrations have fallen to very low values. In contrast to the red cell, other tissues apparently have the capacity to maintain more adequate supplies of intracellular inorganic phosphate despite hypophosphatemia.

In our own studies, dogs were fed a calorie-restricted diet containing abundant phosphorus. When their baseline body weight had been reduced by one-third, hyperalimentation was carried out without adequate phosphorus until their serum phosphorus fell to 1.0 mg/dl or less. Although total muscle P fell rapidly during hyperalimentation, muscle inorganic phosphorus concentration remained normal as also did the concentrations of ATP and ADP. Thus, both the phosphorylation potential and the adenylate pool remained normal. These observations suggest that retention of inorganic phosphorus by muscle despite hypophosphatemia represents a fundamental, vital process to maintain cellular integrity.

Examination of skeletal muscle inorganic phosphorus, ATP, and ADP concentrations in dogs with chronic phosphorus deficiency has shown that each component fell by approximately 50%. The phosphorylation potential became twice normal, indicating that the cell's capacity to produce ATP was reduced. Since the content of ATP is low, such a cell is in a state of peril should there be a demand for energy production. For example, if inorganic phosphorus cannot be maintained in the face of acute hypophosphatemia, ATP would fall further, and disintegration might follow. These findings probably explain why superimposition of severe hypophosphatemia on a cell already injured by chronic phosphorus deficiency causes florid rhabdomyolysis.

It would seem possible that cells injured by a variety of noxious influences such as ethanol, malnutrition, acute starvation, uremia, anoxia, or a host of metabolic derangements could be easily destroyed in the event of severe hypophosphatemia. A preceding injury would only need to compromise those mechanisms responsible for maintaining an optimal concentration of inorganic phosphorus in the cell. Thereby, both energy production and the adenylate pool would become inadequate to sustain vital cellular functions.

III. TREATMENT OF ACUTE SEVERE HYPOPHOSPHATEMIA

In any discussion of treatment, the issue of efficacy should be given first considerations. Thus, what evidence exists showing that treatment of phosphorus deficiency and/or hypophosphatemia is beneficial?

A. Clinical Evidence

1. Diabetes Mellitus

Simultaneous administration of phosphate salts with glucose improves glucose utilization in diabetic patients. Patients with chronic phosphorus deficiency and mild hypophosphatemia resulting from renal tubular disorders or vitamin D-resistant rickets have been shown to have impaired glucose utilization. Employing the glucose clamp technique, it has been shown that glucose intolerance was not the result of impaired insulin secretion but the consequence of impaired tissue sensitivity to insulin. The effect of phosphorus repletion was not examined. Administration of phosphate salts in association with conventional therapy appears to hasten recovery of patients with diabetic ketoacidosis.

Treatment with phosphate salts in the management of diabetic ketoacidosis (DKA) has become exceptionally popular in the United States. This practice has resulted from the fact that nearly all patients with DKA show a decline in serum phosphate following administration of fluids and insulin. Despite the foregoing, recent studies have made routine phosphate therapy in DKA controversial. Keller and Berger compared 12 patients with DKA who were not treated with phosphate with 12 patients who were treated with phosphate. Red cell 2,3-DPG was severely depressed in both groups initially, and although the rate of its recovery was more rapid in those treated with phosphate, recovery also progressed rapidly in the untreated group. In practical terms, the difference was probably not sufficient to be important clinically. In addition, restoration of 2,3-DPG levels in red cells indicates that phosphorus was utilized to synthesize this compound despite moderately severe hypophosphatemia. The lowest average serum phosphorus concentration in those treated without phosphate was 2.2 ± 0.3 mg/dl, whereas in patients treated with phosphate, the lowest average value was 3.6 ± 0.4 mg/dl. Of the 12 patients not receiving phosphate treatment, only three had serum phosphorus levels below 2.0 mg/dl, and these were 1.5, 1.2, and 1.7 mg/dl.

Wilson and his associates have examined the effects of phosphate treatment in 44 patients with DKA. They were unable to show any evidence of clinical benefit in terms of duration of DKA, dose of insulin required to correct the acidosis, abnormal muscle enzymes, glucose disappearance, morbidity, or mortality.

As indicated previously in this section, acute hypophosphatemia does not ordinarily produce severe complications unless serum levels fall below 1.0 mg/dl. In both of the aforementioned studies, serum phosphorus did not fall to such values. Most patients with diabetic ketoacidosis give a history of loss of diabetic control for a period of only 2 to 5 days before they seek treatment. Two studies have reported the effects of experimental insulin withdrawal on previously stable patients. Before it became necessary to resume insulin treatment because of ketoacidosis, the measured net losses of phosphorus corrected for nitrogen balance varied from 20 to 66 mEq (11.5 to 37 mmol). In quantitative terms, such small losses compare with those probably existing in the typical patient whose illness has been of short duration. Such patients nearly always display hyperphosphatemia at the time of admission to the hospital. In contrast, one should be alert for patients who present with normal or low values.

Rarely, patients with diabetic ketoacidosis will develop serum phosphorus values below 1.0 mg/dl during treatment, and although specific studies on such a group have not been reported, it would seem likely that serious effects could well occur. Sometimes, patients whose diabetic ketoacidosis has been long standing and especially severe will show hypophosphatemia on admission despite severe acidosis. Such patients are usually hypokalemic as well. These two findings doubtless indicate severe, simultaneous deficiencies of phosphorus and potassium, and almost certainly, both need to be replaced.

Based on the foregoing, current evidence suggests that phosphate replacement is probably not necessary in the majority of patients with DKA, especially those whose illness has been of short duration and moderate in severity. In all patients with ketoacidosis, serum phosphorus should be measured every 12 hr during the acute illness. If it falls below 1.0 mg/dl, replacement therapy should be initiated (see later discussion for phosphate administration).

2. Central Nervous System

A fair amount of evidence indicates that the central nervous system complications of acute severe hypophosphatemia observed during hyperalimentation of wasted patients do not occur if adequate phosphorus is provided to prevent hypophosphatemia. Brain dysfunction, electroencephalographic abnormalities, and decreased red cell 2,3-DPG content revert to normal if hypophosphatemia is corrected.

3. Fructose Intolerance

Patients with hereditary fructose intolerance show sharp increments in the excretion of inosine and uric acid after challenge with fructose. Administration of phosphate supplements with fructose reduces excretion of both inosine and uric acid. These observations suggest that cystosolic depletion of inorganic phosphate and depletion of the adenylic acid pool are both attenuated in these patients by administration of phosphorus.

4. Metabolic Acidosis

Studies of children with protein–calorie malnutrition resulting from lactase deficiency have shown that administration of calories without adequate phosphorus during refeeding therapy led to the rapid development of severe metabolic acidosis. They showed that phosphorus supplementation resulted in a sharp increase of titratable acidity in the urine and rapid correction of metabolic acidosis.

5. Congestive Cardiomyopathy

Reversal of congestive cardiomyopathy associated with profound hypophosphatemia has been shown following administration of phosphate salts. In two patients, recovery occurred without simultaneous administration of digitalis or diuretics.

6. Selective Phosphorus Deficiency in Man

Phosphorus deficiency studies on human volunteers showed unquestionable improvement in weakness and bone pain following restoration of phosphorus to their diet.

B. Experimental Evidence

1. Fructose-Loading Injury

Parenteral fructose damages the liver and renal cortex. During metabolism of fructose in these tissues, as phosphorus is rapidly utilized to phosphorylate fructose, the decline of cytosolic inorganic phosphate activates adenylate deaminase which, in turn, decomposes the precursors of ATP. When ATP declines, 5'-nucleotidase is activated, further decomposing the nucleotide pool. When cells become critically depleted of ATP, disintegration follows. Fructose loading in the rat leads to a decline of ATP, ADP, and inorganic phosphate in liver and renal cortical tissue which is substantially less if phosphate is given with fructose.

2. Rhabdomyolysis in the Phosphorus-Deficient Hypophosphatemic Dog

In our own studies, the acute florid rhabdomyolysis produced by hyperalimentation of a partially starved phosphorus-deficient dog did not occur if large quantities of inorganic phosphate were added to the hyperalimentation mixture to prevent hypophosphatemia. When hyperalimented without phosphorus, the same animals display marked weakness, tremors, fasiculations, and in many instances convulsions before death. None of these events occurred if adequate phosphorus supplementation was provided.

3. Biochemical Myopathy in the Phosphorus-Deficient Dog

In the chronic phosphorus-deficient dog, studies of skeletal muscle show a rise of sodium chloride content, water, and a decrease of the transmembrane resting electrical potential difference. Restoration of inorganic phosphate to the diet leads to correction of these abnormalities.

4. Myocardial Dysfunction in the Phosphorus-Deficient Dog

Impaired contractile force and decreased left ventricular ejection rates in phosphorus-deficient dogs were effectively reversed by phosphorus repletion.

5. Resistance to Infection

Guinea pigs administered graded doses of *Salmonella* organisms regularly become hypophosphatemic as a result of hyperventilation and respiratory alkalosis. The LD_{50} is reduced by administration of sufficient phosphorus to prevent hypophosphatemia.

The foregoing is considered to be persuasive clinical and experimental evidence that treatment of phosphorus deficiency and hypophosphatemia is not only important but effective. However, in those situations in which tissue destruction has already occurred, benefit would not be expected.

IV. THERAPEUTIC CONSIDERATIONS

The general principles of management for phosphorus deficiency and hypophosphatemia are similar to those for deficiency of many other ions or minerals. First, if an individual can tolerate oral administration of the supplement, it should be administered by this route. Milk is an excellent source of phosphorus as well as potassium and calcium. Its phosphorus content is approximately 33 mmol/qt. Many patients with severe phosphorus deficiency cannot tolerate milk because of its content of lactose or fat. Skim milk may be tolerable, but in the event it is not, one might attempt administration of Fleet's enema solution orally, which is buffered sodium phosphate. The dose is 15–30 cc three or four times daily. In the presence of phosphorus deficiency and otherwise normal intestinal function, the capacity for phosphate absorption may be enhanced so that the usual diarrhea with administration of sodium phosphate salts does not occur.

In most instances of severe hypophosphatemia, it is necessary to administer phosphate salts intravenously. One should select an intravenous preparation and become acquainted with its composition. Commercial preparations are readily available.

Ideally, the compound should be given in a quantity that will not produce hyperphosphatemia. Hypocalcemia and metastatic calcification are distinct hazards incident to intravenous phosphate salts. Infusion of phosphate salts will lower ionized calcium if the product of calcium and phosphorus exceeds $2.4–2.5 \times 10^{-6}$ mM (58 mg/dl). Infusion of 1.8 mmol PO_4/kg body weight into normal subjects produces a fall of serum calcium that averages 0.18 mmol/liter (−0.7 mg/dl). In one patient with hypoparathyroidism, 1.3 mmol PO_4/kg body weight reduced serum calcium from 2.1 to 1.8 mM (−1.2 mg/dl). If serum calcium is low before administration of PO_4 salts, an appreciable fall of serum calcium would not be anticipated if the solubility product were not exceeded. In healthy subjects, a fall of calcium produced by PO_4 infusion would be in part corrected by release of parathyroid hormone. However, if a patient also has hypomagnesemia, release of parathyroid hormone would be suppressed, and, in turn, hypocalcemia could conceivably become more severe and prolonged. Alkalosis could potentiate the tendency for $CaHPO_4$ formation and thereby enhance hypocalcemia.

Patients being treated for diabetic ketoacidosis, alcoholics in withdrawal, and patients with streatorrhea often have hypophosphatemia, hypomagnesemia, hypocalcemia, and hypokalemia. In such patients, electrolyte replacement solutions should include phosphate, magnesium, and potassium. However, lest the conclusion be made that it might be best to avoid phosphate altogether, the natural course of diabetic ketoacidosis should be considered.

Without phosphate treatment, adults treated for diabetic ketoacidosis may become hypocalcemic (73%) or hypomagnesemic (55%). In a study of nine children with diabetic ketoacidosis given phosphate salts, five became hypocalcemic. In the latter study, hypomagnesemia was present in each patient but fell below 1 mEq/liter in only one. The dose of phosphate in those children who had the most severe hypocalcemia was greater than 11 mmol/kg per 24 hr. Serum phosphorus was also high. A 9-year-old child with diabetic ketoacidosis has been described who developed hypocalcemia and hypomagnesemia after administration of more than 5 mmol phosphorus/kg body weight in 29 hr. Administration of intravenous phosphate in adults with diabetic ketoacidosis in doses ranging from 15 to 45 mmol during the first 10 hr of treatment did not result in a significantly greater depression of serum calcium in those receiving phosphate than in those who did not. Keller and Berger infused from 40 to 130 mmol PO_4 into adult patients with diabetic ketoacidosis. The average serum calcium concentration fell from 9.4 to 8.3 mg/dl in those not treated with PO_4 and from 8.7 to 7.8 in those who were treated with PO_4. Based on such data, hypocalcemia occurs in the majority of patients during treatment of diabetic ketoacidosis whether phosphorus is given or not. In addition, if large doses of phosphorus are given, hypocalcemia can be seriously aggravated.

In treating adult patients with hypophosphatemia, a rule of thumb that continues to be successful in our hands has been to administer approximately 20 mmol of sodium phosphate intravenously each 8 hr. Using this formula, the total daily dose is less than 1 mmol/kg body weight. This amount has generally been adequate to maintain serum phosphorus levels at

Table IV. Phosphate Preparations for Intravenous Use[a]

Preparation	Composition (mg/ml)	Phosphate (mmol/ml)	Sodium (mEq/ml)	Potassium (mEq/ml)
K phosphate	236 mg K_2HPO_4 224 mg KH_2PO_4	3.0	0	4.4
Na phosphate	142 mg Na_2HPO_4 276 mg $NaH_2PO_4 \cdot H_2O$	3.0	4.0	0
Neutral Na phosphate	10.0 mg Na_2HPO_4 2.7 mg $NaH_2PO_4 \cdot H_2O$	0.09	0.2	0
Neutral Na,K phosphate	11.5 mg Na_2HPO_4 2.6 mg KH_2PO_4	1.10	0.2	0.02

[a] Adapted from Lentz et al: *Ann Intern Med* 89:941–944, 1978.

or above 1.5 mg/dl. This concentration appears to prevent most of the severe consequences of hypophosphatemia and at the same time should be sufficiently low to prevent hyperphosphatemia and precipitation of calcium phosphate in tissues.

In treating the complex electrolyte derangements described above in the patient with alcohol withdrawal, it is practical to administer phosphorus, magnesium, and potassium in the same solution. For example, we have employed solutions composed of 1 liter of 5% glucose in 0.45% saline to which has been added 20 mmol of potassium phosphate, 20 mEq of potassium chloride, and 4.0 ml of 50% magnesium sulfate (16 mEq of magnesium). This quantity is infused over 8 hr. We have infused this mixture three times daily for several days in many patients with successful results. The three electrolytes are compatible in solution. Used in such quantities, we have not encountered severe hypocalcemia. Obviously, intravenous phosphorus should not be administered in the presence of hyperphosphatemia.

SUGGESTED READINGS

Blachley JD, Ferguson ER, Carter NW, Knochel JP: Chronic alcohol ingestion induces phosphorus deficiency and myopathy in the dog. *Trans Assoc Am Physicians* 93:110–122, 1980.

Darsee JR: Hypophosphatemic myocardial dysfunction: The role of phosphorus and high-energy phosphate compounds in myocardial function and dysfunction, Hurst JW (ed): *The Heart* (update 3). New York, McGraw-Hill, 1979, pp 1–8.

Darsee JR, Nutter DO: Reversible severe congestive cardiomyopathy in three cases of hypophosphatemia. *Ann Intern Med* 89:867–870, 1978.

Farber E: ATP and cell integrity. *Fed Proc* 32:1534–1539, 1973.

Keller U, Berger W: Prevention of hypophosphatemia by phosphate infusion during treatment of diabetic ketoacidosis and hyperosmolar coma. *Diabetes* 29:87–95, 1979.

Knochel JP: The pathophysiology and clinical characteristics of severe hypophosphatemia. *Arch Intern Med* 137:203–220, 1977.

Knochel JP: Hypophosphatemia in the alcoholic. *Arch Intern Med* 140:613–615, 1980.

Knochel JP: Hypophosphatemia. *West J Med* 134:15–26, 1981.

Lentz RD, Brown DM, Kjellstrand CM: Treatment of severe hypophosphatemia. *Ann Intern Med* 89:941–944, 1978.

Martin HE, Smith K, Wilson ML: The fluid and electrolyte therapy of severe diabetic acidosis and ketosis. *Am J Med* 24:376–389, 1958.

O'Connor LR, Klein KL, Bethune JE, et al: Effects of hypophosphatemia on myocardial performance in man. *N Engl J Med* 297:901, 1977.

Sestocft L: Regulatory processes in rat liver induced by sudden changes in fructose concentration, in Lundquist F, Tygstrup N (eds): *Regulation of Hepatic Metabolism*. Copenhagen, Munksgaard, 1974, pp 285–301.

Wilson HK, Keuer SP, Lea AS, Boyd AE III, Eknoyan G: Phosphate therapy in diabetic ketoacidosis. *Arch Intern Med*: 517–520, 1982.

Zipf WB, Bacon GE, Spencer ML, Kelch RP, Hopwood NJ, Hawker CD: Hypocalcemia, hypomagnesemia, and transient hypoparathyroidism during therapy with potassium phosphate in diabetic ketoacidosis. *Diabetes Care* 2:265–268, 1979.

6

Acid–Base Disturbances
Metabolic and Respiratory Acidoses

ROBERT G. NARINS and EDWARD R. JONES

I. INTRODUCTORY TERMS AND CONCEPTS

Wide-ranging and potentially devastating biochemical and physiological effects are attributable to common acid–base abnormalities. It is imperative, therefore, that all physicians gain a comfortable understanding of the pathophysiology, diagnosis, and therapy of these often reversible disorders. It is our purpose to emphasize diagnosis and therapy, basing discussions on key pathophysiological principles established in the introductory paragraphs.

Maintenance of normal acid–base balance results from controlled integration of acid production, buffering, and excretion. Partial oxidation of fat, carbohydrate, and protein causes synthesis of 1.0–1.5 mmol/kg per day of fixed metabolic acids in the form of phosphoric, sulfuric, and various organic acids. Complete oxidation of these foodstuffs yields 15,000–20,000 mmol daily of carbon dioxide, the hydration of which produces the volatile carbonic acid.

A. Acidity

The acidity of body fluid is a function of the availability of hydrogen ions (H^+) which are present in two forms. The *free protons* exist as trace elements in cellular and extracellular fluid (ECF), their nanomolar quantity

ROBERT G. NARINS and EDWARD R. JONES • Departments of Medicine and Physiology, Temple University Health Sciences Center, Philadelphia, Pennsylvania 19140.

being directly measured by glass electrodes; pH is the negative logarithm of the H^+ concentration, defining an inverse relationship between the two terms. Thus, an increasing or decreasing pH corresponds, respectively, to decreasing or increasing concentrations of protons (Fig. 1). The overall curvilinear relationship manifests a linear segment over the biologically significant pH range of 7.10–7.50. The slope of this line indicates that a change of 0.1 pH unit corresponds to a 10 nM change in H^+ concentration. Since the proton concentration at normal pH (7.40) is 40 nM, it becomes a simple matter to interconvert pH and H^+ concentration.

Blood and tissue buffers are admixtures of weak acids (e.g., HX) and their free anions (e.g., X^-). Weak acids hold protons tightly, and when H^+ is absorbed by the anions (X^-), the weak acid (HX) is reformed. The ionization potential of an acid is a measure of the ease with which it gives up protons. The weaker the acid, the more tightly it holds H^+; or in other terms, the weaker the acid, the more readily its anion binds H^+. During periods of acid stress, anions such as bicarbonate, phosphate, or proteins absorb accumulating protons, thereby lessening the impact of the acidifying process. Conversely, during alkaline conditions, when free H^+ concentration is reduced, weak acids donate protons, once again acting to return acidity towards normal. Thus, these buffers may remove or add protons to body fluids, depending on the individual buffer's acid avidity and the prevailing free H^+ concentration. Protons are far more abundant in the *bound* form.

B. Acidosis, Alkalosis, Acidemia, Alkalemia

Pathological *processes*, whether metabolic or respiratory, that increase or decrease the availability of protons are termed *acidoses* and *alkaloses*. When blood acidity actually increases or decreases beyond the normal range

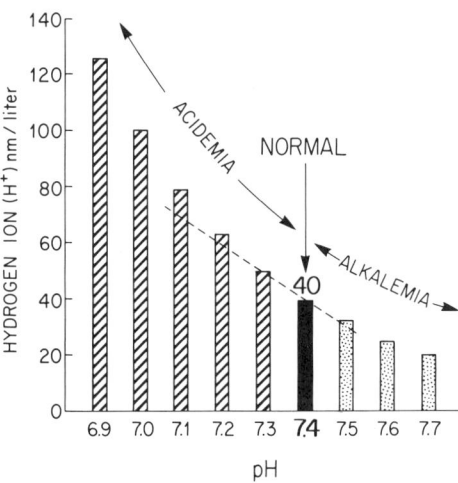

Figure 1. Relationship of pH to hydrogen ion concentration. Broken line is drawn to emphasize the (approximately) linear relationship between hydrogen ion concentration and pH over the pH range of 7.1–7.5. From Narins RG, Emmett M: Simple and mixed acid–base disorders: A practical approach. *Medicine* 59:161, 1980.

(i.e., pH < 7.36, [H$^+$] > 44 nM, or pH > 7.44, [H$^+$] < 36 nM), the patient is said to be *acidemic* or *alkalemic*. Thus, the suffix -*osis* describes the ongoing process acting to generate protons or alkali, whereas the actual quantitative description of blood acidity is defined by terms containing the suffix -*emia*.

C. Bicarbonate Space

The bodily space of distribution available to acid and alkali is a matter of some confusion to most physicians. First, it should be appreciated that the *bicarbonate space* is only an apparent space, artificially constructed to facilitate therapy with acid and alkali. Secondly, the apparent dimensions of this space expand as the acidosis worsens. Brief explanations of these statements follow.

Initially, as the body pool of acid expands, blood pH changes relatively little, since protons are largely absorbed by body buffers. Because the lungs and kidneys actively stabilize H_2CO_3 and HCO_3^- concentrations, respectively, this buffer pair more effectively competes with other buffers for the common pool of incoming protons. As the $HCO_3^- - H_2CO_3$ system becomes overwhelmed, and the H$^+$ concentration progressively increases, nonbicarbonate buffers absorb greater amounts of acid.

Expansion of body alkali stores during any of the metabolic alkaloses increases the concentration of bicarbonate and other buffer anions. In other terms, infused alkali, like infused acid, titrates all body buffers.

It follows that the quantity of accumulating acid or alkali must be proportional to observed changes in serum bicarbonate concentration. Since buffers other than bicarbonate are also titrated, the precise quantitation of added acid or base could be obtained in one of two ways. The product of the change in bicarbonate concentration (in mmol/liter) and its exact space of distribution (in liters) defines the amount of acid or alkali buffered by bicarbonate. If bicarbonate's fractional contribution to the total buffering process were known, then the total acid or alkali amassed could be easily computed. For example, if the serum bicarbonate concentration decreased by 10 mM and bicarbonate's space of distribution were restricted to the ECF, (20% of body weight), a 70-kg man would buffer 140 mmol of acid (10 mM × 14 liters). If, however, it were known that bicarbonate contributed only 50% of the total buffering, then the total acid load would have been 280 mmol, i.e., 140 mmol buffered by bicarbonate and an additional 140 mmol buffered by other cellular and extracellular buffers.

The same answer could be achieved by ignoring the presence of other buffers but attributing to bicarbonate an "apparent" space of distribution twice that of the ECF. Thus, the product of the change in serum bicarbonate concentration (e.g., 10 mM) and its apparent space of distribution (40% of body weight) yields the same 280 mmol acid load in this 70-kg man. This latter approach has been developed from experimental data showing that infusion of 280 mmol of HCl into a 70-kg man resulted in a 10 mM fall in serum bicarbonate concentration. The erroneous but clinically useful assumption was made that only bicarbonate buffered the incoming HCl. The contribution of other buffers was ignored. Thus, if 280 mmol of acid decreased the serum bicarbonate by 10 mM, then the acid and the bicarbonate appeared to distribute in 28 liters or 40% of body weight.

Since the contribution of nonbicarbonate buffers is difficult to measure, this latter method has gained general acceptance. It should be obvious, however, that as acidemia worsens and more nonbicarbonate buffering takes place, bicarbonate's apparent space of distribution progressively expands. Indeed, as the serum bicarbonate concentration decreases below 10 mM, its apparent space may exceed that of body water and approach total body weight.

D. The Acid–Base Equation

Since all buffers communicate with each other and with a common pool of free H^+, knowledge of the buffer's strength (i.e., its pK) and assay of its state of titration define the state of acidity. Since the bicarbonate–carbonic acid system is readily accessible and easily measured, it is used most effectively to define acid–base balance. This relationship between the buffer's three acid–base components is delineated by equation 1.

$$[H^+] = 24 \; P_{CO_2}/[HCO_3^-] \tag{1}$$

This equation, derived from the Henderson–Hasselbalch equation, indicates that blood acidity is a function of the ratio of P_{CO_2} to bicarbonate concentration. Knowledge of any two of these key acid–base parameters allows calculation of the third.

Acidemia develops whenever the $P_{CO_2}/[HCO_3^-]$ ratio increases. Respiratory acidosis primarily increases the numerator, whereas metabolic acidosis increases the ratio by primarily decreasing the denominator. Alkalemia is created by the opposite respiratory and metabolic effects.

E. Compensation, the Anion Gap, and Simple and Mixed Disorders

Conceptualization of *simple and mixed* acid–base disorders is best achieved by briefly defining the pathophysiological and diagnostic roles of *compensation* and the *anion gap* in the analysis of acid–base perturbations. Simple metabolic acidoses and alkaloses are characterized by consumption or accrual of bicarbonate, and the unopposed primary hypobicarbonatemia or hyperbicarbonatemia respectively acidify or alkalinize body fluids (eq. 1). Alterations in the acidity of brainstem centers controlling alveolar ventilation result in secondary changes in P_{CO_2} (i.e., carbonic acid) which lessen the impact of the primary change in bicarbonate concentration on blood acidity.

Thus, the hypobicarbonatemia of metabolic acidosis evokes the carbonic acid-lowering—i.e., alkalinizing—effect of increased ventilation. The hyperbicarbonatemia of metabolic alkalosis depresses respiration, and the resulting increase in P_{CO_2} ameliorates the alkalemia. In other terms, these compensating or secondary changes lessen the impact of primary alterations in the $P_{CO_2}/[HCO_3^-]$ ratio (eq. 1).

Simple respiratory acidosis and alkalosis are characterized by primary changes in P_{CO_2} which stimulate body buffers and the kidney to secondarily increase or decrease bicarbonate availability. The secondary hyperbicarbonatemia elicited by primary respiratory acidosis and the secondary hypobicarbonatemia elicited by primary respiratory alkalosis mitigate pH changes (eq. 1).

The four primary metabolic and respiratory derangements constitute the simple acid–base disorders. A mixed condition exists when two or three primary disorders coexist in a given patient. Recognition of mixed respiratory–metabolic disorders comes about through knowledge of a few simple facts (Table I).

Metabolic and respiratory compensation for primary acid–base disorders do not normalize pH. Rather, the compensating force simply lessens the degree of pH abnormality. A normal pH in the presence of at least one clinically obvious disorder indicates that at least one other offsetting disorder must be present.

Since the pathophysiological demands of normal compensation require that serum bicarbonate concentration increase in respiratory acidosis and decrease in respiratory alkalosis, failure of serum bicarbonate to move in the appropriate direction signals the presence of a mixed disorder. Not only are the directions of the P_{CO_2} and bicarbonate changes predictable, but it is also true that a given degree of primary respiratory or metabolic acidosis or alkalosis elicits a predictable degree of compensatory change in P_{CO_2} or serum bicarbonate concentration. The anticipated compensation for the four simple disorders is outlined in Table II. Failure to obtain appropriate respiratory compensation for primary metabolic disorders or to achieve appropriate metabolic changes for primary respiratory disorders also defines the presence of a mixed acid–base disorder (see below).

Table I. Guidelines for the Diagnosis of Mixed Acid–Base Disorders

1. Compensation for primary acid–base disorders returns blood pH toward but not to normal. Thus, a normal pH with abnormal HCO_3 and P_{CO_2} defines a mixed respiratory–metabolic disorder.

2. Combination of frank hypercapnia with hypobicarbonatemia or frank hypocapnia with hyperbicarbonatemia defines a mixed respiratory–metabolic disorder.

3. Since the degree of compensation is predictable (Table II), lack of appropriate respiratory or metabolic compensation identifies a mixed disorder.

4. When the increment in the anion gap (mM) exceeds the decrease in serum bicarbonate concentration, a mixed metabolic acidosis–alkalosis is present (see text for details).

Table II. Classification and Characteristics of Simple Acid–Base Disorders[a]

	Primary change	Compensatory response	Predicted compensation
Metabolic			
Acidosis	↓ ↓ ↓ HCO_3^-	↓ ↓ P_{CO_2}	P_{CO_2} = 1.5 [HCO_3^-] + 8 ± 2
			P_{CO_2} falls by 1–1.3 mm Hg for each mEq/liter fall in HCO_3^-
			Last two digits of pH = P_{CO_2} (thus, if P_{CO_2} = 28, pH = 7.28)
			HCO_3^- + 15 = last two digits of pH (HCO_3^- = 15, pH = 7.30)
Alkalosis	↑ ↑ ↑ HCO_3^-	↑ ↑ P_{CO_2}	P_{CO_2} increases 6 mm Hg for each 10 mEq/liter rise in HCO_3^-
			HCO_3^- + 15 = last two digits of pH (HCO_3^- = 35, pH = 7.50)
Respiratory			
Acidosis			
Acute	↑ ↑ ↑ P_{CO_2}	↑ HCO_3^-	HCO_3^- increases by 1 mEq/liter for each 10 mm Hg rise in P_{CO_2}
Chronic	↑ ↑ ↑ P_{CO_2}	↑ ↑ HCO_3^-	HCO_3^- increases by 3.5 mEq/liter for each 10 mm Hg rise in P_{CO_2}
Alkalosis			
Acute	↓ ↓ ↓ P_{CO_2}	↓ HCO_3^-	HCO_3^- falls by 2 mEq/liter for each 10 mm Hg fall in P_{CO_2}
Chronic	↓ ↓ ↓ P_{CO_2}	↓ ↓ HCO_3^-	HCO_3^- falls by 5 mEq/liter for each 10 mm Hg fall in P_{CO_2}

[a] From Narins RG, Gardner LB: Med Clin North Am 65:321, 1981.

The *anion gap* (AG) is the difference (in mM) between the serum sodium concentration and the sum of the concentrations of chloride and bicarbonate.

$$\text{Anion gap (AG)} = [Na^+] - ([Cl^-] + [HCO_3^-]) \qquad (2)$$

Under normal conditions the AG is 12 ± 2 mM and reflects the presence of routinely unmeasured anions (albumin, sulfate, organic anions) that normally neutralize sodium's positive charge. Normally 130 mM of sodium's 142 mM of positive charge is offset by chloride and bicarbonate (105 and 25 mM, respectively). The remaining 12 mM, i.e., the anion gap, accounts for the aforementioned unmeasured anions (eq. 2). Hydrochloric acidosis, associated with diarrhea and renal tubular disorders, effectively replaces serum bicarbonate with chloride without altering serum sodium concentration. The entering proton destroys bicarbonate, converting it to H_2CO_3 which rapidly dehydrates and is eliminated as CO_2. Accumulating chloride offsets sodium's cationic charge, and since the sodium concentration and the sum of chloride and bicarbonate do not change, these disorders do not alter the AG.

All other metabolic acidoses increase the AG by replacing bicarbonate with anions other than chloride. Thus, in lactic acidosis, serum chloride concentration remains unchanged while that of bicarbonate decreases,

Table III. Mixed Metabolic Acidosis and Alkalosis

Electrolyte	Normal	Lactic acidosis	Addition of metabolic alkalosis
Na^+	140	140	140
Cl^-	105	105	95
HCO_3^-	25	10	20
Anion gap	10	25	25

thereby resulting in an increased AG. In the pure acidosis, each 1 mM increment in the AG reflects a similar increment in serum lactate concentration. Thus, each mM increase in the AG decreases the serum bicarbonate concentration by 1 mM. Close stoichiometry between the increase in the AG and the decrease in serum bicarbonate concentration is to be anticipated. Disruption of this stoichiometry indicates the presence of a mixed metabolic acidosis–alkalosis.

If a patient with simple lactic acidosis begins to vomit, a metabolic alkalosis becomes superimposed on his preexisting acidosis. His electrolytes reflect this common mixed acid–base abnormality (Table III). The HCl lost in vomitus causes hypochloremia, whereas serum bicarbonate concentration increases, and the serum lactate concentration and AG both remain elevated and unchanged. In the new steady state, the increment in the AG exceeds the decrement in bicarbonate concentration, thereby identifying the superimposed metabolic alkalosis. If a bicarbonate-generating process were not at play (i.e., an alkalosis), the accumulated acid (reflected by the increased AG) would have lowered the serum bicarbonate concentration even further.

Application of these introductory terms and concepts now enables physicians to diagnose even the most complicated acid–base abnormalities. Further amplification follows on the ensuing pages.

II. THE ACIDOSES

Acidification of body fluids is caused by retention of fixed acids with attendant bicarbonate consumption or by retention of the volatile carbonic acid. These disorders appear in pure, simple form or in combinations as mixed respiratory–metabolic disorders (see below).

A. Effects of Metabolic and Respiratory Acidoses

1. Epinephrine Release

The acidoses evoke adrenal medullary release of epinephrine but simulteneously effect selective blockade of its cardiovascular effects (see below).

2. Vascular

Metabolic and respiratory acidoses block the increased peripheral arteriolar resistance induced by catecholamines. "Warm shock" evolves from the ensuing vasodilation, hypotension, and well-perfused extremities. Venoconstriction caused by acid-stimulated epinephrine release persists, thereby reducing venous capacitance and forcing return of more blood to heart and lungs.

3. Cardiac

The direct inhibition of myocardial contraction by low pH is offset by the positive inotropic effect of released epinephrine. Over the pH range of 7.40–7.20, these two countervailing forces approximately neutralize each other, and myocardial function remains largely unchanged. With more profound degrees of acidemia (pH < 7.20), the epinephrine effects are blocked, thereby unmasking negative inotropic effects of acidosis. Concurrence of inhibited myocardial contraction and increased venous return often results in pulmonary edema.

4. Potassium

Organic metabolic acidoses (lactic, ketoacidosis, etc.) do not cause hyperkalemia unless complicated by dehydration, marked deficiency of insulin, or renal failure. Certain of the hyperchloremic acidoses are associated with potassium loss (e.g., diarrhea, renal tubular acidosis; see below), whereas hyperkalemic, hyperchloremic forms are usually associated with disordered adrenal–renal function, causing renal potassium retention. Respiratory acidosis, unless associated with acute or severe hypoxia, is uncommonly associated with hyperkalemia. It follows that although hyperkalemia often complicates the acidoses, its presence is certainly not a simple function of blood pH.

5. Neurological

Only acute and chronic respiratory acidosis regularly cause significant neurological changes. The key pathophysiological event seems to be the cerebral vasodilatation and striking increase in cerebral blood flow caused by hypercapnia. Stupor, confusion, coma, and papilledema may result.

6. Hyperglycemia

Cellular acidification caused by respiratory and metabolic acidoses mildly impairs glycolysis, causing a tendency to mild hyperglycemia.

7. Hyperuricemia

Organic anions (lactate, ketone acids) vie with uric acid for active transport from blood to the renal tubular lumen and ultimately for excretion into the final urine. Organic acidoses competitively exclude uric acid from excretion, thereby effecting hyperuricemia.

8. Calcium Metabolism

Metabolic but not respiratory acidosis enhances calcium resorption from bone. Both forms of acidosis reduce calcium binding to blood proteins, thereby tending to increase glomerular filtration of calcium. Tubular reabsorption of calcium is impaired by metabolic but not respiratory acidosis. For these reasons, hypercalciuria and osteopenia complicate chronic metabolic but not respiratory acidosis.

9. Tissue Oxygenation

Acidoses asynchronously effect two countervailing metabolic events, the algebraic sum of which tends to enhance tissue oxygenation acutely but causes little change chronically. Acute acidification directly reduces hemoglobin's affinity for oxygen, thereby tending to enhance tissue oxygenation (Bohr effect). Within 4–8 hr of induction, acidosis impairs red blood cell (RBC) glycolysis and reduces the cellular concentration of 2,3-diphosphoglyceric acid (2,3-DPG). Oxygen binding by hemoglobin is affected by 2,3-DPG in the same way that it is by acid. Thus, in chronic acidosis, the direct effect of acid on hemoglobin persists but is equally offset by the reduction in RBC 2,3-DPG. Thus, the salubrious effect of acute acidosis on tissue oxygen delivery is lost in the chronic phase.

B. Metabolic Acidosis

1. Pathogenesis

Accumulation of metabolic acids and consumption of alkali stores, the hallmarks of metabolic acidosis (Table IV; Fig. 2), are generated by any combination of three processes.

a. Acid Overproduction

Net overproduction of acid may develop from primary disorders of intermediary metabolism (e.g., lactic acidosis and ketoacidosis) or from exposure to toxic precursors of acid such as the formic acidosis of methanol intoxication or glycolic acidosis caused by ethylene glycol. Certain toxins, e.g.,

Table IV. The Metabolic Acidoses

Pathophysiology	Anion gap	Accumulating acid	Osmolar gap
Acid overproduction			
Ketoacidosis	Increased	Acetoacetic and	Normal
Diabetic		β-hydroxybutyric	
Alcoholic		acids	
Glycogenoses			
Starvation			
Lactic acidosis	Increased	Lactic acid	Normal
Hypoxia-associated			
(type A)			
Hypoxia not clinically			
apparent (type B)			
Toxin-induced	Increased		
Methanol		Formic	>15 mOsm
Ethylene glycol		Glycolic	>15 mOsm
Salicylates		Various organic acids	Normal
Paraldehyde		Unknown	Unknown
Bicarbonate wasting			
Gastrointestinal losses	Normal	Hydrochloric	
Diarrhea			
Biliary/pancreatic fistula			
Renal tubular acidosis	Normal	Hydrochloric	
Proximal type			
Acid underexcretion			
Uremia	Increased	$H_2PO_4^-$, H_2SO_4, organic	Normal
Renal tubular acidosis	Normal	Hydrochloric	
Distal type			
Hypoaldosteronism			
Buffer deficiency			
Low NH_3 excretion			
Low phosphate excretion			

biguanides or salicylates, disrupt intermediary metabolism, causing the host to overproduce endogenous acids.

b. Underexcretion of Acid

Zero metabolic acid–base balance is maintained by the kidneys' ability to excrete an amount of acid equal to production. This process effects renal synthesis and return to the body of an amount of alkali equal to that consumed by normal acid production. Failure of these vital functions during renal failure causes retention of a variable fraction of the 50–100 mmol of acid produced daily. Since acid retention is tantamount to alkali consumption, hypobicarbonatemia ensues.

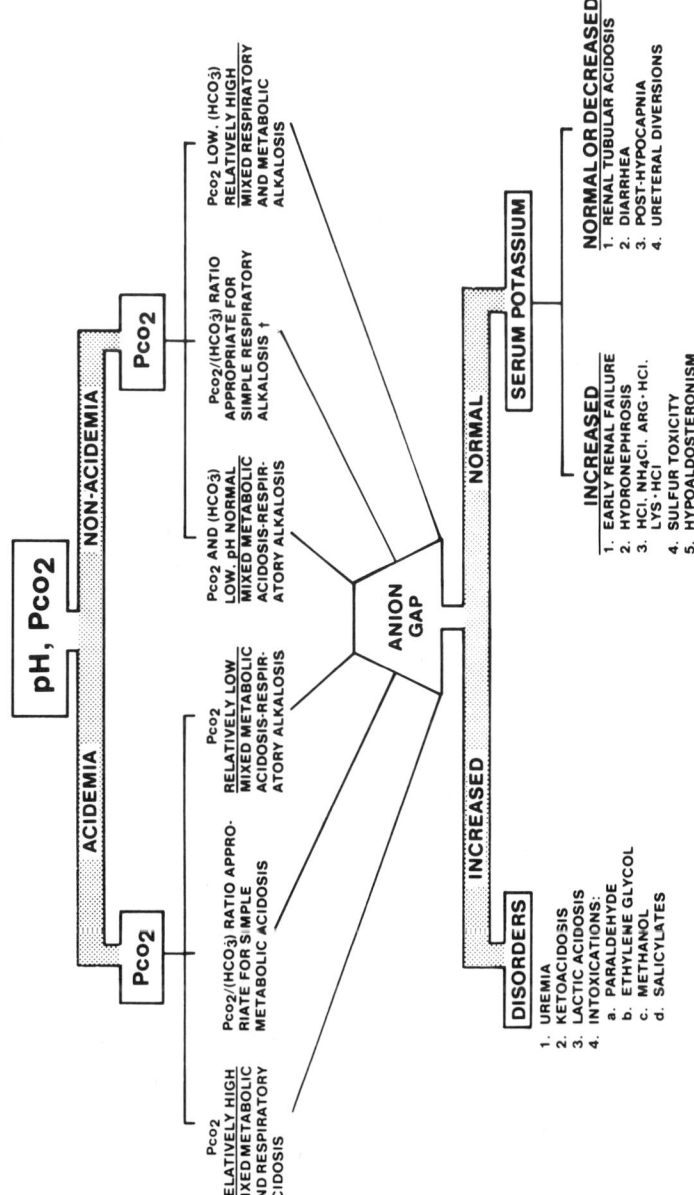

Figure 2. Diagnostic approach to hypobicarbonatemia. $^*P_{CO_2} = 1.5(HCO_3^-) + 8 \pm 2$ (see Table II). $^\dagger HCO_3^-$ decreases 2.5 mM for each 10 mm Hg decrease of P_{CO_2} in acute respiratory alkalosis and 5.0 mM in chronic respiratory alkalosis (see Table II).

c. Bicarbonate Loss

Diarrhea and certain renal tubular diseases—including early chronic renal failure—lead to loss of $NaHCO_3$ which is replenished by NaCl. The net result is replacement of body alkali with chloride.

2. Pathophysiology

a. Respiratory Compensation

Brainstem centers controlling alveolar ventilation respond to acidification by producing hypocapnia. Indeed, the degree of hypocapnia elicited in stable, steady-state metabolic acidosis is directly proportional to the degree of hypobicarbonatemia. In addition to predicting the P_{CO_2} for a given bicarbonate deficit, formulas can predict the last two digits of the pH (Table II).

Should a hypobicarbonatemic subject's P_{CO_2} and pH be substantially removed from these predicted values, a coexisting respiratory acid–base disorder may be diagnosed. In the previous example (serum HCO_3^- of 10 mM), if the subject's P_{CO_2} exceeded 25 mm Hg and pH fell below 7.20, a mixed metabolic and respiratory acidosis would be present; i.e., the P_{CO_2} would be too high for this degree of hypobicarbonatemia. With such metabolic parameters, the physician must seek out causes for respiratory acidosis (see below) as well as causes for metabolic acidosis. Conversely, if this subject's P_{CO_2} were less than 21 mm Hg and pH greater than 7.32, a superimposed respiratory alkalosis would be present; i.e., the P_{CO_2} would be too low and pH too high for the degree of hypobicarbonatemia. Causes for hyperventilation above and beyond appropriate compensation for metabolic acidosis must be sought out.

b. The Anion Gap

The proton from accumulating metabolic acid titrates alkaline stores and, in the process, removes bicarbonate from the ECF. The acid anion replaces bicarbonate which, depending on the anion, either leaves the AG unchanged—as in HCl acidoses (see above)—or increases it—as with all other metabolic acidoses. It is clinically useful to classify all metabolic acidoses in terms of whether they increase the AG or allow it to remain unchanged (Fig. 2).

3. Differential Diagnosis

a. Elevated Anion-Gap Acidoses

i. Renal Failure. Most generalized renal diseases cause progressive and proportional loss of glomerular and tubular functions. When serum creatinine reaches 4.0 mg/dl and BUN reaches 40 mg/dl, some degree of elevated-AG acidosis is usually present. Glomerular failure causes retention of acid anions (PO_4^{3-}, SO_4^{2-}, organic anions), whereas tubular failure prevents re-synthesis of HCO_3^- lost in titration of retained acids. Loss of bicarbonate with the above usually unmeasured anions causes the AG to increase by 1 mM for each 1 mM decrement in serum bicarbonate. Early renal failure, especially with interstitial nephritis, often causes a normal AG acidosis to develop (see below). Serum bicarbonate usually remains at 15 mM or greater, and the AG rarely increases above 20–25 mM.

ii. *Ketoacidosis.* Starvation rarely causes clinically significant ketosis.

False positive qualitative tests for ketones occur in patients ingesting alcohol while taking disulfiram (Antabuse®) and in patients intoxicated with paraldehyde. The new antihypertensive drug captopril also yields false positive ketone tests. Isopropyl (rubbing) alcohol is metabolized to true acetone which gives a positive ketone test without causing an acidosis.

Alcoholism and diabetes mellitus remain the major ketoacidoses causing significant hypobicarbonatemia. Alcoholic ketosis characteristically occurs in the vomiting alcoholic who no longer has measurable ethanol in his blood. These patients, like certain diabetics, often manifest a ketotest (nitroprusside)-negative ketoacidosis. Metabolism of alcohol, like hypoxia, alters the tissue redox potential, effecting a shift in ketone acids from the oxidized, nitroprusside-positive acetoacetate to the reduced, nitroprusside-negative β-hydroxybutyric acid (β-HB).

Regardless of whether the reduced β-HB or oxidized acetoacetate is present, the AG increases by 1 mM, and the serum bicarbonate decreases by 1 mM, for each 1 mM increment in blood ketone concentration.

Acetoacetic acid enhances the intensity of color developed in the creatinine assay, thereby spuriously increasing its serum level. Thus, serum creatinine cannot be truly defined until serum acetoacetate is normalized.

iii. *Lactic Acidosis.* Peripheral conversion of neutral carbohydrates and proteins to lactic acid results in daily production of 1000–2000 mmol of protons and the like consumption of alkali. Hepatic resynthesis of lost bicarbonate from lactate prevents net consumption of alkali despite lactic acid's heavy traffic from muscle to blood to liver. Imbalance between peripheral production and hepatic consumption results in net destruction of bicarbonate and the emergence of clinical lactic acidosis. Tissue hypoxia, whether clinically apparent (type A) or inapparent (type B), stimulates peripheral lactic acid production and simultaneously impairs its hepatic consumption (Fig. 3).

Type A lactic acidosis complicates severe congestive heart failure, states of severe shock, anemia, or hypoxemia and, as such, rarely presents a diagnostic dilemma. Most metabolic acidoses evolve over days to weeks, whereas type A lactic acidosis erupts within minutes of the onset of hypoxemia or hypotension.

With an increased awareness of the disorders listed in Table V, one can also easily recognize Type B lactic acidoses. Indeed, since those causes of

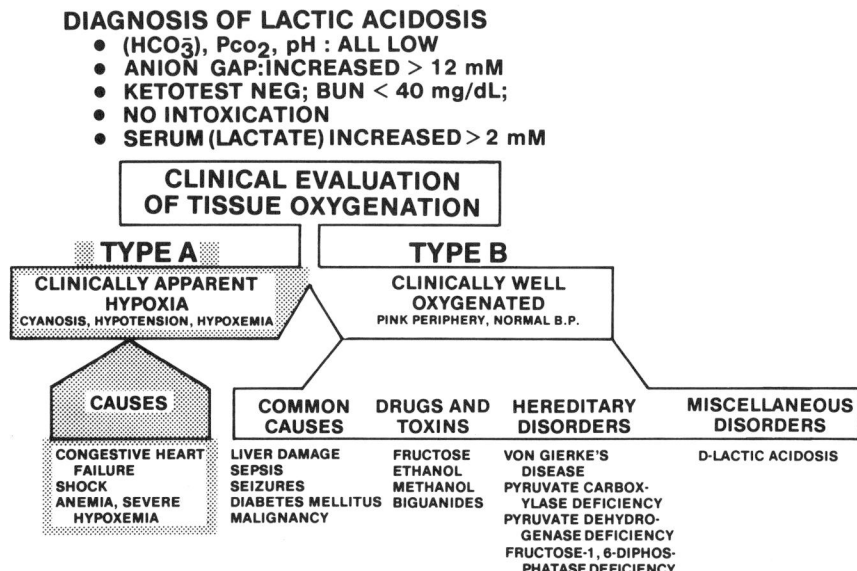

DIAGNOSIS OF LACTIC ACIDOSIS
- (HCO_3^-), Pco_2, pH : ALL LOW
- ANION GAP:INCREASED > 12 mM
- KETOTEST NEG; BUN < 40 mg/dL;
- NO INTOXICATION
- SERUM (LACTATE) INCREASED > 2 mM

Figure 3. Diagnosis of lactic acidosis.

lactic acidosis have been identified, the spontaneous, idiopathic variant has been rarely recognized and has virtually disappeared.

Clinical differentiation of lactic acidosis from ketoacidosis with β-HB as the dominant ketone is difficult. Both disorders present with an increased-AG, appropriately compensated metabolic acidosis with negative serum and urine ketone tests. Two clinically useful differentiating tests may be used. First, lactic acidosis but not β-HB acidosis commonly causes hyperphosphatemia. Indeed, a serum phosphate-to-creatinine ratio greater than 3.2 is strongly supportive of lactic acidosis. Secondly, the addition of a few drops of the oxidizing agent 30% hydrogen peroxide to urine will nonenzymatically convert the nitroprusside (ketotest)-negative β-HB to the reactive acetone. Thus, conversion to positive of an initially negative urinary ketotest

Table V. Mixed Hyperchloremic and High-Anion-Gap Metabolic Acidosis

Serum parameters	Normal (mM)	Diarrhea (mM)	Diarrhea and lactic acidosis (mM)
Sodium	140	140	140
Chloride	105	115	115
Bicarbonate	25	15	5
Anion gap	10	10	20
Change in bicarbonate	0	−10	−20
Change in anion gap	0	0	+10
Lactate	1	1	11

by H_2O_2 suggests the presence of a β-HB acidosis. Ultimately, the diagnosis depends on demonstration hyperlacticemia.

iv. Intoxications. Illicit alcohol ("smoke," "white whiskey," "alley juice") frequently contains cheap, narcotizing wood alcohol or *methanol.* Windshield wiper fluid and Sterno® are other sources of methanol readily available to the less discerning alcoholic. Toxicity of this alcohol derives from its slow conversion to formaldehyde and formic acid by the enzyme alcohol dehydrogenase. These toxic metabolites create the high-AG acidosis and accumulate in the central nervous system, causing characteristic retinal edema, papillitis, and coma.

Desperate alcoholics lustful for self-abuse occasionally ingest antifreeze, the active component of which is *ethylene glycol*. Metabolism of this toxin yields, among other metabolites, glycolic and oxalic acids. The former accounts for the high-AG acidosis, whereas the latter precipitates as calcium oxalate in a variety of tissues, including the kidney. Indeed, the presence of large numbers of calcium oxalate crystals in the urinary sediment in a stuporous alcoholic with a high-AG acidosis strongly favors the diagnosis of ethylene glycol toxicity.

The past 15 years have not produced a single report of *paraldehyde-* induced acidosis. The original seven cases were most likely examples of alcoholic ketosis in subjects taking paraldehyde.

The *osmolar gap* plays a central role in defining diagnosis and directing therapy in nonazotemic alcoholics with high-AG metabolic acidoses. Osmolality is the number of solute particles dissolved in each liter of plasma water. Under normal circumstances, urea, glucose, and sodium with its attendant anions constitute virtually all dissolved plasma solute. Total plasma osmolality may be calculated by converting the concentration of solute in mass units (mg/dl) to osmotic units (mOsm) by dividing the BUN by 2.8 and blood glucose by 18.

$$\text{Calculated osmolality } (Osm_c) = BUN \text{ (mg/dl)}/2.8$$
$$+ \text{ Blood sugar (mg/dl)}/18 + 2 \text{ }[Na^+] \quad (3)$$

The Osm_c and simultaneously measured serum osmolality (Osm_m) should agree within 10 mOsm. If, however, the Osm_m exceeds the Osm_c by more than 10 mOsm, some circulating particle not accounted for by urea, glucose, or sodium and its anions is causing a further increase in plasma osmolality. These added osmols may be accounted for by such low-molecular-weight substances as ethanol, isopropyl alcohol, ethylene glycol, or methanol.

Figure 4 incorporates data and concepts discussed in the text to illustrate a rational diagnostic approach to alcoholics with increasing AGs.

Aspirin toxicity manifests four pathophysiological effects that may variously alter acid–base balance. Aspirin stimulates alveolar ventilation through its action on brainstem centers; it may cause gastritis and vomiting;

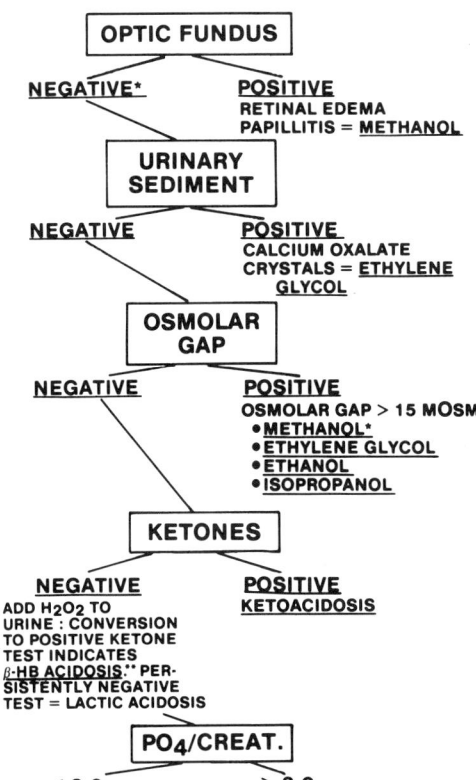

Figure 4. Approach to the non-azotemic alcoholic with high anion gap acidosis. *Methanol: chronic abusers may not show optic changes. **β-HB: β-hydroxy-butyric acid.

it redirects intermediary metabolism, causing overproduction of various organic acids; and, since acetylsalicylic acid's molecular weight is 180, every 18 mg/dl increment in its blood level reflects the addition of 1 mM of acid to the body. It follows that a variety of acid–base abnormalities commonly complicate aspirin toxicity. Toxic blood levels often range from 40–80 mg/dl, and a high-AG acidosis is frequently complicated by an offsetting respiratory alkalosis. In this mixed disorder, Pco_2 is lower than simple compensation for hypobicarbonatemia would demand; the resulting pH is therefore closer to normal and indeed may be frankly alkalemic. A blood salicylate level should be obtained in all patients with unexplained high-AG acidoses, especially in those with a mixed metabolic acidosis–respiratory alkalosis. Children are more prone to pure metabolic acidosis.

b. The Normal-Anion-Gap Acidoses

Replacement of serum bicarbonate with chloride occurs in a variety of disease states that are best characterized by attendant changes in serum potassium concentration. Since serum sodium concentration remains unchanged, and since the sum of the chloride and bicarbonate concentrations remains constant, the AG also remains unchanged and normal.

It should be understood that many clinical situations exist in which an elevated-AG acidosis becomes superimposed on a hyperchloremic acidosis. When, for example, dehydration, sepsis, and hypotension cause a lactic acidosis to erupt in a patient with diarrheal hyperchloremic acidosis, the serum electrolytes assume a characteristic pattern (Table V). With addition of lactic acid to blood, serum bicarbonate is further reduced, but lactate, not chloride, serves as its replacement, thereby increasing the AG. The serum electrolytes in the fully developed mixed disorder (column C, Table V) demonstrate a decrease in bicarbonate concentration of 15 mM that is only partially explained by the 5 mM increment in the AG (i.e., the chemical sign of accumulated but unmeasured lactate). Thus, when the decrement in serum bicarbonate concentration exceeds the increment in the AG, a mixed hyperchloremic–high-AG acidosis is present.

i. *Hyperkalemic Variants.* Potassium excess impairs renal ammonia buffer synthesis, thereby impairing proton excretion. These hyperkalemic, hyperchloremic acidoses are frequently associated with diminished adrenal secretion of aldosterone and reduced renal responsivity to the hormone. Mineralocorticoids not only increase renal sodium reabsorption and potassium secretion but also increase distal tubular H^+ secretion. Thus, these syndromes are characterized by diminished renal buffer synthesis and impaired acid secretion.

Diabetic nephropathy and various interstitial nephritides, including lead nephropathy and hydronephrosis, cause hyporeninemic hypoaldosteronism. Various infections (TBC, fungi, etc.), tumors, and infiltrative disorders (amyloidosis, hemochromatosis) destroy the adrenal glands, causing adrenal insufficiency. Finally, sickle cell anemia, lupus nephropathy, renal transplantation, and certain rare hereditable and acquired disorders are characterized by failure to respond to normally elaborated aldosterone.

Demonstration of impaired secretion of renin and aldosterone in response to hypovolemic stimulation is central to evaluating these patients. Plasma renin and aldosterone are assayed before and after a 1-day furosemide diuresis (40 mg tid) coupled with a low-sodium diet (10 mmol daily). Plasma renin, drawn after 4 hr of upright posture on the morning following dehydration, fails to increase normally. Before results of these analyses are known, we begin patients on 0.2 mg per day of the potent mineralocorticoid, 9α-fluorohydrocortisone. If this high dose stimulates kaliuresis and sustains normokalemia, we seek the lowest effective dose. If 0.2 mg per day is ineffective, however, we increase the dose to 1.0 mg daily. If the higher dose does not enhance potassium clearance after several days, we assume that tubular hormone resistance is the dominant cause of hyperkalemia, and therapy, therefore, must utilize potassium-binding resins and not mineralocorticoids. Because high-dose mineralocorticoid therapy often causes sodium retention regardless of its effect on potassium excretion, potent diuretics are often required. The mixed serum electrolyte pattern that evolves when uremic high-AG acidosis is superimposed on the hyperchloremic acidosis has been described.

ii. Hypokalemic Variants. Gastrointestinal or renal loss of potassium accompanies replacement of body bicarbonate with chloride in these syndromes.

Diarrhea. Stool loss of bicarbonate equivalents with potassium is the most common cause of hypokalemic, hyperchloremic metabolic acidosis. Liquid stool may contain as much as 30–120 mM of potassium.

Renal tubular acidoses (RTA). Sodium, bicarbonate, and potassium wasting characterize proximal RTA (type 2), whereas failure of urinary acidification and potassium wasting characterize distal RTA (classical, type 1). Alkali therapy reverses the kaliuresis of the distal form but worsens that complicating proximal RTA. Patients with proximal RTA reestablish acid balance, albeit at a reduced serum bicarbonate concentration, whereas patients with the distal form remain in positive H^+ balance. This difference seems to underlie the reversible bone resorption and hypercalciuria that complicate distal but not proximal disease. Although both forms of RTA may present with hypokalemic, hyperchloremic acidosis, renal potassium wasting, and relatively alkaline urine, they are easily distinguished. *Proximal* bicarbonate wasting rarely occurs in the absence of some combination of phosphate, glucose, uric acid, or amino acid wasting. The distal form is not complicated by these findings. *Disordered calcium metabolism*—nephrolithiasis, nephrocalcinosis, hypercalciuria, and osteopenic bone disease— are major complications of distal but not proximal RTA.

First morning urinary pH. Following overnight dehydration, patients are instructed to discard accumulated urine, collecting their next specimen in a container with 2.5–5.0 ml of mineral oil. The more dense urine sinks under the mineral oil which retards loss of CO_2. Urine is withdrawn with a needle and syringe, and the pH accurately measured. A pH greater than 6.1 strongly suggests proximal RTA.

Acid loading test. If the first morning pH is above 6.1, patients should be given 0.1 g/kg of NH_4Cl in capsules ingested over 45 min, and hourly urine pHs followed. Urine, collected under mineral oil, is acidified to pH 5.3 or less in normals and patients with proximal RTA but not in those with distal disease.

4. Therapy

a. Indications for Alkali Therapy

Three mechanisms are potentially available for replenishment of lost alkali.

1. *Metabolism of organic anions.* Net conversion of retained lactate, acetoacetate, or β-hydroxybutyrate to bicarbonate rapidly (in hours) corrects organic acidoses.

2. *Renal bicarbonate synthesis.* Ionization of H_2CO_3, formed in tubular epithelial cells from hydrated CO_2, into H^+ and HCO_3^- allows for distal secretion of protons into the urine with concomitant return of HCO_3^- to blood. Renal bicarbonate synthesis, compared to organic anion metabolism, is relatively slow; e.g., it takes several days for complete renal correction of diarrheal acidosis.
3. *Exogenous alkali.* Inorganic acidosis complicating renal failure can only be corrected with exogenous alkali.

The following principles are offered as guides for therapy of metabolic acidosis with exogenous alkali.

i. Hemodynamic Considerations. For reasons outlined above (see Section II.A), we recommend giving enough alkali to maintain arterial pH above 7.20. Below this pH, myocardial contraction and blood pressure are compromised. In most adults with uncomplicated but severe hypobicarbonatemia, two to four ampules (100–200 mmol) of $NaHCO_3$ increases serum bicarbonate to or above 10 mM which, in the absence of pulmonary disease, usually raises pH to or above 7.20. Alkali supplementation should be given to sustain this value. With cessation of organic acid overproduction, anion metabolism and renal alkali synthesis will eventually normalize serum bicarbonate concentration.

ii. Sensitivity of pH to Additional Small Changes in Serum Bicarbonate or P_{CO_2}. The mathematical constraints of the acid–base equation (eq. 1) demand that with severe hypobicarbonatemia and appropriate hypocapnia, H^+ concentration (pH) become exquisitely sensitive to further change in serum bicarbonate concentration or P_{CO_2} (Table VI). The precarious acid–base status of patients with simple severe metabolic acidosis is illustrated in Table VII. A mere 2.5 mM decrease in serum bicarbonate or a trivial 16 mm Hg increase in P_{CO_2} drives the pH below 7.0. Physicians may capitalize on this sensitivity, since a 2.5 mM increase in bicarbonate concentration raises pH to the safer value of 7.29.

iii. Inorganic Acidoses and Renal Failure. As noted, the combined lack of circulating organic anion—i.e., bicarbonate precursor—and impaired renal alkali synthesis make these patients vitally dependent on exogenous alkali.

Table VI. Metabolic Acidosis Sensitizes pH to Small Changes in Bicarbonate and P_{CO_2}

Acid–base parameter	Simple, severe metabolic acidosis (SMA)	SMA plus mild respiratory acidosis	Further 2.5 mM decrease in serum HCO_3^-	2.5 mM increase in serum HCO_3^-
HCO_3^- (mM)	5.0	5.0	2.5	7.5
P_{CO_2} (mm Hg)	16.0	32.0	16.0	16.0
$[H^+]$ (nM)	76.8	153.6	153.6	51.2
pH	7.11	6.81	6.81	7.29

iv. Bones, Stones, and Growth. Chronic renal acidoses (uremic and RTA) damage bones, retard growth in children, and predispose to hypercalciuric nephrolithiasis. Alkali therapy prevents and reverses these complications.

b. Complications of Alkali Therapy

i. Hypernatremia and Volume Overload. Aggressive use of excessive amounts of hypertonic $NaHCO_3$ can cause hypervolemia and hypertonicity. "Space" may be created for needed isotonic $NaHCO_3$ by inducing a brisk NaCl diuresis with furosemide. Hourly replacement of NaCl losses with an equal number of millimoles of $NaHCO_3$ maintains sodium stores unchanged while effecting exchange of parenteral bicarbonate for excreted chloride.

ii. Hypokalemia. Alkalinization of blood causes translocation of extracellular potassium to the intracellular space. Patients depleted of potassium (RTA, diarrhea, diabetes) are particularly prone to this problem. Frequent serum electrolyte analyses coupled with appropriate infusions of KCl easily avoid significant degrees of hypokalemia.

iii. Tissue Hypoxia. As outlined above (see Section II.A), chronic metabolic acidosis simultaneously reduces RBC 2,3-DPG and acidifies hemoglobin. Depletion of the RBC metabolite enhances hemoglobin–oxygen binding, but acidification of hemoglobin (Bohr effect) has the opposite effect. These offsetting vectors leave hemoglobin–oxygen binding and, therefore, tissue oxygen delivery, unchanged. Therapy with alkali, by rapidly erasing the Bohr effect but only slowly stimulating replenishment of RBC 2,3-DPG, could transiently increase hemoglobin–oxygen binding and consequently diminish tissue oxygen delivery. At this writing, there exists little evidence to give clinical credibility to this interesting *in vitro* observation.

iv. Overshoot Alkalosis. During repair of organic acidoses, the final serum bicarbonate concentration evolves from metabolized lactate and ketone and from infused and retained exogenous alkali. Overzealous use of bicarbonate may ultimately result in hyperbicarbonatemia. Renal excretion of bicarbonate and organic anion usually minimizes this complication.

c. Use of Alkali

Sodium bicarbonate is clearly the *parenteral* alkali of choice. Sodium lactate offers no advantage and has the significant disadvantage of requiring metabolic conversion to bicarbonate before its alkaline potential is realized. Hypotensive states and liver disease may impair this conversion. Generation of CO_2 from titrated *oral* $NaHCO_3$ by gastric HCl causes abdominal distension and frequent eructations. Shohl's solution is a sodium citrate-containing oral alkalinizing agent that avoids this complication. Absorbed citrate is converted to bicarbonate in the liver without causing gastric discomfort. Each milliliter of solution contains 1 mmol of Na and 1 mmol of alkali.

The quantity and rate at which $NaHCO_3$ is infused is dictated by the unique demands presented by each patient. The rate of ongoing acid production and the patient's bicarbonate space are variables that can only be roughly assessed. Effective therapy therefore requires frequent measurements of pH, PCO_2, and HCO_3^- to evaluate the effects of alkali therapy.

For example, to increase serum bicarbonate from 5 mM to 10 mM in a 70-kg acidotic man, one must provide 5 mmol of alkali for each liter of "apparent" bicarbonate space (see above). At this severe degree of hypobicarbonatemia, the apparent alkali space represents 50% or more of body weight. Infusion of 175 mmol of $NaHCO_3$ (35 liters × 5 mM) therefore represents a minimum dose to be amended by subsequent blood tests. Enough alkali should be given to maintain pH above 7.20.

Once their acid production has normalized, patients with organic acidoses will increase their serum bicarbonate concentration by catabolizing organic anions and through renal mechanisms. Patients with inorganic acidoses and normal renal function (largely accounted for by diarrhea) will repair their alkali deficit by renal synthesis over several days. Those with renal insufficiency require exogenous alkali to replenish losses and for continuing normal acid production (50–100 mmol per day). Thus, the 70-kg patient with renal failure whose serum bicarbonate concentration has diminished to 10 mM requires 450 mmoles of $NaHCO_3$ (15 mM deficit × 30 liters). Depending on individual exigencies, this could be replaced over 3 days. If there were complete absence of renal acid excretion and bicarbonate synthesis, an additional 50–100 mmol per day (mean 75 mmol) of alkali should be added to cover daily alkali losses. Thus, this patient would receive 675 mmol of $NaHCO_3$ over 3 days or 225 mmol per day. This could be accomplished by taking 75 ml of Shohl's solution every 8 hr for 3 days. Thereafter, only continuing daily needs (75 mmol of alkali) need be replaced.

d. Some Specific Therapies

i. Ketoacidosis. Alcoholic subjects usually do not require insulin, and the amount of alkali required to sustain their pH above 7.20 is usually small. Infusion of dextrose-containing solutions rapidly reverses the ketogenic stimulus and allows for metabolic normalization of serum bicarbonate concentration. Saline, insulin, and judicious use of $NaHCO_3$ are effective in the great majority of patients with uncomplicated *diabetic* ketoacidosis. The importance of parenteral phosphorus repletion in this disorder has yet to be documented. Urinary loss of ketone anions coupled with retention of parenteral saline effectively rids the body of alkali precursor and simultaneously converts a high-AG acidosis to a hyperchloremic acidosis. Loss of metabolizable anions shifts the full weight of bicarbonate replenishment to the kidney. This slows the reparative process.

ii. Methanol, Ethylene Glycol. Ethanol therapy and hemodialysis should be initiated in symptomatic patients poisoned with either of these toxins. Ethanol, which blocks metabolism of methanol and ethylene glycol to toxic metabolites, should be given in a loading dose to achieve a blood level of 100 mg/dl. Since ethanol distributes throughout body water, 35–50 g (350–500 ml of 10% ethanol) should be given over 1–2 hr and followed by a sustaining dose of 10 g hourly. The sustaining dose must be increased to cover the additional losses through dialysis. Alcohol therapy should not be discontinued until neurological signs have cleared.

iii. Salicylism. An alkaline diuresis (200–300 ml/hr) leads to urinary trapping and removal of salicylate. Diuresis should be initiated with mannitol, and a 50 mM $NaHCO_3$, 20 mM KCl solution of dextrose infused to replace urinary losses. Dialysis is only needed if renal function is severely compromised.

iv. Lactic Acidosis. Removal of the underlying cause of lactic acid over-production remains the key to effective therapy. Treatment of CHF, anemia, hypotension, or hypoxia and removal of toxins are crucial for survival. Sodium bicarbonate should be given at rates required to sustain arterial pH at or above 7.20. Diuretics or dialysis may be required to create space for the large loads of $NaHCO_3$ often required. Despite initial indications of its effectiveness, methylene blue has long since been discarded as a treatment for this disorder. Dichloroacetate remains an experimental treatment for type B lactic acidosis. An occasional patient with reduced peripheral perfusion responds to vasodilator therapy with nitroprusside.

C. Respiratory Acidosis

1. Pathogenesis

The 15,000–20,000 mmol of CO_2 produced daily from the complete oxidation of fats, carbohydrates, and proteins is buffered by blood and carried to the lungs where it is efficiently excreted. The partial pressure of CO_2 (P_{CO_2}) is the driving force moving the gas from relatively hypercapneic cellular sites of production to the relatively hypocapneic blood where a trivial fraction is dissolved in plasma, and the remainder enters RBCs where it temporarily changes form. A small fraction combines with hemoglobin, forming carbamino compounds, and the remainder undergoes catalytic hydration by carbonic anhydrase to H_2CO_3. The H^+ ion moiety of H_2CO_3 is buffered by hemoglobin, and HCO_3^- leaves the RBC in exchange for plasma Cl^-. The relatively high P_{CO_2} in tissues drives these transformations of CO_2, thereby increasing venous blood CO_2-carrying capacity. These processes are reversed in the low-P_{CO_2} environment of the pulmonary alveolus, thereby allowing for efficient excretion of CO_2.

Carotid body and brainstem chemoreceptors recognize and translate changes in blood P_{CO_2} and acidity into alterations in alveolar ventilation. This biofeedback mechanism allows hypercapnia and acidemia to stimulate ventilation and thereby normalize blood P_{CO_2} and hydrogen ion concentration.

Accumulation of CO_2 increases cellular and extracellular H_2CO_3 concentrations. This increased acidity titrates blood and cellular buffers and stimulates renal acid excretion and bicarbonate generation. These facts are important in our understanding of the pathophysiology and diagnosis of acid–base disorders (see below).

Any factor that reduces alveolar ventilation reduces the efficiency with which the lungs excrete CO_2, i.e., reduces CO_2 clearance, thereby causing hypercapnia. In a given subject, the P_{CO_2} continues to increase because normal production exceeds excretion. The higher the P_{CO_2}, however, the more favorable is the alveolar excretory gradient. A point is ultimately reached at which CO_2 production once again equals excretion; i.e., a new steady state is achieved at this stable, higher blood P_{CO_2}.

Any disorder that impairs brainstem control of ventilation or disturbs neural transmission of regulatory impulses to muscles of respiration or somehow disrupts normal function of these muscles or of the chest wall may cause respiratory acidosis (Table VII). Similarly, the myriad disorders directly affecting the lungs also may cause acute or chronic hypercapnia (Table VII).

2. Pathophysiology

The clinically relevant effects of respiratory acidosis have been noted (see above). Of key diagnostic and therapeutic importance are the questions of whether acute or chronic hypercapnia is present and whether appropriate metabolic compensation has taken place.

Equation 1 demands that without any change in serum bicarbonate concentration (24 mM), an increase in P_{CO_2} from 40 mm Hg to 60 mm Hg must increase the $[H^+]$ from 40 nM (pH 7.40) to 60 nM (pH 7.22). Titration of cellular and extracellular buffers by H_2CO_3, however, generates 1 mmol of HCO_3^- for each acute increase of 10 mm Hg of P_{CO_2}. Thus, 20 mm Hg of acute hypercapnia increases serum bicarbonate concentration from 24 mM to 26

Table VII. Etiologies of Respiratory Acidosis

Acute acidosis	Chronic acidosis
Drugs: Narcotic, sedative overdose; general anesthesia	Neurological: Cerebral disease (tumor, degenerative, vascular); spinal disorders (poliomyelitis); peripheral neuropathies
Trauma and physical disorders: Pneumothorax; ventilator malfunction; aspiration of foreign bodies	Myopathies
Cardiac: Pulmonary edema; cardiac arrest	Thoracic disorders: Severe physical deformities, scleroderma
Metabolic: Tetany (hypocalcemic or hypomagnesemic)	
Primary pulmonary: Bronchospasm, severe pneumonia	Primary pulmonary: Severe, chronic pneumonia; progressive obstructive or parenchymal diseases

mM, thereby yielding a [H^+] of 55 nM (pH 7.26). Sustained hypercapnia stimulates renal acid excretion (mostly increasing ammonium chloride excretion and bicarbonate generation). The recruitment of renal bicarbonate synthesis causes serum bicarbonate concentration to increase by 3.5 mM for each 10 mm Hg increase in P_{CO_2} in chronic respiratory acidosis. Thus, the patient with a sustained P_{CO_2} of 60 mm Hg will have a serum bicarbonate concentration of 31 mM and a [H^+] of 46 nM (pH 7.33).

Based on anticipated compensation, one can identify acute and chronic, simple and mixed respiratory disorders.

3. Diagnosis

The diagnosis of simple acute and simple chronic respiratory acidosis is predicated on the demonstration of hypercapnia coupled with an appropriate increment in serum bicarbonate concentration (Table II). Important examples of mixed respiratory acid–base disorders are given.

a. Combined Chronic and Acute Respiratory Acidosis

Suppose a patient with a chronic compensated hypercapnia of 60 mm Hg, serum bicarbonate of 31 mM, and [H^+] of 46 nM (pH 7.33) suddenly developed pneumonia and acutely increased his P_{CO_2} to 80 mm Hg. This further acute increment of 20 mm Hg caused his serum bicarbonate to increase to 33 mM and his [H^+] therefore to become 58 nM (pH 7.24). This new bicarbonate concentration is less than would obtain with a chronic hypercapnia of 80 mm Hg but is too high for an acute hypercapnia of 80 mm Hg (i.e., a 40 mm Hg increase in P_{CO_2}). Appreciation of the limits of acute and chronic compensation and knowledge of the clinical history allow correct interpretation to be made of the chemical findings. Indeed, even in the absence of historical data, the observed HCO_3^-, P_{CO_2}, and pH, for stated reasons, would strongly suggest acute worsening of respiratory disease.

b. Mixed Respiratory and Metabolic Acidosis

Superimposition of severe hypoxemia, anemia, hypotension, or any other cause of lactic acidosis in a patient with preexisting respiratory failure combines two simple disturbances into a mixed acidosis. Rarely, the potassium deficiency accompanying certain of the hyperchloremic metabolic acidoses (e.g., RTA) is so severe as to cause paralysis of respiratory muscles and hypercapnia. In these mixed disorders, the serum bicarbonate concentration is either frankly depressed or not as high as uncomplicated hypercapnia would otherwise dictate. The finding of an increased AG could be a further clue to the presence of this mixed disorder.

c. *Mixed Respiratory Acidosis and Metabolic Alkalosis*

Diuretics are commonly employed in managing many patients with chronic lung disease, thereby subjecting them to the risk of metabolic alkalosis. Serum pH increases and may normalize or become frankly alkalemic depending on whether hypercapnia or hyperbicarbonatemia dominates. The more alkaline pH tends to reduce respiratory drive and worsen hypoxia. Recognition of this mixed disturbance is based on the relative or absolute hyperbicarbonatemia vis-à-vis the demands of compensation (Table II).

d. *"Triple" Disorder: Respiratory Acidosis Combined with Metabolic Acidosis and Alkalosis*

Superimposition of respiratory acidosis on a mixed metabolic acidosis–alkalosis is rather common. One example of this triple disorder is diuretic-induced metabolic alkalosis in a patient whose respiratory failure is so advanced as to cause hypoxia, hypotension, and lactic acidosis. The diagnosis of mixed metabolic acidosis and alkalosis has been described (Table III). In this case, serum bicarbonate concentration falls less than the AG increases. Hypobicarbonatemia may be mild. Hypercapnia in the face of a low serum bicarbonate concentration completes the picture.

4. Management

Patients with acute, reversible respiratory acidosis urgently need correction of the underlying cause, reduction of hypercapnia, and improvement of hypoxia. Intubation and ventilation are usually required. If moderate to severe hypercapnia (60–80 mm Hg) has been present for days, compensatory hyperbicarbonatemia will also be found. Normalization of PCO_2 prior to that of bicarbonate may produce a striking posthypercapnic metabolic alkalosis. Maintenance of ECF volume and prevention of hypokalemia prevent sustained renal retention of bicarbonate and alkalemia. Blood pH must be closely followed as PCO_2 is normalized, since developing alkalemia may require induction of bicarbonaturia with acetazolamide (Diamox®). Oral or parenteral use of 250–500 mg of acetazolamide is useful if hyperbicarbonatemia causes pH to increase above 7.50.

Patients with compensated chronic respiratory acidosis usually tolerate their hypercapnia quite well and maintain a pH of 7.30–7.35. Judicious use of antibiotics, bronchodilators, and physiotherapy reflects good conservative medical management. Intubation and ventilation are best avoided until clearly indicated.

Superimposed metabolic alkalosis should be watched for and treated. Acidemia helps to drive respiration; thus, inappropriate hyperbicarbonatemia may induce worsening hypercapnia and hypoxia. Maintenance of normokalemia in patients on diuretics is helpful in avoiding alkalosis.

Occasional addition of acetazolamide may be needed to avoid hyperbicarbonatemia.

SUGGESTED READINGS

Cohen JJ, Madias NE: Acid–base disorders of respiratory origin, in Brenner BM, Stein JH (eds): *Contemporary Issues in Nephrology*, vol. 2: *Acid–Base and Potassium Homeostasis.* New York, Churchill Livingstone, 1978, pp 137–167.

Emmett M, Narins RG: Clinical use of the anion gap. *Medicine* 56:38–59, 1977.

Garella S, Dana CL, Chazan JA: Severity of metabolic acidosis as a determinant of bicarbonate requirement. *N Engl J Med* 289:121–126, 1973.

Kassirer JP, Bleich HL: Rapid estimation of plasma carbon dioxide from pH and total carbon dioxide content. *N Engl J Med* 272:1067–1070, 1965.

Kassirer JP, Madias NE: Respiratory acid–base disorders. *Hosp Pract*, December 1980, pp 57–71.

Narins RG, Bastl CP, Rudnick MR: Lactic acidosis and the elevated anion gap, Part I. *Hosp Pract*, May 1980, pp 125–136.

Narins RG, Bastl CP, Rudnick MR: Lactic acidosis and the elevated anion gap, Part II. *Hosp Pract*, June 1980, pp 91–98.

Narins RG, Bastl CP, Rudnick MR, et al: Acid–base metabolism, in Gonick HC (ed): *Current Nephrology*, vol 5. New York, John Wiley & Sons, 1981, pp 79–130.

Narins RG, Emmett M: Simple and mixed acid–base disorders: A practical approach. *Medicine* 59:161–187, 1980.

Narins RG, Gardner LB: Simple acid–base disturbances. *Med Clin North Am* 65:321–346, 1981.

Narins RG, Goldberg M: Renal tubular acidosis: Pathogenesis, diagnosis and treatment. *DM*, March 1977, pp 1–65.

7

Acid–Base Disturbances
Metabolic and Respiratory Alkaloses

ROBERT G. NARINS, MARY C. STOM, and
THOMAS R. BECK

I. EFFECTS OF ALKALOSIS

The increased risk of digitalis intoxication, prolonged QT internal, and U waves are well known complications of alkalosis. Cerebral vascular resistance is quite sensitive to P_{CO_2}, and hypocapnia is a potent cerebral vasoconstrictive force. Diminished cerebral blood flow in respiratory alkalosis may underlie many of the observed neurological signs and symptoms.

Alkalosis increases neuromuscular excitability by several mechanisms: replacement of titrated protons on albumin with calcium, citrate overproduction binding calcium to tissue, and alkalosis enhancing release of acetylcholine. Severe alkalemia (pH > 7.55) may therefore precipitate tetany.

Several *metabolic* effects of alkalosis are well recognized: mild stimulation of organic acid overproduction (serum lactate may increase 1–2 mM), mild increase in the AG (rises by 3–5 mM) because of lactate accumulation and titration of protons on albumin, thereby replacing HCO_3^- with protein anions, increased potassium excretion but enhanced calcium reabsorption, stimulation of the entry of extracellular potassium and phosphorus into cells, and mild stimulation of glycolysis, causing a tendency toward hypoglycemia.

ROBERT G. NARINS, MARY C. STOM, and THOMAS R. BECK • Department of Medicine, Temple University Health Sciences Center, Philadelphia, Pennsylvania 19140.

II. METABOLIC ALKALOSIS

A. Pathogenesis

Rational therapy of metabolic alkalosis cannot be developed until one understands the underlying mechanisms by which hyperbicarbonatemia is generated and sustained. Under normal circumstances, the kidney reabsorbs 24 mmol of bicarbonate from each liter of glomerular filtrate, allowing excess alkali to escape into the urine. Thus, for chronic hyperbicarbonatemia to develop, a source of new alkali must be provided, and the kidney must be signaled to reclaim this alkali lest bicarbonaturia normalize the serum level.

1. Source of Alkali

Hyperbicarbonatemia may derive from four sources.

a. Contraction

Loss of sodium, chloride, and water from the ECF leaves the body content of bicarbonate unchanged but causes its concentration to increase by suspending it in a lesser volume. Only very edematous patients can lose enough ECF to become significantly hyperbicarbonatemic.

b. Renal Synthesis

By hydrating CO_2 to H_2CO_3 and then independently transporting its ionization products, H^+ and HCO_3^-, into the urine and blood, respectively, the cells of the distal nephron simultaneously excrete H^+ and return new HCO_3^- to the body. Sodium, from filtered NaCl, is reabsorbed in exchange for secreted H^+ and is ultimately returned to the blood as $NaHCO_3$ while HCl is excreted. Actually, the HCl is not excreted as such but rather in association with titrated ammonia (NH_3) buffer, being excreted as NH_4Cl. Enhanced distal delivery of NaCl—as caused by most diuretics—stimulates this exchange process, thereby causing the kidney to synthesize new alkali. Mineralocorticoids directly stimulate distal H^+ secretion and thereby synthesize alkali.

c. Gastrointestinal Synthesis

Parietal cells in the stomach, like renal tubular cells, also separate H^+ from HCO_3^-, acidifying the gastric lumen while alkalinizing the blood. Reabsorption of secreted H^+ eventually neutralizes HCO_3^- added to blood, thereby preventing systemic alkalosis. It follows that removal of gastric H^+ by vomiting or nasogastric suction allows for retention of new alkali.

d. Exogenous Alkali

Ingestion of sodium bicarbonate (baking soda), various absorbable antacids (calcium carbonate, Tums®, Alka Seltzer®), or exposure to metabolizable salts of strong acids such as sodium lactate, sodium citrate, etc. provide a source for hyperbicarbonatemia.

2. Renal Reclamation of Bicarbonate

a. Hypovolemia

Hypovolemia is a potent stimulus for renal reabsorption of sodium with its attendant anion. Thus, bicarbonate added to the blood from the stomach or distal nephron is reclaimed from the glomerular filtrate under stimulation by ECF volume contraction, thereby sustaining hyperbicarbonatemia. By far the most common forms of metabolic alkalosis—gastric and diuretic induced—are sustained by ongoing hypovolemia and reversed by volume reexpansion with saline. Relieved from the constraints of volume contraction, renal reabsorption of $NaHCO_3$ is reduced, allowing bicarbonaturia to normalize serum bicarbonate concentration.

b. Hypercapnia

An elevated P_{CO_2} acidifies renal tubular cells, thereby enhancing bicarbonate reabsorption. It is the high P_{CO_2} that stimulates bicarbonate synthesis and allows for its retention in compensation for chronic respiratory acidosis.

c. Hyperaldosteronism

Mineralocorticoids stimulate distal sodium reabsorption and H^+ and potassium secretion. The new bicarbonate, returned to blood as acid is excreted, is conserved as a consequence of the alkali-retaining effect of potassium depletion. Hypokalemia prevents the bicarbonaturia that would otherwise accompany the sodium retention and ECF volume expansion attending primary hyperaldosteronism. Most forms of secondary hyperaldosteronism, e.g., CHF, cirrhosis, nephrosis, however, do not cause metabolic alkalosis unless diuretic therapy has been used. The increased proximal sodium reabsorption that characterizes these disorders limits distal sodium delivery and thereby renders ineffectual hormonal stimulation of distal Na^+/H^+ exchange. Diuretics insure distal delivery of sodium and thereby allow for effective distal hormone action.

d. Potassium Depletion

Hypokalemia mildly stimulates proximal bicarbonate reabsorption and enhances renal ammonia synthesis while simultaneously sensitizing the distal tubule to the alkalinizing effects of mineralocorticoids. Through uncertain mechanisms, severe potassium depletion (500–1000 mmol) impairs renal chloride reabsorption. These alkalinizing effects of potassium depletion tend to be offset by the inhibition of aldosterone secretion caused by the direct effects of hypokalemia on the adrenal gland. On balance, potassium depletion tends to be mildly alkalinizing in man.

e. Parathyroid Hormone and Calcium

Parathyroid hormone inhibits proximal bicarbonate reabsorption; therefore, the parathyroprival state tends to enhance bicarbonate reabsorption, increasing the tendency of patients with hypoparathyroidism to alkalosis. Hypercalcemia, however, stimulates bicarbonate reabsorption. Thus, hypercalcemic hyperparathyroidism does not frequently yield acid–base disturbances by consequence of the countervailing effects of the hormone and calcium. Hypercalcemic, hypoparathyroid states like sarcoidosis, however, are not uncommonly associated with hyperbicarbonatemia.

B. Pathophysiology

1. Respiratory Compensation

Alkalinization of peripheral and brainstem chemoreceptors by hyperbicarbonatemia suppresses respiration, allowing the acidifying effect of hypercapnia to compensate for the alkalosis. In uncomplicated metabolic alkalosis, the PCO_2 ought to increase by 6 mm Hg for every 10 mM increase in serum bicarbonate concentration. Indeed, the constraints of this mathematical relationship dictate that the addition of "15" to elevated serum bicarbonate concentration yields the last two digits of the pH (Table II of Chapter 6). Thus, a serum bicarbonate concentration of 35 mM (10 mM above normal) ought to be associated with a pH of 7.50 (15 plus 35) and a PCO_2 of 46 mm Hg (40 plus 6).

2. Mixed Disorders

It now appears that metabolic alkaloses are commonly associated with disorders that stimulate respiration and thereby prevent appropriate compensation from occurring. Thus, coexisting respiratory alkalosis is diagnosed when hyperbicarbonatemia is associated with a frankly low PCO_2 or when the degree of elevation of serum bicarbonate concentration demands a higher PCO_2 than is actually found. A superimposed respiratory acidosis is diagnosed when the PCO_2 is higher than predicted.

The means of diagnosing a mixed metabolic acidosis and alkalosis have been discussed previously (Chapter 6).

C. Differential Diagnosis

The metabolic alkaloses are most practically classified on the basis of their therapeutic response to expansion of the ECF space (Fig. 1). Saline-responsive metabolic alkaloses are characterized by signs of ECF volume contraction and urinary chloride concentration less than 20 mM. Hyperbicarbonatemia is not improved with volume expansion in the saline-unresponsive group whose urinary chloride concentration is greater than 20 mM. It is helpful to further subdivide these patients on the basis of whether their blood pressure is normal or elevated.

1. Saline-Responsive Metabolic Alkaloses

a. Contraction Alkaloses

These are seen primarily in overdiuresed previously edematous patients. Loss of NaCl without $NaHCO_3$ creates hyperbicarbonatemia by contracting the space in which the alkali is dispersed.

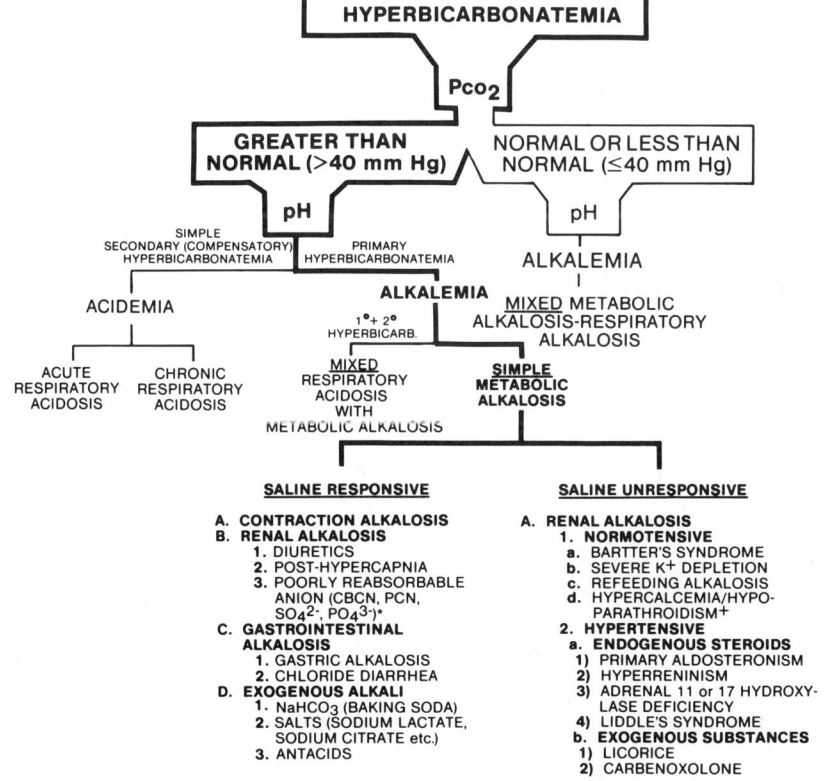

Figure 1. Differential diagnosis of hyperbicarbonatemia. *CBCN, carbenicillin; PCN, penicillin; $SO_4{}^{2-}$, sulfate; $PO_4{}^{3-}$, phosphate.

b. Renal Alkaloses

The edematous patient often has secondary hyperaldosteronism which causes the distal nephron to vigorously secrete H^+ and potassium when such diuretics as furosemide, ethacrynic acid, thiazides, and metolazone provide large amounts of sodium for distal reabsorption. The long-acting thiazides tend to be most commonly associated with alkalosis. Sodium-depleted patients treated with large doses of carbenicillin, penicillin, sulfate, or phosphate often develop hyperbicarbonatemia. The salt-avid tubule reabsorbs the sodium associated with these compounds, leaving the poorly reabsorbable anions in the lumen. This negative charge accumulating in the tubule stimulates secretion of potassium and H^+, causing excessive synthesis of bicarbonate.

c. Gastrointestinal Alkalosis

Gastric secretions contain only 5–10 mM potassium, making direct loss of stomach contents an unlikely means of losing potassium. The hypokalemia attending vomiting and nasogastric suction evolves from alkalemia driving extracellular potassium into cells and concomitantly impairing renal potassium reabsorption. Thus, the combination of translocation from ECF to ICF and kaliuresis depresses serum potassium in these disorders.

d. Exogenous Alkali

Exposure to alkaline salts only causes chronic hyperbicarbonatemia when renal bicarbonate retention has been stimulated by such phenomena as ECF volume contraction, hypercapnia, hypokalemia, hypercalcemia, or hypoparathyroidism. Salts of strong acids as found in Ringer's lactate, peritoneal dialysis bath, etc. are alkalinizing by consequence of their metabolism to bicarbonate. "Hidden" sources of alkali include baking soda, which is routinely used by some patients to "settle their stomach." Vomiting, hypovolemic patients abusing $NaHCO_3$ develop striking degrees of hyperbicarbonatemia. Transfusion products contain sodium citrate which is rapidly metabolized to HCO_3^-. Each unit of whole blood contains 17 mmol of potential bicarbonate, and each unit of packed RBC contains 5 mmol. Infusion of 10 units of whole blood into a hypotensive postoperative patient whose kidney cannot clear alkali well adds 170 mmol of $NaHCO_3$, thereby increasing serum bicarbonate concentration by 6 mM in a 70-kg man. Since surgical trauma stimulates respiration, the patient whose serum bicarbonate increased from 24 mM to 30 mM would also be likely to sustain a decrease in P_{CO_2} from 40 mm Hg to 30 mm Hg, thereby increasing his pH from 7.40 to 7.62. Various proprietary antacids contain generous amounts of alkali. Tums® contains 5.25 mmol (10.5 mEq) of $CaCO_3$ per tablet, and Alka Seltzer® contains 22.6 mmol of $NaHCO_3$ per tablet. Rolaids® contains $Al_2(CO_3)_2$ which, unlike $CaCO_3$ and $NaHCO_3$, is a nonabsorbable alkali.

2. Saline-Unresponsive Metabolic Alkaloses

a. Renal Alkaloses

The various disorders that cause excessive renal acid excretion and, therefore, excessive bicarbonate synthesis and addition to the body are best classified according to their effect on systemic blood pressure.

b. Normotensive Variants

i. *Bartter's Syndrome.* The major features of this rare syndrome include a hypokalemic, hypochloremic metabolic alkalosis, urinary chloride and potassium wasting, striking hyperreninemia, and hyperaldosteronism despite normotension and reduced responsivity to exogenous pressor agents. Although many theories have been proffered in explanation of these findings, on balance it appears that permanently impaired NaCl reabsorption by the thick ascending limb of Henle's loop accounts for virtually all of the observations. Potassium depletion and excessive bicarbonate synthesis follow from hormonal responses to salt depletion and continued increased distal sodium delivery. These patients behave "as if" they were chronically taking a "loop-acting" diuretic such as furosemide. Renal prostaglandin synthesis seems to nonspecifically evolve from potassium depletion. The prostaglandins worsen the underlying problem by stimulating the renin–angiotensin–aldosterone cascade and thereby enhancing the kaliuresis and hyperbicarbonatemia. Inhibitors of prostaglandin synthesis help but do not fully erase the problem.

ii. *Severe Potassium Depletion.* Most hypokalemic subjects suffer losses of 100–300 mmol, and their alkalosis is associated with urinary chloride retention. More severe degrees of depletion appear to inhibit chloride reabsorption along the entire nephron, causing chloruresis along with the continuing kaliuresis. The exact pathogenesis of this unusual disorder remains to be clarified.

iii. *Refeeding Alkalosis.* Many starved patients develop striking hyperbicarbonatemia during the first week of refeeding. Sodium retention and edema are commonly associated. The pathogenesis of this cause of metabolic alkalosis is uncertain.

iv. *Hypercalcemia.* Through uncertain mechanisms, hypercalcemia stimulates renal H^+ secretion and bicarbonate reabsorption while simultaneously stimulating ammonia synthesis. Increased acid excretion and bicarbonate synthesis and retention produce chronic hyperbicarbonatemia. Since parathyroid hormone antagonizes these effects, only disorders such as vitamin D intoxication and sarcoidosis, which couple hypercalcemia with hypoparathyroidism, commonly produce sustained hyperbicarbonatemia.

c. Hypertensive Variants

i. *Primary Aldosteronism.* Potassium depletion is intrinsically more important in this disorder than in those noted above. The cation must be replaced if serum bicarbonate is to be normalized prior to surgical treatment of the adrenal lesion. The ECF is already expanded as part of the underlying disease process, thereby negating any helpful effect of parenteral saline. Bicarbonate synthesis is stimulated distally by hormone action, whereas ECF volume expansion and potassium deficiency offset each other proximally. Unopposed ECF volume expansion would prevent retention of alkali generated distally, thus establishing the important role of potassium depletion.

ii. *Hyperreninism, 11- and 17-Hydroxylase Deficiencies, Licorice and Carbenoxolone.* These all stimulate distal tubular acid and potassium excretion while causing mild sodium and bicarbonate retention. *Hyperreninism* is seen in renovascular hypertension and in subjects with accelerated or malignant hypertension. Renin secreted by certain malignancies—hemangiopericytoma, Wilm's tumor—also creates this syndrome. Unrestricted secretion of ACTH secondary to the cortisol deficiency caused by *11- and 17-hydroxylase deficiencies* stimulates the adrenal cortex to overproduce mineralocorticoids. A heroic degree of precocious puberty is seen in hypertensive males with 11-hydroxylase deficiency, whereas females manifest the stigmata of masculinization. Gonadal failure attends 17-hydroxylase deficiency. *Liddle's syndrome* is a very rare familial disorder characterized by secretion of a nonaldosterone mineralocorticoid causing hypertension, kaliuresis, and a hypokalemic alkalosis. The disorder responds to triamterene but not spironolactone.

Licorice and *carbenoxolone* contain glycyrrhizinic acid which is a nonsteroidal mineralocorticoid. American licorice, unless imported, contains little or none of the active principle. Ingestion of 20–200 g per day causes this syndrome. *Carbenoxolone* is an oral antiulcer therapy not yet released for use in the United States. *Lydia Pinkham's Tablets* ® (for menstrual cramps) and *chewing tobacco* also contain derivatives of glycyrrhizinic acid and have been incriminated in this mineralocorticoid syndrome.

D. Management

1. General Principles

Most metabolic alkaloses do not require immediate correction. The urgency usually relates to the degree of ECF volume contraction or associated digitalis intoxication and not the hyperbicarbonatemia and hypokalemia *per se. Volume depleted,* hypovolemic, hypotensive subjects obviously need saline primarily to reestablish the integrity of their circulation and simultaneously to allow bicarbonaturia to normalize hyperbicarbonatemia. The presence of increased *neuromuscular excitability* also signals the need for more rapid repair of the alkalosis. It is essential that physicians remember that many of the causes of metabolic alkalosis also cause *magnesium depletion*. The alkalotic, hypokalemic patient may also be hypomagnesemic, and his tetanic symptoms and signs may be more a function of divalent cation depletion than alkalosis. Magnesium deficiency stimulates kaliuresis and, by impairing parathyroid hormone secretion and its effect on bone, also causes hypocalcemia. We routinely measure serum magnesium in all alkalotic patients.

2. Specific Disorders

a. Contraction Alkalosis

When diuresing very edematous patients, it is often helpful to briefly discontinue therapy with furosemide or thiazide (alkalinizing diuretics) and use a short, 1- to 2-day course of acetazolamide (Diamox®). Use of 500–1000 mg of this bicarbonaturic diuretic often helps to avoid or erase contraction alkaloses.

b. Saline-Responsive Alkaloses

i. Saline. Most patients with relatively normal renal function respond to replacement of 1–2 liters of normal saline given over 24–36 hr. Although each case must be assessed separately, giving saline at this rate is a reasonable first approach. More mild alkaloses may be treated with oral sodium chloride. It must, of course, be remembered that ongoing water and salt losses must be replaced as deficits are repaired.

ii. Potassium. Although saline-responsive alkaloses may be repaired without potassium, KCl should be added to the therapeutic prescription. Most hypokalemic subjects are depleted of 100–300 mmol, but patients may have lost as much as 1000 mmol. The presence of U waves on their electrocardiograms adds to the urgency of replacement, and development of muscle (hypokalemic) paralysis is a medical emergency.

iii. Cimetidine. Gastric loss of HCl is markedly reduced (90%) by this H_2-histamine-receptor blocker. Patients undergoing nasogastric suction or vomiting benefit from intravenous use of 600 mg of cimetidine every 6 hr. The dose is halved when advanced renal failure is present.

iv. Acidifying Agent. As long as renal function is intact, patients with saline-responsive alkaloses rarely require an acidifying agent.

c. Saline-Unresponsive Alkaloses

i. Mineralocorticoid-Induced Alkaloses. Addition of spironolactone (300–600 mg daily), salt restriction (20–30 mmol daily), and KCl induce potassium retention and normalize serum bicarbonate concentration in most patients with Conn's syndrome. Permanent correction is ultimately accomplished by surgical extirpation of the adrenal adenoma.

ii. Use of an Acidifying Agent. The ECF volume expansion associated with most saline-unresponsive metabolic alkaloses limits the extent of hyperbicarbonatemia and therefore renders an acidifying agent unnecessary. Adequate renal function is obviously required if saline infusion and KCl are to repair a metabolic alkalosis. Severe hyperbicarbonatemia in association with advanced renal failure, therefore, is the most common setting in which an acidifying agent is required. Asymptomatic metabolic alkalosis, when associated with renal failure, need not be treated aggressively (or at all), since the kidney's inability to excrete the normal daily acid production allows the retained acid to titrate body alkali. Symptomatic alkalosis, i.e., with signs of heightened neuromuscular excitability and electrocardiographic abnormalities, in the azotemic patient often demands therapy with an acidifying agent.

Available oral and parenteral acidifying agents contribute protons by different mechanisms (Table I). Calcium chloride acidifies by interaction with certain of the pancreatic secretions and therefore is only effective when given orally. The pancreas, like the nephron and the gastric mucosa, forms H_2CO_3 by hydrating CO_2. Unlike the other organs that secrete acid and alkalinize blood, the pancreas secretes HCO_3^- into the lumen while transiently acidifying the ECF by adding H^+ to blood leaving it.

Eventual reabsorption of intestinal HCO_3^- and its recombination with blood H^+ prevent development of net acidification. Ingested calcium binds secreted HCO_3^-, preventing neutralization of pancreas-derived blood H^+. Net acidification therefore occurs. Ammonium chloride, lysine, and arginine hydrochloride acidify by consequence of their metabolism to urea and HCl. These agents worsen azotemia when used in patients with renal failure. Patients with advanced liver disease may not metabolize the cationic amino acid arginine. In this setting, intracellular accumulation of the positively charged arginine displaces cellular potassium and may cause life-threatening hyperkalemia. Ammonium chloride therapy transiently causes hyperammonemia and is therefore contraindicated in patients with liver disease. Calcium chloride is a reasonable substitute for ammonium chloride in this setting.

Parenteral HCl seems to be the safest acidifying agent. When it is given via a large vein as a 100–200 mM solution, very few complications have been encountered. Infusion of 200–300 mmol may be given in 24 hr without significant hemolysis or azotemia. Calculation of the amount of acid required to produce a specific decrement in serum bicarbonate concentration and pH is complicated by coexisting differences in intracellular and extracellular alkalinization. Cellular potassium losses accompanying most metabolic alkaloses are partially replaced with protons from the ECF. This maldistribution of protons intensifies the extracellular alkalosis while rendering the ICF more acid. We therefore calculate the amount of acid to be given on the conservative impression that only the ECF bicarbonate is to be titrated.

For example, a hypokalemic 70-kg man in renal failure has a symptomatic hyperbicarbonatemia of 40 mM, a PCO_2 of 50 mm Hg and a pH of 7.52. To reduce his serum bicarbonate by 10 mM requires that 10 mmol of H^+ be

Table I. Commonly Used Acidifying Agents

Agent	Formula	Formula weight	mEq (mmol)/g	Comments	Complications
Calcium chloride	$CaCl_2$	111	18 (9)	Oral only	Hypercalcemia
Ammonium chloride	NH_4Cl	53	19 (19)	Oral: Avoid tablets, use capsule or liquid IV: Given as 0.9% or 2% (170 or 277 mM) solution	Azotemia, high blood ammonia Avoid when liver disease coexists
Lysine · HCl	$C_6H_{14}N_2O_2HCl$	182	5.5 (5.5)	Oral: 40% solution; each Tsp contains 2g (11 mmoles)	Azotemia
Arginine · HCl	$C_6H_{14}N_4O_2HCl$	210	4.8 (4.8)	IV	Azotemia, hyperkalemia
Hydrochloric acid	HCl	36	28 (28)	IV: 0.1–0.2 M, given via large vein.	Hemolysis, tissue necrosis with extravasation

given for each liter of ECF. Since ECF space is 20% of body weight (14 liters), a total of 140 mmol of HCl should be given. Infusion of 700 ml of 0.2 M HCl over 12–24 hr suffices. The rate and quantity of the infusion should be readjusted on the basis of frequent (every 3 hr) measurements of pH, PCO_2, and HCO_3^-. If this patient's serum bicarbonate concentration decreased to 30 mM, and if his PCO_2 was reduced to 45 mm Hg, his pH would become the more acceptable 7.44.

III. RESPIRATORY ALKALOSIS

A. Pathogenesis

A wide range of physiological, pharmacological, and noxious stimuli act on brainstem respiratory control centers, the chest wall, and the pulmonary parenchyma to increase alveolar ventilation (Table II). Although deep-seated anxiety may cause striking degrees of hyperventilation, the pain and trauma inherent in the routine drawing of arterial blood usually do not significantly stimulate alveolar ventilation. Measurements of pH, PCO_2, and HCO_3^- from blood drawn via indwelling vascular lines, when compared with that obtained via arterial puncture, have clearly established this point.

Virtually any disease process (tumor, trauma, infection, vascular disease, etc.) is capable of interacting with medullary centers in causing pathological hyperventilation. Salicylates and endotoxin are two particularly common metabolic causes of central hyperventilation. Mild congestive heart failure (CHF), pulmonary emboli, and early interstitial lung disease initiate local reflexes that stimulate respiration. Severe CHF or advanced interstitial disease commonly overwhelm the lung's capacity to clear CO_2, thereby causing respiratory acidosis. Many disorders stimulate respiration by several mechanisms. The fever, endotoxemia, and local irritation associated with pneumonia are an example of a multifactorial cause of hyperventilation.

B. Pathophysiology

1. Metabolic Buffering

Within minutes of lowering PCO_2, tissue and blood buffers donate protons which consume bicarbonate, thereby lessening the alkalinizing impact of acute hypocapnia. Indeed, serum bicarbonate decreases by 2.5 mM for each 10 mm Hg decrease in PCO_2 (Table II of Chapter 6). As in respiratory acidosis, the kidney's regulatory role is trivial in acute respiratory alkalosis.

Table II. Etiologies of Respiratory Alkalosis

CNS diseases	Liver failure
Vascular	Drugs, hormones
Tumor	Salicylates
Infection	Catecholamines
Anxiety	Progesterone
Fever, sepsis	Analeptic drugs
Endotoxemia	Early pulmonary edema
Hyperthyroidism	Pulmonary disease
Pregnancy	Mild restrictive diseases
Hypoxia	Pulmonary emboli
Respirator malfunction	Pneumonia (mild)

Within days, hypocapnia suppresses renal acid excretion, thereby allowing retained metabolic acids to further lower serum bicarbonate concentration. In chronic respiratory alkalosis, i.e., after 48–72 hr, serum bicarbonate reaches its nadir, falling by a total of 5 mM for each 10 mm Hg fall in P_{CO_2}. In sharp contrast to all other simple acid–base disorders, prolonged respiratory alkalosis (i.e., more than 2 weeks) often is associated with a *normal pH*. The reasons why this disorder manifests total compensation is unknown. Most causes of respiratory alkalosis are treatable or self-limited, making it unusual to achieve the chronicity required for normalization of pH.

Lost bicarbonate is replaced with retained chloride. Serum electrolytes therefore manifest hypobicarbonatemia and hyperchloremia, and serum potassium is often mildly depressed. Viewed in isolation, this electrolyte pattern cannot be distinguished from the hyperchloremic, hypokalemic acidosis caused by diarrhea or RTA. The clinical history and blood pH, however, readily distinguish these disorders. Serum bicarbonate rarely falls below 15 mM in respiratory alkalosis but commonly does so in metabolic acidosis. The AG may be slightly increased (3–5 mM) secondary to stimulation of organic acid production and protein buffering (see Section II. B).

C. Diagnosis

Respiratory alkalosis is recognized by the clinical setting in which it occurs, the hypobicarbonatemia and hyperchloremia found on serum analysis, and finally proven by measurement of arterial pH and P_{CO_2}. A simple, uncomplicated respiratory alkalosis is present when clinical history, serum electrolytes and pH, and bicarbonate assays exclude other disorders. A proper reduction of serum bicarbonate (Table II of Chapter 6) and stability of the AG defines the simple disorder. Bicarbonate concentrations higher or lower than anticipated indicate coexisting metabolic alkalosis or acidosis, respectively.

D. Management

Therapy should be primarily aimed at removing the underlying cause of hyperventilation. Certain clinical disorders, however, require brief review.

1. Anxiety

Attempts should be made to help subjects cope with their problem, but in addition, the simple expedient of carrying a rebreathing bag can be quite helpful. By rebreathing exhaled air from a paper bag, patients can maintain a relatively normal Pco_2 and avoid troublesome symptoms of alkalemia.

2. Neurological Disease

Patients suffering midbrain strokes may develop severe hyperventilation and alkalemia. The elevated pH lowers seizure threshold, and hypocapnia further compromises cerebral blood flow. When pH exceeds 7.50, thought should be given to using a rebreathing mask, increasing ventilator dead-space, and, as a final resort, to paralyzing the patient and creating a normal Pco_2.

SUGGESTED READINGS

Narins RG, Bastl CP, Rudnick MR: Metabolic alkalosis, in Franklin S (ed): *Practical Nephrology.* New York, John Wiley & Sons, 1981, pp 409–445.

Rudnick MR, Bastl CP, Narins RG: Diagnostic approaches to hypertension, in Brenner BM, Stein JH (eds): *Contemporary Issues in Nephrology, Hypertension,* vol 7. New York, Churchill-Livingstone, 1981, pp 270–338.

Seldin DW, Rector FC Jr: The generation and maintenance of metabolic alkalosis. *Kidney Int* 1:306–315, 1972.

8

Disturbances of Uric Acid Metabolism

EDWIN MEJÍAS and MANUEL MARTÍNEZ-MALDONADO

I. INTRODUCTION

Interest in the role of purines in human disease began with the observation that uric acid was a component of some renal calculi. Thereafter it was noted (1) that in its ionized form, monosodium urate was a major constituent of tophi and (2) that uric acid was elevated in the serum of gouty patients, and that in its crystalline form it was present in synovial fluid during acute attacks of gouty arthritis. In this chapter we discuss: the synthesis and degradation of uric acid in man; the renal and extrarenal disposition of uric acid; a rational approach to the evaluation of uric acid disorders; and modalities used in the treatment of uric acid disorders in man.

II. REGULATION OF PURINE METABOLISM IN MAN

The pathways by which purine nucleotides are synthesized and degraded are shown in Fig. 1. The purine nucleotides, adenylic (AMP), inosinic (IMP), and guanylic acid (GMP), represent the end products of purine biosynthesis. They can be synthesized directly from purine bases (e.g., guanine to GMP, hypoxanthine to IMP, and adenine to AMP), or they may be synthesized de novo beginning with nonpurine precursors and progressing through

EDWIN MEJÍAS • Rheumatology Section, Department of Internal Medicine, Veterans Administration Hospital, San Juan, Puerto Rico 00936.   MANUEL MARTÍNEZ-MALDONADO • Medical Service, Veterans Administration Hospital, San Juan, Puerto Rico 00936; and Departments of Internal Medicine and Physiology, University of Puerto Rico School of Medicine, San Juan, Puerto Rico 00931.

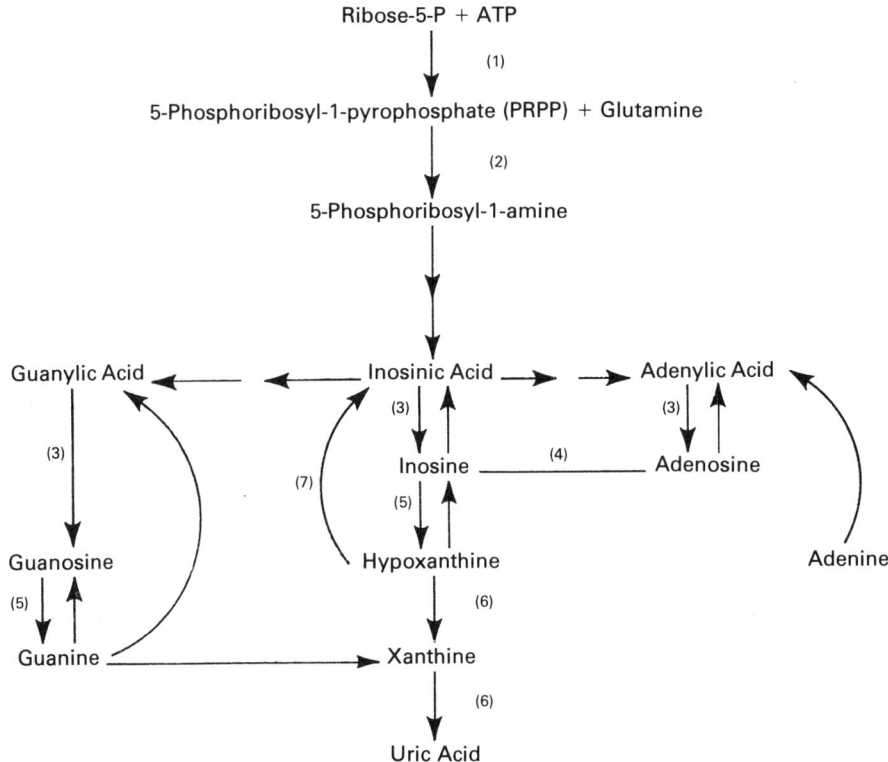

Figure 1. Purine metabolism in man: (1) PRPP synthetase, (2) amidophosphoribosyltransferase, (3) 5'-nucleotidase, (4) adenosine deaminase, (5) purine nucleoside phosphorylase, (6) xanthine oxidase, (7) hypoxanthine–guanine phosphoribosyltransferase.

a series of steps to the formation of inosinic acid (IMP), which is the common intermediate nucleotide. Inosinic acid may be converted either to AMP or to GMP. Once the purine nucleotides are formed, they are utilized for the synthesis of nucleic acids, cyclic AMP, cyclic GMP, ATP, and important cofactors.

The purine components of nucleic acids and cyclic nucleotides are degraded to purine nucleotide monophosphates (Fig. 1). Guanylic acid is then degraded via guanosine, guanine, and xanthine to uric acid. Inosinic acid is degraded directly through inosine, hypoxanthine, and xanthine to uric acid. Adenylic acid may be deaminated to form IMP and further catabolized through inosine to uric acid in a way similar to IMP or it may be degraded to inosine by an alternate pathway with the intermediate formation of adenosine. The enzymatic components of those reactions are listed at the bottom of Fig. 1.

The main step in the *de novo* synthesis of purine nucleotides is catalyzed by the enzyme amidophosphoribosyltransferase (Fig. 1). This enzyme is thought to be the rate-limiting step in the *de novo* pathway of uric acid formation. In man, this enzyme appears to be under the regulation of intracellular purine nucleotides and phosphoribosylpyrophosphate (PRPP). The intracellular concentration of PRPP will determine, to a great extent, the rate of synthesis of uric acid. Although exceptions may exist, in general, when the concentration of PRPP is elevated, uric acid synthesis is elevated; when the concentration of PRPP is reduced, the synthesis of uric acid is reduced. This concept may apply to most clinical situations.

III. ORIGIN OF URIC ACID IN MAN

A. Exogenous

Unless an individual is fasting or ingesting a purine-free diet, the exogenous intake of purine is sufficient to maintain urinary excretion of uric acid. The excretion will depend on both the amount and type of purine in the diet. When young healthy males are placed on a purine-free diet, serum urate falls approximately 37% in 10 days, and urinary excretion declines about 33%. The difference between the amounts of purine administered and excreted may result from partial hydrolysis, incomplete absorption, gastrointestinal decomposition, suppression of purine synthesis *de novo*, or a combination of some or all of these factors.

B. Endogenous

After 5 to 7 days of severe dietary purine restriction, urine excretion of uric acid declines to constant low values. Mean values range from 300 to 400 mg/24 hr. These values reflect the continued synthesis and turnover of endogenous purines. It should be pointed out that the urine uric acid excretion accounts for only a part of the daily disposition of uric acid. Another part is disposed of by extrarenal routes. Thus, assessment of the true rate of endogenous purine turnover requires the use of isotope dilution techniques in subjects in whom the exogenous contribution has been reduced to a minimum by severe dietary purine restriction.

IV. DISPOSITION OF URIC ACID

A. Extrarenal

A normal man on a purine-free diet has a urate pool of about 1200 mg. The pool size in a normal woman is half as large. In the normal person, approximately 50–60% of the urate pool turns over each day. Thus, on a purine-free diet, an average man synthesizes and disposes of about 600 to 700 mg of uric acid in 24 hr. Of that amount, 450 mg of uric acid is excreted in the urine, and about 200 mg is eliminated through the gastrointestinal tract. Colonic bacteria possess uricase, allantoinase, allantoicase, and urease which act sequentially in the degradation of uric acid to carbon dioxide and ammonia as the end products. Very little uric acid, however, will be present in the stool. Nevertheless, in pathological states such as renal failure, gastrointestinal excretion of uric acid can increase several times.

B. Renal Handling of Uric Acid in Man

Except for approximately 5% of plasma urate which may be protein bound, uric acid is freely filtered across the glomerulus. In the early part of the proximal tubule, 90 to 100% of the filtered urate is reabsorbed. A variable percentage of the filtered load is secreted back into the tubular lumen in a more distal region of the proximal tubule. This three-component mechanism—filtration, reabsorption, and secretion—has been expanded to include a fourth component, postsecretory reabsorption, which may occur in the late part of the proximal tubule or in the distal tubule (Fig. 2). The final urine concentration of uric acid will be a function of the relative amounts of tubular secretion and postsecretory reabsorption. Normally, the tubular secretory capacity of uric acid is very high and may account for as much as 85% of the tubular load of urate. Since only about 12% of the filtered urate load appears in the urine, the postsecretory reabsorption of uric acid must be of a magnitude similar to that of the secretory component.

To summarize, the most widely accepted model of urate handling by the kidney is a four-component system which includes: (1) filtration; (2) reab-

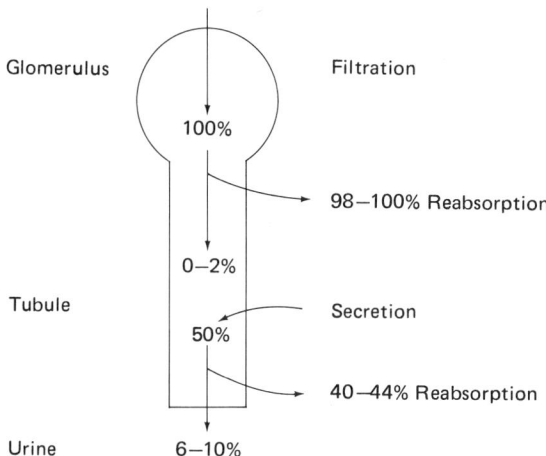

Figure 2. Renal handling of uric acid in man.

sorption in the proximal tubule; (3) secretion in the proximal tubule possibly coexisting with reabsorption; and (4) reabsorption in the distal nephron, possibly the collecting duct, which represents the postsecretory reabsorptive site.

V. EVALUATION OF HYPERURICEMIC STATES

A. Etiology of Hyperuricemia

Hyperuricemia may be defined as primary or secondary (Fig. 3). In the secondary form, hyperuricemia develops in the course of another disease or as a consequence of its treatment. Whatever the etiology of hyperuricemia, it may reflect overproduction of purines, reduced renal clearance of uric acid, or a combination of the two mechanisms (Fig. 4).

In most patients with hyperuricemia, an underlying etiology can be defined from history and physical examination. In addition, it may be the first clue to the presence of a previously unsuspected disorder and should not go unexplored in any patient.

Figure 5 summarizes the evaluation of hyperuricemia. It seems reasonable to use as guidelines for the work-up the initial history and physical examination. For example, acquired hyperuricemia may be associated with normal uric acid excretion and its cause known (e.g., diuretics). Under most circumstances, further evaluation of such patient is probably not warranted. Quantification of the 24-hr urinary uric acid is useful to determine if the patient presents an underlying disorder associated with an overproduction of uric acid. The higher the urine uric acid in these patients, the higher the incidence of renal calculi and of acute uric acid nephropathy; therefore, the greater is the need for treatment.

Some authorities have suggested that 24-hr urine uric acid should be measured only in those patients with a serum uric acid above 13 mg/100 ml, particularly if no secondary causes are clearly detectable.

B. Work-up for Hyperuricemia

1. History

Once a patient with elevated serum uric acid is encountered, it is necessary to formulate questions that may help our understanding of the problem.

1. Is the hyperuricemia primary or secondary?
2. Is the patient overweight?
3. Is the patient an alcoholic?
4. Does the patient take diuretics or any other drugs?

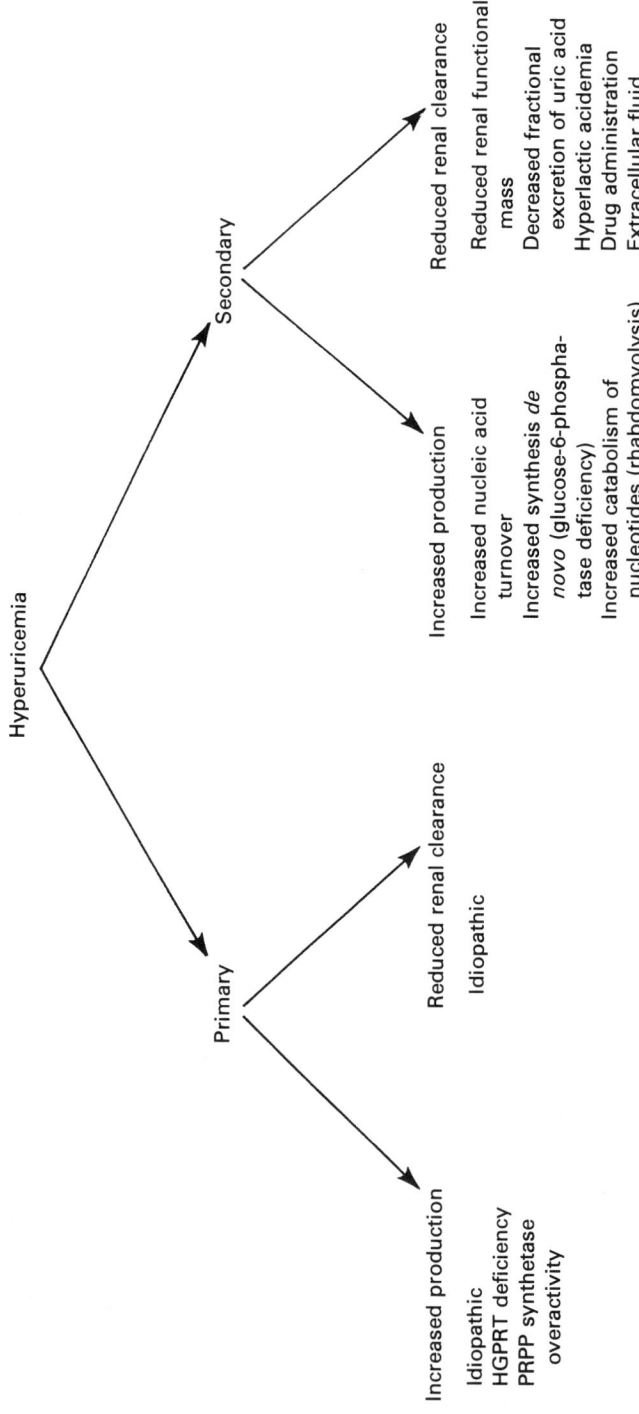

Figure 3. Classification of hyperuricemia.

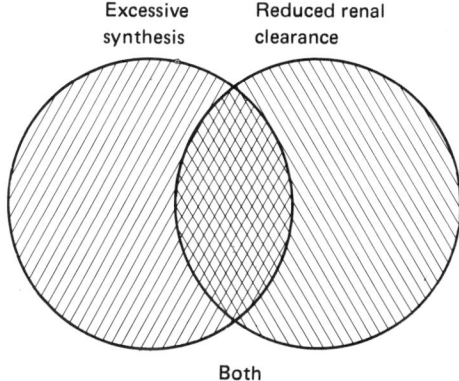

Excessive synthesis

Reduced renal clearance

Both

Figure 4. Mechanisms of hyperuricemia.

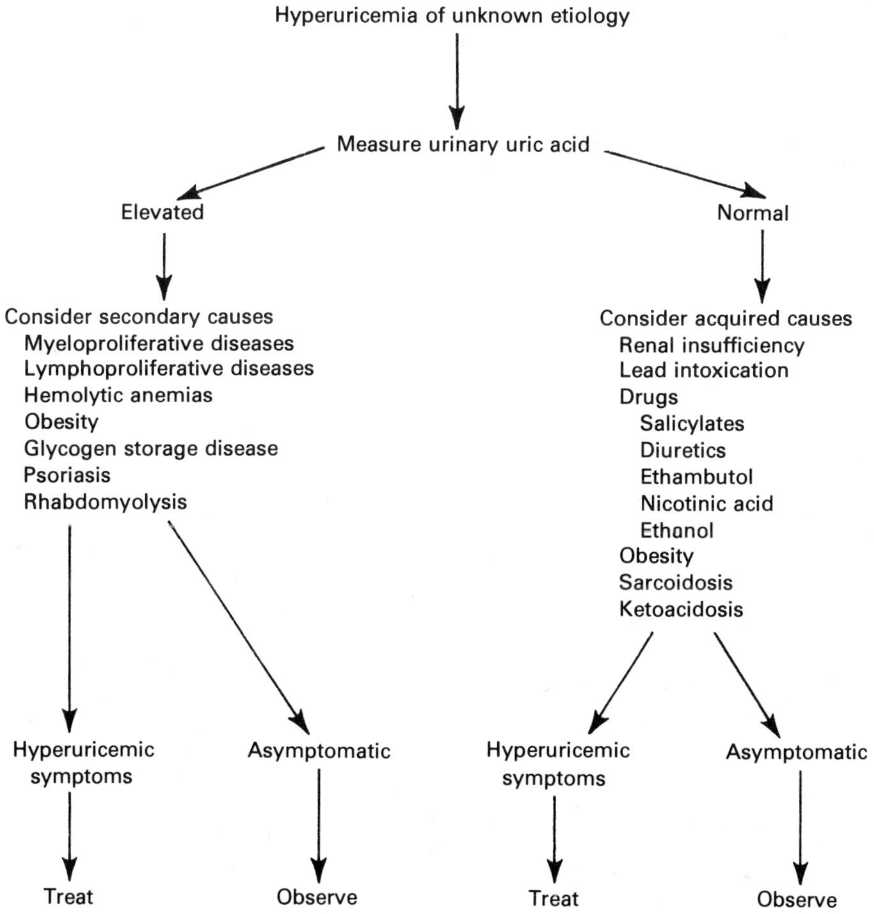

Hyperuricemia of unknown etiology

Measure urinary uric acid

Elevated

Normal

Consider secondary causes
  Myeloproliferative diseases
  Lymphoproliferative diseases
  Hemolytic anemias
  Obesity
  Glycogen storage disease
  Psoriasis
  Rhabdomyolysis

Consider acquired causes
  Renal insufficiency
  Lead intoxication
  Drugs
    Salicylates
    Diuretics
    Ethambutol
    Nicotinic acid
    Ethanol
  Obesity
  Sarcoidosis
  Ketoacidosis

Hyperuricemic symptoms

Asymptomatic

Hyperuricemic symptoms

Asymptomatic

Treat

Observe

Treat

Observe

Figure 5. Investigation of hyperuricemic states.

5. Does the patient have kidney disease?
6. Is there a history of a myeloproliferative disease?
7. Is there any history of acute arthritis suggestive of gout?
8. Is there a history of kidney stones?
9. Is there family history of hyperuricemia, gout, nephrolithiasis, or renal disease?
10. Is there a history of hypertension or heart disease?

2. Physical Examination

Once we have answered those questions, we should look for findings in the physical examination that may help to clarify the cause of hyperuricemia. Special attention should be given to the weight and height of the patient. Other important findings to look for are lymphoadenopathy, hepatospleno-megaly, hypertension, and the presence of tophi or joint disease.

3. Laboratory Studies

The next steps in evaluation of a patient with hyperuricemia include urinalysis and determination of hemoglobin, hematocrit, white blood cell count, creatinine clearance, and 24-hr excretion of uric acid. The patient should not be taking drugs capable of influencing serum or urine uric acid values. Some special tests that are helpful include: (1) synovial fluid analysis in the patient with arthritis and hyperuricemia; (2) needle aspiration or biopsy of suspected tophi for urate crystal identification; and (3) analysis for uric acid and other constituents of any recovered kidney stones.

4. Assessment of Tissue Damage

After the initial work-up is completed, an assessment of tissue damage attributable to hyperuricemia should be made. This includes patients with arthritis, subcutaneous nodules, bone erosions demonstrable on X-ray, kidney stones, or renal insufficiency.

5. Presence of Kidney Stones

A history or laboratory findings indicative of a renal calculus provides information important to the future management of the patient. A typical uric acid stone is radiolucent and therefore may not be visible on routine films of the abdomen. It will appear as a filling defect with the use of radioopaque contrast material and may be confused with other radiolucent stones such as cysteine and the rare xanthine stones or with blood clots or tumors.

It is important to evaluate the patient who presents with hyperuricemia and radioopaque stones, since the initial nidus for opaque stones in this setting is frequently uric acid. It has been recommended that patients with hyperuricosuria who form calcium-containing stones be given a trial with allopurinol.

6. Renal Insufficiency

In the evaluation of hyperuricemia, we may face the difficult problem of assessing the relationship of hyperuricemia to renal insufficiency in the patient who presents with both abnormalities. Hyperuricemia may be of etiologic importance in the patient with gout and renal insufficiency in whom the cause for the renal disease is not apparent. In the patient with acute renal failure, acute uric acid nephropathy should be considered. In this setting, the uric acid/creatinine ratio (times 100) in a spot urine may help in the diagnosis. The finding of a ratio in excess of 1.0 in a patient with acute renal failure is indicative of a substantial increase in urate production and increases the possibility that uric acid deposition in the collecting duct system may be contributing to the renal insufficiency.

In acute uric acid nephropathy vigorous therapy is indicated as outlined below. It should be pointed out that the more common finding in acute renal failure of other origin is a ratio of less than 1.0 and that the hyperuricemia in those cases may be entirely a result of the renal disease (fall in GFR) and associated factors such as dehydration or acidosis.

VI. RENAL COMPLICATIONS OF HYPERURICEMIA

Individuals with hyperuricemia may present two types of renal damage: chronic gouty nephropathy and uric acid nephropathy. Chronic gouty nephropathy is caused by deposition of sodium urate crystals in the renal interstitial tissue and by the associated inflammatory reaction. This condition is most commonly seen with longstanding hyperuricemia. Uric acid nephropathy is secondary to the formation of crystals in the collecting tubules, pelvis, or ureters, with the resulting blockade of urine flow. This second type of renal damage associated with hyperuricemia is related to hyperuricosuria and is subdivided in two types, acute uric acid nephropathy and uric acid stones. Each type of renal lesion appears in a sufficiently distinctive setting to allow a presumptive diagnosis on clinical grounds, and only rarely do both lesions coexist in the same kidney.

A. Chronic Gouty Nephropathy

As the name implies, this condition is most commonly associated with gout and chronic hyperuricemia. In fact, significant urate nephropathy is rare in the absence of gouty arthritis. Chronic renal disease may account for

20 to 25% of deaths in the gouty population. A common manifestation of urate nephropathy is *albuminuria* which is present in 20 to 40% of patients with gout. It is usually mild and intermittent. An early manifestation may be inability to generate a maximally concentrated urine after 18 hr of water deprivation ($U_{max} < 800$ mOsm/kg).

Hypertension, which occurs in about 33% of the gouty population, may contribute to the renal disease, or, in turn, urate nephropathy may aggravate the hypertensive state. As the renal disease progresses, azotemia and renal failure appear. At this stage, it may be difficult to determine whether renal disease is a consequence of hyperuricemia and urate nephropathy or whether the hyperuricemia is secondary to the renal disease. Nevertheless, as mentioned previously, a history of gout suggests that urate nephropathy is the underlying disease, since gout is rarely seen in chronic renal disease of other etiologies. This type of renal disease has a characteristic histological finding, namely, the deposit of urate crystals with a giant-cell reaction in the interstitium of the medulla and pyramids. It has been concluded by different investigators that the initial lesion is damage of the tubular epithelium of the loop of Henle and juxtaposed interstitial tissue. In addition to the changes in the tubules and interstitium, hyalinization of the glomeruli and hypertrophy of the intima and portions of the media of the arterioles may be prominent.

B. Uric Acid Nephropathy

1. Acute

This condition results from tubular obstruction as a result of urate and uric acid deposits in the tubular system. The disease is usually found in association with neoplastic disorders in which there are rapid cellular turnover and elevated plasma levels of urate from nucleic acid catabolism. It may also occur in patients with gout and accelerated purine synthesis and rhabdomyolysis, the latter producing marked hyperuricemia, uricaciduria, and strongly acid urines.

The pathogenesis of acute uric acid nephropathy is intimately related to the fact that uric acid exists at concentrations approaching or exceeding saturation under normal conditions. When filtered urate is at very high concentrations, it is further concentrated as water abstraction occurs. In the latter portions of the tubule, the acid environment may lead to tubular precipitation and obstruction. This precipitation occurs predominantly within the collecting duct system and results in increased intratubular pressure, an overall increase in intrarenal pressure, and extrinsic compression of the small renal venous network. The compression of the venous system leads to an increase in renal vascular resistance and a subsequent fall in renal blood flow. The elevated tubular pressure and decreased renal blood flow diminish the glomerular filtration, leading to renal failure. The majority of the deposition of urate material is located within the collecting duct system, and occasionally, ureteral calculi may form and contribute to the problem.

Acute uric acid nephropathy is a preventable condition and, furthermore, may be reversed by prompt, aggressive management. This condition occurs almost exclusively in the setting of an underlying malignancy in which there is rapid turnover of cells and loss of nuclear proteins into the plasma. In addition, patients with such disorders as leukemias or lymphomas are likely to receive radiation therapy or chemotherapy which, by its tumor lysis effect, increases the load of uric acid presented to the kidneys. Furthermore, many of those patients have extracellular fluid volume depletion as a result of anorexia and vomiting, a condition that results in low urine volumes of high concentration, and low urine pH is not uncommon under these circumstances.

There are several features of this syndrome that are distinctive. The hyperuricemia is usually between *20 and 90 mg/100 ml* at the onset of renal dysfunction. *Oliguria and azotemia* are common features. However, the most distinctive feature of this syndrome is the amount of uric acid excreted in the urine in patients who are not anuric. In most cases of renal failure from other etiologies, the urinary uric acid excretion is normal or reduced and the urine-to-plasma uric acid ratio divided by the urine-to-plasma creatinine ratio in a spot urine specimen is usually less than 1.0. In acute uric acid nephropathy, this ratio is greater than 1.0 and helps to confirm the diagnosis in patients who present with acute renal failure and hyperuricemia. Once the diagnosis is confirmed, therapy should be initiated at once.

2. Uric Acid Nephrolithiasis

Uric acid stones account for approximately 5 to 10% of all stones in the United States, but in countries such as Israel, they may account for up to 40% of all stones. In patients with gout, the prevalence ranges from 10 to 25% or approximately 1000 times greater than in the general population. Uric acid stones may occur in patients without a history of gouty arthritis, and about 20% of the patients in this group are hyperuricemic. Other conditions that may lead to uric acid stones are shown on Fig. 6.

Several factors that may predispose toward uric acid stones in gout are: (1) increased urinary excretion of uric acid; (2) undue acidity of the urine; (3) increased urine concentration; and (4) perhaps qualitative abnormalities of other urinary constituents which may affect solubility of uric acid. However, the most important factor leading to uric acid stones in such patients appears to be an increased concentration of uric acid in urine.

Hormones such as estrogens and corticosteroids increase uric acid excretion. Dehydration resulting from excessive extrarenal loss of water by way of the skin or gastrointestinal tract leads to a reduced urine volume and to an increased urinary concentration of uric acid. This may explain the high prevalence of uric acid stones in hot dry climates such as Israel or in patients

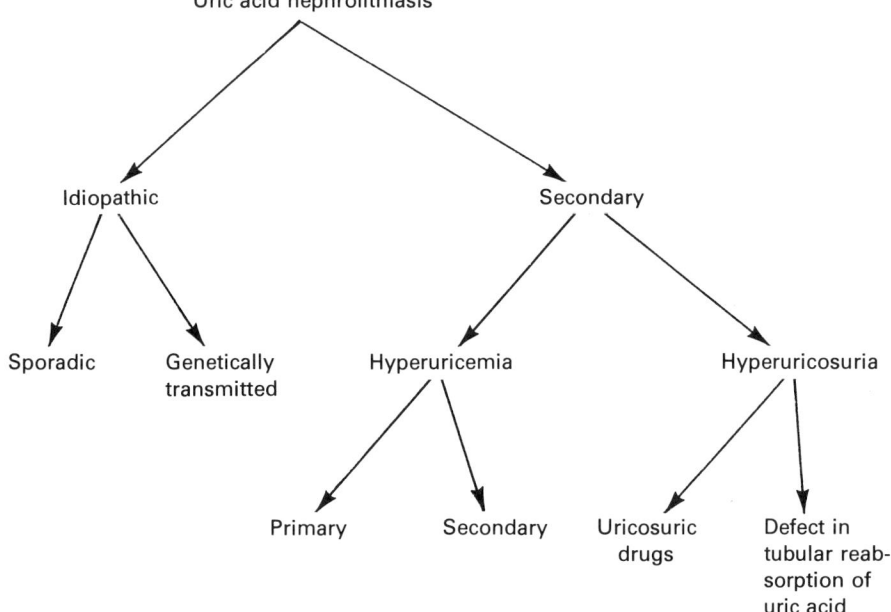

Figure 6. Uric acid nephrolithiasis.

with ileostomies who exhibit increased renal conservation of sodium, a decreased urinary Na^+/K^+ ratio, increased urinary acid excretion, low urinary pH values, and low urine volumes.

An idiopathic form of uric acid lithiasis has been described. It may be sporadic or familial (Fig. 6). Both groups have normal plasma and urinary uric acid concentrations and a tendency toward acid urines in the absence of other abnormalities of renal function. Both conditions are rare causes of uric acid lithiasis.

VII. THERAPY OF HYPERURICEMIC STATES

Every patient who presents with symptoms related to hyperuricemia should be treated with antihyperuricemic agents. Controversy as to therapy is encountered when hyperuricemia is uncomplicated by gout, as is asymptomatic hyperuricemia. Figures 5 and 7 summarize the approach to hyperuricemia.

A. Asymptomatic Hyperuricemia

Asymptomatic hyperuricemia is defined as that stage in which the serum uric acid level is elevated but arthritis, tophi, or nephrolithiasis have not occurred (Fig. 5). In most subjects with asymptomatic hyperuricemia, this stage lasts throughout life without evidence of serious complications. Although there are conflicting notions as to when to treat asymptomatic hyperuricemia, our recommendations are not to treat unless (1) the patient presents with a 24-hr urinary uric acid in excess of 1000 mg or (2) a serum uric acid level greater than 13 mg/100 ml. Both of these suggest a substantial uric acid overproduction with its potential complications.

It is not reasonable to treat hyperuricemia with the goal of preventing gout, since gout therapy is reserved for the onset of arthritis. Most studies have shown that renal function is not adversely affected by asymptomatic hyperuricemia and that correction of hyperuricemia has no apparent effect on renal function. In fact, hyperuricemia is a reflection of the renal disease that accompanies uncontrolled hypertension rather than the cause of the renal disease.

B. Uric Acid Nephrolithiasis

In patients who present with hyperuricemia and uric acid stones, the first therapeutic rule is to maintain a large urinary volume by the liberal ingestion of fluids, about 2–3 liters per day if the cardiovascular status permits it. This is very important in those patients whose daily urinary uric acid excretion is augmented. Besides liberal fluid intake, drug therapy with allopurinol, 300–600 mg per day, should be given. This will lower serum

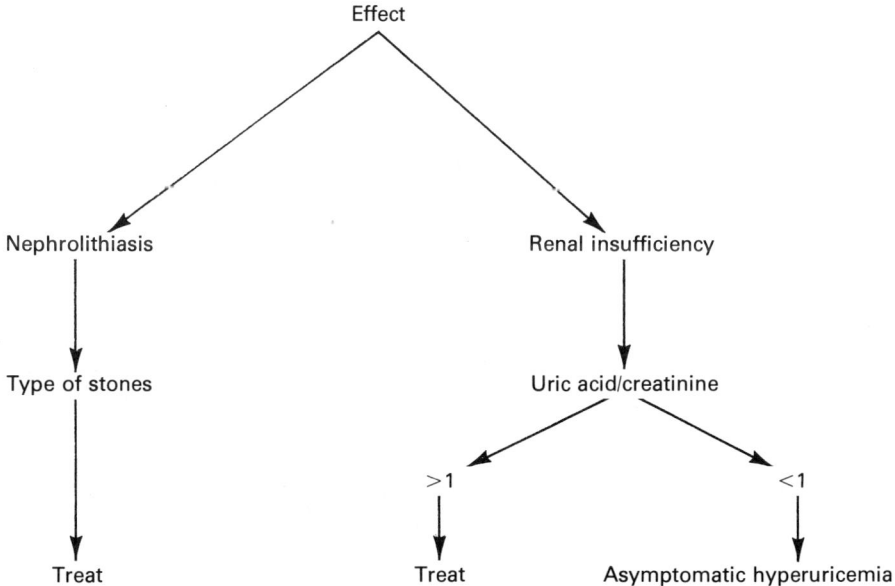

Figure 7. Treatment decision for hyperuricemia and renal disease.

and urinary uric acid. Uricosuric agents such as probenecid should not be given to patients with hyperuricosuria and uric acid stones and are, in fact, contraindicated.

C. Acute Uric Acid Nephropathy

1. Conservative Management

All severely hyperuricemic patients should undergo the procedures indicated below. Moreover, any subject about to receive chemotherapy and/or radiotherapy for lympho- or myeloproliferative disorders should be handled similarly.

a. Forced Diuresis

If the patient is not anuric or oliguric, intravenous fluids should be administered to achieve a urine output of 100 ml/hr. Saline, 0.45% and 0.9%, with and without 5% glucose are satisfactory as intravenous fluids. In addition, diuretics such as furosemide or ethacrynic acid may be used to maintain an adequate urine output and reduce tendencies for fluid retention (Fig. 8).

b. Urine Alkalinization

This can be achieved with azetazolamide, 250 to 1000 mg per day, given orally or by the use of one to four ampules of sodium bicarbonate (7.5%) added to 5% glucose in water and administered intravenously to produce a urine pH of 7.0. The urine should be checked hourly for pH changes. Fluid balance should be carefully monitored. In cases in which acetazolamide is used, therapy should not last longer than necessary, since it will lead to systemic acidosis. If tolerated and absolutely necessary, a combination of bicarbonate infusion and acetazolamide administration may be tried in an

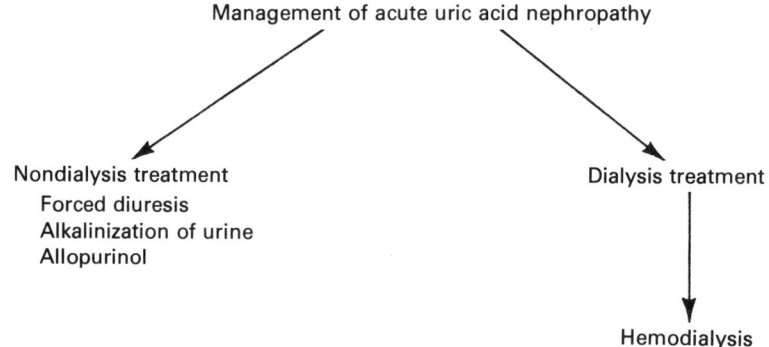

Figure 8. Management of acute uric acid nephropathy.

attempt to avoid acidosis. One should watch for hypokalemia and replace urine K^+ losses secondary to the sodium–bicarbonaturia.

c. Allopurinol

This inhibitor of xanthine oxidase is given orally in doses ranging from 300 to 1000 mg daily in subjects with acute uric acid nephropathy. Because of its long half-life, it may be given as a single dose. A potential complication of the therapy outlined above may result from the use of xanthine oxidase inhibitors. Allopurinol leads to accumulation of xanthine, hypoxanthine, and oxipurinol, all of which have the potential to precipitate in the tubules. Nevertheless, such a complication has only been reported (for xanthine) in patients with lymphomas of large tumoral mass receiving chemotherapy and allopurinol. Renal stones composed of xanthine and oxipurinol have also been described.

2. Dialysis

When, despite urine alkalinization, high urine flow rates, and allopurinol, acute renal shutdown supervenes, dialysis would be the treatment of choice. This procedure not only removes large amounts of urate from the ECFV but controls the metabolic complications of acute renal failure.

Hemodialysis is the more effective procedure for urate dialysis. Clearances of up to 150 ml/min can be obtained with blood flows of 300–400 ml/min, a value that is ten times the clearance observed by peritoneal dialysis. The higher urate clearances are found with large parallel-plate dialyzers. Smaller clearances are obtained with hollow fibers and coil dialyzers. Reductions of up to 50% of the original plasma concentration can be achieved in 6 hr.

VIII. HYPOURICEMIC STATES

The definition of hypouricemia is arbitrary, and its significance has been elucidated only recently. However, most investigators have defined hypouricemia as a serum acid value of 2.0 mg/100 ml or less. This may result from a decreased production of urate or from enhanced elimination of this compound (Fig. 9).

A. Decreased Production of Uric Acid

Several potential mechanisms for a reduced production of uric acid can be adduced from Fig. 1. Xanthinuria, which results from a marked reduction of xanthine oxidase activity, is associated with the most profound hypouri-

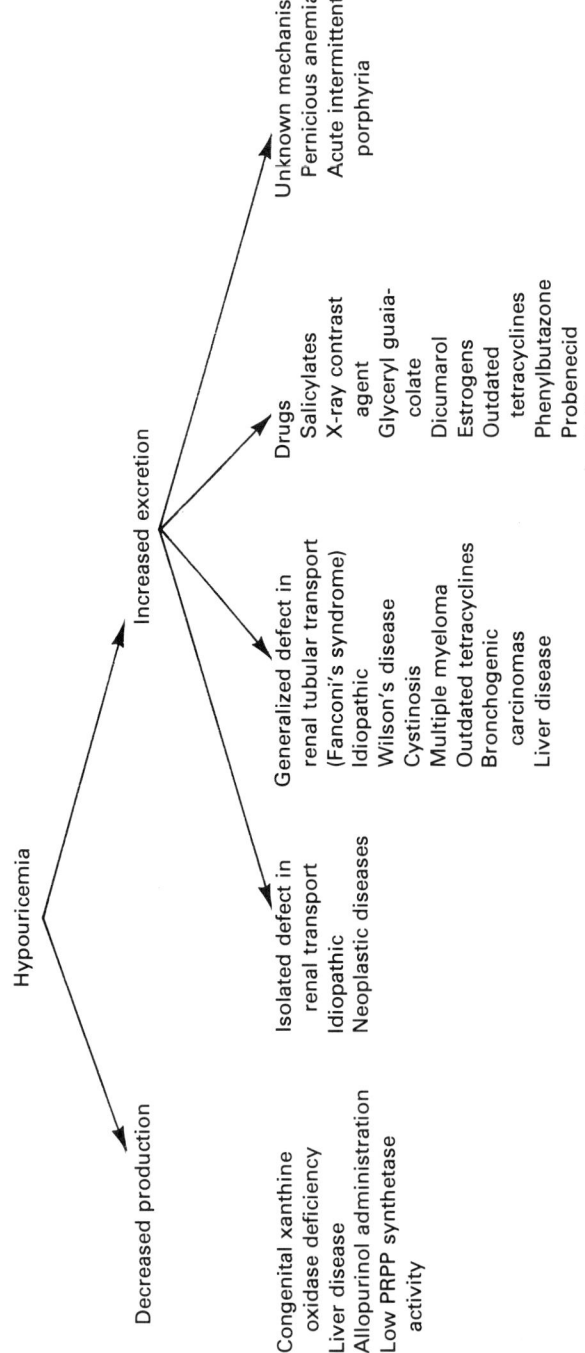

Figure 9. Causes of hypouricemia.

cemia in man. This enzyme defect leads to a reduced synthesis of uric acid and causes an accumulation of the precursors, hypoxanthine and xanthine. The serum urate concentration in xanthinuria is usually less than 1.0 mg/ 100 ml.

Hypouricemia may be seen in patients with hepatic disease. The mechanism may involve reduced xanthine oxidase production by the liver; however, other factors such as acquired renal tubular defects may also play a role. Allopurinol and its major metabolite oxipurinol are potent inhibitors of xanthine oxidase and lead to a prompt reduction in the serum urate concentration in most subjects.

B. Increased Excretion of Uric Acid

Theoretically, hypouricemia could also result from an increased degradation of uric acid, increased secretion through the gastrointestinal tract, or an increased renal excretion of uric acid. However, only the last mechanism has been shown to be important as a cause of hypouricemia.

An isolated defect in the renal transport of uric acid has been described. This may be idiopathic or associated with neoplastic disorders (Hodgkin's disease and pulmonary tumors) or liver diseases. In the idiopathic isolated defect, all patients demonstrate a high uric acid clearance with no other evidence of tubular dysfunction present. Hypouricemia has also been associated with a generalized defect in the transport of solutes in the proximal tubule (Fanconi syndrome) (Fig. 9). Besides hyperuricosuria, patients with the complete syndrome exhibit phosphaturia, hypophospatemia, glucosuria, low serum glucose, aminoaciduria, bicarbonate wasting, and metabolic acidosis. The increased clearance of uric acid is perhaps one of the most sensitive indices of tubular dysfunction in the Fanconi syndrome.

The most common cause of hypouricemia is drug administration, and drugs are implicated in about 66% of the cases of hypouricemia. The most important uricosuric drugs are salicylates in high doses, glyceryl guaiacolate, and X-ray contrast agents (Fig. 9). Drugs may induce uricosuria by decreasing urate binding to proteins, inhibiting the reabsorption of filtered urate, or enhancing urate secretion.

SUGGESTED READINGS

Barrientos A, Pérez-Díaz V, Díaz González R, et al: Hypouricemia by defect in tubular reabsorption. Arch Intern Med 139:787–789, 1979.
Boss GR, Seegmiller JE: Hyperuricemia and gout. N Engl J Med 300:1459–1468, 1979.
Conger JD: Acute uric acid nephropathy. Sem Nephrol 1:69–74, 1981.
Kelton J, Kelley WN, Homes EW: A rapid method for the diagnosis of acute uric acid nephropathy. Arch Intern Med 138:612–615, 1978.

Lian MH, Fries JF: Asymptomatic hyperuricemia: The case for conservative management. *Ann Intern Med* 88:666–670, 1978.

Perry MC, Hoagland C, Wagoner R: Uric acid nephropathy. *JAMA* 236:961–962, 1976.

Steele TH, Rieselbach RE: Renal urate excretion in normal man. *Nephron* 14:21–32, 1975.

Warnock DG: Uric acid, diuretics and the kidney. *West J Med* 129:407–411, 1978.

Wyngaarden JB, Kelley WN: *Gout and Hyperuricemia.* New York, Grune & Stratton, 1976.

Yü TF, Berger L, Dorph D, et al: Renal function in gout. V. Factors influencing the renal hemodynamics. *Am J Med* 67:766–771, 1979.

9

Management of Glomerulonephritis and Nephrotic Syndrome

CECIL H. COGGINS

I. PATHOGENESIS OF GLOMERULONEPHRITIS

Antigens stimulating antibody formation with a subsequent train of events have been documented in the development of several kinds of glomerulonephritis (GN). This once straightforward immunologic picture has become complicated in recent years, with T and B lymphocytes, macrophages, complement, granulocytes, and fibrin playing prominent roles in addition to antigen and antibody (Fig. 1).

Antigens from both within and outside the body participate in these processes. Hepatitis, malarial, schistosomal, and other infective antigens have been demonstrated in glomeruli, as have tumor surface components, DNA, thyroglobulin, and other naturally occurring antigens. Under the influence of "helper" T lymphocytes and despite the action of "suppressor" T cells, B lymphocytes are stimulated to produce and release antibodies specific for the inciting antigen. Abnormalities in these subpopulations of lymphocytes, genetic or acquired, may influence the type, number, and timing of the resulting antibodies and determine the type of resulting glomerular damage or, indeed, whether any damage occurs.

Initially, the immunopathology of glomerulonephritis was considered in two broad divisions: (1) that in which the induced antibodies reacted

CECIL H. COGGINS • Department of Medicine, Harvard Medical School; and Renal Unit, Massachusetts General Hospital, Boston, Massachusetts 02114.

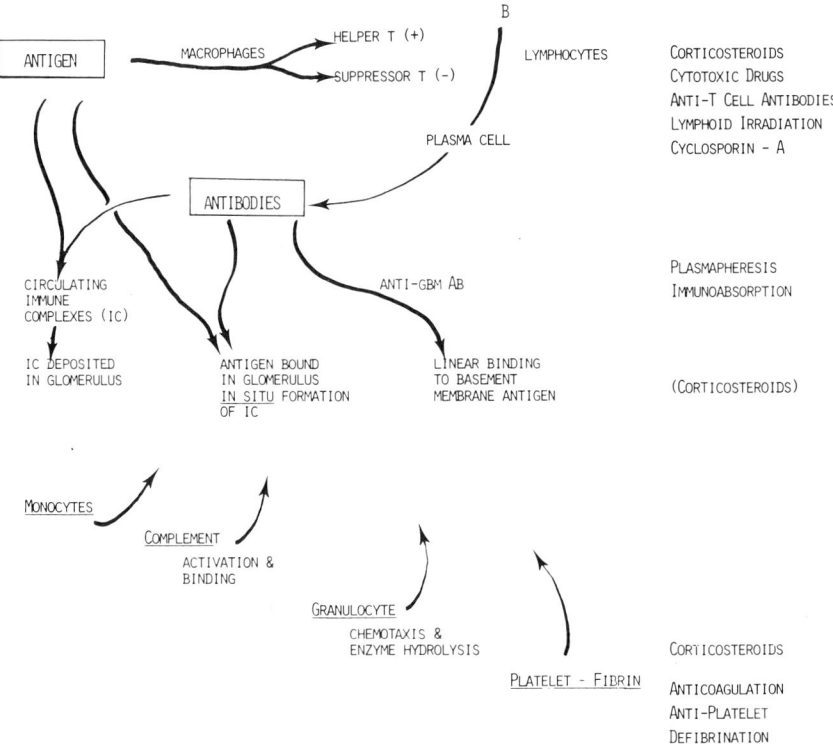

Figure 1. Schematic representation of the immunopathogenesis of glomerular disease indicating where therapy might interrupt the process.

directly with receptors in the glomeruli; and (2) that in which circulating complexes of antigen and antibody become lodged in the glomeruli, producing damage.

In the first type, anti-glomerular-basement antibodies can be found in the blood, and immunofluorescence microscopy shows a linear deposition of antibody along the glomerular capillary wall. Some patients with rapidly progressive, crescentic GN (RPGN) show this pathology, as do those with Goodpasture's syndrome. It is not clear whether the antigenic stimulus in these cases is a component of the glomerulus, or whether some nonglomerular antigen shares some characteristic of the glomerular capillary wall and initiates the process.

The second mechanism with circulating immune complexes has been demonstrated in some types of naturally occurring glomerulonephritis as well as in animal models. In the "serum sickness model," following the administration of a single dose of foreign protein antigen, glomerular damage occurs after antibody production begins but before a great excess of antibody removes all antigen from the circulation. Not all glomerulonephritides have demonstrable circulating immune complexes, however, and recent work shows other means by which antibody can become deposited in glomeruli. Immune complexes may form *in situ* when antigen first becomes fixed in glomeruli and later binds antibody. Antibody may also bind to glomerular receptors without any demonstrable antigen present.

However the antibody comes to rest in the glomeruli, activation and fixation of complement, attraction of granulocytes with release of their lysosomal enzymes, and, often, the deposition of fibrin contribute to ensuing glomerular damage. In some animal models, a foreign antigen initiates the disease process, and injured components of kidney then become new antigens that sustain the chronic disease. This could occur in human disease as well but has not been clearly demonstrated to date.

The complex series of events offers a number of points at which outside influence might alter the outcome. Corticosteroids, which suppress the attraction of granulocytes and the release of their enzymes, also affect localization of antibody in the glomerulus. Steroids may also change the relative numbers and activities of lymphocyte subsets, as do cyclophosphamide, chlorambucil, and azathioprine. Anticoagulants and platelet inhibitors affect the formation of thrombi and fibrin. Plasmapheresis can remove circulating immune complexes as well as complement components, clotting factors, and other plasma components. In addition, plasmapheresis can improve the efficiency of the monocytic phagocyte system. The mechanism of this effect is not clear. Extracorporeal immunoabsorption may offer a more specific means to remove some of these components. Unfortunately, present therapy, empirically chosen, barely begins to tap these possibilities. Perhaps in the near future "shotgun immunosuppression" will be supplemented by more specific agents with fewer harmful side effects.

II. PATHOPHYSIOLOGY OF NEPHROTIC SYNDROME

When glomerular disease results in severe protein loss, whether the glomerular damage results from primary kidney disease or from a systemic illness, the group of abnormalities known as nephrotic syndrome appears.

A list of diseases that may manifest nephrotic syndrome is presented in Table I. The elements of nephrotic syndrome include hypoalbuminemia, edema, hyperlipidemia, and lipiduria, together with large quantities of proteinuria (usually defined as more than 3 g/day in adults and proportionate amounts in children). Many glomerular diseases pass through a nephrotic stage, and skillful management of the elements of the nephrotic syndrome will go far toward relieving the patient's symptoms. Indeed, it will often be all we have to offer.

A. Proteinuria

One of the earliest and most characteristic clinical abnormalities occurring in patients with glomerulonephritis is proteinuria. Instead of the 50

Table I. Nephrotic Syndrome

	Relative incidence	
	Adults	Children
Primary glomerular diseases (75%)		
Membranous	30%	

Proliferative and focal
   Acute (poststreptococcal) glomerulonephritis (rare)
   Rapidly progressive (subacute) glomerulonephritis
   "Focal" and mesangial proliferative glomerulonephritis
   Focal sclerosis
	20%	

Membranoproliferative, including dense deposit disease	7%	
Minimal-lesion (lipoid) nephrosis	18%	80–90%
Other disorders (25%)		

Relatively common
   Diabetes mellitus
   Systemic lupus erythematosus
   Amyloid (including multiple myeloma)		

Uncommon causes
   Associated with malignancy
     Hodgkin's, lymphoma, usually minimal change
     Other tumors, usually membranous
   Heavy metals, drugs, allergens, gold, mercury,
     probenecid, penicillamine, triparamethadione,
     "street" heroin
   Infections
     Bacterial endocarditis and shunt infections,
     malaria, hepatitis, 2° and congenital syphilis,
     schistosomiasis
   ? Immunologic disease (in addition to SLE)
     Polyarteritis, dermatomyositis, scleroderma,
     Takayasu's disease, Sjogren's disease,
     Henoch–Schonlein purpura, serum sickness,
     transplant rejection, sarcoid, mixed
     cryoglobulinemia
   Congenital or familial (including Fabry's,
     Alport's, nail–patella)
   Pregnancy-associated		

mg/day or so of small proteins and peptides that appears in normal urine, the patient with glomerular disease will have pronounced proteinuria. The major component of this proteinuria is albumin, and its quantity is usually more than 1 or 2 g per day. In nephrotic syndrome, proteinuria of 4–15 g per day is typical, but even 50 g per day or more may be excreted (a remarkable demonstration of our capacity to synthesize albumin).

The normal glomerular capillary wall restricts the passage of proteins while allowing almost free filtration of water, salts, and smaller molecules into Bowman's space. Studies of the filtration of uncharged neutral dextran molecules demonstrate that restriction of glomerular filtration occurs with increasing molecular size. The smaller dextran particles pass across the capillary wall and into the urine together with water, salt, and markers of glomerular filtration such as inulin and creatinine. Larger dextran particles pass less freely until a size is reached at which no filtration occurs.

Similar studies using negatively charged dextran sulfate showed that the sulfate forms were filtered less freely than the uncharged neutral dextrans of the same molecular size. Thus, in addition to a size limitation, filtration is limited by electrical charge. Fixed negative charges on structures of the glomerular capillary wall are thought to repel and hence impede the filtration of negatively charged dextran. Since most plasma proteins are also negatively charged at physiological pH, it is probable that both charge and size normally restrict the passage of plasma proteins into the urine.

In glomerulonephritis, changes in the glomerular capillary wall alter this normal sieving action. In particular, the charge restriction seems to be lost, and negatively charged albumin and other proteins may pass from capillary into Bowman's space and the renal tubules.

The severity of the damage to the basement membrane may determine the nature and size of proteins that pass into the urine. With relatively mild abnormalities, the proteinuria may consist almost completely of albumin, whereas in more severe disease, a variety of larger proteins appear as well. This difference provides the basis for a diagnostic test, the "selectivity index." The test is most simply accomplished by measuring the blood and urine concentrations of immunoglobulin G (molecular weight about 160,000) and transferrin (molecular weight 88,000, only a little larger than albumin). The clearances of these proteins from the blood are calculated and, when expressed as the ratio of IgG clearance to transferrin clearance, constitute a "selectivity index." Values of 0.1 or less suggest relatively mild damage to the glomerular basement membrane, whereas values over 0.3 suggest more severe changes. Unfortunately, there is only a loose correlation between the different selectivities and specific histological diagnosis.

B. Hypoproteinemia

Hypoalbuminemia accounts for most of the reduction in total plasma protein concentration, although a degree of hypoglobulinemia may occur as globulins of smaller molecular weights are lost in the urine. The major cause of hypoalbuminemia is the loss of albumin into the urine, but when metabolic turnover rate is calculated, losses of albumin from the plasma and storage pools often exceed that appearing in the urine. This discrepancy may be explained by noting that some of the albumin that is filtered through the diseased glomerulus is subsequently reabsorbed by renal tubular epithelial cells and broken down into peptides or their constituent amino acids. There is also some evidence of increased loss of albumin elsewhere in the body.

Some nephrotic patients seem capable of remaining in albumin balance (with low serum albumin concentration) despite urinary protein losses of 20–30 g per day or more. Others, however, are severely hypoproteinemic with measured urinary losses of only a few grams. Poor appetite, ill-advised dietary protein restriction, or malabsorption as a result of edematous bowels may account for some limitations in albumin synthesis, but it seems likely that some impairment of liver protein synthesis may be present as well in some nephrotic patients.

C. Edema

Edema formation requires the movement of fluid from plasma into the interstitial space and the retention by the kidney of salt and water. The redistribution of salt and water into the interstitial space is the result of the reduced plasma oncotic pressure which follows from reduced plasma albumin concentration. There is little evidence to suggest that abnormalities of capillary permeability, surface area, or pressure lead to this edema formation. The renal retention of salt and water appears to be secondary to reduced plasma volume in most nephrotic patients, particularly those with minimal change disease. In some edematous nephrotics, however, plasma volume and circulating renin and aldosterone levels have been found to be normal even prior to their use of diuretics. Presumably, the salt and water retention in this latter group of patients result from some intrarenal abnormality accompanying the glomerular disease.

D. Hyperlipemia

Cholesterol, phospholipids, and triglycerides all tend to be elevated in the nephrotic syndrome in a roughly inverse relationship to the serum albumin concentration. Triglyceride elevation may not occur until albumin concentration is very much reduced but may then rise to extremely high levels, producing a lactescent serum.

Infusing dextran, PVP, or albumin itself to elevate plasma oncotic pressure leads to a reduction of hyperlipemia. It would appear that when the liver increases albumin synthesis in response to the stimulus of low plasma albumin concentration and low oncotic pressure, lipoprotein synthesis occurs as well.

E. Lipiduria

Droplets of lipid in casts, in cells, or as free fat droplets are a frequent finding in nephrotic urine sediment. Droplets of cholesterol esters form an optically active liquid crystal which is birefringent and appears as four bright quadrants of light separated by a dark cross-shaped area ("Maltese Cross") when they are viewed between crossed Nicol prisms or Polaroid® disks (Fig. 2). The source of the lipid appears to be lipoprotein filtered through the permeable glomerular membrane. Much of this filtered lipoprotein is taken up by tubular cells where it is partially degraded. The cells may slough into the tubular lumen and appear in the urine where they are seen as lipid-packed cells ("oval fat bodies").

III. GENERAL MANAGEMENT OF NEPHROTIC SYNDROME AND GLOMERULONEPHRITIS

A. Edema

Edema is most characteristic in nephrosis and may occur as well in acute glomerulonephritis or in chronic renal failure, especially when heart failure is present. It will respond to the same therapy used for nonrenal edema—

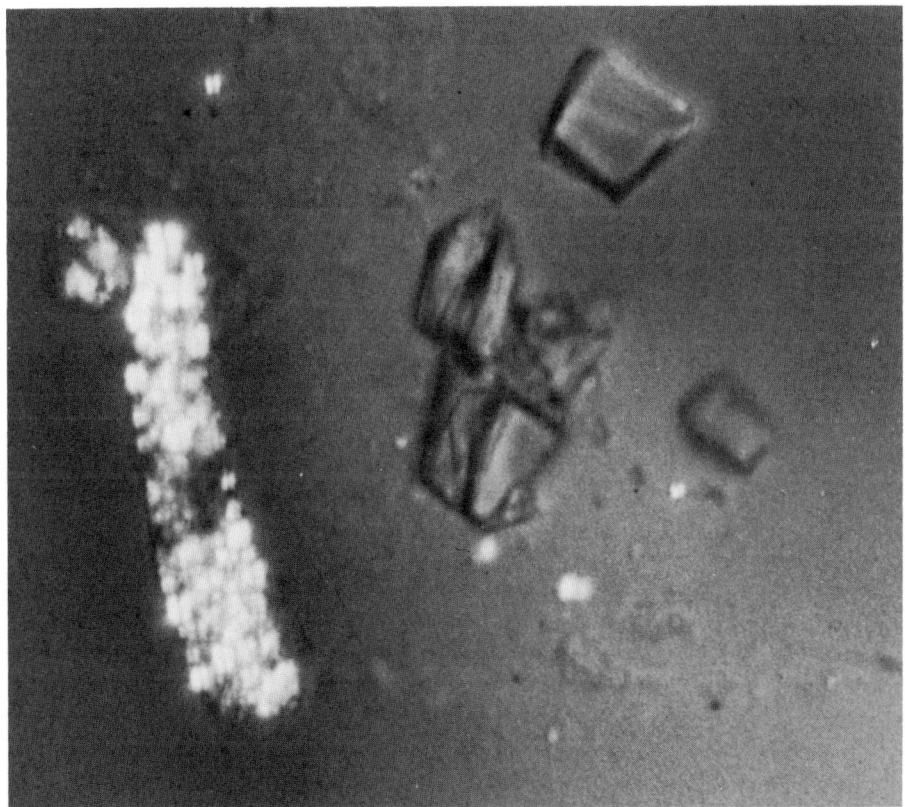

Figure 2. Maltese crosses in a fatty cast.

dietary salt restriction and diuretics. Note that a reduced plasma volume will be diminished even more by diuretics. Severe postural hypotension, "prerenal azotemia," or even shock may be produced by diuretics when the serum albumin concentration is particularly low. Since removal of the edema is symptomatic relief and has no effect on the underlying renal disease, the benefits of diuresis should be weighed against the hazards of further reduced plasma volume, glucose intolerance, hyperuricemia, and potassium depletion that may be induced by the diuretic. Mild edema need not require treatment at all. Life-threatening edema with ascites and pleural effusions may require a careful program of powerful diuretics and even the temporary use of simultaneous albumin infusions to sustain the plasma volume.

B. Hypoalbuminemia

The infusion of albumin to expand plasma volume ordinarily increases the proteinuria considerably above the baseline rate, so the effect on serum protein concentration lasts only a few days. It is therefore not practical for the management of chronic nephrotic syndrome but may tide the patient over short periods of intensive therapy. Generous dietary protein will insure that amino acids will be available for albumin synthesis.

C. Hyperlipemia

Although hypercholesterolemia is a potent risk factor for atherosclerosis in patients without renal disease, the story in nephrotics is not so clear. Although severe coronary artery narrowing was reported in one series of nephrotic patients, this group predominantly included patients with systemic lupus erythematosus and diabetes mellitus. These underlying diseases may have influenced the coronary artery disease. A recent study of nephrotic patients in southeast England showed no increased mortality from ischemic heart disease or increased angina or claudication in nephrotic patients relative to age-matched controls. Although this question remains open, it would appear reasonable to attempt dietary treatment of hyperlipemic nephrotics but to refrain from the use of clofibrate, which appears to have increased toxicity in these patients (see below).

D. Drug Metabolism in the Nephrotic Syndrome

Acidic drugs that are positively charged at pH 7.4 usually circulate bound to plasma proteins, including albumin. It is the small unbound fraction of these drugs that is pharmacologically most active and most quickly metabolized. With hypoproteinemia, the quantity of total circulating drug may be reduced to one-half of normal, although the unbound concentration remains relatively normal. When possible, it is wise to plan therapy by measuring unbound rather than total plasma concentration of drug. When the rate of metabolism of the drug is proportional to the unbound concentration (as in phenytoin), it may not be necessary to alter the dosage for a nephrotic patient. With other drugs (clofibrate), the reduction in binding seems to lead to an increase in toxicity and to a need to reduce the normal dose.

E. Vitamin D, Thyroid, and Iron

The vitamin D precursor 25-OH cholecalciferol normally circulates in the plasma bound to "vitamin D binding protein." In nephrotic patients, this protein and vitamin D itself may be abnormally low because of urinary losses. Although evidence for impaired calcium absorption from the GI tract has been found in occasional nephrotic patients, others do not seem to have obvious abnormalities of calcium metabolism.

Although triiodothyronine and thyroid binding globulin may be reduced in nephrotic patients because of urinary losses, TSH levels are generally normal, and the patients are probably euthyroid and do not require thyroid supplements.

Iron transport may be impaired by hypoproteinemia, but it is not clear whether this significantly impairs hemoglobin synthesis.

When in doubt, a vitamin–mineral supplement containing small quantities of vitamin D and iron (such as a "prenatal formula") may be prescribed.

F. Thrombosis

Deep venous thrombosis, renal vein thrombosis, and pulmonary emboli are rather frequent in nephrotic patients. Although the use of corticosteroids may aggravate this occurrence, an increased tendency to thrombosis may be a part of the nephrotic syndrome itself. Levels of antithrombin III may be low in the nephrotic syndrome, especially in patients with thromboses. This deficiency may be related to urinary losses or to hyperlipemia. Lipid-induced platelet abnormalities may also be present. Routine prophylactic anticoagulation of nephrotic patients would not seem wise, but treatment of thrombosis once it occurs is important. The length of adequate treatment of renal vein thrombosis is unknown. Resolution and recanalization will occur within a few weeks, so that subsequent renal venograms may show no clot. If the nephrotic syndrome persists when anticoagulation is discontinued, however, the thrombosis may recur.

G. Infection

The loss of serum immune globulins into the urine is thought to be responsible for the susceptibility of nephrotic patients to gram-positive infections. Nephrotics treated with corticosteroids should probably avoid live vaccines and postpone immunizations.

H. Proteinuria

The proteinuria itself is, of course, a basic manifestation and ordinarily cannot be eliminated without successful treatment of the underlying disease. Reduction in proteinuria through the use of indomethacin, which also diminishes glomerular filtration rate, is possible, but this drug seems to have no effect on the underlying disease. In patients whose glomerular disease has progressed to renal failure but in whom proteinuria, hypoalbuminemia, and edema remain severe and disabling symptoms, even nephrectomy has been performed. Destruction of the kidneys by intentional embolization of clots or other material through the renal arteries or by surgical nephrectomies will stop the proteinuria at the cost of the remaining renal function.

I. Hypertension and Renal Failure

Hypertension and renal failure may occur during the course of glomerulonephritis or nephrotic syndrome, just as in other types of renal disease. The management will be the same as in patients with hypertension or renal failure of other cause.

J. Renal Biopsy

In young nephrotic children, the likelihood of minimal-lesion nephrosis is so high that a trial of corticosteroids is warranted without renal biopsy. If the proteinuria completely disappears in response to treatment, this diagnosis is even more certain. In adults and other children, however, or when proteinuria is "nonselective," some other histological diagnosis is likely. Since some of the diseases underlying nephrotic syndrome benefit from steroid or immunosuppressive therapy whereas others do not, and since their courses and prognoses vary considerably, it is very useful to have a biopsy-confirmed histological diagnosis. When biopsies are done, it is of great importance that facilities for adequate fluorescence microscopy be available for the analysis of the tissue. When this form of examination is not performed, much of the value of the biopsy may be lost.

IV. TREATMENT OF GLOMERULAR DISEASES

Curing disease is vastly preferable to suppressing symptoms as a goal of therapy. Let us examine this possibility for some major types of glomerular disease.

A. Minimal-Lesion Nephrosis

This histological type includes most childhood nephrosis, although the disease may occur in adults of any age as well. The peak incidence is in 2- to 3-year-old boys. Minimal-lesion nephrosis (MLN) is responsible for more than 90% of nephrotic syndrome cases in young children and for perhaps 20% of nephrotic syndrome in adults. It often has a rapid onset, sometimes following a respiratory infection, and may result in massive edema with extremely low serum albumin levels.

The clinical course is most commonly treatment–remission–relapse, the cycle occurring several times over a period of a few years. Patients with MLN rarely if ever progress to renal failure, although it is debated whether focal sclerosis represents a stage of progression in MLN in some patients. In the preantibiotic era, however, many nephrotic children died of infection.

The characteristic pathological lesion is seen on electron microscopic examination of the glomeruli and consists of fusion of the foot processes of the glomerular epithelial cells over the surface of the basement membrane. This epithelial cell change, which is visible only on electron microscopy, is responsible for the name "minimal lesion." Light microscopy ordinarily shows no proliferation of cells. The cause and pathogenesis remain obscure.

When ACTH and cortisone first became available, the treatment of MLN was one of their first applications. As many as 95% of children with MLN will achieve complete remission within 4 weeks of corticosteroid treatment. The response rate in adults may be lower but is still probably above 80%. The exact response rate is unknown because of the difficulty of excluding focal glomerular sclerosis (see below). Unfortunately, most initial MLN responders relapse, and some undergo a long series of prednisone-induced remissions alternating with relapses. Sometimes continuous corticosteroids are required to maintain remissions ("steroid dependence") with resulting severe drug side effects and toxicity. Although it is clear that corticosteroids benefit some patients with MLN, it is not clear in the long run what the balance between benefit and toxicity may be.

Immunosuppressive agents such as cyclophosphamide and chlorambucil have also been proven effective in the treatment of MLN. These agents have sometimes been chosen to induce longer remissions in patients who relapse frequently on corticosteroid treatment. In well-designed controlled clinical trials, these agents have produced long-lasting remissions in such patients. It is not so clear that they are effective in "steroid-dependent" patients.

Unfortunately, the hazardous side effects of cyclophosphomide can include bladder fibrosis, hemorrhagic cystitis, alopecia, bone marrow suppression, sterility in both sexes, and possibly increased incidence of malignancies of certain types in the years following treatment. It appears that courses of therapy as short as 8 weeks in children may have a measurable effect on germ cell production in the adult, although sterility has generally been observed to follow courses of 6 months' duration or longer. The toxic effects of chlorambucil have not been so extensively described at present, but there is little documentation that it is much safer.

Prolonged corticosteroid, cyclophosphamide, and chlorambucil therapies are all potentially hazardous. Their use in therapy of MLN usually produces a prompt remission of proteinuria, but there is no solid evidence that they change the final outcome of the renal disease. It is necessary, therefore, to balance the dangers of the therapy against the morbidity from proteinuria and the accompanying edema. If the nephrotic symptoms are not extremely severe, it may be wiser to wait for a spontaneous remission that will likely occur (though it may take years) rather than subject the patient to potentially hazardous therapy.

Many programs of prednisone and cytotoxic treatment have been proposed, but the following are reasonable regimens:

1. Prednisone, 2 mg/kg per day (but not more than 80 mg/day) divided into three oral doses and continued for 28 days or for 2 weeks after a complete response occurs (signalled by a diuresis and confirmed by a negative urine protein test). After the initial daily schedule, the patient is switched to an alternating-day schedule of 4 mg/kg in a single dose every second day for a month followed by a slow reduction in alternate-day doses over a period of 4–6 months.
2. For a patient who relapses within 4 months of the initial treatment, this program can be repeated, except that the 4 mg/kg alternating-day dose, if well tolerated, could be continued for 6 months prior to tapering.
3. If these measures do not result in satisfactory control of the nephrotic syndrome (either persisting nephrosis or appreciable corticosteroid side effects), then consideration should be given to stopping prednisone therapy and treating the nephrotic syndrome only symptomatically. If diuretics, diet, etc. produce adequate comfort and function, then it may be prudent not to proceed further with corticosteroids or immunosuppressive agents. Only if the patient is severely disabled or in danger of serious complications of the nephrotic syndrome should immunosuppression be used. In such cases, cyclophosphamide in a single oral daily dose of 3 mg/kg can be used after remission has been achieved with corticosteroids, and the 8-week cyclophospha-

mide course can be accompanied by a tapering course of steroids. Chlorambucil has been found to be effective at 0.3 mg/kg per day accompanied by prednisone over a period of 12 weeks. In each case, close attention to differential white blood cell counts as well as a close watch for drug toxicity (alopecia, hemorrhagic cystitis or pyelitis, infection, etc.) will be necessary and will guide direct drug dosage.

B. Focal Segmental Glomerular Sclerosis

Clinically this disease at first resembles MLN, presenting with the signs and symptoms of nephrotic syndrome. Unlike MLN, however, there is usually no response to corticosteroid therapy, and persisting nephrosis gradually progresses to renal failure. Compared to MLN, there is a relatively higher incidence in older children and adults. Hypertension is common, microscopic hematuria is frequent and persistent, and proteinuria tends to be nonselective with an IgG/transferrin ratio above 0.3. Biopsies in patients with focal segmental glomerular sclerosis (FGS) show a glomerulosclerosis beginning in the juxtamedullary region and progressing over time to involve glomeruli further out in the cortex. It is not certain whether FGS is a severe form of progression of MLN or whether it is a distinct disease entity. Since the pathological process early in the disease involves only a minority of glomeruli, it would always be possible for a biopsy to show only "minimally damaged" glomeruli and, hence, to be read as MLN. Since there are no features of either FGS or MLN that are invariable identifying characteristics, we remain unable at present to resolve whether they are the same or distinct diseases.

Occasional patients resolve spontaneously or respond to corticosteroid or immunosuppressive treatment and may go on to a cure or to a relapsing course more characteristic of MLN. This relatively benign course is seen more frequently in younger children. More commonly, however, there is no response, and the patient gradually progresses to renal failure. If renal transplantation is performed, there is considerable likelihood of redeveloping FGS in the allograft, sometimes within days or hours of transplantation. This recurrence in the setting of the intense immunosuppression accompanying transplantation confirms the poor responsiveness of FGS to corticosteroid and immunosuppressive therapy.

Since there is no clear demonstration that any therapy benefits patients with this disease, it would appear reasonable either to treat such patients symptomatically for the nephrotic syndrome from the beginning or to try a brief course of prednisone or immunosuppressive therapy but not to persist with such therapy in the absence of a clear-cut remission.

C. Membranous Nephropathy

Membranous nephropathy is the most frequent cause of nephrotic syndrome in adults of all ages. It may occur in children as well, although in younger children it is much less common than MLN. The usual presenting signs and symptoms are proteinuria and edema, with a full-blown nephrotic syndrome in most of the patients. In idiopathic membranous nephropathy, the usual course is one of persisting proteinuria and relatively stable or slowly declining renal function over a period of many years. A smaller fraction of patients have a complete recovery or a remitting and relapsing course similar to that of MLN, whereas another minority progress more rapidly over a few years to end-stage renal failure.

The characteristic pathological change, as seen on light microscopy, consists of thickening of the capillary wall. Electron microscopy shows electron-dense deposits in the subepithelial side of the membrane with an increase in basement membrane material extending between and sometimes around the deposits. Fluorescence microscopy shows that the deposits contain immunoglobulins (particularly IgG) and complement. Deposits are thought to represent antigen—antibody complexes that either were formed in the circulation and became deposited in the capillary wall or were formed in situ in their subepithelial position.

Although this type of glomerular pathology has been considered the example of an immune-complex-mediated glomerular nephritis, the specific antigen responsible for the formation of the complex is infrequently identified. Identified in some patients with membranous nephropathy have been antigens associated with infectious agents (hepatitis B, quartan malaria, leprosy, schistosomiasis, syphilis), drugs (penicillamine, gold, mercury), tumor surface antigens (lung, stomach, colon, breast), and other endogenous antigens including thyroglobulin and DNA.

Some physicians vigorously promote the use of corticosteroids in the treatment of membranous nephropathy, noting stabilization of renal function and frequent remissions in patients on prolonged high-dose therapy. Recently, a controlled prospective study of the use of alternate-day prednisone (120 mg qod for 2 months) suggested that prednisone benefits some patients with this disease. Although most patients in both treatment and control groups had stable courses, a larger minority of patients in the control group progressed to renal failure than was seen in the prednisone-treated group. Although benefits of cyclophosphamide have also been claimed in treating this disease, no controlled study of this agent has appeared. The combined use of cyclophosphamide, warfarin, and dipyridamole has been compared to no therapy in an Australian study. To date, there has been a relatively high incidence of side effects of therapy and no demonstrated difference in glomerular filtration rates between the groups. The levels of proteinuria, however, are reduced in the treated group. It would seem reasonable to treat most patients with membranous nephropathy with a 2-month course of alternate-day (125 mg) prednisone therapy.

In membranous nephropathy, as in other types of nephrotic syndrome, a fall in proteinuria to 1 g per day or less seems to signal a good prognosis for continued normal renal function. This appears to be true whether this reduction is achieved as a result of therapy or spontaneously. Patients with membranous nephropathy who have a fall in proteinuria to 1 g per day or less at any time during their course, therefore, may not require prednisone therapy.

D. Membranoproliferative Glomerulonephritis (Mesangiocapillary Glomerulonephritis, Chronic Hypocomplementemic Glomerulonephritis, MPGN)

This disease occurs most commonly in older children and teenagers, although it may be seen in adults. Clinical symptoms and signs are usually those of nephrotic syndrome, often accompanied by microscopic hematuria and hypertension. At some time in the disease course almost all such patients have low serum C′3 complement levels.

The nephrotic syndrome in these patients is generally persistent and the course steadily downhill, resulting ultimately in renal failure. A tendency for the histological abnormality to reoccur in a kidney transplant is frequent, although the recurrence of the nephrosis is less common.

Biopsies in such patients demonstrate proliferation in the glomeruli as well as changes in the capillary walls. Several variants are recognized. Type 1 shows mesangial hypercellularity and interposition of mesangial cytoplasm between the endothelial cell and underlying capillary wall. Subendothelial deposits may be present, probably reflecting the presence of immune complexes. In type II (dense deposit disease), extensive, extremely electron-dense deposits are distributed within the basement membrane itself. The deposits generally include complement, with or without accompanying immunoglobulins in Type I. In Type II, however, immunoglobulins are usually not present.

Claims have been made for prolonged alternate-day prednisone therapy or for a combination anticoagulation–antiplatelet therapy. Effectiveness of such therapies has not been demonstrated in satisfactorily controlled trials.

E. Rapidly Progressive Glomerulonephritis

Proteinuria, hematuria, and impairment of renal function are often apparent at the time of presentation of this disease. In addition, systemic signs such as fever, anemia, and hypertension are commonly present. Sometimes this clinical picture is part of an obvious systemic disease such as disseminated lupus, vasculitis, or other connective tissue disease. When no systemic disease is obvious, it is called "idiopathic." Biopsies in such patients show marked proliferation of the epithelial cells lining Bowman's capsule and often of cells of the glomerular tufts as well. Fibrin deposition is seen by fluorescence microscopy. A variant of RPGN is Goodpasture's syndrome, in which circulating antibodies against both glomerular basement (anti-GBM) and alveolar basement membrane can be demonstrated, and pulmonary hemorrhage with respiratory failure may be prominent clinical findings. The course is usually one of rapid deterioration, especially for patients showing extensive crescent formation.

It is not surprising that a variety of therapies have been tried. Heparin, warfarin, dipyridamole, sulfinpyrazone, cyclophosphamide, azathioprine, and plasmapheresis have been used in addition to oral or intravenous corticosteroids alone and in various combinations. Each combination has its advocates, but no solid evidence supports any one program. Oral use of prednisone, when combined with cytotoxic agents such as cyclophosphamide and azothiaprine, has shown little evidence of success. Programs including anticoagulants and antiplatelet agents have appeared to be effective in some patients but are not usable in patients with active pulmonary hemorrhage and have not been proven by controlled trial.

Plasmapheresis (in which approximately 4 liters of plasma are removed from the patient with replacement of a smaller volume of albumin solution as well as the patient's red cells) has achieved some popularity in treating RPGN. This therapy presumably removes circulating immune complexes as well as complement components and clotting factors. It has also been shown to improve the effectiveness of the monocyte phagocytic system. The plasma exchanges are often three or four times a week for 3 or 4 weeks or until circulating immune complexes or anti-GBM antibodies have fallen to low levels. The plasma exchange is usually combined with prednisone, cyclophosphamide, and sometimes azathioprine to prevent the formation of new antibodies. Reports of this treatment have been most enthusiastic, especially in Goodpasture's syndrome or RPGN mediated by anti-GBM antibodies. Good results are generally seen only when the initial serum creatinine is below 6 or 7 and the patient is nonoliguric. The incidence of side effects, including sudden death from infection in a sizable fraction of patients over age 40, emphasizes the danger inherent in this form of treatment. To date, the effectiveness of plasmapheresis for RPGN has not been demonstrated in controlled trials.

Corticosteroid "pulse" therapy (in a frequently used protocol, 1 g of methylprednisolone is administered intravenously over a period of an hour on alternate days for a total of three doses) is usually followed by more conventional oral prednisone therapy. This program also has enthusiasts but has not been shown to be clearly effective in treating RPGN. It may be somewhat safer than the plasmapheresis–immunosuppressive program mentioned above, although sudden deaths and deaths from opportunistic infections have been noted here as well.

In the absence of more certain knowledge of the effectiveness of these treatment programs, the physician might elect to try "pulse" therapy or plasmapheresis–immunosuppressive therapy in a patient with severe, clearly progressive RPGN or with Goodpasture's syndrome. When pulmonary hemorrhage is not threatening, the physician should remember the option of no therapy, which will at least offer the patient the maximum opportunity of remaining alive until such time as dialysis or transplantation may be required.

F. Acute Proliferative Glomerulonephritis

These varieties of glomerulonephritis show proliferation of glomerular endothelial and mesangial cells and are generally characterized by microscopic hematuria with or without substantial proteinuria. The prototype is acute poststreptococcal glomerulonephritis which follows group A streptococcal infections of the throat or skin. Clinically, 1 to 3 weeks following the infection, hematuria is noted, sometimes followed by oliguria, edema, hypertension, and azotemia. Acute proliferative glomerulonephritis may less commonly follow other acute bacterial infections and perhaps certain viral infections as well. In mild cases, no treatment is necessary other than eradication of the infective organism if this is possible. In severe cases with oliguria or anuria, careful fluid restriction and management of hyperkalemia and of other manifestations of acute renal failure will be necessary. No specific treatment for the glomerulonephritis is known.

G. Mesangial Proliferative Glomerulonephritis [Including IgA Nephropathy (Berger's Disease), Benign Hematuria, and Some Varieties of Hereditary Glomerular Nephritis]

These diseases are characterized by microscopic hematuria on routine urinalysis or the presence of gross hematuria accompanying fever, upper respiratory infections, or other acute illnesses. Proteinuria may vary from none to massive, but most commonly only slight proteinuria is present. By light microscopy biopsies show either a focal or a diffuse proliferation of mesangial cells, but in most cases immunofluorescence shows diffuse deposition of IgA (with or without other immunoglobulins and complement) in the mesangium. Most patients with this disease follow a benign course, but in 20–25%, there may be a gradual deterioration of renal function and eventual renal failure. This deteriorating course is more common among patients who have nephrotic range proteinuria. There is no known effective treatment for this condition.

V. CONCLUSION

With increasing understanding of the immunopathogenesis of glomerular disease, and with improved specificity in our manipulation of the immune response, we may be approaching an era of successful treatment or prevention of glomerular disease.

At present, however, most of our therapies are puny antagonists of glomerular disease, yet powerful toxins to the healthy body. We must usually be content to treat symptoms rather than causes.

SUGGESTED READINGS

Coggins CH, Pinn V: Collaborative study of the adult idiopathic nephrotic syndrome. *N Engl J Med* 301:1301–1306, 1979.

Glassock RJ, Cohen AH, Bennett CM, Martínez-Maldonado M: Primary glomerular diseases, in Brenner B, Rector F (eds): *The Kidney* (ed 2). Philadelphia, WB Saunders, 1981, pp 1351–1492.

Kim Y, Michael A: Idiopathic membranoproliferative glomerulonephritis. *Annu Rev Med* 31: 273–288, 1980.

Levy M, Seely: Pathophysiology of edema formation, in Brenner B, Rector F (eds): *The Kidney* (ed 2). Philadelphia, WB Saunders, 1981, pp 723–776.

Lockwood C, Peters D: Plasma exchange in glomerulonephritis. *Annu Rev Med* 31:167–79, 1980.

McPhaul J: IgA-associated glomerular nephritis. *Annu Rev Med* 28:37–42, 1976.

Wilson C, Dixon F: Renal response to immunological injury, in Brenner B, Rector F (eds): *The Kidney* (ed 2). Philadelphia, WB Saunders, 1981, pp 1237–1350.

10

Drugs and the Kidney
Renal Contribution to
Handling of Drugs

D. CRAIG BRATER

I. INTRODUCTION

Renal function can permute the relationship between drug dose and effect in a variety of ways. Effects on absorption, distribution volume, and elimination influence the concentration of drug attained in blood. Consequently, such effects can often be detected and/or prevented by monitoring of serum concentrations of drugs. However, the relationship between the concentration of drug in serum and response may also be changed. Monitoring serum concentrations alone, therefore, is insufficient for optimal therapeutics and must be accompanied by clinical monitoring of the endpoints of efficacy and toxicity. In addition, accumulation of active metabolites that are not measured by conventional assays makes interpretation of serum concentrations of some drugs particularly hazardous. Since renal function can affect drug disposition in so many different ways, the astute clinician must be aware of these potential mechanisms and call on his clinical skills and laboratory armamentarium to best care for his patients. This section will discuss principles of the effects of renal disease on response to drugs using specific examples for illustration. This will then provide a framework for more detailed consideration of individual drugs but, more importantly, will provide a set of principles applicable to any therapeutic setting.

D. CRAIG BRATER • Departments of Pharmacology and Internal Medicine, Southwestern Medical School at the University of Texas Health Science Center at Dallas, Dallas, Texas 75235.

In simplest terms, one must consider each of the different ways in which changes in renal function can affect the relationship between the administered dose of a drug and the response to that drug. Figure 1 depicts a general scheme by which one can subdivide the determinants of the relationship between dose and response and analyze them separately. Even though the pharmacological role of the kidney can be analyzed with respect to each of the determinants indicated in the scheme, one must be aware that changes in the relationship between dose and response can occur by permutations of any one or a combination of the determinants.

II. DETERMINANTS OF THE RELATIONSHIP BETWEEN THE DOSE OF A DRUG AND ITS CONCENTRATION IN BLOOD

A. Absorption

Changes in absorption can occur by affecting rate and/or extent of absorption. The rate of absorption determines the time at which the peak concentration of drug is reached in blood and its magnitude. The extent of absorption determines how much of the drug enters the system and, consequently, contributes only to the magnitude of its concentration.

The effects of renal dysfunction on gastrointestinal absorption have not been examined. However, one might speculate that uremia itself, changes in potassium homeostasis, administration of phosphate binders, etc. could affect rate and/or extent of absorption. One clear example of an effect of the kidney on absorption is the decreased intestinal absorption of calcium caused by insufficient 1-hydroxylation of 25-OH vitamin D_3 which occurs with decreased nephron mass and in renal tubular acidosis. One group reported that the bioavailability of propranolol increased in patients with renal disease, presumably because of a secondary effect decreasing presystemic elimination. However, a more detailed study did not support these

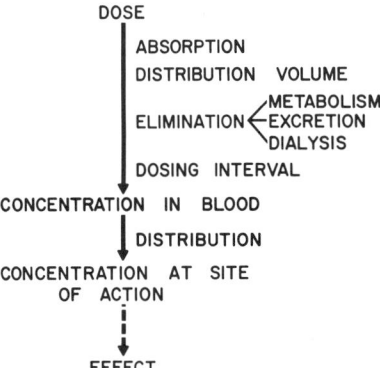

Figure 1. General scheme relating dose of a drug to its clinical effect.

findings. It does appear, however, that presystemic elimination of propoxyphene decreases in end-stage renal failure, resulting in greater bioavailability. It behooves the astute clinician to be cognizant of possibilities for abnormal absorption of drugs in caring for his patients.

Rate and extent of absorption from intramuscular or subcutaneous sites can also be changed by a variety of factors. For example, phenytoin and some of the benzodiazepines precipitate in muscle and, consequently, are absorbed erratically over prolonged periods of time. Patients in shock perfuse peripheral sites poorly and absorb parenterally administered drugs unpredictably. Again, although studies in patients with renal dysfunction have not been reported, acidemia, disrupted volume and electrolyte homeostasis, etc. could cause changes in absorption from intramuscular or subcutaneous sites.

B. Distribution

Effects of renal dysfunction on drug distribution are considered in two separate parts of this discussion. This section includes effects on distribution that change the total concentration of drug (free plus protein bound) in blood, and a later section describes distribution effects in which the concentration of drug in blood remains the same but its access to its site of action changes.

It is clear that systemic pH, degree of protein binding, disease states, and other diverse factors can affect the distribution of a drug into tissues (Table I). The mechanism of these effects, their consequences, and their clinical relevance are poorly defined. Renal dysfunction can result in changes in systemic pH such as the acidemia of uremia or of renal tubular acidosis or the alkalemia of potassium depletion; these pH changes can affect distribution of drugs to tissues. The hypoalbuminemia of nephrotic syndrome, the displacement of protein-bound drugs by endogenous organic acids that accumulate in uremia, and the altered albumin with decreased capacity to bind drugs in uremia all can affect distribution. Over and above these described changes in distribution that occur in renal dysfunction, renal disease per se by unknown mechanisms may affect how drugs distribute to tissues.

Table I. Potential Mechanisms of Effect of
Renal Dysfunction on Drug Distribution

Changes in systemic pH
   Acidemia of uremia
   Acidemia of renal tubular acidosis
   Alkalemia of potassium depletion
Hypoalbuminemia
Displacement of drugs from protein
   By accumulated endogenous compounds
   By other drugs
Altered binding characteristics of protein

With the exception of digoxin, changes in distribution are important only with drugs that are highly protein bound ($\sim$90% or more of the drug normally being bound), and with renal disease, one is only concerned with acidic drugs. A list of drugs of potential concern would include penicillins, cephalosporins, sulfonamides, thiazide and loop diuretics, sulfonylureas, nonsteroidal antiinflammatory drugs, etc., but no clinically important changes in distribution have been reported with these drugs. Quantitatively important distribution-related effects have been described with phenytoin, valproic acid, coumadin, salicylates, thiopental, and diazoxide. Phenytoin, valproic acid, and coumadin represent drugs in which effects on distribution cause a change in the concentration of drug in blood. With salicylates, thiopental, and diazoxide, changes occur in the relationship between the concentration of drug in blood and its effect. These drugs will be considered subsequently.

In both hypoalbuminemia and uremia, phenytoin, valproic acid, and coumadin are displaced from albumin, increasing the amount of drug free in plasma. This displacement from binding in itself would cause an increased pharmacological effect, since the amount of drug accessible to its site of action is related to the amount of free drug in plasma. However, this free drug is also available for elimination and for distribution into tissue in which the drug is not active. The overall result is that a steady state is reached in which the concentration of drug free in plasma is virtually the same as in the unperturbed condition; the pharmacological effect is the same, but the total concentration of drug in blood (that free plus that bound) is less than that before displacement. This consequence is illustrated schematically for phenytoin in Fig. 2.

The clinical importance of this phenomenon is that the amount of drug administered to the patient remains the same, i.e., for phenytoin approximately 300 mg/day. The "therapeutic" concentration of phenytoin in blood in patients with the nephrotic syndrome or uremia, however, is one-half to one-third that in normals. Consequently, the importance of this effect is in interpretation of measurements of phenytoin concentrations in blood. "Low" total concentrations of phenytoin or valproic acid in a uremic or nephrotic patient should not be misinterpreted as subtherapeutic. This interpretive problem does not occur with coumadin, for one monitors the response to the anticoagulant rather than its blood concentration.

Free	1.0		5.5		1.0
		Displacement → From Protein		Steady → State	
Bound	9.0		4.5		4.5
	—		—		—
TOTAL	10.0		10.0		5.5

Figure 2. Schematic representation of the influence of uremia or hypoalbuminemia on the disposition of phenytoin (values for phenytoin expressed in μg/ml).

As noted above, digoxin is the exception to the general rule regarding changes in distribution. In end-stage renal failure, by unknown mechanisms, the volume of distribution of digoxin is decreased, and a smaller loading dose is needed to achieve a given concentration in blood. This dose adjustment is in addition to the reduced maintenance dose of digoxin required in end-stage renal disease caused by the decreased ability of the kidney to eliminate digoxin.

C. Elimination

Drugs are eliminated by metabolism and/or excretion or, in special circumstances, by dialysis.

1. Metabolism

Metabolism occurs predominantly in the liver, and the kidney's metabolic pathways for drugs, though present, are relatively inconsequential. A considerable amount of insulin is metabolized by the kidney. This observation may account in part for the decreased insulin requirement that occasionally occurs in a diabetic as renal function deteriorates.

The most important aspect of metabolism relating to the kidney is that by the liver in which metabolites of drugs are pharmacologically active and dependent on the kidney for elimination. For example, procainamide is acetylated to N-acetylprocainamide (NAPA) which is itself an antiarrhythmic and which is eliminated by the kidney. Consequently, in renal failure, NAPA accumulates preferentially to procainamide and may do so in amounts that become toxic. Interpretation of serum concentrations of procainamide in a patient with azotemia becomes difficult, for both procainamide and NAPA contribute to the pharmacological effect, although only the former is measured in many assays, and "therapeutic" concentrations for the latter have not been well defined. One must emphasize the need for clinical assessment of pharmacological effect rather than reliance on and possible misinterpretation of serum concentration measurements. Some of the oral sulfonylureas are converted to active metabolites which accumulate in uremia, potentially causing prolonged and long-lasting hypoglycemia. Meperidine (pethidine) and propoxyphene are metabolized to normeperidine and norpropoxyphene which depend on the kidney for elimination. Accumulation of the metabolite can result in seizures or cardiovascular collapse, respectively. Oxypurinol, the active metabolite of allopurinol, also accumulates in uremia, though the clinical importance is unclear.

By uncertain mechanisms, renal disease appears in some circumstances to secondarily decrease hepatic elimination of some drugs. For drugs that can be eliminated by both the liver and the kidney, one would expect a decrease in the renal component to result in a compensatory increase in the hepatic. One cannot, however, make this assumption.

2. Excretion

Some drugs such as paraldehyde and anesthetic gases are excreted by the lungs, others have important biliary excretion, but by far the most important excretory route when considering both parent drug and metabolites is the kidney. It is easiest to consider renal modes of elimination in terms of the kidney's physiological functions of filtration, active transport, metabolism, and passive transport. Metabolism has been discussed previously. The other modes of elimination will be discussed in sequence.

a. Filtration

The determinants of a drug's capacity to be filtered are protein binding, molecular size and charge, glomerular integrity, and the number of filtering nephrons.

Since only that amount of drug free in plasma can pass through a normal glomerulus, displacement of highly bound drugs from serum proteins can increase the amount eliminated in the urine. As discussed previously, the clinical importance of this phenomenon with phenytoin, valproic acid, and coumadin relates to proper interpretation of their concentration in blood.

Effective molecular size has been shown to be a limiting factor for excretion of mixed and high-molecular-weight dextrans. The dextran 40 used clinically is actually a mixture of different molecular weight species; the high-molecular-weight species ($\sim$70,000) is selectively retained because it cannot be filtered. Consequently, these preparations remain in patients for extended periods of time. Other drugs are small enough that there are essentially no size limitations to filtration.

The integrity of the glomerulus as a sieve is disrupted in nephrotic syndrome. Drugs bound to albumin could be carried with the protein into the urine, enhancing renal elimination. This phenomenon has been shown to occur with phenytoin and clofibrate, but in the four patients studied, the excretion rate was not increased enough compared to overall elimination to be important.

Most studies and clinical attention are directed at influences of decreased numbers of functioning nephrons on the renal elimination of drugs. The effect of decreased creatinine clearance on the elimination of digoxin and aminoglycoside antibiotics is particularly well known. In general, if 50% or more of the administered drug (or its active metabolites) is eliminated unchanged in the urine, decreased renal function will importantly change handling of the drug and require dose adjustment. An approach to dose adjustment is presented in Chapter 11.

b. Active Transport

The renal tubule can both actively secrete and actively reabsorb a variety of substrates. Active reabsorption appears to be inconsequential except for iodipamide (a cholecystographic agent) which can induce marked uricosuria, presumably by decreasing the active reabsorption of uric acid in the proximal tubule. The same mechanism accounts for the uricosuria caused by probenecid, high-dose salicylates, and high-dose phenylbutazone. The uricosuria could induce the acute renal failure occasionally reported with this contrast agent.

The uptake by pinocytosis from the proximal tubular lumen of gentamicin and other aminoglycoside antibiotics might be considered another example of active reabsorption. Originally it was felt that different capacities for uptake or egress from the tubular cells after uptake determined the potential for nephrotoxicity of aminoglycosides, those that tended to accumulate within the cell being most toxic. More recent evidence has indicated that the potential for nephrotoxicity is more related to the ability of the particular aminoglycoside to disrupt lysosomal function once it has gained access to the interior of the cell.

The pars recta (straight segment) of the proximal tubule actively secretes into the tubular lumen a variety of organic acids and bases. The pathways for acids and for bases appear to be separate, but within a group there is lack of specificity such that a variety of organic acids can compete with each other for transport, as can a variety of organic bases.

A clinically important drug transport that is not of acids or bases is a secretory component of digoxin and digitoxin elimination which can be competed for by spironolactone and quinidine. Patients coadministered these drugs will develop higher serum levels of cardiac glycoside.

i. Organic Acid Transport. Table II shows a list of organic acids with potentially important renal secretion. The different compounds in this table can compete with each other for secretion. This fact is used to therapeutic advantage in the treatment of gonorrhea, in which probenecid pretreatment causes the subsequently administered penicillin to be secreted more slowly, resulting in higher and more sustained concentrations of penicillin in blood. Although all of the drugs listed in Table II have the potential to compete with each other, the degree to which they will compete is impossible to predict *a priori*. Most clinicians are aware of the need to decrease the dose of methotrexate if probenecid is administered. Few are aware, with potentially disastrous consequences, of a possible similar need if other drugs listed in Table II are administered with methotrexate. "Idiopathic sensitivity" to methotrexate might well be a result in some cases of coadministration of inhibitors of the active secretion of methotrexate. A similar scenario could be postulated for combinations of any of the drugs listed in Table II.

Another clinically important example of competition for transport is that which occurs between a variety of drugs and the accumulated endogenous organic acids of uremia. In fact, in mild to moderate renal failure, this

Table II. Organic Acids with a Clinically
Important Component of
Active Transport

p-Aminohippurate
Cephalosporins
Diphylline
"Loop" diuretics
Methotrexate
Nonsteroidal antiinflammatory agents
Penicillins
Probenecid
Salicylates
Sulfonamides
Sulfonylureas
Thiazide diuretics

mechanism is probably more important than is decreased nephron mass for the decreased elimination of a number of organic acids. Organic acid diuretics such as furosemide, ethacrynic acid, thiazides, metolazone, etc. reach their site of action by secretion into the lumen by the organic acid transport pathway. Accumulated organic acids in uremia block the access of these diuretics to their active site, accounting for the requirement for larger doses of organic acid diuretics to attain amounts within the tubular lumen sufficient to cause a diuresis.

  ii. Organic Base Transport. The active transport system for organic bases and its importance in man are less well understood than that for organic acids. Table III lists bases that have been shown to undergo potentially clinically important active secretion. It has been assumed that organic bases can compete with each other for secretion as do acids, but such an interaction has never been documented clinically. Consequently, its importance in man is unknown. Recent evidence indicates that there may be several different base transport systems that do not cross compete. Because our understanding of the base transport system is so rudimentary, it is impossible to speculate about its importance, though clinicians should be aware of the potential for interactions of drugs within this group.

Table III. Organic Bases with a Clinically
Important Component of
Active Transport

Amantadine
Cimetidine
Ethambutol
Mecamylamine
Mepacrine (quinacrine)
N-Methylnicotinamide
Procainamide
Pseudoephedrine
Tetraethylammonium

c. Passive Transport

Weak acids and bases can be passively reabsorbed in the collecting duct. For this to occur, these drugs must gain entry to the tubular lumen in the proximal portion of the nephron either at the glomerulus or by active secretion by the proximal tubule. Even drugs with high rates of proximal entry can be almost completely reabsorbed in the collecting duct. Passive reabsorption is modulated by urinary pH and flow rate.

i. Urinary pH. The effect of urinary pH is related to the principle of passive nonionic diffusion which is based on the premise that a nonionized molecule passes more readily across a lipid membrane than does its ionized congener. Consequently, the effect of urinary pH on the relative amount of ionized component decreases, and excretion decreases. Not all weak acids and bases demonstrate urine pH-dependent elimination; one cannot assume that these principles will apply to all weak acids and bases. Part of the lack of effect with some drugs probably relates to the drug's pK_a and the lipid solubility of the congeners. For example, if even the nonionized species is poorly soluble in lipid, its ability to cross the tubular plasma membrane would not be enhanced. In this setting, changes in urinary pH would not cause changes in renal elimination.

Another modulator of the ability of the nonionized congener's ability to pass across the lipid membrane may be antidiuretic hormone which can increase by 50–100% the ability of lipophilic compounds to pass across the toad urinary bladder, a structure functionally analogous to the mammalian collecting duct. These findings have not been extrapolated to studies in man. Other modulators of the effects of urinary pH on drug reabsorption are less well defined.

Urinary pH has been shown to be a clinically important determinant of elimination for the drugs shown in Table IV. This importance for the weak

Table IV. Compounds with Clinically
Important Urine pH-Dependent
Elimination

Weak acids
Phenobarbital
Salicylates
Sulfonamide derivatives
Trimethoprim
Weak bases
Amphetamine
Ephedrine
Mexiletene
Pseudoephedrine
Phencyclidine (PCP)
Quinine
Tocainide
Tricyclic antidepressants

acids, particularly phenobarbital and salicylates, is well known; that for weak bases less so. Alkalinization of the urine, by favoring excretion of the ionized congener of phenobarbital or salicylates, is a mainstay of therapy for toxicity caused by these agents. It has also been demonstrated that the small changes in urinary pH caused by modest doses of antacids can enhance the elimination rate of salicylate sufficient to prevent attaining concentrations in blood necessary for their antiinflammatory effect.

The effect of urinary pH on the elimination of amphetamine may be better known to abusers of this drug than to clinicians. Since amphetamine is a weak base, alkalinizing the urine increases the amount un-ionized, favoring reabsorption. Amphetamine abusers regularly ingest baking soda before "shooting" to prolong the "high." Therapeutically, it would be important to acidify the urine of a patient with an overdose of amphetamines. Recently, a similar importance of urinary pH has been demonstrated with phencylcidine (PCP, "angel dust," etc.). The supposedly nontoxic pseudoephedrine has been shown to accumulate to toxic levels in children with renal tubular acidosis in whom a persistently alkaline urine favored passive reabsorption of the drug. A similar phenomenon occurs with tocainide, an orally available lidocainelike agent, for which the administration of bicarbonate decreased the elimination rate.

    ii. Urinary Flow Rate. Urinary flow rate can affect excretion of some drugs by decreasing the concentration gradient for reabsorption because the urine is dilute and by decreasing the time for drug to diffuse out of the urine.

Urinary flow rate has been shown to be an important determinant of elimination for chloramphenicol, ephedrine, phenobarbital, pseudoephedrine, and theophylline. This phenomenon would probably be clinically important only in patients with high urinary flow rates for prolonged periods of time.

Clinicians seem to pay little attention to the importance of urinary pH and flow rate except in the case of salicylate or barbiturate overdose. As discussed above, more thought should be given to the importance of the urine pH for excretion of a broader gamut of drugs as well as for clinical diagnosis.

    iii. Dialysis. Space does not allow discussion of the elimination of drugs by dialysis in great detail, but some of the more pertinent determinants of a drug's dialyzability are discussed.

Molecular size can importantly influence a drug's dialyzability. In general, compounds of molecular weight less than 500 have flow-dependent dialyzability, whereas elimination of larger drugs depends on dialyzer surface area. Vancomycin, with a molecular weight of 1800, is too large to be dialyzable. Other drugs for which molecular size is clinically important are amphotericin B, erythromycin, morphine, digoxin, and digitoxin, all of which have poor dialyzability which is limited by membrane surface area. All other drugs are small enough that their dialysance is determined by flow rate of blood and dialysate and by other determinants to be discussed subsequently.

For a drug to be dialyzable, it must be water soluble (this does not apply to resin hemoperfusion). Many of the sedative–hypnotics that are often seen in overdose settings such as glutethimide, methaqualone, meprobamate, ethchlorvynol, tricyclic antidepressants, etc., although of small molecular weight, are relatively insoluble in water and are poorly dialyzable by conventional hemodialysis. Resin or charcoal hemoperfusion is not dependent on water solubility and therefore can remove these drugs effectively. In addition, drugs highly bound to serum proteins, in general, are poorly dialyzable. Protein binding does not appear to be a limiting factor with sorbent hemoperfusion.

Whether or not dialysis can contribute importantly to a drug's removal from the body relates to that drug's intrinsic plasma clearance, namely, how fast the body can eliminate the drug exclusively of dialysis. For dialysis to add a clinically important increment to overall drug elimination, clearance by dialysis should increase overall clearance by approximately 30%. Some general principles can be appreciated by considering the determinants of the clearance of a drug. Clearance is equal to the product of the elimination rate constant and the volume of distribution:

$$Cl = K_e \times V_d$$

but K_e is related to half-life such that

$$Cl = 0.693 \, V_d / T_{1/2}$$

From this relationship, it is clear that if the volume in which a drug distributes is large, clearance is large, and for dialysis to add an important increment to clearance, dialyzability would have to be great. This also makes intuitive sense in that a large volume of distribution means that much of the body burden of the drug is in the peripheral tissues. Dialysis can only remove the amount in the blood; consequently, drug in the tissues is not accessible to the dialyzer, and the body burden of the drug is not importantly decreased by dialysis. The converse is true for a drug with a small volume of distribution unless it is highly protein bound and thereby does not cross the dialysis membrane.

Similarly, if the half-life is short (i.e., elimination is fast), the intrinsic clearance is great, and dialysis would be less likely to have an important effect. The converse is also true. The effect of dialysis on the clearance of aminoglycosides illustrates the validity of this concept. In a patient with normal renal function, the half-life of an aminoglycoside antibiotic is relatively short (2 or 3 hr). Therefore, clearance is large, and dialyzing such a patient would not remove important amounts of the drug. However, aminoglycosides have long half-lives in patients with end-stage renal failure. Therefore, clearance is low, and dialysis can eliminate enough of the antibiotic to require dosing after each dialysis.

When to use hemodialysis or hemoperfusion (*vide infra*) for patients with drug overdoses is often debated and must be highly individualized to both patient status and the capacities of one's hospital. For example, an identical patient might be treated differently depending on whether one's local expertise were pulmonary care versus technical skill in performance of dialysis. We suggest in Table V a modification of guidelines proposed by Schreiner, all of which are predicated on the ability of dialysis to contribute importantly to elimination of the drug.

Methanol and ethylene glycol ingestion warrant more detailed comments, for poisoning with either of these two agents is a clear indication for hemodialysis. Toxicity of massive doses can be completely prevented by appropriate treatment. Both methanol and ethylene glycol are benign, and their toxicity is mediated by metabolic byproducts. The first step in the metabolism of both of these compounds is alcohol dehydrogenase for which ethanol is a preferred substrate. Consequently, adequate therapy entails not only hemodialysis to remove the parent methanol and ethylene glycol and any metabolites that may have formed but also administration of sufficient ethanol to block further formation of the toxic metabolites. The latter can be complicated, for ethanol itself is dialyzable, and its infusion rate must be adjusted to maintain enzyme-blocking serum concentrations of ethanol (target concentration is 100 to 200 mg/dl). In addition, chronic drinkers have a higher capacity to metabolize ethanol and require higher maintenance infusion rates, unless, of course, they have liver disease. Clearly, the ethanol dose must be individualized and followed with serum concentrations if possible. Table VI presents recommendations as a first approximation of the required ethanol dose. Hemodialysis for 4 to 6 hr appears sufficient for treatment of even massive overdoses. Ethanol infusion should probably be continued for up to 24 hr.

Recently, attempts have been made to increase the dialyzability of water-insoluble drugs that are severely toxic in overdose settings. Resins or activated charcoal have been used to bind these drugs and irreversibly extract them from the patient's blood. It is clear that these drugs can be removed

Table V. Guidelines for Dialysis of the Poisoned Patient

1. Severe clinical intoxication with life-threatening cardiovascular instability despite adequate volume replacement.
2. Ingestion and probable absorption of a potentially lethal dose.
3. A blood level of the drug that is in a range resulting in considerable mortality.
4. Impaired ability to eliminate the drug by endogenous routes either by disease itself, toxicity of the drug, or by saturation of pathways of elimination.
5. Prolonged coma in a setting in which expertise in hemodialysis exceeds expertise in respiratory care.
6. Methanol or ethylene glycol ingestion.

Table VI. Dose of Ethanol for Achieving a Target
Concentration of 100 mg/dl in the Treatment of
Methanol or Ethylene Glycol Ingestions

Loading dose	0.6	g/kg
Maintenance dose		
Nondrinkers	66	mg/kg per hr
Chronic drinkers	154	mg/kg per hr
During hemodialysis[a]	170	mg/kg per hr

[a] The same results can be achieved by maintaining a dialysate
ethanol concentration of 100 mg/dl.

efficiently by resin hemoperfusion. In fact, dialysis clearance for many of
them is equal to blood flow through the dialyzer. Unfortunately, however,
these drugs have large volumes of distribution so that the maximal reduction
in blood concentrations of many or most of these drugs is only short-lived,
and the drug stores in peripheral tissues serve as a reservoir to refill the blood
with drug as soon as hemoperfusion is stopped. In addition, the procedure
itself causes decrements in circulating formed elements in the blood. Although newer generation columns appear to be safer, one can still anticipate
a 30 to 40% decrease in platelet count after 4 hr of hemoperfusion. It is likely
that clearer indications for use of resin hemoperfusion will evolve. At present, the general indications for dialysis for poisoning listed in Table V would
also apply for hemoperfusion, since hemoperfusion has been demonstrated
to remove important amounts of the drugs listed in Table VII in overdose
settings.

D. Dosing Interval

Dosing interval and dosing regimens are discussed in Chapter 11.

Table VII. Drugs for Which Resin
Hemoperfusion Has Been Demonstrated
to Remove Clinically Important Amounts

Barbiturates
Chloral hydrate (trichlorethanol)
Chloroquine
Digitalis glycosides
Ethchlorvynol
Glutethimide
Meprobamate
Methaqualone
N-Desmethylmethsuximide
Salicylate
Theophylline
Tricyclic antidepressants

III. EFFECT OF THE KIDNEY ON THE DISTRIBUTION OF DRUGS TO TISSUES

Changes in the distribution of a drug that affects the relationship between dose and its concentration in blood were discussed previously. In other circumstances, there occur changes in distribution of a drug in which the concentration in blood is the same but the response to that concentration is altered. This phenomenon should not be construed as a change in "sensitivity" to the drug, for it probably represents a change in distribution of drug in peripheral tissues that favors more drug reaching its site of action, the relationship between concentration at the site of action and effect remaining the same.

Uremia or alterations in systemic pH appear capable of changing access of a drug to its site of action. In uremia, the change in albumin binding of diazoxide increases the antihypertensive effect although the total concentration of diazoxide in blood remains the same as in nonuremic patients. A similar phenomenon occurs with thiopental anesthesia. The dose needed to attain a certain level of anesthesia is less in subjects after urea infusion, or, considered in another light, the same concentration of anesthetic causes more depression of consciousness in subjects administered urea than in normals.

Changes in systemic pH can also affect distribution of a drug to a site of activity without changing concentrations in blood, as has been demonstrated with salicylates and phenobarbital. Salicylates and phenobarbital demonstrate increased distribution into the central nervous system during acidemia. Central nervous system toxicity is increased during acidemia at any given blood concentration of either of these drugs. It appears that acidemia favors the nonionized species, allowing diffusion of more drug into the CNS. This phenomenon has been documented in pediatric patients in whom acidemia causes increased delivery of salicylate into the cerebrospinal fluid. Consequently, an important part of therapy of salicylate or phenobarbital toxicity would be correction of a systemic acidemia.

IV. EFFECT OF RENAL FUNCTION ON SENSITIVITY TO DRUGS

Whether renal function can modulate "sensitivity" to drugs is unclear. Supposed instances of increased "sensitivity" may, in fact, represent changes in distribution or access of drug to its site of action. For example, the effect described earlier of thiopental in patients with uremia was originally felt to represent changes in sensitivity, but further scrutiny showed the effect to be one of distribution rather than of changing the relationship between drug concentration at the active site and response.

The acidemia of uremia and/or renal tubular acidosis may cause resistance to the pressor effects of catecholamines. This phenomenon may be a true example of changes in sensitivity.

Electrolyte and acid–base abnormalities resulting from renal dysfunction can affect "sensitivity" to drugs that affect the cardiovascular system. Hyperkalemia slows conduction throughout the heart and predictably increases the similar effects on conductivity of digitalis glycosides, quinidine, procainamide, disopyramide, phenothiazines, and tricyclic antidepressants. Alkalosis, magnesium or potassium depletion, and hypercalcemia increase the sensitivity to the toxic effects of digitalis glycosides. Some investigators feel that decreased potassium increases digoxin availability to its site of action; if this does occur, sensitivity has not changed, but the relationship has changed between the concentration of digoxin in blood and that at the active site. Whether the other conditions predisposing to digitalis toxicity represent true changes in sensitivity is unclear. Uremia appears to increase the sensitivity to pindolol in that blockade of exercise-induced increases in heart rate occurs at lower serum concentrations of pindolol than those required in normal subjects.

The exact mechanism by which changes occur in response to a given amount of drug in blood is moot compared to the importance of realizing its occurrence in clinical settings. If the drug concentration in blood may not closely relate to response, clinicians cannot rely on measures of drug levels as therapeutic guidelines. One must follow clinical endpoints to assess response.

The kidney can influence the disposition and response to drugs in many ways. Categorizing and cataloguing these effects are helpful in sorting out the complexities of the kidney's role in handling of drugs. A better understanding of the multiplicity of effects of the kidney should help clinicians to better recognize and be more able to anticipate changes from "normal" in response to or handling of drugs. By so doing, they should be able to improve drug efficacy and decrease toxicity. Since changes in renal function can affect handling of a drug in many different ways, the clinician must understand not only the pathophysiology of his patient's disease but also the pharmacology of the drugs being used so he can assess clinical endpoints of efficacy and toxicity as a guide to therapy.

SUGGESTED READINGS

Anders MW: Metabolism of drugs by the kidney. Kidney Int 18:636–647, 1980.

Bennett WM: Principles of drug therapy in patients with renal disease. West J Med 123:372–379, 1975.

Boobis WM: Alteration of plasma albumin in relation to decreased drug binding in uremia. Clin Pharmacol Ther 22:147–153, 1977.

Brater DC: The pharmacological role of the kidney. Drugs 19:31–48, 1980.

Brater DC, Thier SO: Renal disorders, in Melmon KL, Morrelli HF, (eds): *Clinical Pharmacology* (ed 2). New York, Macmillan, 1978, pp 349–387.

Garrett ER: Pharmacokinetics and clearances related to renal processes. *Int J Clin Pharmacol Biopharm* 16:155–172, 1978.

Gibson TP: Dialyzability of common therapeutic agents. *Dialysis Transplant* 8:24–40, 1979.

Gibson TP, Nelson HA: Drug kinetics and artificial kidneys. *Clin Pharmacokinet* 2:403–426, 1977.

Greenblatt DJ, Koch-Weser J: Clinical pharmacokinetics. *N Engl J Med* 293:702–705, 964–970, 1975.

Greenblatt, DJ, Koch-Weser J: Intra-muscular injection of drugs. *N Engl J Med* 295:542–546, 1976.

Jelliffe RW, Brooker G: A nomogram for digoxin therapy. *Am J Med* 57:63–68, 1974.

Kunin CM: A guide to use of antibiotics in patients with renal disease. *Ann Intern Med* 67:121–158, 1967.

Lee SC, Marbury TC, Benet LZ: Clearance calculations in hemodialysis. Application to blood, plasma, and dialysate measurements for ethambutol. *J Pharmacokinet Biopharm* 8:69–81, 1980.

Le Sher DA: Considerations in the use of drugs in patients with renal failure. *J Clin Pharmacol* 16:570–576, 1976.

Peters L: Renal tubular excretion of organic bases. *Pharmacol Rev* 12:1–35, 1960.

Prescott LF: Mechanisms of renal excretion of drugs (with special reference to drugs used by anaesthetists). *Br J Anaesth* 44:246–251, 1972.

Prescott LF: Limitations of haemodialysis and forced diuresis. *CIBA Found Symp* 26 (New Ser):269, 1974.

Prescott LF: Drug overdosage and poisoning, in Avery GS, (ed): *Drug Treatment* (ed 2). Sydney, New York, ADIS Press; Edinburgh, Churchill-Livingstone, 1980, pp 263–281.

Rennick BR: Renal excretion of drugs; tubular transport and metabolism. *Annu Rev Pharmacol Toxicol* 12:121–156, 1972.

Rosenbaum JL: Hemoperfusion for acute drug intoxication. *Kidney Int* 18(Suppl 10):S106–S108, 1980.

Scribner BH, Crawford MA, Dempster WJ: Urinary excretion by nonionic diffusion. *Am J Physiol* 196:1135–1140, 1959.

Weiner IM, Mudge GH: Renal tubular mechanisms for excretion of organic acids and bases. *Am J Med* 36:743–762, 1964.

11

Drugs and the Kidney
Adjusting Drug Regimens in Patients with Renal Disease

D. CRAIG BRATER

I. INTRODUCTION

The medical literature is replete with guidelines for dose calculation in patients with renal disease. Several different methods have been proposed, with advocates and criticisms of all. At one extreme are publications testifying to the accuracy and predictability of a particular nomogram in allowing the attainment of a desired concentration of drug. At the other extreme are examples of inaccuracies and poor predictability, leaving the clinician with little confidence in the ability of nomograms to allow attainment of desired concentrations in his individual patient. As a result, the clinician is left with the dilemma of not knowing which guideline to use and, if he uses one, how much he can trust it. Clearly, measuring concentrations of the drug facilitates the attainment of desired concentrations in individual patients. However, obtaining such measures is impractical or impossible in many settings. Following clinical endpoints of pharmacological effect, both efficacious and toxic, is invaluable in guiding drug therapy, but in many circumstances, the clinician must place his faith in and entrust his patient's well-being to one or another guideline of drug dosage.

In this chapter, we shall briefly discuss pharmacokinetic terms and principles which will be used in a more detailed analysis of the goals and

D. CRAIG BRATER • Departments of Pharmacology and Internal Medicine, Southwestern Medical School at the University of Texas Health Science Center at Dallas, Dallas, Texas 75235.

principles of design of dose adjustment in patients with renal disease. If used with an understanding of their limitations, dosing guidelines can be extremely useful. The goal of this chapter is to clarify the characteristics of a dosing regimen that make it useful or not by focusing on methods of dose adjustment for aminoglycoside antibiotics, because their narrow therapeutic index, kinetic characteristics, and total dependence on the kidney for elimination dictate the greatest amount of precision of dose adjustment of any drugs in our armamentarium. The reader may then apply these principles in assessing current and future dosing guidelines.

II. TERMINOLOGY

Although the mathematical derivation of pharmacokinetic parameters can be quite complex, the concepts are relatively simple. Most clinicians are comfortable with the concept of a drug's half-life, $t_{1/2}$, which is the time required for the concentration of drug to decrease by half (Table I). Many dosing guidelines use half-life in their terminology, but others use elimination rate constant, K_e. These two parameters can be used interchangeably, since they are reciprocally related:

$$t_{1/2} = 0.693/K_e \text{ or } K_e = 0.693/t_{1/2}$$

Both of these parameters are determined by graphic or computer analysis of the linear, terminal segment of a plot of the logarithm of the concentration of drug versus time. The slope of this segment is equal to $K_e/2.303$ when the

Table I. Terminology

$t_{1/2}$	Half-life. The amount of time required for the concentration of drug to decrease by ½.
K_e	Elimination rate constant, determined by the slope of the terminal log-linear phase of a plot of concentration of drug versus time.
K_r	Elimination rate constant for the renal component of drug elimination.
K_{nr}	Elimination rate constant for the nonrenal component of drug elimination.
V_d	Volume of distribution which relates to the concentration of drug achieved by a given dose.
Cl	Clearance. The amount of blood, plasma, or serum from which all drug is removed per unit time.
f_e	Fraction of dose excreted unchanged in the urine.
F	Fraction of dose absorbed after oral administration.
τ	Dosing interval. The time between doses.
Cp_{ave}	Average concentration of drug at steady state.
Cp_{max}	The maximum or peak concentration of drug at steady state.
Cp_{min}	The minimum or trough concentration of drug at steady state.
GFR	Glomerular filtration rate.
Cl_{Cr}	Creatinine clearance.

serum concentrations are plotted as logarithm to the base 10 in the graphic analysis.

The volume of distribution of a drug, V_d, is an experimentally derived value without physiological meaning. It relates the concentration of drug achieved to the amount of drug in the body:

$$V_d = \text{amount of drug in the body} / \text{drug concentration}$$

The clearance of a drug, Cl, is analogous to the use of the term clearance in any other medical or scientific application. Clearance represents the amount of blood, plasma, or serum from which drug is totally removed per unit time. Consequently, a blood clearance of 100 ml/min means all of the drug is removed from 100 ml of blood in 1 min. Clearance, then, represents the ability of the body to remove the drug and is a function of both the volume in which the drug distributes (or dissipates from the blood) and the elimination rate of the drug:

$$Cl = K_e \times V_d$$

These parameters, along with the dose of drug that enters the body, determine the concentration achieved and the rate of its decline. If a drug is administered repeatedly, the dosing interval, τ, also becomes important.

It may be easiest to conceptualize the interrelationships of these factors by considering the situation in which a patient has been receiving a drug for a sufficient period of time that he is at steady state. This occurs quickly if he has received a loading dose of drug and is then placed on a maintenance regimen. Otherwise, the time to reach steady state is four to five times the elimination half-life. At steady state, the rate of drug entering the body is equal to the rate at which it is leaving:

$$\text{Rate in} = \text{Rate out}$$

The rate of drug entering is, in turn, a function of the dose administered, the fraction, F, of that dose absorbed if the drug is administered orally or intramuscularly, and the time interval over which it is administered:

$$\text{Rate in} = F \times \text{Dose}/\tau$$

The rate of drug leaving the body is a function of its steady-state concentration (Cp_{ave}) and its clearance:

$$\text{Rate out} = Cp_{ave} \times Cl$$

Therefore, at steady state,

$$F \times \text{Dose}/\tau = Cp_{ave} \times Cl$$

or, rearranging the equation:

$$Cp_{ave} = F \times Dose / \tau \times Cl$$

Clearly, the steady-state concentration of drug is an inverse function of dosing interval and clearance and directly related to dose. If drug clearance decreases as a result of decreased renal function as illustrated schematically in Fig. 1, a new steady state is attained after four to five times the new elimination half-life in which Cp_{ave} is increased by the same order of magnitude as the decrease in clearance. Changes in dose, in dosing interval, or in both can be used to compensate for changes in clearance and maintain Cp_{ave} the same as in patients with normal drug clearance. Dosing guidelines suggest changes in dose and dosing interval, but additionally many guidelines attempt to quantitatively correlate an index of renal function such as serum creatinine or creatinine clearance with drug clearance at that level of renal function.

Two other pharmacokinetic parameters are important in considering dosing regimens, namely, Cp_{max}, the maximum or peak, and Cp_{min}, the minimum or trough concentration. Both can be important determinants of efficacy and toxicity, as will be discussed in more detail subsequently. Additionally, in a patient receiving intermittent multiple dosing, Cp_{max} and Cp_{min} are the usual values measured when the patient is monitored with determi-

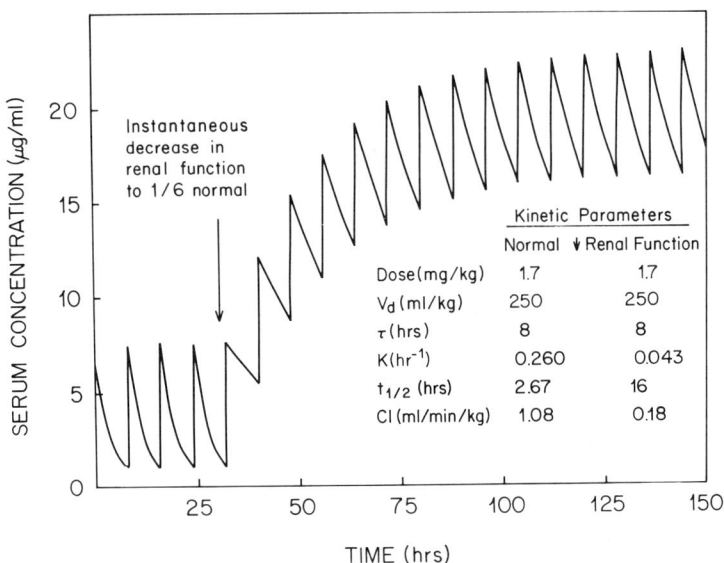

Figure 1. Schematic representation of the serum concentration-vs.-time profile for a hypothetical patient administered gentamicin in whom an instantaneous decrease in renal function to 1/6 normal occurs (arrow). Kinetic parameters for gentamicin are listed in the figure. Volume of distribution was assumed to remain constant. Intravenous bolus administration is depicted for illustrative purposes only.

nations of concentrations of drug in serum. The average serum concentration, Cp_{ave}, on the other hand, is a theoretically calculated value which is not the geometric or arithmetic mean of maximum and minimum concentrations. It can only be directly measured if a patient is receiving a continuous intravenous infusion. Dosing nomograms can be designed to obtain a desired Cp_{max} or Cp_{min} as well as Cp_{ave}.

III. QUANTITATIVE DOSE ADJUSTMENT

As demonstrated in Fig. 1, drug accumulation occurs in patients with renal failure and may cause toxicity. Quantitative dose adjustment is mandatory to avoid toxicity from a drug with a low therapeutic index and involves three steps: (1) evaluation and quantitative estimation of renal function, i.e., glomerular filtration rate (GFR); (2) estimation or prediction of the half-life of the chosen drug in that patient based on the estimated GFR and data from the literature relating drug half-life to renal function; (3) choice of an appropriate dosing regimen of the drug with selection of dose and dosing interval to produce the desired predicted concentrations of drug in serum and time course of these concentrations.

A. Determination of Creatinine Clearance as an Index of Renal Function

The most reliable way to determine creatinine clearance is by a carefully collected, timed urine specimen with a serum creatinine determined at the midpoint of the collection. However, because of the inherent difficulties and errors of urine collection, serum creatinine, rather than direct measurement of creatinine clearance, has been commonly used to estimate renal function. Several nomograms and formulas that consider age, sex, and body weight are available to convert serum creatinine to creatinine clearance. Other nomograms have not considered these variables and, not surprisingly, are less accurate predictors of creatinine clearance than the nomograms accounting for age and weight of patients.

A simple nomogram for bedside use to obtain creatinine clearance based on serum creatinine, age, sex, and weight of a patient was published by Siersbaek-Nielsen and colleagues. This nomogram is widely used and appears to be very reliable. Cockcroft and Gault have published a formula estimating creatinine clearance from serum creatinine in an adult male:

$$C_{Cr} + (140 - age) \times wt(kg)/72 \times [creat] \ (mg/dl)$$

The creatinine clearance for females is 85% of that for males. Creatinine clearances from this method are almost identical to those from the Siersbaek-

Nielsen nomogram. The variability of values derived by this method compared to those from creatinine clearance determined with a urine collection was no greater than the variability between two separate, direct measurements of creatinine clearance. This formula has been tested by other groups and found to be extremely reliable.

A limitation of using serum creatinine in these nomograms is that serum creatinine can correctly relate to renal function only during steady state with a stable serum creatinine. For practical purposes, one can assume stable renal function when clinical evaluation so indicates and if two separate determinations of serum creatinine obtained at least 12 hr apart have values within 0.2 mg/dl.

It is important to note that many clinicians may need to somewhat reorient their thinking regarding magnitudes of change in creatinine clearance. For example, when considering the patient whose creatinine clearance decreases by 50% from 100 to 50 ml/min per 1.73 m², the clinician readily recognizes the magnitude of this decrement and its importance to therapy and drug dosing. On the other hand, a comparable percent decrease from 10 to 5 ml/min per 1.73 m² may be less readily appreciated, for both levels of renal function represent severe impairment, and therapy would differ only a small amount if at all. However, such a change when used in a dosing nomogram mandates a large change in recommended dose or dosing interval, the neglect of which could result in toxicity or inadequacy of treatment.

In summary, by using the Siersbaek-Nielsen nomogram or the Cockroft and Gault formula, one may estimate creatinine clearance from serum creatinine with a degree of reliability sufficient for clinical settings, assuming serum creatinine is at steady state. If renal function is changing, one should directly measure creatinine clearance, realizing that in such a setting any estimate is inherently less accurate. Despite creatinine clearance in many circumstances not being an accurate measure of GFR, this flaw may be relatively unimportant, since changes in creatinine clearance have been accurately and predictably correlated with changes in pharmacokinetics of specific drugs in patient populations.

B. Choice of an Appropriate Dosing Regimen with Selection of Dose and Dosing Interval

After the elimination rate constant or half-life of the drug in an individual patient is predicted from a nomogram or tabulation, one must select a dosing regimen to produce the desired predicted concentration and the time course of the concentration of drug for that patient.

As with any dosing regimen, the objective is to achieve efficacy without toxicity. Precisely defining the pattern of concentration of drug versus time that accomplishes this objective is difficult, for with some types of drugs the goal is not well defined, even in patients with normal renal function. For example, it is debated in the infectious disease literature whether the objective of a dosing regimen is to maintain concentrations of antibiotic continually above the minimum inhibitory concentration (MIC) or to allow wide swings in concentrations from peak to trough with periods of time in which concentrations of antibiotic are less than the MIC. With cardiac glycosides, antiarrhythmics, antiepileptics, and theophylline, the objective is more clearly to maintain trough concentrations within the therapeutic range.

Most nomograms attempt to provide patterns of concentrations of drug in patients with renal dysfunction similar to those achieved in subjects with normal renal function. However, a change in the elimination rate of a drug causes a change from normals in the slope of the descent from peak to trough concentration. Consequently, a dosing regimen in a patient with decreased renal function will never produce a serum concentration-vs.-time curve identical to that of a subject with normal renal function (with the exception of a continuous intravenous infusion).

1. Variable Frequency Regimen

Several methods have been used to accomplish the objective of obtaining a serum concentration profile close to that in uncompromised patients. One method of dose adjustment is commonly referred to as the variable frequency regimen. This method in particular has been widely used for aminoglycoside dosage adjustment. A commonly cited nomogram used this method by recommending the same dose of gentamicin in patients with decreased renal function as in the uncompromised patient but administered at an increased dosing interval in direct relation to the prolongation of half-life of elimination. By so doing, Cp_{max}, Cp_{ave}, and Cp_{min} remain the same as in patients with normal renal function (Figs. 2–4). In these schematics, we have assumed pharmacokinetic parameters identical to those in Fig. 1 in a patient with normal renal function and proportional changes in a patient with varying levels of renal function.

This method of dosing interval adjustment prevents toxicity caused by accumulation of drug in serum in patients with renal impairment, since the total dose administered is decreased in proportion to the decrease in renal function. However, as can be seen in the figures, as renal function decreases, the amount of time during the dosing interval increases in which the serum concentration of the drug is below the minimally effective concentration. This phenomenon occurs with aminoglycosides and other drugs that have a dosing interval considerably less than their half-life. Using this method of dose adjustment, the duration of time in which the concentration is below the effective concentration increases with increasing half-life. As one can see, in patients with the worst renal impairment, serum concentrations remain below the effective concentration for prolonged periods of time. Despite an increased absolute amount of time with serum concentrations above the effective level, the very long continuous time at subtherapeutic concentrations must be of concern to the clinician. Clearly, a longer period of time

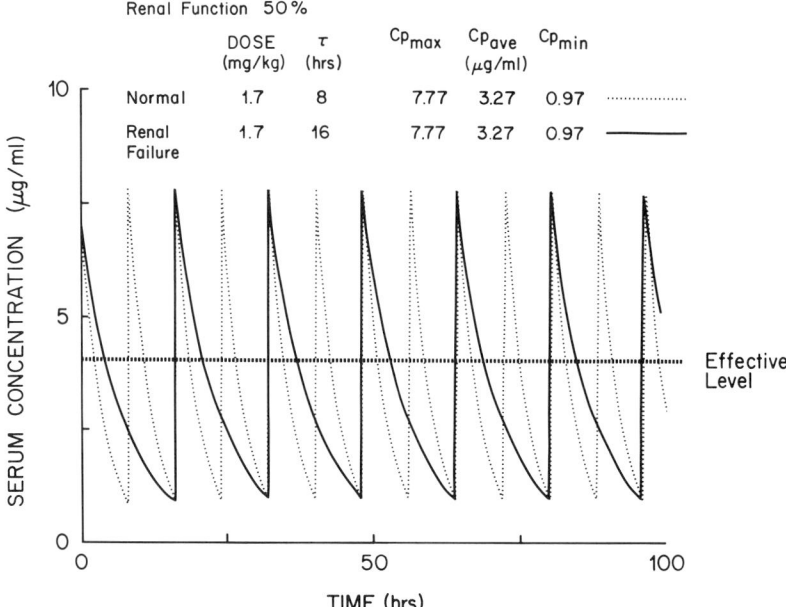

Figure 2. Schematic representation of the serum concentration profile for gentamicin in a patient with normal renal function (stippled curve) and in a patient with renal function 50% of normal in whom the variable frequency regimen has been used for dose adjustment (solid curve). A serum concentration of 4 μg/ml was selected as the "effective level." Derived values for each hypothetical patient assuming intravenous bolus administration are shown.

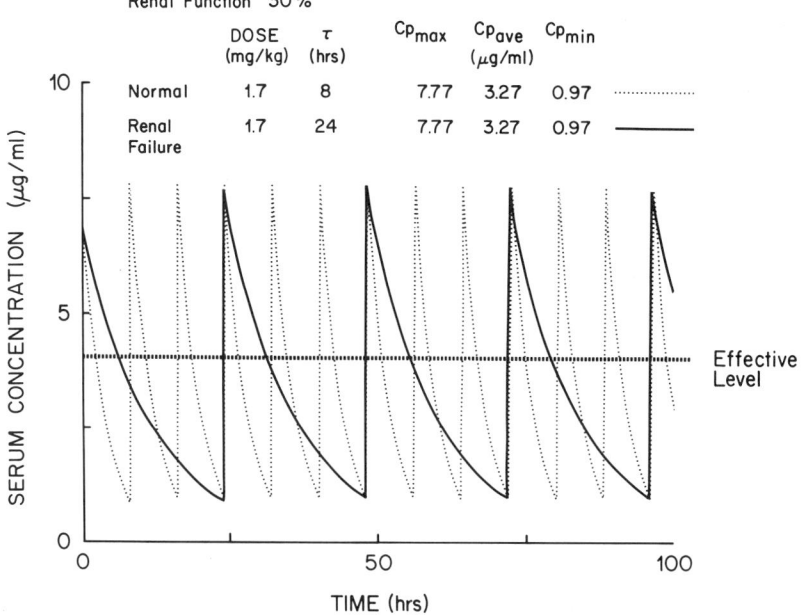

Figure 3. Schematic representation of the serum concentration profile in a patient with renal function 30% of normal in whom the variable frequency regimen has been used for dose adjustment. The format is as in Fig. 2.

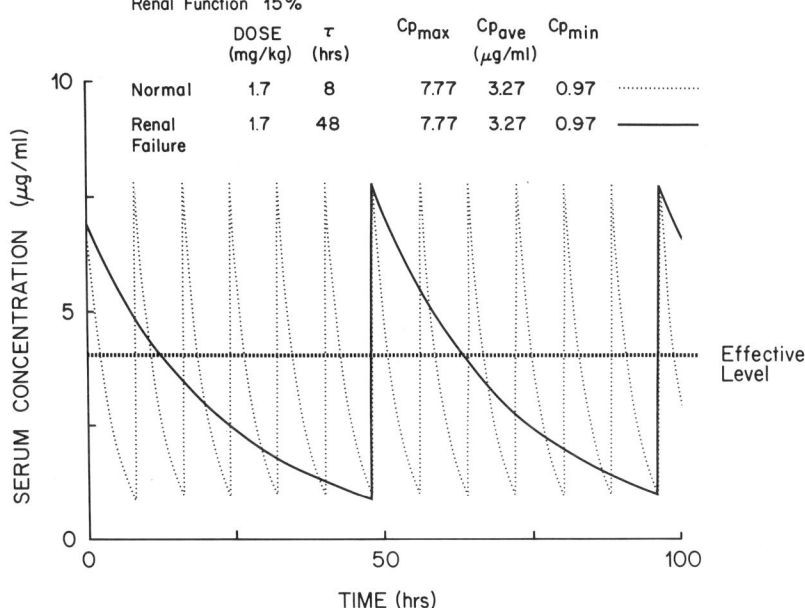

Figure 4. Schematic representation of the serum concentration profile in a patient with renal function 15% of normal in whom the variable frequency regimen has been used for dose adjustment. The format is as in Fig. 2.

"subtherapeutic" might increase the likelihood of persistent infection in the case of antibiosis or of exacerbation of signs and symptoms of disease in use of other agents.

As a basic pharmacokinetic principle, the time during which the serum concentration is higher or lower than a fixed effective level is not only a function of half-life but also of dose. Increasing the dose of a drug will not only increase absolute serum concentrations but will also increase the amount of time spent above a chosen concentration. However, increasing the dose to vary the amount of time above a selected effective level is limited by the narrow therapeutic ratio of many drugs including the aminoglycosides. For other drugs such as pencillins, we have considerably greater latitude for increasing dose, and the precision of dose adjustment can be less. It is not known what duration of subeffective concentrations becomes critical for continued efficacy of the regimen. Clearly, however, most clinicians would feel uncomfortable with the prolonged subtherapeutic concentrations of drug that occur in patients with wide dosing intervals.

2. Variable Dosage Regimen with Fixed Average Concentration of Drug in Blood

In constrast to the variable frequency method, several authors have suggested a variable dosage regimen by maintaining the dosing interval as in patients with normal renal function and by compensating for the decreased clearance of drug by decreasing the dose. This regimen results in the same Cp_{ave}, but Cp_{max} is lower and Cp_{min} higher than in patients with normal renal function. This regimen, as does the variable frequency regimen, prevents drug accumulation, but in contrast, it avoids great fluctuations of serum concentration and theoretically could thereby avoid the prolonged duration of subeffective serum concentrations. However, as illustrated in Figs. 5–7, with decreasing renal function, the serum concentration may actually remain below the effective concentration at all times. This phenomenon occurs with a drug like gentamicin in which the dosing regimen in patients with normal renal function produces wide swings of serum concentration with a Cp_{ave} below the effective concentration.

Another important consideration when using a variable dose regimen is that a "loading dose" is necessary to avoid a delay in time before the serum concentration reaches steady state. Figure 7 demonstrates a serum concentration profile of this regimen when administration is begun with a maintenance dose (lower curve) as opposed to a first dose identical to the dose used in patients with normal renal function, a "loading dose" (upper curve). It is important to note that with a loading dose there will be a delay before the patient becomes "subtherapeutic."

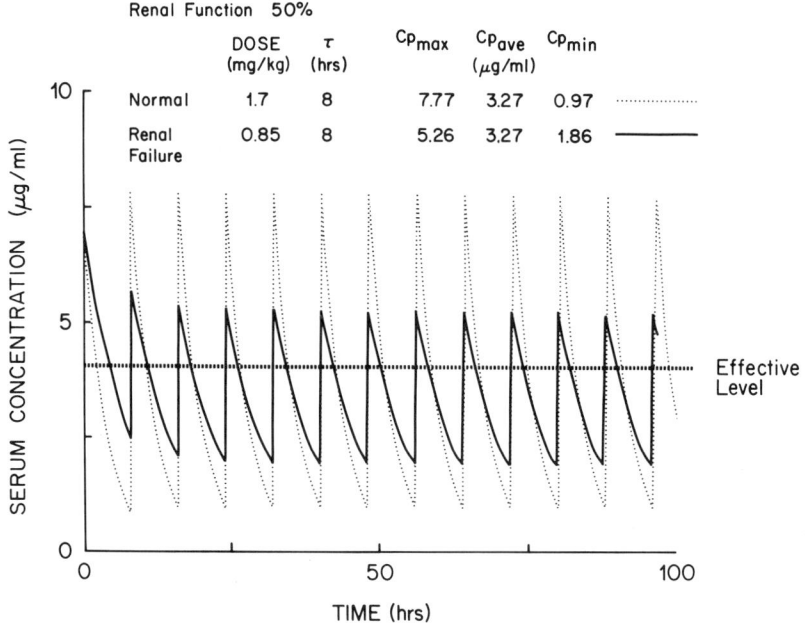

Figure 5. Schematic representation of the serum concentration profile of gentamicin using the variable dose regimen for dose adjustment in a patient with renal function 50% of normal. The format is as in Fig. 2.

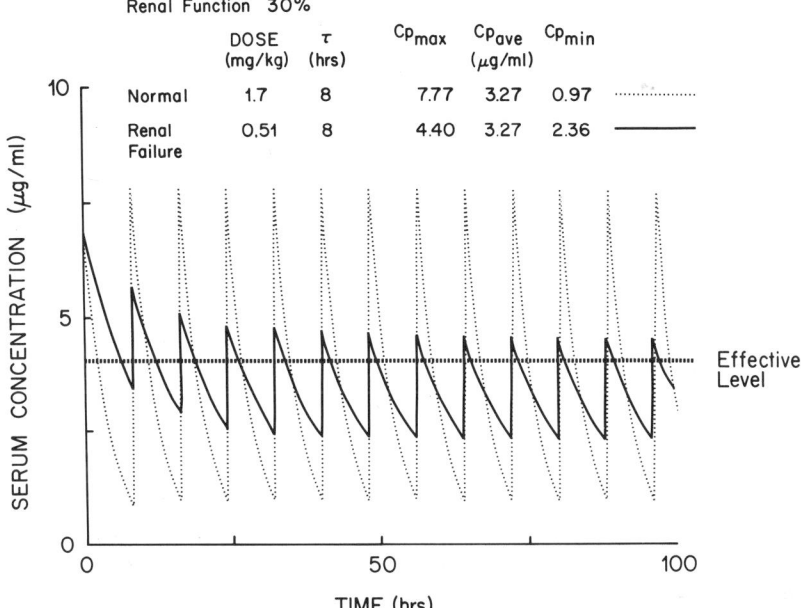

Figure 6. Schematic representation of the serum concentration profile of gentamicin using the variable dose regimen for dose adjustment in a patient with renal function 30% of normal. The format is as in Fig. 2.

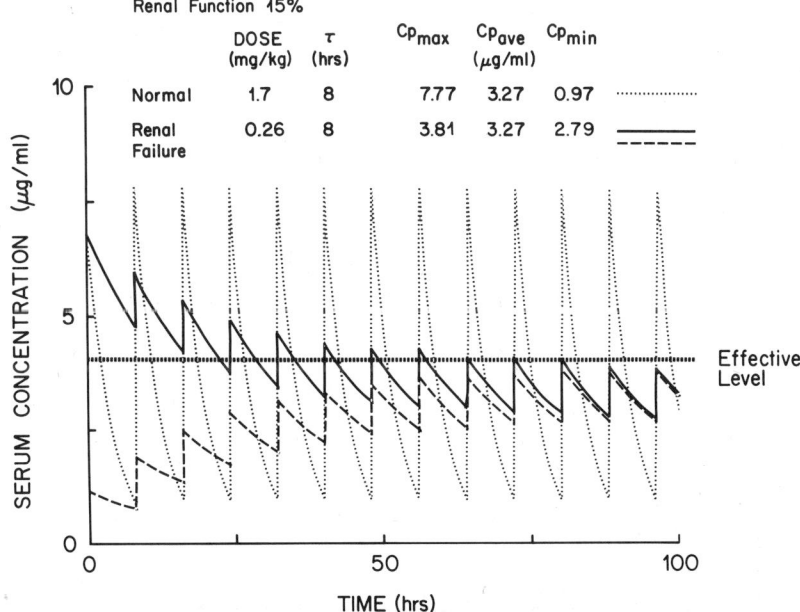

Figure 7. Schematic representation of the serum concentration profile of gentamicin using the variable dose regimen for dose adjustment in a patient with renal function 15% of normal. The format is as in Fig. 2. The solid curve represents the profile when a "loading dose" is administered to the patient with renal impairment; the dashed curve represents the profile when the patient receives a maintenance dose throughout.

3. Variable Dosage Regimen with Fixed Peak Concentration of Drug in Blood

In another so-called variable dosage regimen, one can calculate a dose that will attain a serum concentration of Cp_{max} in patients with renal disease similar to that of a patient with normal renal function. Many nomograms, in fact, are calculated to achieve the same Cp_{max} in patients with decreased renal function as in those without renal impairment. In this situation, the dose used in patients with renal failure will not decrease in proportion to decreased clearance of the drug, because the dose also depends on the magnitude of the chosen dosing interval relative to half-life.

Figures 8–10 depict serum concentration-vs.-time curves for a dosing regimen calculated to obtain a Cp_{max} similar to that of patients with normal renal function and maintaining the same dosing interval. Again, the importance of "loading dose" is depicted in Fig. 10. Using this regimen, one can avoid subtherapeutic serum concentrations for patients with severe renal failure. However, using this regimen, the patient with the most compromised renal function is exposed to a progressively greater concentration of drug over time, because the higher the Cp_{min} the worse the patient's renal function. Consequently, to increase the amount of time with therapeutic concentrations of drug, one may have to subject the patient to greater risk, assuming

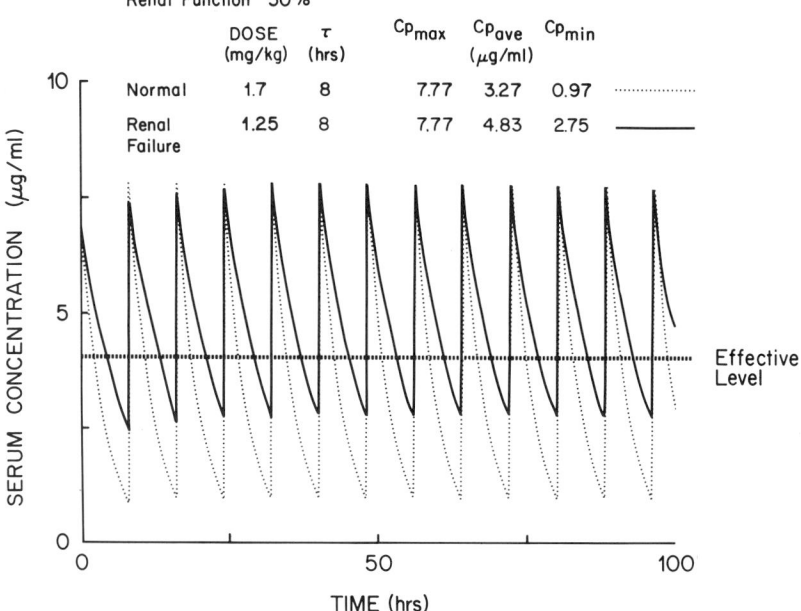

Figure 8. Schematic representation of the serum concentration profile of gentamicin in a patient with renal function 50% of normal using a variable dose approach to dose adjustment but maintaining Cp_{max} in the patient with decreased renal function the same as in the "normal" patient. The format is as in Fig. 2. Note the difference in this profile compared to the variable dose regimen which targeted the same Cp_{ave} in both sets of patients (Fig. 5).

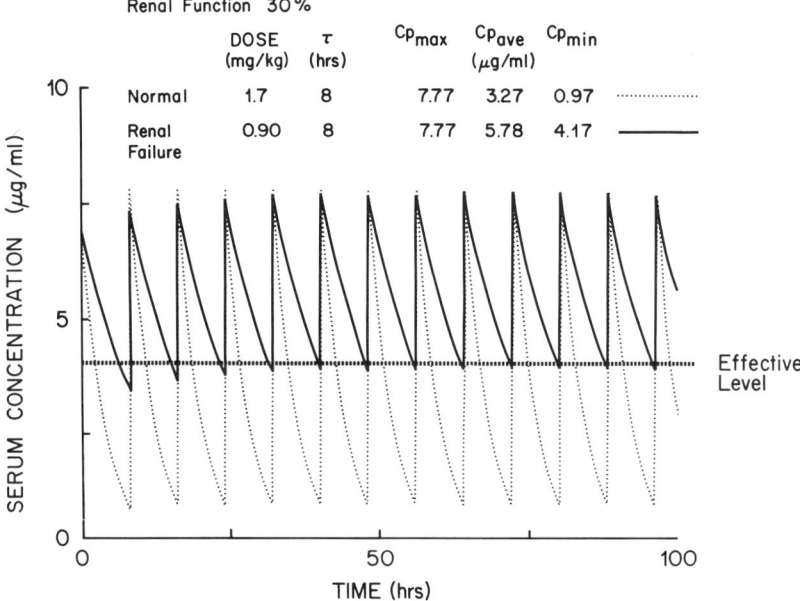

Figure 9. Schematic representation of the serum concentration profile of gentamicin in a patient with renal function 30% of normal using a variable dose approach to dose adjustment but with maintenance of Cp_{max} in the patient with decreased renal function the same as in the "normal" patient. The format is as in Fig. 2. Note the difference in this profile compared to the variable dose regimen which targeted the same Cp_{ave} in both sets of patients (Fig. 6).

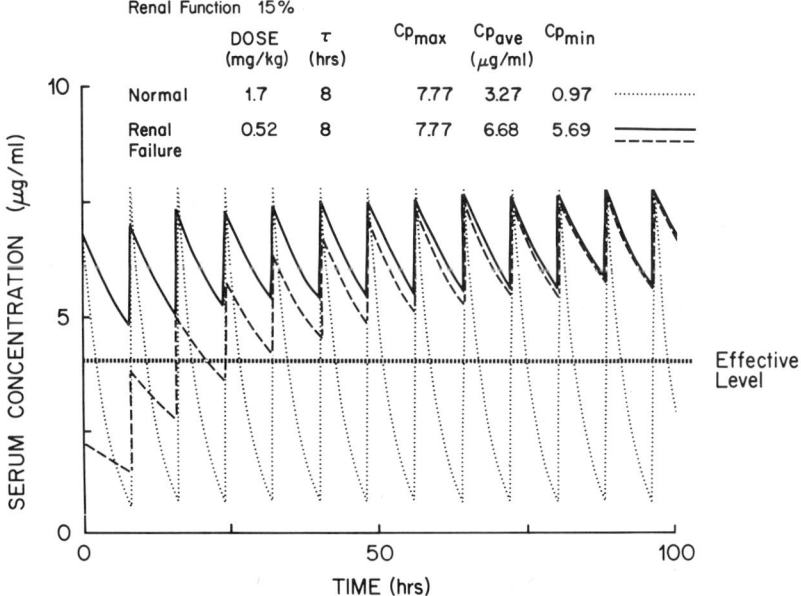

Figure 10. Schematic representation of the serum concentration profile of gentamicin in a patient with renal function 15% of normal using a variable dose approach to dose adjustment but with maintenance of Cp_{max} in the patient with decreased renal function the same as in the "normal" patient. The format is as in Fig. 7. Note the difference in this profile compared to the variable dose regimen which targeted the same Cp_{ave} in both sets of patients (Fig. 7).

risk is related to total drug exposure or related to cumulative trough concentration of drug in serum.

4. Kunin Method for Dose Adjustment

Another method of dosing, originally proposed by Kunin, suggests that one-half of the dose usually administered to patients with normal renal function be given to the patient with renal failure at a dosing interval equal to the drug half-life. Figures 11–13 show serum concentration-vs.-time curves using this method with the first dose of the drug being similar to that of normal subjects, i.e., a modified loading dose. For a drug such as gentamicin, which is normally given every third half-life, Kunin's method provides total doses higher than those in the variable frequency regimen. This may result in increased toxicity. A potential problem with Kunin's method is the "odd" dosing interval which may be impractical from a nursing point of view, particularly in patients with mild renal dysfunction. Overall, however, with severe renal disease, Kunin's method is practical and simple.

5. Combination Method for Dose Adjustment

A combination approach has also been suggested for a number of drugs by Dettli and by Hull and Sarubbi, suggesting a variable dose regimen for

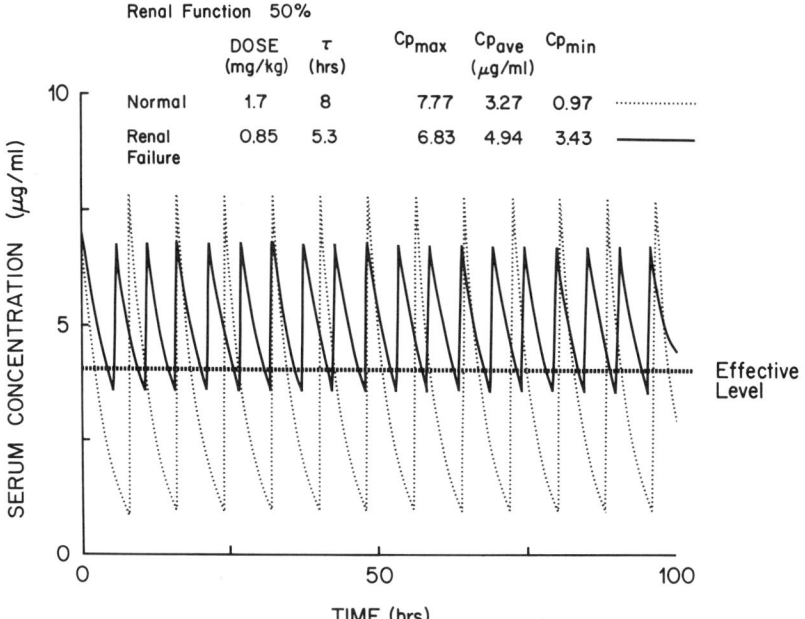

Figure 11. Schematic representation of the serum concentration profile of gentamicin for a patient with renal function 50% of normal using Kunin's method of dose adjustment in which one-half of the dose used normally is administered every half-life. The format is as in Fig. 2.

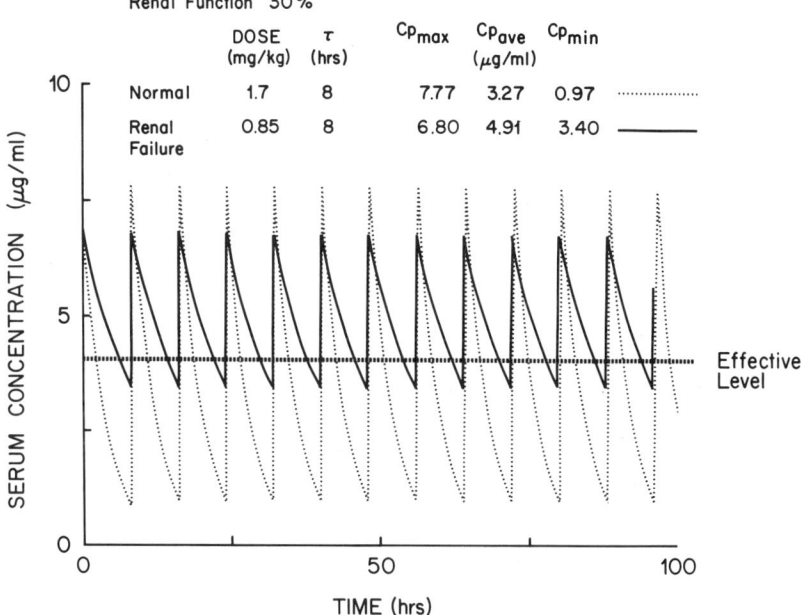

Figure 12. Schematic representation of the serum concentration profile of gentamicin for a patient with renal function 30% of normal using Kunin's method of dose adjustment in which one-half of the dose used normally is administered every half-life. The format is as in Fig. 2.

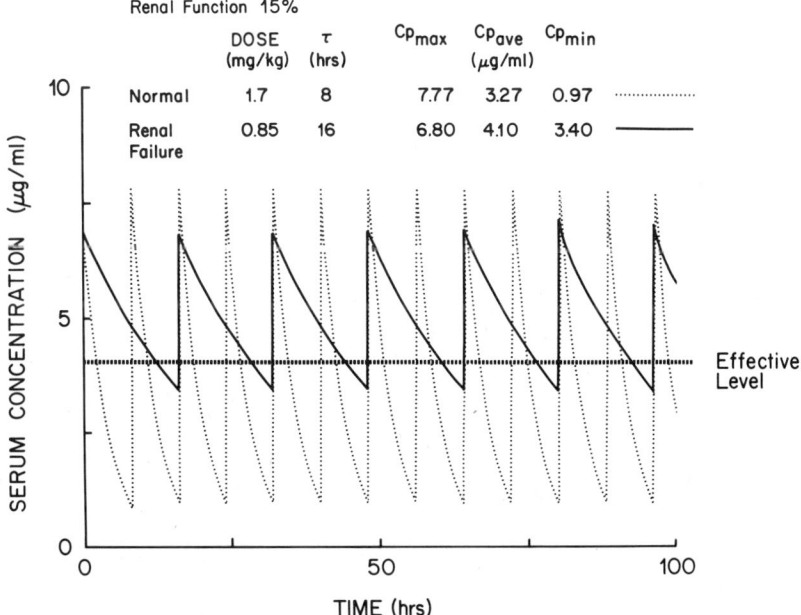

Figure 13. Schematic representation of the serum concentration profile of gentamicin for a patient with renal function 15% of normal using Kunin's method of dose adjustment in which one-half of the dose used normally is administered every half-life. The format is as in Fig. 2.

mild renal dysfunction to obtain a similar Cp_{max} to that in normals and a modified regimen in patients with more severe renal failure by increasing dosing interval, still maintaining Cp_{max} but avoiding sustained high trough levels of drug that may cause toxicity. For a patient with renal function 50% of normal, these guidelines would produce a pattern of response identical to that in Fig. 8. For worse renal function, this approach as shown in Figs. 14 and 15 changes both dose and dosing interval to minimize the sustained trough concentrations (compare to Figs. 9 and 10).

The Hull and Sarubbi recommendations provide that as renal function worsens, the magnitude of difference between Cp_{max} and Cp_{min} becomes less, but Cp_{max} remains the same as in patients with normal renal function. The authors appropriately recommend increasing the dosing interval at severe degrees of renal impairment to avoid sustained high trough concentrations. This feature of the Hull and Sarubbi guidelines is its main advantage for aminoglycosides. The dosing interval should not be greater than 24 hr to avoid long durations of subtherapeutic serum concentrations.

In summary, different dosage regimens have advantages and disadvantages. There is no one universal dosing method that is applicable to all situations. A regimen is the best regimen for one drug at one renal function. Table II lists some of the advantages and disadvantages of the various general approaches. Dosing nomograms are subject to the errors of their assumptions

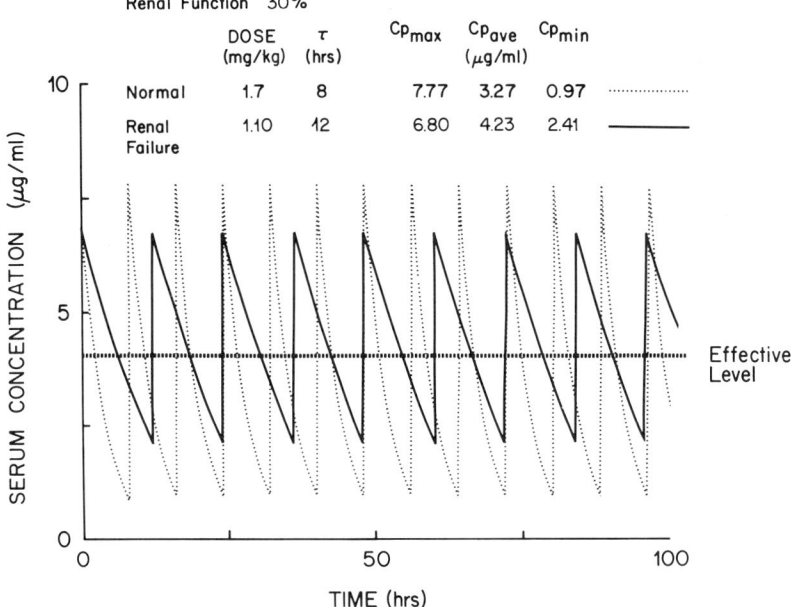

Figure 14. Schematic representation of the serum concentration profile of gentamicin for a patient with renal function 30% of normal using the combination approach of Hull and Sarubbi. The format is as in Fig. 2.

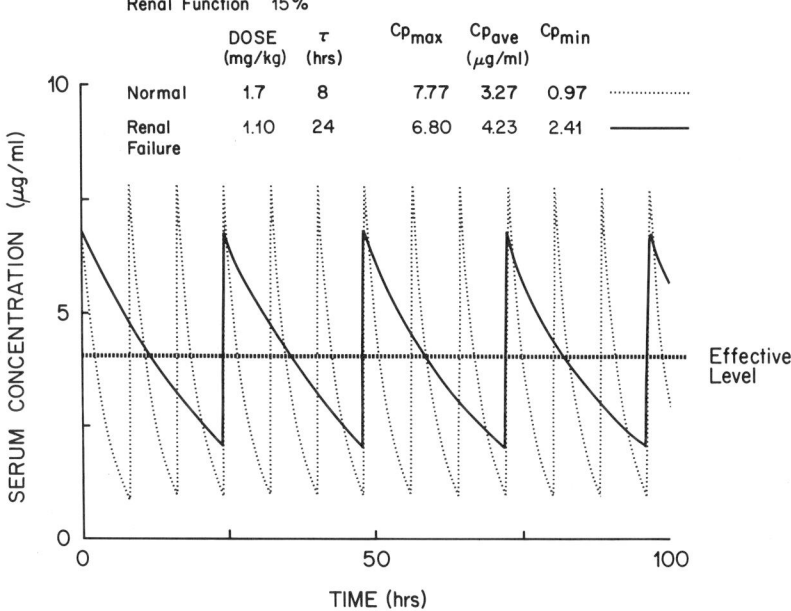

Figure 15. Schematic representation of the serum concentration profile of gentamicin for a patient with renal function 15% of normal using the combination approach of Hull and Sarubbi. The format is as in Fig. 2.

and data base, emphasizing the need for close following of individual patients with measures of serum concentrations of drugs and evaluation of clinical endpoints of pharmacological effect.

IV. CONCLUSIONS

This section has attempted to assess dosing guidelines, particularly those specifically designed for aminoglycosides, in a manner that will allow use of principles of regimen design in evaluation of other current or future guidelines. We feel that the approaches of Dettli in general and that of Hull and Sarubbi for aminoglycosides are preferable, for they "individualize" therapy at different levels of renal dysfunction in an effort to maximize theoretical benefit and lessen the risk of potentially toxic serum concentrations. The clinician must be aware of the limitations of dosing guidelines. Nomograms cannot be used to relieve the clinician of the responsibility of evaluating clinical endpoints of pharmacological effects in each patient. He must realize that nomograms should be used as approximations. Their usefulness has limits, particularly in the patient with severe renal failure or in the patient with changing renal function who may never be at steady state.

Table II. Advantages and Disadvantages of General Approaches of Dosing Nomograms

Method	Advantages	Disadvantages
Variable frequency (Figs. 2–4)	Same Cp_{ave}, Cp_{max}, Cp_{min} "Normal" dose Ease of calculation	Possibly deleterious length of time subtherapeutic "Odd" dosing interval causes potential for administration errors
Variable dose with fixed Cp_{ave} (Figs. 5–7)	Same Cp_{ave} "Normal" dosing interval Ease of calculation	Decreased Cp_{max} which may be continually subtherapeutic "Odd" doses may lead to medication errors Increased Cp_{min}; ? increased toxicity
Variable dose with fixed Cp_{max} (Figs. 8–10)	Same Cp_{max}; attains therapeutic concentrations "Normal" dosing interval	Increased Cp_{ave}, Cp_{min}; ? increased toxicity More difficult to compute dose
Kunin method (Figs. 11–13)	Same Cp_{max}; attains therapeutic concentrations Ease of calculation of both dose (fixed as ½ normal) and of dosing interval (every half-life)	"Odd" dosing interval Increased dose for drug with half-life shorter than dosing interval in subjects with normal renal function Decreased dose for drug with half-life longer than dosing interval in subjects with normal renal function
Combination (Figs. 14, 15)	Can target same Cp_{max} Can simultaneously change dosing interval and lessen impact of increased Cp_{ave} and Cp_{min} and possible toxicity	Need specific regimen for level of renal function and for each drug

When available, serum concentrations of drugs should be measured frequently but judiciously, for their use can clearly facilitate attaining a desired serum concentration. What concentration is desired may be yet another question and may vary among patients, thereby mandating frequent clinical assessment.

SUGGESTED READINGS

Bennett WM, Porter GA, Bagby SP, McDonald WJ: *Drugs and Renal Disease.* New York, Churchill Livingstone, 1978, pp 9–10.

Bjornsson TD: Use of serum creatinine concentrations to determine renal function. *Clin Pharmacokinet* 4:200–222, 1979.

Chennavasin P, Brater DC: Nomograms for drug use in renal disease. *Clin Pharmacokinet* 6:193–214, 1981.

Dettli L: Multiple dose elimination kinetics and drug accumulation in patients with normal and with impaired kidney function. *Adv Biosci* 5:39–54, 1969.

Dettli L: Individualization of drug dosage in patients with renal disease. *Med Clin North Am* 58:977–985, 1974.

Dettli L: Drug dosage in renal disease. *Clin Pharmacokinet* 1:126–134, 1976.

Fabre J, Balant L: Renal failure, drug pharmacokinetics and drug action. *Clin Pharmacokinet* 1:99–120, 1976.

Kunin CM, Finland M: Restrictions imposed on antibiotic therapy by renal failure. *Arch Intern Med* 104:1030–1050, 1959.

O'Grady F: Antibiotics in renal failure. *Br Med Bull* 27:142–147, 1971.

Riff LJ, Jackson GG: Pharmacology of gentamicin in man. *J Infect Dis* 124(Suppl 1):98–113, 1971.

Spring P: Calculation of drug dosage regimens in patients with renal disease: A new nomographic method. *Int J Clin Pharmacol* 11:76–80, 1975.

Tozer TN: Nomogram for modification of dosage regimens in patients with chronic renal function impairment. *J Pharmacokinet Biopharm* 2:13–28, 1974.

Wagner JG: Relevant pharmacokinetics of antimicrobial drugs. *Med Clin North Am* 58:479–492, 1974.

Wagner JG, Metzler CM: Prediction of blood levels after multiple doses from single-dose blood level data: Data generated with two-compartment open model analyzed according to the one-compartment open model. *J Pharm Sci* 58:87–92, 1969.

12

Infections and Antibiotic Usage in Patients with Renal Diseases

GERALD B. APPEL and HAROLD C. NEU

I. INTRODUCTION

Infections are a major cause of morbidity and mortality in patients with renal dysfunction. Infections remain the leading cause of death in acute renal failure. Sepsis, arteriovenous access site infections, and viral hepatitis continue to be major problems for patients with chronic renal failure on maintenance hemodialysis. Other modalities to treat patients with end-stage renal disease (ESRD), including peritoneal dialysis and organ transplantation, are associated with unique and significant infectious complications. In patients with ongoing intrinsic renal diseases (whether glomerular, tubulointerstitial, or vascular in nature), intercurrent systemic infections or infections localized to the urinary tract often lead to further deterioration in renal function and may prove life threatening. At times, the very antimicrobial agents used to treat these infections may contribute further to renal damage. Finally, the treatment of infections of the urinary tract, whether uncomplicated or in patients with structural deformities of the urinary system, poses a constant therapeutic challenge to the clinician.

Many patients with kidney dysfunction have a unique predisposition to infections. In some patients, the renal disease *per se* may predispose to certain infectious complications. In other patients, the predisposition to infection relates equally to the mode of therapy used to treat the disease (e.g.,

GERALD B. APPEL and HAROLD C. NEU • Hemodialysis Unit, Columbia Presbyterian Medical Center; and Departments of Pharmacology and Medicine, Divisions of Nephrology and Infectious Diseases, College of Physicians and Surgeons, Columbia University, New York, New York 10032.

hemodialysis, peritoneal dialysis, corticosteroids, and immunosuppressives in transplant recipients). Finally, other patients have a predisposition to infection related to the primary systemic disease that contributes to their renal dysfunction (e.g., diabetes mellitus).

Although the diagnosis of infection may be obvious in some patients, in others it may be exceedingly difficult to establish early. Thus, the signs and symptoms of uremia may obscure those of an underlying infection. Likewise, corticosteroid and other immunosuppressive therapies may mask the expression of a life-threatening infectious process. The accurate and rapid diagnosis of infections in the population with renal disease requires a high index of suspicion, appropriate use of both routine and more exotic laboratory tests, and, at times, invasive procedures to define the offending organism.

Even the treatment of an established infection with a known organism can prove challenging in patients with renal disease. Knowledge of the pharmacokinetics of antimicrobial agents, the special renal and electrolyte problems they can induce, and the general principles of antibiotic therapy in this population can be crucial in delivering adequate care to such patients. A lack of this knowledge will lead to low cure rates and toxic side effects in patients who are least able to overcome such insults.

II. THE PREDISPOSITION TO INFECTION

Patients with a variety of nephrologic diseases have a predisposition to infections. Knowledge of these predisposing factors can lead to a better understanding of the pathophysiology of infections in patients with renal diseases. This may lead to appropriate preventive measures as well as to rapid diagnosis and a logical choice of antimicrobial therapy.

A. Renal Failure and Dialysis

Infections remain the major cause of mortality in acute renal failure and are a leading cause of mortality and morbidity in chronic renal failure. Although renal failure *per se* leads to a number of defects in host defenses against infections, the use of either hemodialysis or peritoneal dialysis to treat the renal insufficiency adds additional predispositions to infectious complications. In part, the numerous conflicting reports in the literature clearly relate to a failure to distinguish these features and to the varying populations studied (e.g., acute renal failure, chronic renal failure before initiation of dialysis, chronic renal failure on maintenance dialysis).

1. Defects in the Mucocutaneous Defenses against Infection

The mucocutaneous barrier, the first line of host defense against the environment, is defective in patients with renal failure. Uremia may be associated with dermatological abnormalities leading to excessive dryness of the skin, ichthyosis, and atrophy of the epidermis and sweat glands. Pruritis is a common problem which resists simple forms of therapy in patients with renal failure. This may lead to multiple skin excoriations and the potential for penetration of the dermal barrier by skin flora. Minor trauma to the extremities is common in patients with uremic sensory neuropathy and may lead to abrasions and lacerations. Impaired wound healing prevents the rapid recovery from these minor lesions. Likewise, in patients with renal failure who have recently undergone a surgical procedure or trauma, impaired wound healing will exacerbate any primary defect in the host's barrier to infection.

Hemodialysis patients are commonly found to harbor *Staphylococcus aureus* organisms in their nares as well as cutaneously at a much higher frequency than several control populations. Highest staphylococcal carriage rates are found in chronic hemodialysis patients, with intermediate rates found in nondialyzed uremic patients and dialysis unit employees. In a number of studies, both sepsis and vascular access site infections, most often caused by S. *aureus* in the dialysis population, have been found to correlate with prior staphylococcal carriage by phage typing. The host and environmental factors that cause this high carriage rate of staphylococci are unclear.

There are a number of other alterations in host mucocutaneous defenses in renal failure. Respiratory tract abnormalities include retention of fluid within alveoli because of "uremic lung" and congestive heart failure, defective pulmonary clearance of small particles, as well as changes induced by either hemodialysis or peritoneal dialysis (Sections II.A.4, II.A.6). Abnormalities of the gastrointestinal tract in uremia include stomatitis, parotitis, and ulcerative lesions of the mucosal surface predisposing to invasion by intestinal bacteria or fungi. Decreased gastric acidity in some patients may also be a factor in the overgrowth and invasion by some intestinal organisms. In acute and chronic renal failure, a high incidence of urinary tract infections has been noted (as high as 15% of patients with chronic renal failure and 33–90% of patients with acute renal failure studied). Bladder catheterizations, oliguria, urinary stasis, and structural abnormalities of the urinary tract contribute to this incidence of infection. Finally, the techniques of peritoneal and hemodialysis themselves bypass the host's mucocutaneous defenses (Sections II.A.4, II.A.6).

2. Leukocyte Abnormalities in Renal Failure

There are a number of leukocyte functional abnormalities in patients with renal failure. These patients often have a mild to moderate leukocytosis, and the defects noted relate more to inadequate function than to diminished numbers of cells. Morphological and biochemical abnormalities include hypersegmentation of neutrophils, abnormally enlarged neutrophils, neutrophils with excessive vacuolation or prominent granulation, leukocytes with altered electrolyte composition, and neutrophils with increased intracellular enzymes.

Leukocyte function has been reported to be subnormal, normal, or supranormal in patients with renal failure. Locomotion and chemotactic abnormalities appear to be related to the uremic environment, since leukocytes from uremic patients migrate normally when placed in the serum of normal individuals. Whether this is because of inhibitors that decrease the generation of chemotactic factor or another mechanism is unclear. Although some studies indicate that neutrophils from patients with uremia are defective in phagocytosing foreign particles, the majority of evidence indicates that phagocytosis proceeds normally with neutrophils from uremic patients. Uremic serum does not appear to cause defects in opsonization or phagocytosis by neutrophils.

Studies of the intracellular bactericidal activity of neutrophils from patients with renal failure have given variable results, with decreased intracellular bactericidal activity for some organisms and not for others. Studies of monocytes in this population have shown either decreased or normal phagocytosis. Uremic plasma may also cause altered macrophage adhesiveness and phagocytosis. Lymphopenia is common in both acute and chronic renal failure.

3. Defects in Humoral and Cell-Mediated Immunity

Despite abnormalities in the numbers of B lymphocytes in chronic renal failure, this defect is corrected by dialysis, and most studies show normal levels of circulating immunoglobulins. Patients with chronic renal failure have shown adequate antibody response to immunization with a number of exogenous antigens including tetanus toxoid, diphtheria toxoid, and influenza vaccine. However, diminished antibody response to a number of primary immunizing antigens (e.g., typhoid antigen, pneumococcal capsular polysaccharide, staphylococcal teichoic acid antigen following bacteremia) has been documented. Thus, although immunoglobulin levels and synthesis are normal, there may be defects in humoral immunity, especially involving antigens evoking an initial primary response in patients with chronic renal failure. Whether this is a major predisposing factor in the serious bacterial and viral infections the patients with chronic renal failure suffer remains to be defined.

Cell-mediated immunity is depressed in uremic patients. In patients with both acute and chronic renal failure, there is impaired lymphocyte stimulation and decreased macrophage migration inhibition in response to a number of mitogens. Uremic plasma may depress the ability of normal human lymphocytes to undergo transformation and blastogenesis in response to mitogens; this is reversed by dialysis. Dermal reactivity to tuberculin, histoplasmin, mumps, and *Candida* antigens are all markedly depressed in acute and chronic renal failure versus control populations. Tuberculin skin reactivity becomes progressively more and more depressed as renal function worsens, and positive reactors may convert to negative in uremia. The incidence of cutaneous anergy increases with the duration of dialysis.

This generalized defect in cell-mediated immunity is attested to by the prolonged survival of skin and renal homografts in uremic animals and man. It may also explain the predisposition to infections by a number of organisms that are normally partially destroyed by cell-mediated immunity: tuberculosis, fungal infections, listeriosis, and hepatitis B infections.

The reticuloendothelial system appears to function normally in renal failure as shown by normal clearance of microaggregated human serum albumin in humans and normal clearance of staphylococci from the blood of nephrectomized rabbits. However, it is likely that numerous other factors contribute to the predisposition to infection in acute and chronic renal failure; these include acidosis, nutritional deficiencies, electrolyte abnormalities, and the effect of medications on the host defenses.

4. Hemodialysis and the Predisposition to Infection

The dialytic process, while correcting many of the abnormalities of uremia, imposes additional factors that render patients with renal failure susceptible to infection. Most patients undergoing maintenance hemodialysis now have an internal arteriovenous fistula created for angioaccess. However, some patients still rely on external silastic arteriovenous shunts or on prosthetic devices linking the arterial and venous systems internally (e.g., Gore-Tex® grafts). In both of the latter cases, the presence of a foreign body provides a site for bacteria to lodge and multiply during transient bacteremias. Even patients with internal fistulae on maintenance hemodialysis have two needles cannulating their fistulae thrice weekly for 4 to 6 hr at a time. This clearly bypasses the normal mucocutaneous barriers and provides a potential entry route for invading organisms if absolutely sterile procedures are not followed. Although the duration and frequency of hemodialysis in acute renal failure are variable, they often exceed those of chronic maintenance hemodialysis, and it is often performed under less optimal circumstances. It is likely that the majority of access-site infections in hemodialyzed patients relate to improper access site preparation and cannulation. Although S. aureus remains the primary offending organism, an increasing number of access-site infections are caused by gram-negative organisms.

The hemodialysis dialysate in batch-type dialyzers provides an excellent culture medium for bacteria. Although only the upper delivery cannister is warmed to body temperature, nevertheless, with its high glucose content and good oxygenation, the dialysate bath readily allows bacterial colony counts to progressively increase during dialysis. Outbreaks of sepsis in dialysis units have been attributed to contaminated water supply. In general, however, bacterial organisms cannot pass through the dialyzer membrane. Even with blood leaks, the pressure gradient from blood to bath should prevent infection of the patient by bacteria colonizing the dialysate bath. On the other hand, bacterial products and endotoxin may enter the patient's circulation from the bath, leading to febrile episodes during or shortly after dialysis.

Alterations of the body's defense system against infection occur immediately at the onset of contact of the host's blood with the hemodialysis lines and dialyzer. Granulocytes adhere to the hemodialysis membrane and are subject to disruption and destruction. Although complement levels are typically normal in renal failure, there is a rapid decrease in complement levels during hemodialysis as a result of activation of the alternate complement pathway by contact of blood with dialyzer membrane. This activation of the complement system is associated with a transient but relatively profound neutropenia during the initial hours of each hemodialysis procedure. Circulating granulocytes become sequestered in the pulmonary vasculature, leading to intense capillary leukostasis. Although leukocyte counts typically return towards normal levels within several hours of hemodialysis, this is because of release of band forms from the bone marrow.

Whether complement activation is crucial for this "granulocytopenia of dilaysis" and whether this pulmonary capillary sequestration of neutrophils is related to the transient hypoxemia noted so commonly during the early hours of the dialytic procedure remain unclear. The findings of complement activation, pulmonary sequestration of leukocytes, granulocytopenia, and early hypoxemia are all well documented and reproducible. However, reuse of dialyzers typically leads to an absence of the leukopenia with no effect on the transient hypoxemia, supporting the alternate role of dialysis of HCO_3^- and alterations in ventilation as a cause of the hypoxemia. Likewise, when dialyzer membranes are made of polyacrylonitrile and polycarbonate rather than the routine cellulose, complement activation and neutropenia can be dissociated. The interaction of these events and their influence on the susceptibility of the dialysis patient to infection will require further study.

5. The Viral Hepatitis Problem

A major infectious problem common to the hemodialysis population is that of viral hepatitis transferred by blood products and other body fluids. At any one time, 6–15% of chronic hemodialysis patients possess hepatitis B antigen. The impaired immunologic response of dialysis patients may account for their typically mild anicteric response with only slight elevations of liver enzymes and the attainment of the carrier state for hepatitis B. However, outbreaks of hepatitis B among dialysis personnel have led to fatalities and major morbidity. Among the dialysis population itself, there is considerable variability in response to this viral infection, with some patients exhibiting as vigorous a symptomatic infection as dialysis staff members. Screening of blood products for hepatitis-associated antigen and antibody to it, isolation of patients who are hepatitis B carriers, and care in handling all blood products and secretions of this population have clearly decreased the risk of outbreaks of hepatitis B infections. Nevertheless, it remains a persistent problem in dialysis units. More recently non-A, non-B hepatitis has increased in frequency and in many dialysis facilities has become the leading form of viral hepatitis. This poses new challenges in detection as well as questions concerning isolation of these patients and the joint use of isolation facilities with patients who are positive for hepatitis B antigen.

6. Peritoneal Dialysis

The patient undergoing peritoneal dialysis, although untroubled by the problems of extracorporeal circulation of his blood and its interaction with artificial membranes, has unique susceptibilities to infection of his own. Peritonitis is by far the most common infectious complication of peritoneal dialysis. In acute renal failure, peritoneal dialysis is often performed through a temporary catheter inserted percutaneously at the bedside. Lack of sterile technique in insertion and during subsequent catheter care are major factors involved in the induction of peritonitis. It has been stated that the duration of such acute peritoneal dialyses is directly related to the incidence of peritonitis, with dialyses lasting over 48 hr leading to a high incidence of infection. This does not appear to be true if truly aseptic technique and optimal catheter care are used.

Insertion of a temporary prosthesis (Dean prosthesis) to provide easy access for future insertion of a subsequent catheter may provide the access route for infection in the interdialytic period unless absolutely sterile techniques are utilized. With chronic peritoneal dialysis, a "permanent" indwelling catheter is tunneled under the skin and sewn within the peritoneal cavity. The risk of infection here probably relates not to insertion, which is done sterilely in the operating room, but rather to the technique with which the catheter lines are connected to the dialysate lines. With either acute or chronic dialysis, lack of sterile techniques in these connections surely leads to a high incidence of peritonitis. This clearly is the major problem facing patients on chronic ambulatory peritoneal dialysis who must make a number of connections and disconnections of the dialysate reservoir each day. Aerobic gram-negative enteric organisms and staphylococcal species are the most common organisms causing peritonitis, whether in the setting of acute or chronic peritoneal dialysis.

There are additional problems for patients receiving peritoneal dialysis which render them susceptible to infection. The reservoir of fluid within the peritoneal cavity may elevate the diaphragm, leading to poor ventilation of the lower lung fields, atelectasis, and pneumonia. Peritoneal dialysis also leads to a constant loss of protein from the body (approximately 0.5 g albumin lost per liter of dialysate removed). This may contribute to protein malnutrition and decreased host resistance to infection.

B. Renal Transplant Recipients and Other Patients with Renal Disease Receiving Immunosuppressive Medications

The patient receiving a transplanted renal allograft is the prototype of a group of renal patients who have an acquired, drug-induced susceptibility to infection. Although the successful kidney transplant corrects a number of the predispositions to infection caused by uremia and the dialytic process, the immunosuppressive agents and cytotoxic drugs used to prevent the rejection of the foreign organ render the patients more susceptible to a number of opportunistic and mundane infecting organisms. Although the transplant patient in general will be discussed in Chapter 22, an overview of this predisposition to infection is clearly warranted here. This is especially true since infection remains a common cause of graft failure and death in the transplant population.

Corticosteroids, a mainstay of transplant immunosuppression, exert a number of deleterious effects on the host's ability to resist infections. They impair chemotaxis of neutrophils and monocytes, alter the phagocytic and bactericidal activity of neutrophils, and appear to diminish the bactericidal and fungicidal activity of monocytes. Lymphopenia and monocytopenia are predictable results of corticosteroid therapy, and immunoglobulin synthesis is also somewhat impaired. A major effect of steroid treatment is to diminish cell-mediated immunity as evidenced by decreased delayed skin test reactivity to a number of immunogens.

Azathioprine, a maintenance drug for all transplant patients other than identical twins, impairs both humoral and cell-mediated responses to a number of new antigens. Its effects on the primary immune response exceed that on the secondary response. In addition to these effects, a common side effect of azathioprine therapy is myelosuppression leading to neutropenia and enhanced susceptibility to infection. Cylophosphamide, although used less frequently in transplant patients, has equally profound effects on humoral and especially cell-mediated immunity. It also shares the risk of myelosuppression and neutropenia. Other drugs now used experimentally for transplant immunosuppression include antithymocytic globulin (ATG), antilymphocytic globulin (ALG), and cyclosporin A. All have potent lympholytic activity and will probably achieve major roles in transplant immunosuppression in the future. Patients receiving ATG appear to have a higher incidence of cytomegalovirus infections compared to transplant patients treated under routine protocols. Patients receiving high doses of cyclosporin A appear to be predisposed to a number of serious opportunistic infections.

Most drugs used in transplant immunosuppression are associated with major defects in cell-mediated immunity and lesser effects on the humoral system. This is confirmed by altered delayed skin test reactivity in the transplant population, although acceptable antibody responses are achieved against a number of foreign antigens. A number of factors clearly enhance the transplant patient's risk of acquiring a serious infection. These include: age over 40 years, neutropenia, diabetes mellitus, persistent renal failure, and, most important, excessive treatment with multiple courses of high-dose corticosteroids in an attempt to reverse transplant rejections. The use of prophylactic antibiotics at the time of transplantation may contribute to decreased wound infections and sepsis and to the improved survival of cadaveric transplant recipients.

A great many other patients with renal disease are treated with corticosteroids and other immunosuppressive and cytotoxic drugs. These include certain patients with idiopathic nephrotic syndrome, systemic lupus erythematosus, Wegener's granulomatosis, periarteritis nodosa and other vasculitides, and Goodpasture's syndrome to mention only a few. In general, the host defects produced by these medications are similar to those in the transplant population, with additional presdisposition to infection imposed by the specific underlying disease.

C. Other Renal Diseases with a Predisposition to Infection

A number of other patterns of renal dysfunction render patients more susceptible to infectious diseases. The nephrotic syndrome with its constant loss of protein in the urine may lead to protein deprivation. Prior to antibiotic therapy, both pulmonary and peritoneal infections were major causes of death in nephrotic patients. The strong predisposition to infection by encapsulated bacteria (e.g., *Streptococcus pneumoniae*, *Haemophilus influenzae*) may relate to acquired immunoglobulin deficiency caused by massive proteinuria. This may lead to defective opsonization of organisms. Pneumococcal vaccine, prophylactic antibiotics, and hyperimmune γ-globulin have all been used to decrease the risk of infection in high-risk patients with the nephrotic syndrome.

Other patients whose renal disease in only one manifestation of a systemic disease may have unique susceptibilities to infection. Patients with diabetes generally have a decreased resistance to infection and a high incidence of pyelonephritis. This is in part because glycosuria provides a good culture medium for bacterial growth, in part because of frequent obstructive problems in association with autonomic neuropathy and bladder dysfunction, and in part because of impaired renal blood flow. Likewise, patients with multiple myeloma commonly have significant renal dysfunction because of a number of factors; they also commonly have significant infectious complications caused by the immunologic impairment associated with multiple myeloma.

Finally, it is crucial to be aware of certain iatrogenic factors that may predispose patients with renal disease to infection. The use of indwelling catheters, endotracheal tubes, respiratory assist devices, and hyperalimentation lines in many hospitalized patients bypasses the first lines of host defense. The indiscriminant use of prophylactic antibiotics may destroy natural host flora and select out invasive pathogens. The very act of hospitalization may lead to host colonization with less susceptible gram-negative organisms.

Although these features are true equally for patients with or without renal disease, this added predisposition to infection superimposed on that of the renal patient who already has impaired host defenses may be crucial in leading to serious infectious complications.

D. Pathogenesis of Urinary Tract Infections

1. Uncomplicated Urinary Tract Infections

It has been estimated that 10–20% of normal women will have at least one urinary tract infection, and many have recurrent infections. In patients with prior renal dysfunction, urinary infections can lead to further functional impairment and be extremely difficult to eradicate.

Although bacteria might enter the urinary tract either by ascending spread from the perineal region or by hematogenous or lymphatic routes, in man, ascending infection is by far the most common pathway. The bladder is normally sterile, and a number of host factors inhibit the initiation of infection here. High urinary flow rates dilute and wash out bacterial organisms. The high concentration of urea and other solutes, frequent changes in osmolality of the urine, and the low urinary pH tend to inhibit many bacterial organisms. Thus, fastidious organisms and anaerobes, the major fecal bacterial organisms, will not readily grow in urine. Prostatic secretions contain substances that inhibit bacterial growth, and the urinary bladder mucosa has antibacterial activity. The low pH of vaginal secretions may inhibit colonization by fecal bacteria.

Despite these protective mechanisms, urinary tract infections are exceedingly common, especially in females. This supports the concept of ascending infection with colonic bacteria that have colonized the anterior vagina, vulvar region, and distal urethra. The normal distal urethral flora in patients who rarely develop urinary infections does not include colonic gram-negative organisms but rather diphtheroids, lactobacilli, and *Staph. epidermidis*. The short female urethra facilitates contamination from the perirectal region. With trauma to the urethra, as in sexual intercourse, there is migration of bacteria into the bladder. Failure to clear this initial colonization by adequate urine flow permits multiplication of bacteria and subsequent clinical infection.

Infections are more common with certain bacterial organisms even within the same species. For example, the serotypes of *E. coli* that most commonly cause urinary infections have been shown to possess K antigens that allow these strains to adhere to vaginal epithelial cells more readily. Likewise, the presence of pili (short projections) on the surface of some *E. coli* and *Proteus* sp. favors bacterial uroepithelial cell attachment. The introital epithelial cells of females who develop frequent urinary infections commonly have bacteria attached to their surfaces. Thus, a combination of bacterial affinity for colonization and host predisposition (absence of low pH, vaginal epithelial cells of glycocalyx type with high affinity for bacteria) may lead to symptomatic infection. Motility of some bacteria facilitating ascent along the ureters and urease production by others favoring renal medullary tissue injury may both enhance the opportunity for upper urinary tract infection.

2. Complicated Urinary Tract Infections

Although many factors lead to urinary infections in women, it is uncommon even for the female patient with recurrent uncomplicated lower urinary tract infections to develop significant damage to the upper urinary tract. A number of genitourinary abnormalities, however, greatly enhance the susceptibility to both lower and upper tract infection as well as rendering the infection more difficult to eradicate. Obstruction to urine flow with stasis anywhere in the urinary tract is prominent among these factors. The obstruction may be localized anywhere from the distal urethra to the renal pelvis; it may be partial or complete, anatomic or functional in nature. Thus, incomplete emptying of the bladder, whether because of urethral stricture or neurogenic bladder dysfunction, will predispose to multiplication of any organism that enters the bladder.

Vesicoureteral reflux predisposes to infection by a number of mechanisms. It delivers organisms from the lower urinary tract to the upper, forms initial sterile foci of parenchymal damage for bacteria to lodge in, and, finally, allows stasis of the urine. Other intrarenal anatomic deformities and foreign bodies such as calculi and scars provide a nidus for bacteria to colonize and multiply on within the upper urinary tract.

Certain additional factors render certain patients more susceptible to urinary infections. Thus, pregnancy, because of hormonal changes and physical obstruction, leads to ureteral dilatation, decreased peristalsis, and a high incidence of urinary tract infections. Diabetes mellitus leads to enhanced urinary infections through an enhanced medium for bacterial growth with a high urinary glucose concentration, fixed urinary osmolality because of impaired urine-concentrating ability, and pH alterations. Frequent catheterization and urinary stasis in the bladder because of autonomic neuropathy no doubt contribute to this predisposition. The enhanced susceptibility of patients with chronic renal failure has been mentioned previously.

Urethral catheterization is a major cause of urinary tract infections. With one "straight" catheterization in a healthy female patient, the risk of infection is small (1–2%). This risk dramatically increases if the patient is pregnant (5–15% risk) or if the patient is hospitalized and has an underlying disease (10–20%). The risk of infection increases with the duration of time the catheter is left in place. Although some initial infections may be associated with the "pushing" of organisms into the bladder, the majority of catheter-related infections arise from ascent of bacteria along the catheter sheath. The risk of bacteremia from catheterization is small but significant. Careful technique at catheter placement, use of a closed drainage system, use of catheters that do not allow organisms to encrust on them, and the use of intermittent straight catheterization several times daily (as opposed to indwelling catheters in patients with neurological bladder problems) will reduce the incidence of infections.

III. THE DIAGNOSIS OF INFECTIONS IN PATIENTS WITH RENAL DISEASE

In general, the diagnostic techniques used to document active infection in patients with renal dysfunction are similar to those used in patients with normal kidney function. However, crucial in the population with impaired host defenses are a high index of suspicion for certain infectious organisms, meticulous care in obtaining and handling specimens, and the rapid use of procedures that allow a specific etiologic diagnosis. The onset of infection may be quite subtle. Thus, the uremic patient or the patient receiving transplant immunosuppression may not exhibit a normal febrile response to a life-threatening infection. Likewise, the source of infection may prove cryptic. Localizing the site of infection in the uremic patient with altered mental status, pulmonary congestion, a systolic and "diastolic flow murmur of uremia," and bony changes resulting from renal osteodystrophy can be a major challenge to the clinician. Nevertheless, in the vast majority of cases, prompt and accurate diagnosis is possible, allowing specific antimicrobial treatment when indicated and thus avoiding indiscriminate use of broad-spectrum antibiotics. The following brief guidelines will prove useful in the diagnosis of most infections in patients with renal dysfunction.

A. Skin, Mucosal, and Soft Tissue Infections

Superficial bacterial infections of the skin and soft tissues are commonly caused by gram-positive cocci, staphylococci and streptococci. Dialysis patients whose skins are colonized by *Staph. aureus* are likely to have soft tissue infections with this organism. However, many hospitalized patients with renal disease become colonized by the local gram-negative flora of their environment and present with soft tissue infections caused by aerobic gram-negative bacilli.

Three specific sites of soft tissue infection with unusual features include the oropharyngeal region, decubitus ulcers, and the perirectal area. Oropharyngeal and gingival infections are usually caused by gram-positive organisms and anaerobes. Hospitalized patients are prone to orophyaryngeal colonization by the gram-negative flora of their local environment. These infections commonly respond to local hygiene, dental repair, and systemic antibiotics. Decubitus ulcers, a major problem in chronically debilitated patients, can be a frequent source of sepsis. Gram-negative aerobic and anaerobic bowel organisms predominate in decubiti of the sacral region. Local therapy with appropriate debridement and relief of pressure are especially important in the care of these ulcers. Perianal infections are a common source of "fever of unknown origin" and sepsis in patients with impaired host defenses. In leukopenic patients, many of the local findings of a perirectal abscess will be absent. Aerobic gram-negative rods, gut anaerobes, and enterococci are the predominant organisms. Surgical drainage combined with systemic antibiotics will cure the majority of these infections.

At times, the site of the infection and characteristic clinical finding may suggest the nature of the offending organism in soft tissue infections. Thus, the characteristic sweet odor and greenish color of a purulent exudate may suggest a *Pseudomonas* sp. infection, whereas localized gas formation and foul-smelling pus may suggest the presence of an anaerobic infection. Despite these clinical guides, a firm diagnosis rests on appropriate culture of the organism. Usually there is adequate purulent material for gram stain, routine bacterial cultures, and anaerobic cultures. In patients with impaired host defenses, cultures for fungi and other opportunistic organisms should be obtained. In nonpurulent infections, as cellulitis, sterile saline can be injected with a 25-gauge needle into the margin of the area of inflammation and aspirated for culture and gram stain. It is wise to perform blood cultures whenever systemic symptoms accompany a localized soft tissue infection. Blood cultures should be performed routinely in immune-compromised hosts with any evidence of infection.

B. Respiratory Infections

Upper respiratory infections in patients with renal disease are usually similar to those in the general population and require no special diagnostic procedure. Most are mild, self-limited, and respond rapidly to appropriate antimicrobial therapy. An occasional patient who fails to respond to therapy for otitis media or sinusitis will need aspiration or drainage procedures for specific diagnosis as well as symptomatic pain relief. Gram stains of upper respiratory secretions are often unreliable, and the specific diagnosis rests on appropriate culture.

Lower respiratory infections continue to be a common cause of morbidity and mortality in many groups of patients with renal disease. Pulmonary infections are the most common cause of death in the renal transplant population and are a significant cause of death in patients with both acute and chronic renal failure. Diagnostic maneuvers are aimed at determining the extent of the pulmonary infection and the nature of the offending organism(s). The extent of the infection can usually be determined from clinical symptomatology (e.g., presence of high fever, dyspnea, etc.), physical examination, chest X-ray, and arterial blood gases. However, some immunosuppressed patients with suspected infectious pneumonias may have no infiltrate on chest X-ray despite impressive symptomatology and hypoxemia. With correction of their leukopenia and hydration, an infiltrate often becomes apparent. One must also consider a number of noninfectious etiologies for pulmonary infiltrates in patients with renal diseases. These include allergic drug reactions, pulmonary vascular congestion, uremic pneumonitis, and emboli with pulmonary infarction. It is crucial to rapidly distinguish these conditions from treatable infectious pneumonias in which early specific antimicrobial therapy can prove life saving.

The clinical presentation, physical examination, and chest X-ray are of some value in determining the nature of the offending organisms in lower respiratory infections. For example, an acute onset with fever, chills, and purulent sputum might suggest a bacterial infection, whereas a more indolent course may suggest a more chronic infectious agent. Nevertheless, accurate diagnosis must rest on culture of secretions and/or tissue obtained from the lower respiratory tract. To obtain an adequate sputum specimen for smears and culture, expectoration may be induced by a respiratory nebulizer, and secretion may be obtained by nasotracheal or pharyngotracheal suctioning or transtracheal aspiration avoiding oropharyngial contamination. Poorly collected specimens will often grossly reveal saliva mixed with mucus and the presence of numerous epithelial cells on microscopic examination. In leukopenic hosts, however, it is not unusual to see very few inflammatory cells despite adequate sputum collection. Smears should be prepared for gram stain, acid-fast staining, as well as mucicarmine and silver stain if opportunistic organisms are suspected. Cultures should routinely be processed for mycobacterium, fungi, and anaerobic bacteria as well as for routine culture. Although a "best guess" antibiotic regimen based on the results of clinical findings and smears is reasonable initial therapy, treatment should be specifically redirected at the organism cultured as soon as possible in accord with sensitivities as determined by the laboratory.

In many immune-compromised febrile patients, therapy will be started empirically with an antibiotic regimen. If the routine culture fails to provide a specific diagnosis, and the patient shows no clinical response to the regimen in several days or is clinically deteriorating, an opportunistic or resistant organism may be responsible. More invasive procedures including bronchoscopy and transbronchial and open lung biopsy should be considered. These invasive procedures designed to diagnose rapidly the specific offending organism are especially crucial in immune-compromised hosts. At the time of the procedure, appropriate smears and culture specimens for aerobic bacteria, mycobacteria, anaerobic bacteria, fungi, viruses, and Pneumocystis should be obtained.

In renal transplant and immunosuppressed patients, several exotic organisms causing lower respiratory infections are common. The patient with fever, dyspnea, cough, hypoxemia, and infiltrate on chest X-ray may harbor Pneumocystis carinii. Legionella pneumophila and similar organisms can cause pneumonias resistant to empirical therapy with commonly used antibiotics (cephalosporins, aminoglycosides). Mycoplasma infections and viral pneumonias with herpes virus and especially cytomegalovirus are also common in immunocompromised hosts.

C. Endovascular Infections

Endovascular infections are especially common in the hemodialysis population. They usually arise from local infection at the arteriovenous hemodialysis access site. In patients with infections of both external silastic arteriovenous shunts and internal arteriovenous fistulae, the bacterial organism most commonly isolated is *Staphylococcus aureus*. Dialysis patients, with their high rate of nasal and dermal colonization with this organism, are autoinfected at the time of cannulation for dialysis. Although the incidence of local infections with external shunts ranges from one to three episodes per patient per dialysis year, it is less than 0.15 episodes per patient per dialysis per year for internal fistulae. However, two-thirds of the episodes of septicemia in the dialysis population still arise from access site infection. In older reports, virtually all of these infections were attributed to *Staph. aureus*. In a recent review, however, 70% were reported caused by *Staph. aureus* and 25% by gram-negative bacilli.

Patients with infected external shunts often present with localizing findings of thrombosis, bleeding, cannula extrusion, or purulence at the shunt site. Although local findings are far less common in patients with infected arteriovenous fistulae, infections here, especially when caused by *Staph. aureus*, may present with localized swelling, pain, purulent discharge, or frank abscess formation along the arteriovenous fistula. As an aid to diagnosis in subtle cases, cultures may be obtained from the access site itself and compared with venous blood cultures from elsewhere in the body. Positivity at the access site alone confirms the localization of the infection, whereas positive cultures at both sites is nondiagnostic.

The mortality from sepsis related to access site infections remains high, between 10 and 20%. In the absence of a localized abscess, infected fistulae can often be treated with prolonged antibiotic therapy without removal or surgical repair of the fistula. This is fortunate, since new access sites are limited in the chronic dialysis population, and since many patients may be adequately treated with once-a-week intravenous vancomycin therapy (this drug, which is excellent against *Staph. aureus*, is renally excreted and not dialyzed; thus, prolonged effective serum levels are achieved by one injection per week). Patients with infected external shunts require removal of the foreign body to eradicate the infection. In general, infected bovine heterografts and prosthetic vascular access devices (e.g., Gore-Tex®) also require removal for sterilization of the infection. An unfortunate but increasingly common problem occurs in heroin addicts who develop renal failure as a result of heroin nephropathy and then suffer repeated bouts of septicemia and access-site infections as they utilize their fistulas for the injection of illicit drugs.

Bacterial endocarditis is commonly caused by staphylococci or streptococci in dialysis patients. Often it is difficult to distinguish true endocarditis from an access-site infection, since the latter may present only with sepsis and no localizing findings, and since systolic and diastolic murmurs, cardiac valve abnormalities, and anemia are common in the dialysis population in general.

D. Gastrointestinal Infections

Enteric infections in patients with renal disease are similar to those of the general population. Several diagnostic techniques along with appropriate stool cultures are of value. Thus, the presence of numerous fecal leukocytes on methylene blue staining of a diarrheal specimen is suggestive of invasive gastroenteritis (secondary to salmonella, shigella, and some *E. coli*) rather than toxin-induced gastroenteritis (caused by noninvasive *E. coli* or staphylococcal food poisoning). Gram stain of the stool is also useful to diagnose the sheets of positive cocci in *Staph. aureus* superinfection of the gut in patients receiving broad-spectrum antimicrobial therapy. A more common cause of diarrhea in patients receiving antibiotics is pseudomembranous colitis. When this condition is suspected, the stool should be assayed for toxin produced by *Clostridium difficile*.

In immune-compromised hosts and especially renal patients receiving corticosteroids and other immunosuppressive drugs, a number of less common gastrointestinal infections may occur. With the use of broad-spectrum antibiotics, superficial overgrowth of the gut flora by *Candida* is common. This may at times lead to deeper invasion of the gastrointestinal tract mucosa; for example, *Candida* esophagitis is characterized by fever, dysphagia, substernal pain, and distinctive shaggy lesions on barium swallow. Renal transplant patients may also develop overwhelming infestations with gastrointestinal parasites such as strongyloides.

E. Urinary Tract Infections

In some patients, both the diagnosis of infection within the urinary tract and the differentiation between upper and lower tract infection may be obvious. The patient with frequency, dysuria, painful voiding of small volumes of blood-tinged urine, and suprapubic tenderness who has a positive urine culture and responds to antimicrobial therapy has a classic bacterial cystitis. Likewise, the patient with fever, chills, costovertebral angle tenderness, leukocyte casts on urinalysis, and a positive urine culture has a classic case of acute bacterial pyelonephritis. In other patients, the diagnosis may be more subtle. This is especially true for immunosuppressed transplant recipients who frequently present with fever as their only manifestation of a urinary tract infection and patients with chronic renal failure who chronically have pyuria and may have low back pain as a result of renal osteodystrophy. The following section is a guide to accurate diagnosis of infections of the urinary tract in patients with or without prior renal disease.

In young females, over 85% of outpatient urinary tract infections are caused by *E. coli*, with the remainder caused by *Proteus mirabilis*, *Staph. saphrophyticus*, and enterococci. In hospitalized patients, especially following urethral instrumentation, infections occur commonly with *Pseudomonas aeruginosa*, *Morganella*, *Enterobacter*, or *Citrobacter*. Infection is usually caused by a single organism but may be caused by multiple species in patients with indwelling catheters and/or recent urethral instrumentation.

Urinary tract infections are the most common specific infection in patients with acute and chronic renal failure. From 30 to 90% of patients with acute renal failure and from 10 to 20% of patients with chronic renal failure will develop such infections, often with enterobacteraceae other than *E. coli*. Up to three-quarters of the renal transplant population will also have urinary infections. Most are easily treated; however, some become chronic problems in patients with scarred, deformed bladders or other structural abnormalities of the urinary system. It is worth noting that infections caused by *Staph. epidermidis* occur in the transplant population and deserve treatment.

1. Definitions

Certain definitions are valuable in avoiding confusion when referring to infections in the urinary tract. Cystitis, as described by the symptom complex above, implies a significant number of pathogenic microorganisms limited to the bladder and/or urethral region. Acute bacterial pyelonephritis indicates bacterial invasion of the kidney and upper urinary tract. Recurrent urinary tract infections are those in which the infection is with the same organism as isolated previously, as opposed to reinfection of the urinary tract which indicates repeated infection by different organisms. Abacteriuric dysuria refers to lower tract symptoms similar to those found with classic bacterial cystitis but in the absence of any cultured organism. Abacteriuric dysuria may be caused by difficult-to-culture organisms as *Chlamydia trachomatis*, *Ureoplasma ureolyticum*, or viral agents, or it may be caused by noninfectious irritation of the bladder or urethra. Asymptomatic bacteriuria implies that despite the absence of symptoms the patient has a significant number of pathogenic organisms in the urine (see Section III. E). Chronic pyelonephritis is a pathological diagnosis indicating longstanding tubulointerstitial disease which may or may not be associated with bacterial infections.

2. Confirming the Diagnosis

In the patient who does not present with obvious bacterial cystitis or acute pyelonephritis, the clinician is faced with a double task: first to confirm or deny the presence of infection within the urinary system; second to differentiate lower tract disease from the involvement of the upper urinary system. The diagnosis of a "significant" infection of the urinary tract by pathogenic organisms rests on examination of the urine. Proper collection of a freshly voided midstream specimen of urine, after thorough cleansing of the periurethral region is crucial to obtaining accurate results when urine is examined for the presence of infection. Although the bladder is normally sterile, the distal urethra is not, and a midstream specimen is necessary to wash out the distal urethral flora.

Once the urine specimen has been obtained, 15 ml is centrifuged at 2000 rpm for 5 min and then examined under the "high dry" (440×) lens of the microscope for leukocytes. Over five to ten leukocytes per high-power field represents significant pyuria and may indicate active infection. Likewise, leukocyte casts indicate renal parenchymal injury which may be caused by bacterial pyelonephritis. Unfortunately, relying on pyuria as an indication of active urinary tract infection results in many false positives and negatives. This is especially true in the population of patients with preexistent renal disease who often chronically have pyuria and/or leukocyte casts in their urine sediment. More useful in the presumptive diagnosis of urinary infection is the presence of bacteria on a smear of a clean midstream urine specimen. In an unstained uncentrifuged specimen, the presence of one or more bacteria per oil-immersion field indicate $>10^6$ bacteria per milliliter of urine. If the unspun urine is gram stained, the finding of one or more bacteria per field indicates $>10^5$ organisms per milliliter of urine which is significant bacteriuria and implies the presence of active infection. It is obvious that a fresh urine specimen is necessary to prevent multiplication of any contaminating bacteria.

A number of other criteria have been suggested for the rapid diagnosis of active urinary tract infections. These include subnormal amounts of glucose in the urine because of bacterial metabolism of the small amount of glucose normally present, a urine pH over 7.5 suggesting the presence of urea-splitting organisms, and the reduction of nitrates to nitrites in the urine by bacteria. None of these criteria provide a more accurate indication of the presence or absence of urinary tract infection than microscopic examination of the urine. Obviously, culturing the urine to provide a definite diagnosis of infection and the sensitivities of the bacterial organisms is mandatory in all cases of suspected urinary tract infection.

3. Localization within the Urinary Tract

Once the presumptive or definitive diagnosis of infection within the urinary tract has been established, there are a number of methods to help localize the infection to the upper or lower urinary system. Ureteral catheterization clearly indicates whether the upper tract harbors pathogenic microorganisms, but this is obviously too invasive a procedure to recommend routinely. Another technique involves bladder catheterization, wash-out with an antibiotic solution to sterilize the bladder, and subsequent collection of urine specimens over time. Increasing numbers of bacteria in subsequent samples implies delivery of significant numbers of bacteria from the upper tract. A third technique uses a single large dose of an oral antibiotic, e.g., amoxicillin, which will eradicate any bacteria within the bladder but not within the kidney itself. The presence of bacteria at 48 hr indicates upper tract disease. Finally, the urine may be examined for antibody-coated bacteria by adding fluorescein-conjugated antihuman globulin to the urine containing bacteria and examining the specimen for fluorescence. This appears to be a sensitive, reliable technique when properly performed, although false positive results have been noted in a number of groups of patients (e.g., those with bladder irritation from indwelling urethral catheters, those with chronic bacterial prostatitis, those with hemorrhagic cystitis).

All bacterial urinary tract infections should be followed with a posttreatment urine culture to guarantee eradication of the infection. Repeated infections in females should warrant radiological investigation of the urinary tract (IVP and/or voiding cystourethrogram) to check for structural abnormalities predisposing to infection. Many clinicians would favor radiological studies in male patients after the first infection unless there is an obvious source of infection (e.g., manipulation of the urethra with insertion of a foreign body, rectal intercourse in homosexuals).

F. Central Nervous System Infections

These infections pose a great problem for patients with compromised host defenses. A rapid, specific diagnosis often leads to the speedy institution of appropriate antimicrobial therapy which may be life saving. Lumbar puncture is indicated in patients with suspected meningitis. Cerebrospinal fluid samples should be sent for leukocyte and erythrocyte cell count, glucose, protein, and cultures for bacterial organisms, mycobacteria, and fungi. In addition, gram stain, acid-fast stains, and techniques for the rapid detection of fungi (e.g., India Ink preparation) should be performed on all specimens from immunocompromised patients with suspected meningitis. It is worth emphasizing that the finding of even one gram-positive rod on gram stain of the cerebrospinal fluid may indicate an active infection with *Listeria monocytogenes*. Likewise, even a few isolated encapsulated organisms on India ink preparation may mean that there is an active cryptococcal infection. Ancillary procedures such as CAT scan, sinus films, and mastoid X-rays may be indicated when the diagnosis of brain abscess or a parameningeal focus of infection is suspected.

The mortality for CNS infections is especially high in the immunosuppressed renal transplant population and in most series exceeds 50%. Cryptococcal infections are most common, but infections with *Aspergillus* sp., *Nocardia* sp., *Candida* sp., and *Listeria* are not rare. Other opportunistic organisms such as *Toxoplasma gondii*, viral meningitis, tuberculous meningitis, and other bacterial meningitides are far less common.

G. Other Sites of Infection

Bone and joint infections may present as "fevers of unknown origin" in the immunosuppressed renal transplant population. They are most commonly caused by *Staph. aureus*. Appropriate X-rays and bone scans may lead to a presumptive diagnosis which can be confirmed by aspiration and culture.

Peritonitis in patients with renal diseases may occur spontaneously in patients with ascites (e.g., the nephrotic patient), be secondary to inflammatory disease or perforation of an intraabdominal organ (e.g., diverticulitis in a dialysis patient, perforated ulcers in the renal transplant recipient), or be related to the process of peritoneal dialysis. Most patients will have fever, localized or diffuse abdominal tenderness, and signs referable to the peritoneal inflammation (rebound tenderness). An exception is the renal transplant patient receiving corticosteroids who may have only mild temperature elevation and minimal abdominal pain despite a major abdominal catastrophe. The incidence of peritonitis in patients receiving peritoneal dialysis is very variable but usually <5% and often <1% when good sterile technique at catheter insertion and use is observed. Peritoneal infections remain a problem in patients receiving chronic ambulatory peritoneal dialysis despite a decreasing frequency of infection in good centers as techniques are improved. Most episodes of peritonitis are caused by aerobic gram-negative bacilli, although a number are caused by *Staph. aureus*.

Among infections in renal patients, hepatitis deserves special mention. Infectious hepatitis remains a major problem in the dialysis population. At any given time, it has been estimated that 6–15% of the hemodialyzed patients have positive tests for hepatitis B surface antigen. Although the incidence of hepatitis B infection may be decreasing in this population, many investigators feel the incidence of non-A, non-B hepatitis may be increasing in dialysis units. Clinical illness with viral hepatitis in the dialysis population is typically mild, with most patients anicteric and asymptomatic. This probably relates to the defects in cell-mediated immunity in dialyzed patients, and these defects may account for the high rate of chronic carriage of the antigen. Massive outbreaks of hepatitis B that proved a major threat to staff workers as well as the patients have fortunately been infrequent. The isolation of hepatitis B surface-antigen-positive patients, avoidance of contamination with blood and other body fluids, and a greater awareness of the risks of transmitting the hepatitis B virus have all led to a declining incidence of such outbreaks.

Infectious hepatitis also continues to be a persistent problem in the renal transplant population. Of the viral organisms isolated, cytomegalovirus and hepatitis B are most common. Although Herpes simplex is occasionally isolated, EB virus and *Toxoplasma gondii* are rarely the cause of posttransplant hepatitis. A significant number of cases of hepatitis following renal transplantation have no clear etiology and have been attributed to medications (e.g., azathioprine) and non-A, non-B viral hepatitis. Although fulminant viral hepatitis can occur in transplant patients, a milder course is more common. Progression to chronicity and cirrhosis may occur with CMV or hepatitis B infection.

IV. GENERAL GUIDELINES TO ANTIBIOTIC USE IN PATIENTS WITH RENAL DISEASE

A. Pharmacodynamic Principles

Patients with kidney disease, in general, suffer from a greater number of adverse drug reactions than do patients with normal renal function. This is related in part to the patient's requirement for a great number of therapeutic drugs concurrently and in part to alterations in absorption, metabolism, and excretion that occur with altered renal function. For those antibiotics and their active metabolites that are excreted by the kidney, appropriate dose adjustments are obviously necessary to avoid toxicity. However, other therapeutic drugs have unique absorption, tissue end-organ sensitivity, serum protein binding, metabolism, or drug–drug interactions in the patient with abnormal renal function. The appropriate use of antibiotics is particularly critical in this population with its predisposition to infection and altered host defenses. Although the pharmacology of drug use in this group of patients is dealt with extensively elsewhere in this text, a review of several pharmacokinetic principles is useful for the proper administration of antibiotics to this population.

1. The Serum Half-Life Concept

Although a number of pharmacological concepts are useful in describing drug elimination from the body, the most commonly used term is the serum half-life ($T_{1/2}$) of the drug, which is defined as the time required for the amount of drug in the body to decrease by one-half. For drugs with first-order kinetics (i.e., those in which the rate of elimination is directly proportional to the serum concentration at any give time), the $T_{1/2}$ is readily calculated by obtaining timed serum levels following drug administration after the initial absorption and tissue distribution phase of the drug (α phase). During the elimination phase of the drug (β period), the $T_{1/2}$ is the time required for the serum level to decline by half. Thus, if a patient's serum level of the aminoglycoside gentamicin is 10 μg/ml following the IV administration and rapid tissue distribution of the drug, the $T_{1/2}$ will be the time required to reach a serum level of 5 μg/ml. If this is found to be 8 hr, for example, then it will likewise take an additional 8 hr for the serum level to decline from 5 μg/ml to 2.5 μg/ml and an additional 8 hr to reach 1.25 μg/ml. In other words, 50% of the drug remains in the body after one $T_{1/2}$, 25% after two $T_{1/2}$s, 12.5% at three $T_{1/2}$s. Virtually all (97%) of a drug has been eliminated from the body at five $T_{1/2}$s. This occurs regardless of the route of elimination, whether by metabolism, renal excretion, or nonrenal mechanisms. The shorter the $T_{1/2}$ of a drug, the more rapid its rate of elimination, and *vice versa*.

Although the biological $T_{1/2}$ for a given drug may not correlate well with its measured serum $T_{1/2}$, for most antibiotics, there is usually excellent correlation between free serum levels and biological activity. For antibiotics that are purely renally excreted, the $T_{1/2}$ is inversely related to the GFR. Thus, knowledge of the change of $T_{1/2}$ for a given change in GFR allows accurate dose adjustment of the antibiotic for any level of renal function. The $T_{1/2}$s of commonly used antibiotics in patients with normal and reduced renal function are given in Table I along with appropriate dose adjustments for the level of renal function.

2. The Measurement of Renal Function

It is clear that appropriate administration of an antibiotic to patients with renal disease requires some reproducible, consistent measure of "renal function." In general, an assessment of glomerular filtration rate serves as the basis for determining the adequacy of renal excretory function. Although this is not always ideal in that a number of antibiotics are eliminated predominantly by secretion across proximal tubular epithelium rather than by filtration (e.g., penicillins and many cephalosporins), it does provide some reproducible measurement of functioning renal mass.

The two most common values used to assess the GFR are the serum creatinine concentration and the endogenous creatinine clearance. The use of the BUN alone to assess renal function is hazardous, since this value may be altered by changes in hydration status, changes in urine flow rate, catabolic states, dietary protein intake, gastrointestinal bleeding, and a number of medications (corticosteroids, tetracyclines).

On the other hand, the serum creatinine concentration is not significantly affected by variation in hydration status, urine flow rate, diet, exertion, or protein metabolism. As an end product of creatine metabolism by skeletal muscle, the serum creatinine level reflects the patient's muscle mass (rate of production) and GFR (rate of excretion). The endogenous creatinine clearance indicates the volume of serum totally cleared of creatinine in a given time interval (expressed as ml/min or liters/day). The creatinine clear-

Table I. The Use of Antimicrobial Agents in Patients with Renal Dysfunction

Drug	$T_{1/2}$ (hr) Normal	$T_{1/2}$ (hr) ESRD	Normal dose[a]	Dose, ESRD	Dialysis
Amikacin	2	30–50	15–20 mg/kg per day	[b]	H-Y P-Y
Amoxicillin	1	6–18	0.25–0.5 g/8 hr	0.25–0.5 g/16–24 hr	H-Y P-N
Amphotericin	24	24	1 mg/kg per 48 hr	0.5–1 mg/kg per 48 hr	H-N P-N
Ampicillin	1	6–20	0.5–1 g/4–6 hr	0.5–1 g/8–12 hr	H-Y P-N
Azlocillin	0.8	4–6	2–3 g/4 hr	1 g/8 hr	H-Y P-sl
Aztreonam	1.6	?	1 g/6–8 hr	?	H-Y P-?
Carbenicillin	1.2	10–20	4–5 g/4 hr	2 g/12 hr[c]	H-Y P-Y
Cefaclor	0.75	3	0.25–0.5 g/6 hr	0.25–0.5 g/6 hr	H-N P-?
Cefadroxil	1.4	20–25	0.25–0.5 g/8 hr	0.25–0.5 g/12–24 hr	H-Y P-?
Cefamandole	0.7	7–10	1 g/4–6 hr	1 g/24 hr	H-Y P-N
Cefazolin	2	20–30	0.5 g/8 hr	0.5 g/24 hr	H-Y P-N
Cefoperazone	2	2	2 g/12 hr	2 g/12 hr[c]	H-N P-N
Ceftazidime	2	27	1 g/8–12 hr	1 g/24 hr	H-Y P-N
Cefotaxime	1	2.5–3	1–2 g/6–8 hr	0.5–1 g/8–12 hr[c]	H-Y P-?
Desacetyl derivative	1.6	11			
Cefsulodin	1.6	18	1 g/6 hr	1 g/24 hr	? ?
Cefoxitin	0.7	7–10	1 g/6 hr	1 g/12–24 hr	H-Y P-N
Ceftizoxime	1.4	29	1–2 g/6–8 hr	1 g/12–24 hr	H-Y P-N
Cefuroxime	1.2	10–24	0.75–1.5 g/6–8 hr	1.5 g/12–24 hr	H-Y P-?
Cephalexin	1	20–30	0.25–0.5 g/6–8 hr	0.25–0.5 g/24–36 hr	H-Y P-Y
Cephalothin	0.5	3–8	1–2 g/4–6 hr	1 g/12 hr	H-Y P-Y
Cephapirin	0.5	3–8	1–2 g/4–6 hr	1 g/12 hr	H-Y P-?
Cephradine	1.3	10–15	0.25–0.5 g/6–8 hr	0.25–0.5 g/24–36 hr	H-Y P-Y
Chloramphenicol	1	3–7	50–75 mg/kg per day	50 mg/kg per day	H-Y P-N
Clindamycin	2–2.5	3–10	0.3–1.2 g/6–8 hr	0.3 g/8–12 hr	H-N P-N
Cloxacillin	0.4–0.6	0.8	0.5–1 g/6 hr	0.5–1 g/6 hr	H-N P-N
Colistemethate	3–8	10–20	Avoid		

(continued)

Table I. The Use of Antimicrobial Agents in Patients with Renal Dysfunction (Continued)

Drug	$T_{1/2}$ (hr) Normal	$T_{1/2}$ (hr) ESRD	Normal dose[a]	Dose, ESRD	Dialysis
Dicloxacillin	0.5–0.9	1–1.6	0.5–1 g/6 hr	0.5–1 g/6 hr	H-N P-N
Doxycycline	14–25	15–35	0.1–0.2 g/12–24 hr	0.1–0.2 g/12–24 hr	H-N P-N
Erythromycin	1–3	4–6	0.5–1 g/6 hr	0.5–1 g/6 hr	H-N P-N
Ethambutol	4	8	15 mg/kg per day	5–10 mg/kg per day	H-Y P-Y
5-Fluorocytosine	3–6	70	150 mg/kg per day	25–50 mg/kg per 24–36 hr	H-Y P-Y
Gentamicin	2	30–60	3–6 mg/kg per day	b	H-Y P-Y
Isoniazid	0.5–2	4	0.3–0.6 g/day	Do not exceed 0.3 g/day	H-Y P-Y
Kanamycin	2	35–50	15–20 mg/kg per day	b	H-Y P-Y
Ketoconazole	8	8	100–400 mg/day	No change	H-N P-N
Lincomycin	4–5	10	0.6 g/8–12 hr	0.3 g/12 hr	H-N P-N
Methenamine mandelate	3–6	Avoid	Avoid		H-? P-?
Methicillin	0.5–1	4	1–2 g/4–6 hr	1–2 g/8 hr	H-N P-N
Metronidazole	6–14	8–15	7.5 mg/kg per 6 hr	7.5 mg/kg per 6 hr	H-Y P-?
Mezlocillin	0.8	4–6	3 g/4–6 hr	1 g/8 hr	H-Y P-sl
Miconazole	20–24	20–24	0.2–0.4 g/8–12 hr	0.2–0.4 g/8–12 hr	H-Y P-N
Minocycline	12–15	15–30	0.1 g/12 hr	0.1 g/24 hr	H-N P-N
Moxalactam	2	19	0.5–1 g/8–12 hr	1 g/24 hr[c]	H-Y P-?
Nafcillin	0.5	1.2	1–2 g/6 hr	1–2 g/8 hr[c]	H-N P-N
Nalidixic acid	1.5	21	Avoid		H-? P-?
Neomycin	2	12–24	Avoid		H-Y P-Y
Netilmicin	2	35–50	3–5 mg/kg per day	b	H-Y P-Y
Nitrofurantoin	0.3	1	Avoid		H-Y P-?
Oxacillin	0.5	1–2	1–2 g/4–6 hr	1 g/8 hr	H-N P-N
Penicillin G	0.5	4–20	Variable	0.6×10^6 U/8–12 hr	H-Y P-sl
Piperacillin	1	2–3	1–2 g/6–8 hr	1–2 g/8 hr	H-Y P-N
Polymyxin B	7	72	Avoid		H-Y P-N

Rifampin	1.5–5	2–7	0.6 g/day	0.3 g/day	H-? P-?
Sisomicin	2	35–50	3–4.5 mg/kg per day	b	H-Y P-Y
Streptomycin	2–2.5	35–100	1–2 g/day	0.5 g/3 days	H-Y P-?
Sulfadiazine	2–5	12–25	4–8 g/day	Avoid	
Sulfamethoxazole	9	25	0.5 g/6–12 hr	0.5 g/24 hr	H-Y P-?
Sulfasoxazole	3–7	12	0.5 g/6 hr	0.5 g/24 hr	H-Y P-Y
Tetracyclines	8.5	100	Avoid (use doxycycline)		
Ticarcillin	1.1	15	2–3 g/4 hr	2 g/12 hr^c	H-Y P-Y
Tobramycin	2	35–50	3–6 mg/kg per day	b	H-Y P-Y
Trimethoprim	10–15	20–25	40 mg/12 hr	40 mg/24 hr	H-Y P-?
Vancomycin	6	240	1–2 g/24 hr	0.5–1 g/5–7 days	H-N P-N

a Dose for serious infections.

b The basic methods of adjusting the dose of aminoglycoside antibiotics in patients with renal failure are discussed in the text. For gentamicin or tobramycin, a loading dose of 2 mg/kg is given. If the variable-frequency regimen is used, this is followed by 1 mg/kg every eight times the serum creatinine (in hours). Thus, for a 70-kg patient with a serum creatinine of 2 mg/dl, a loading dose of 140 mg would be followed by 70 mg every 16 hr. If the variable-dose regimen is used, the loading dose is followed by a maintenance dose calculated as 1 mg/kg body weight divided by the serum creatinine (in mg/dl) given every 8 hr. When the serum creatinine is less than 1 mg/dl or greater than 10 mg/dl, the maintenance dose is divided by one or ten, respectively. Thus, a 70-kg patient with a serum creatinine of 2 mg/dl would receive 140 mg as a loading dose of gentamicin or tobramycin (70 kg × 2 mg/kg) and then 35 mg (1 mg/kg × 70 kg ÷ 2 mg/dl) every 8 hr. If the creatinine clearance is known or if it is calculated from a formula (see Section IV.A.2), the following table from Neu H.C., Antimicrobial Prescribing, may be used.

	Creatinine clearance ml/min	Percent of dosage		
		8 hr	12 hr	24 hr
Gentamicin, tobramycin Loading dose: 2 mg/kg Maintenance dose: 1–1.5 mg/kg	80	80	90	—
	70	75	88	—
	60	70	85	—
	50	65	80	—
	40	55	70	95
	30	45	65	85
Amikacin, kanamycin Loading dose: 7.5 mg/kg Maintenance dose: 5 mg/kg	20	35	50	75
	15	30	40	65
	10	25	35	55

Blood levels should be obtained whenever renal function is changing rapidly and to validate use of this table.

c Further dose reduction is necessary in patients with combined renal and liver failure.

ance is calculated by dividing the amount of creatinine excreted per given unit of time (urine concentration of creatinine times the urine flow rate) by the serum creatinine concentration, $U_{cr} \times \dot{V}/P_{cr}$. Over a broad range, it reflects an accurate estimation of glomerular filtration rate and renal function. However, 10–15% of the urinary creatinine derives from tubular secretion. Thus, the creatinine clearance overestimates the true GFR (as measured by inulin clearance) by 10–15% in patients with normal renal function. As renal function declines, the contribution of this secretory component becomes a greater fraction of the total creatinine excreted. The creatinine clearance can, thus, exceed true GFR by 50–100% in severe renal failure. Despite this caveat, the creatinine clearance in most situations provides a relatively accurate estimation of renal function.

A major difficulty in using the creatinine clearance as a measure of renal function realtes to obtaining accurate timed collections of urine. A common error is to include both first morning voidings of a 24-hr collection (each containing the highly concentrated creatinine of the previous night) and obtaining a supranormal creatinine clearance; likewise, excluding both first morning voidings will give a false low value for the creatinine clearance. Careful instructions to the nursing staff and the patient when possible should prevent these inaccuracies.

In an effort to obviate problems related to timed collection of the urine, a number of formulas and nomograms relating the serum creatinine to the creatinine clearance have been devised. These include adjustments for age, sex, and weight. An example is the Cockroft–Gault formula:

$$C_{cr} = (140 - \text{age}) \times \text{wt (kg)}/72 \times [\text{creat}] \text{ (mg/dl)}$$

with the value for females being 85% that of males. Although helpful, such formulas should not substitute for a careful clinical evaluation of the patient's renal status.

A number of common errors in using the serum creatinine or creatinine clearance to assess renal function are worth noting. First, a serum creatinine "within normal limits" for the laboratory does not necessarily exclude a major reduction in GFR for a given patient. Since creatinine formation is dependent on muscle mass, a value of 1.5 mg/dl may indicate a normal GFR for a New York Jet linebacker, but a value of only 30% of normal for the football player's tiny grandmother.

Second, it is obvious from the formula for creatinine clearance that each time the serum creatinine (in the denominator of the equation) doubles, the GFR is halved. Thus, a rise in serum creatinine from 1 mg/dl to 2 mg/dl represents a halving of GFR (assuming no change in muscle mass and thus production rate of creatinine), as does an increase from 2 mg/dl to 4 mg/dl and from 4 mg/dl to 8 mg/dl. Clearly, a small change in serum creatinine at values within the normal range (e.g., 0.6 mg/dl to 1.2 mg/dl) can reflect a major change in GFR and in the potential excretion of an antibiotic. Likewise, a greater absolute change in serum creatinine concentration at higher values (e.g., 9 mg/dl to 11 mg/dl) may reflect only a small change in GFR and require minimal changes in antibiotic dosing.

A third point is that serum creatinine is of most value in assessing renal function in the steady state. The patient who suddenly becomes anuric may well have a normal serum creatinine that day despite the fact that GFR has been reduced to minimal levels. Basing the dose of an antibiotic on this normal value can easily lead to drug toxicity. Although this appears obvious, it is not uncommon for physicians to calculate the dose of an aminoglycoside such as gentamicin or tobramycin on the basis of a morning serum creatinine that is progressively rising each day, guaranteeing overdosing with the drug. Thus, assessment of renal function by P_{cr} or C_{cr} requires observation of the patient's clinical status, especially if renal function is felt to be changing.

B. Route of Administration: Pharmacological and Drug Interactions

In the choice of the route of antibiotic administration for patients with renal disease, a number of potential problems should be considered. Does the patient have vomiting or diarrhea, precluding adequate oral administration of the antibiotic? Is there edema of the gastrointestinal tract (as in the nephrotic syndrome) or altered absorption of an orally administered drug (e.g., antacids binding to tetracyclines)? Likewise, the nephrotic patient with anasarca may absorb intramuscular and subcutaneous injections only slowly and erratically. In general, for any serious infection, the intravenous route of administration insures adequate delivery of the antibiotic.

Even though the intravenous route guarantees an adequate dose of administered antibiotic, some patients may experience altered serum levels as a result of abnormal protein binding (e.g., nephrotic hypoalbuminemic patients). Likewise, occasionally drug–drug interactions that are not significant in patients with normal renal function will cause major alterations in serum antibiotic levels in patients with renal failure. Penicillins are capable of inactivating aminoglycosides (both tobramycin and gentamicin) by physicochemical binding of their B-lactam ring to amino groups of the aminoglycoside. This interaction requires high levels of both the penicillin and aminoglycoside simultaneously. Although such conditions might be met by placing both drugs in the same IV bottle, no knowledgeable nurse or pharmacist would ever allow this to occur. In the patient with renal failure, however, high circulating levels of both classes of antibiotics can occur, leading to a low measured and effective level of the aminoglycoside. Awareness of this interaction can lead to separation of the administration of the antibiotics in time or to the addition of a larger dose of aminoglycoside (based on serum levels) to insure effective serum concentrations.

C. Method of Drug Administration and Serum Concentrations

Patients with a variety of renal diseases commonly have a reduced GFR. The goal of antibiotic therapy in these patients is to achieve serum concentrations of the antibiotic similar to those in patients with normal renal function after a similar time interval.

Although the use of a "loading dose" is generally important, it is especially crucial in administering renally excreted antibiotics to patients with decreased renal function. If multiple maintenance doses of a drug are given at constant time intervals, the plasma concentration will rise until a steady state is achieved. This requires three to five $T_{1/2}$s of the drug. Since for renally excreted antibiotics, the $T_{1/2}$ is greatly prolonged in renal failure (see Table I), it may require days of drug administration before a steady-state therapeutic level of the antibiotic is reached. This is clearly unacceptable in critically ill patients with life-threatening infections. Thus, a loading dose of the antibiotic is mandatory to achieve rapidly bacteriocidal levels of the drug. The loading dose depends on body size, distribution, and protein binding of the antibiotic but is independent of renal function as long as these other factors remain unchanged.

Although the loading dose of an antibiotic is generally the same for patients with reduced and normal renal function, the maintenance dose of a renally excreted antibiotic must be adjusted for the level of renal function. This is especially true for antibiotics such as the aminoglycosides which have a low therapeutic margin. There are a number of methods of adjusting the maintenance dose of such antibiotics in patients with decreased renal function. In one method, the variable frequency regimen (VFR), a constant maintenance dose is administered at different time intervals. The interval between doses administered varies inversely with the level of renal function remaining (GFR). As renal function declines, the intervals between drug administration would be prolonged. For example, a patient with normal renal function might receive a maintenance dose of the aminoglycoside gentamicin every 8 hr, whereas the patient with a reduced GFR (as reflected by an increased serum creatinine and decreased creatinine clearance) might receive the same amount of gentamicin every 12 or 24 hr. This method gives similar peak serum concentrations and minimal (trough) serum concentrations of the drug as in patients with normal renal function. The total dose delivered is reduced in proportion to the degree of renal dysfunction. However, serum concentrations may be below minimum effective levels for a prolonged period of time if doses of the antibiotic are widely spaced in time.

A second method of administering maintenance antibiotic therapy is to give a variable amount of the drug at a constant time interval (variable dose regimen, VDR). As renal function decreases, the amount given at each set time interval is decreased. Thus, if 1 mg/kg body weight of gentamicin is given every 8 hr to the patient with normal renal function, then ½ mg/kg or ⅓ mg/kg body weight might be given every 8 hr to the patient with reduced renal function. The VDR method avoids the high peaks and prolonged low trough serum levels of the VFR method. Although the mean serum antibiotic concentration and total dose administered are the same with both regimens, the VDR method avoids big fluctuations in serum concentrations. The absence of prolonged low serum levels of an antibiotic with the VDR method may be advantageous in life-threatening infections.

Other methods of maintenance antibiotic administration combine the VDR and VFR methods to some extent through the use of nomograms based on the degree of the patient's renal dysfunction. Finally, antibiotics may be administered by continuous infusion, achieving a constant therapeutic level. Which of these various methods will give greater bacterial cure rates at lower drug toxicity is unclear at this time, and each is championed by different workers in the field. What is agreed on by all is the need for an awareness of dose adjustment as renal function declines.

Since all formulas and nomograms for dose adjustments have limitations, it is best to individualize therapy in patients with significant renal dysfunction. Serum levels may be of value in several ways. Peak serum levels drawn 20–30 min after IV infusion or 30–60 min after IM injection will be of value in guaranteeing that a bacteriocidal drug concentration has been achieved. Rising trough levels of renally excreted antibiotics, drawn just before the next dose of the drug is to be given, may be of value in indicating accumulation of the antibiotic and declining renal function. Whether increased peak or trough serum levels of certain nephrotoxic antibiotics (aminoglycosides) actually correlate with renal damage is debated.

Many antibiotics are cleared by either hemodialysis or peritoneal dialysis. Although estimates can be made from the known effects of dialysis on similar antimicrobials, it is safest to rely on published studies concerning the actual drug used. For antibiotics that are rapidly cleared by hemodialysis, an additional maintenance dose can be given following the dialysis, or the next dose of the antibiotic can be arranged to coincide with the end of the hemodialysis procedure (see Table I). Since peritoneal dialysis may go on for several days, such a dosing method becomes impractical, and either additional doses of the antibiotic must be administered or the desired serum concentration of the antibiotic may be added to the peritoneal dialysate (see Table II). For example, if in a patient receiving tobramycin a serum level of 5 μg/ml is desired, then 5 mg/liter of tobramycin can be added to the dialysate solution. A number of antimicrobial agents are best avoided in patients with marked renal dysfunction. These drugs are listed in Table I.

V. CLINICAL USE OF ANTIBIOTICS IN PATIENTS WITH RENAL DISEASE

A number of general principles of antibiotic use apply equally well to patients with either impaired or normal renal function. Antibiotics should be

Table II. Intraperitoneal Dose of Antimicrobial Agents to Maintain Therapeutic Serum Levels[a]

Drug	Intraperitoneal dose
Amikacin	10 mg/liter
Amphotericin B	2 mg/liter
Ampicillin	50 mg/liter
Carbenicillin	200 mg/liter
Cefazolin	125 mg/liter
Cephalothin	100 mg/liter
Clindamycin	10 mg/liter
Gentamicin	4–8 mg/liter
Kanamycin	10–15 mg/liter
Lincomycin	5–10 mg/liter
Oxacillin	10 mg/liter
Penicillin G	1000–1500 U/liter
Tobramycin	4–8 mg/liter
Vancomycin	15 mg/liter

[a] Patients should be given a routine intravenous loading dose of the antimicrobial agent initially. Serum levels should be followed subsequently. For details see Rubin et al., 1976, 1980; Black et al., 1974; Tenkhoff, 1974.

used only for specific indications: for documented bacterial infections, as established prophylaxis against certain bacterial and other microorganisms, and as empirical therapy for febrile, neutropenic, or immunosuppressed hosts while the results of cultures are pending. Appropriate cultures and diagnostic specimens should always be obtained prior to the start of therapy. The antimicrobial agent most likely to be beneficial in a given circumstance will depend on the patient's predisposition to infection, the presumed site of infection, the patient's prior exposure to antibiotics, and the nature of the flora common in a given hospital locale.

In choosing an antibiotic, certain pharmacological and toxicological features of the drug should be considered. Will this antibiotic be difficult to administer to a given patient with renal insufficiency? Are the pharmacokinetics of the antibiotic during hemodialysis and/or peritoneal dialysis known? Is the drug itself nephrotoxic and likely to further damage the kidney of a patient with renal dysfunction? When should available synergistic drug combinations be used? The use of bactericidal drugs is preferred over bacteriostatic antibiotics in patients with markedly impaired host defenses. Finally, it is crucial to use an adequate amount of the antibiotic for an adequate amount of time to insure effective therapy in patients with host defects in resistance to infection. In the immunosuppressed transplant patient, this often translates into standard doses of the antibiotic but a more prolonged course than would be necessary in other patients.

Causes for antibiotic treatment failure are diverse. The primary infection may not be bacterial but viral or parasitic in nature. The dose or route of administration of the antibiotic may be inadequate to achieve therapeutic serum levels. The antibiotic may be unable to penetrate or eradicate certain areas of infection (e.g., abscesses, foreign bodies). The bacteria may have become resistant to the given antibiotic. The patient may have developed a superinfection with another organism. Finally, the patient may have a drug reaction to the antibiotic, and this febrile episode may simulate resurgence of infection.

Although a detailed discussion of antimicrobial therapy for all types of infection is beyond the scope of this chapter, Table III lists frequently encountered microorganisms and a reasonable choice for initial antimicrobial therapy. Final choice will obviously depend on the results of culture and the pattern of antibiotic sensitivity of the organisms.

Table III. Pathogenic Microorganisms and Recommended Antimicrobial Therapy[a]

Pathogen	Type[b]	First choice[c]	Supplemental therapy needed	Alternatives[c]
Acinebacter	−, R	Aminoglycoside		Ticarcillin
Actinomyces	+, R	Penicillin G		Clindamycin, minocycline
Aeromonas hydrophila	−, R	Cefotaxime		TMP/SMX, moxalactam
Arizona	−, R	Ampicillin		TMP/SMX
Bacteroides fragilis	−, R	Clindamycin		Carbenicillin, cefoxitin, chloramphenicol, moxalactam
Bacteroides melaninogenicus	−, R	Pencillin G		Carbenicillin, cefoxitin, clindamycin, tetracycline
Bordetella	−, C −B	Erythromycin		Ampicillin
Borrelia	−, R	Tetracycline		Chloramphenicol
Brucella	−, R	Tetracycline	Streptomycin	TMP/SMX
Campylobacter	−, R	Erythromycin		Gentamicin
Chlamydia	−, C −B	Tetracycline		Sulfonamides
Citrobacter diversus	−, R	Cefotaxime		Aminoglycoside
Citrobacter freundii	−, R	Cefotaxime		Moxalactam, aminoglycoside
Clostridium botulinum	+, R	Antitoxin		
Clostridium difficile	+, R	Vancomycin		Bacitracin
Clostridium perfringens	+, R	Pencillin G		Cephalosporin, tetracycline
Clostridium tetani	+, R	Antitoxin	Immunization	
Corynebacterium acnes	+, R	Tetracycline		Clindamycin
Corynebacterium diphtheriae	+, R	Antitoxin	Erythromycin	
E. coli (hospital acquired)	−, R	Cefotaxime, moxalactam		Aminoglycoside, TMP/SMX

(continued)

Table III. Pathogenic Microorganisms and Recommended Antimicrobial Therapy[a] (Continued)

Pathogen	Type[b]	First choice[c]	Supplemental therapy needed	Alternatives[c]
E. coli (urine)	−, R	Amoxicillin		TMP/SMX
Eikenella corredens	−, R	Tetracycline		Ampicillin
Enterobacter	−, R	Aminoglycoside		Carbenicillin
Eubacteriae	+, R	Penicillin		Clindamycin, tetracycline
Flavobacteriae	−, R	Aminoglycoside		Carbenicillin
Francisella tularensis	−, C −B	Streptomycin	Tetracycline	Chloramphenicol
Fusobacteriae	−, R	Penicillin G		Clindamycin, tetracycline
Haemophilus influenzae	−, R	Ampicillin, cefotaxime, moxalactam		Chlorampnenicol, TMP/SMX
Haemophilus parainfluenzae	−, R	Ampicillin		Chloramphenicol, TMP/SMX
Haemophilus vaginalis	−, R	Metronidazole		
Klebsiella pneumoniae	−, R	Cephalosporin		Aminoglycoside
Leptospira	−, S	Penicillin		Tetracycline
Listeria monocytogenes	+, R	Ampicillin, mezlocillin	Aminoglycoside	Chloramphenicol
Mycoplasma pneumoniae		Erythromycin		Tetracycline
Neisseria gonorrhoeae	−, C	Penicillin G ampicillin		Spectinomycin, cefoxitin
Neisseria meningitidis	−, C	Penicillin G		Chloramphenicol
Nocardia asteroides	+, R, A, F	Sulfonamide		Minocycline, TMP/SMX
Pasteurella multocida	−, R	Penicillin G		Tetracycline
Peptococcus	+, C	Penicillin G		Clindamycin, tetracycline
Peptostreptococcus	+, C	Penicillin G		Vancomycin
Proteus (indole positive)	−, R	Cefotaxime, moxalactam		Cefoxitin, aminoglycoside
Proteus mirabilis	−, R	Ampicillin		Aminoglycoside, cephalosporin
Providencia	−, R	Cefotaxime, moxalactam		Cefoxitin, aminoglycoside, ticarcillin
Pseudomonas aeruginosa	−, R	Aminoglycoside	Ticarcillin	Cefoperazone
Pseudomonas cepacia	−, R	TMP/SMX	Polymyxin	
Rickettsia	−, C −B	Tetracycline		Chloramphenicol
Salmonella	−, R	Ampicillin		TMP/SMX

(continued)

Table III. Pathogenic Microorganisms and Recommended Antimicrobial Therapy[a]
(Continued)

Pathogen	Type[b]	First choice[c]	Supplemental therapy needed	Alternatives[c]
Salmonella typhi	−, R	Amoxicillin		Chloramphenicol, TMP/SMX
Serratia	−, R	Aminoglycoside, moxalactam		Cefoxitin, cefotaxime
Shigella	−, R	Ampicillin		Tetracycline, TMP/SMX
Spirillum	−, R	Penicillin		Tetracycline
Streptococcus agalactiae (Group B)	+, C	Penicillin G		Erythromycin
Staphylococcus aureus	+, C	PRP[c]		Cephalosporin, vancomycin
Stephylococcus epidermidis	+, C	PRP[c]		Cephalosporin, vancomycin
Streptococcus bovis (D)	+, C	Penicillin G		Cephalosporin
Streptococcus faecalis (enterococcus)	+, C	Ampicillin, amoxicillin	Aminoglycoside	Erythromycin
Streptococcus pneumoniae	+, C	Penicillin G		Erythromycin
Streptococcus pyogenes (A)	+, C	Penicillin		Erythromycin, cephalosporin
Streptococcus viridens	+, C	Penicillin G		Cephalosporin, vancomycin
Treponema pallidum	−, S	Penicillin G		Erythromycin, tetracycline
Ureaplasma urealyticum		Tetracycline		Erythromycin
Yersinia enterolitica	−, R	Ampicillin		
Yersinia pestis	−, R	Streptomycin	Tetracycline	Chloramphenicol

[a] Modified and undated from Neu, 1979.
[b] −, Gram negative; +, gram positive; R, rod or bacillus; C, coccus; A, acid fast; F, filamentous; S, spiral; B, bacillary.
[c] First drug listed is not necessarily drug of choice.
[d] PRP, Penicillinase-resistant penicillin.

VI. THERAPY OF URINARY TRACT INFECTIONS

A. Uncomplicated Acute Urinary Tract Infections

Most patients with acute uncomplicated urinary tract infections are women of a sexually active age. No single antimicrobial agent has been proven to be the unequivocal drug of choice. Indeed, there is not even evidence to support the superiority of bactericidal agents over bacteriostatic agents. However, there is a good correlation between the concentration of antimicrobial agent in the urine and both the clinical and bacteriological cure of the patient. Inhibitory urinary concentrations are achieved in normal individuals after oral administration of many antimicrobial agents.

The conventional treatment of acute uncomplicated urinary tract infection has been a 7- to 14-day course of an antimicrobial to which the bacterial organism is susceptible. The antimicrobial agents used have included sulfonamides, ampicillin, and oral cephalosporins. Recently, however, single-dose therapy has been advocated for these lower urinary tract infections. Compared to conventional therapy, the advantages of single-dose therapy include lower cost, better compliance, convenience of administration, smaller number of adverse effects, and decreased chance of altering intestinal flora and thereby selecting drug-resistant perineal flora.

The earliest single-dose therapy, by Ronald and associates, consisted of a single intramuscular dose of 500 mg kanamycin which achieved a cure in 93% of uncomplicated urinary infections. Similar studies have now been done with other aminoglycosides including amikacin, sisomicin, netilmicin, and dibekacin. However, these agents should be used only if oral therapy is not feasible.

Sulfisoxazole at an oral dose of 200 mg/kg in children or 1 or 2 g in adults is effective. Amoxicillin at a single dose of 3 g, trimethoprim as a single 200-mg dose, or one double-strength tablet of trimethoprim–sulfamethoxazole have all proven effective. Hemorrhagic cystitis, as opposed to uncomplicated urinary infections, requires a 3- to 7-day course of therapy for adequate cure rates.

B. Symptomatic Female Patient with No Bacteria Seen on Urinary Gram Stain

These patients probably have the acute urethral syndrome if they have greater than 20 white cells/hpf. The etiology often is *Chlamydia*. Thus, oral tetracycline, 250 mg to 500 mg four times daily for 7 days, should be the first drug of choice. Alternative forms of therapy would include sulfisoxazole, 1 g four times a day, or sulfamethoxazole, 1 g administered twice daily, for 7 to 10 days.

C. Pyelonephritis, Upper Tract Disease

Although the optimal duration of therapy for pyelonephritis is not established, there is a 30 to 50% failure rate in patients with renal parenchymal bacteria if they are treated for only 7 to 14 days. Thus, it is advisable in many of these patients to continue therapy for 4 to 6 weeks with an agent that achieves good concentrations not only in the bladder but also in the renal parenchyma. Although there are only limited data to support this, it is clear that failure of therapy after 2 weeks of aminoglycoside therapy is less than 10% versus 30 to 40% failure rates after use of β-lactam agents. The aminoglycosides concentrate in the renal parenchyma and are continually "released" into the medullary area and renal pelvis for several weeks after therapy has ended. Because of the risk of potential aminoglycoside nephrotoxicity, it is preferable to use a less toxic antimicrobial whenever feasible. Thus, a 6-week course of amoxicillin, trimethoprim–sulfamethoxazole, or cephalexin would be reasonable agents of first choice.

D. Asymptomatic Bacteriuria

Most patients with asymptomatic bacteriuria are women. Even though cure can be achieved in some patients, relapse and reinfection are common. In the absence of urinary tract obstruction, treatment of asymptomatic bacteriuria is unnecessary unless the potential for urosepsis is high. Therapy should not be initiated until the susceptibilities of the organisms are known and not until the bacteriuria has been reconfirmed by a second culture. Therapy preferably should be for a short period, 7–14 days, with a repeat culture 48 hr after therapy has ended.

Asymptomatic bacteriuria in the pregnant female, children with reflux, and individuals with obstructive uropathy should always be treated with an appropriate agent, depending on susceptibilities, for at least 7–14 days.

E. Prophylaxis

Often females with recurrent urinary tract infections will benefit from prophylactic antimicrobial therapy. Current studies have indicated that use of trimethoprim–sulfamethoxazole (1 tablet thrice weekly) or trimethoprim alone (100 mg thrice weekly) will prevent recurrence of urinary infection in the susceptible female. Although nitrofurantoin, 100 mg orally daily, has also proven useful, recent concern about the toxic side effects of this agent, including interstitial pneumonitis and chronic active hepatitis, suggest that trimethoprim–sulfamethoxazole is preferable. The ideal length of suppressive therapy, whether 4, 6, or 12 months, is unknown. The physician should be alert to the fact that recurrence after this period of prophylaxis is common.

Prophylaxis in the presence of foreign bodies such as calculi or catheters has not been shown to be effective.

SUGGESTED READINGS

Al-Sawwaf M, Pancoast SJ, Hardy MA, et al: Antimicrogbial agents for immune compromised patients. *Compr Ther* 6:18–27, 1980.

Appel GB: Vascular access infections with long-term hemodialysis. *Arch Intern Med* 138:1610, 1978.

Appel GB, Neu HC: Antimicrobial agents in patients with renal diseases. *Med Times* 105:109–129, 1977.

Appel GB, Neu HC: Gentamicin in 1978. *Ann Intern Med* 89:528–538, 1978.

Appel GB, Neu HC: The use of drugs in renal failure. *DM* 25:1–44, 1979.

Axelrod JL: Infections complicating uremia and organ transplantation, in Grieco MH (ed): *Infection in the Abnormal Host.* Yorke Medical Books, New York, 1980, pp 521–546.

Bennett WM, Muther RS, Parker RA, et al: Drug therapy in renal failure: Dosing guidelines for adults. *Ann Intern Med* 93:62–89, 1980.

Black HR, Findelstein FO, Lee RV: Treatment of peritonitis. *Trans Am Soc Artif Int Org* XX:115–119, 1974.

Blagg CR, Tenckhoff H: Microbial contamination of water used for hemodialysis. *Nephron* 15:81–86, 1975.

Cockroft DW, Gault MH: Prediction of creatinine clearance from serum creatinine. *Nephron* 16:31–41, 1976.

Craddock PR, Fehr J, Brigham KL, et al: Complement and leukocyte-mediated pulmonary dysfunction in hemodialysis. *N Engl J Med* 295:769–774, 1977.

Cross AS, Steigbigel RT: Infective endocarditis and access site infections in patients on hemodialysis. *Medicine* 55:453–446, 1976.

Dobkin JF, Miller MH, Steigbiegel N: Septicemia in patients on chronic hemodialysis. *Ann Intern Med* 88:28–33, 1978.

Eknoyan G, Olivero J: The kidney in infectious disease, in Suki WN, Eknoyan G (eds): *The Kidney in Systemic Disease.* New York, Wiley, 1981, Part 6, pp 556–566.

Goldblum SE, Reed WP: Host defences and immunologic alterations associated with chronic hemodialysis. *Ann Intern Med* 93:597–613, 1980.

Greenblatt DJ, Koch-Weser J: Drug therapy—clinical pharmacokinetics. *N Engl J Med* 293:702, 1973.

Kirmani N, Tuazon CU, Murray HW, et al: *Staphylococcus aureus* carriage rate among chronic hemodialysis patients. *Arch Intern Med* 138:1657–1659, 1978.

Kunin CM: *Detection, prevention, and management of urinary tract infections.* Philadelphia, Lea & Febiger, 1979.

Lauver GL, Hasan FM, Morgan RB, et al: The usefulness of fiberoptic bronchoscopy in evaluating new pulmonary lesions in the compromised host. *Am J Med* 66:580–585, 1979.

London WT, Drew JS, Lustbader ED, et al: Host responses to hepatitis B infection in patients in a chronic hemodialysis unit. *Kidney Int* 12:51–58, 1977.

Miller RB, Tassistro CR: Peritoneal dialysis. *N Engl J Med* 281:945–949, 1969.

Neu HC: *Antimicrobial Prescribing.* Princeton, Antimicrobial Prescribing, 1979.

Nolph KD, Sorkin M, Rubin J, et al: Continuous ambulatory peritoneal dialysis: Three-year experience at one center. *Ann Intern Med* 92:609–613, 1980.

Revillard JP: Immunologic alterations in chronic renal insufficiency. *Adv Nephrol* 8:365–382, 1979.

Rubin J, Oreopoulos DG, Lio TT, et al: Management of peritonitis and bowel perforation during chronic peritoneal dialysis. *Nephron* 16:220–225, 1976.

Rubin J, Rogers, WA, Taylor HM, et al: Peritonitis during continuous ambulatory peritoneal dialysis. *Ann Intern Med* 92:7–13, 1980.

Rubin RH, Wolfson JS, Cosimi AB, et al: Infections in the renal transplant recipient. *Am J Med* 70:405–411, 1981.

Tenkhoff H: *University of Washington Chronic Peritoneal Dialysis Manual.* Seattle, University of Washington, 1974.

Valenti W, Trudell R: Factors predisposing to oropharyngeal colonization with gram-negative bacilli in the aged. *N Engl J Med* 298:1108–1111, 1978.

Williams DM, Krick JA, Remington JS: Pulmonary infection in the compromised host. *Am Rev Respir Dis* 114:359–394, 1976.

13

Management of Hypertension
Management of Essential and Secondary Hypertension

C. VENKATA S. RAM

I. INTRODUCTION

Hypertension is the most common cardiovascular disorder encountered by medical practitioners and is an important cause of morbidity and mortality. Although notable advances have taken place in the diagnosis and management of hypertension, it still remains the major risk factor for coronary, renal, and cerebrovascular disease. The incidence of hypertension varies with the definition, but it is estimated that approximately 20% of the U.S. adult population is affected by hypertension (i.e., diastolic blood pressure greater than 90 mm Hg). The majority of hypertensives (approximately 95%) have so-called "essential hypertension" for which there is no cure. Since reduction of blood pressure prevents most of the complications attending this disorder, the treatment strategy is aimed at reducing the blood pressure to "normotensive" levels by pharmacological or other means. Until a few years ago, the indication for treating those patients with diastolic blood pressures above 105 mm Hg was generally accepted, based on the results of the Veterans administration Cooperative Studies and observations from the Framingham Study. But, at the present time, we are witnessing a major effort to utilize as an indication for therapy a diastolic pressure of 90 mm Hg. This recommendation stems from the results of two important studies on the therapy of

C. VENKATA S. RAM • Department of Internal Medicine, Southwestern Medical School at the University of Texas Health Science Center at Dallas, Dallas, Texas 75235; and St. Paul Hospital, Dallas, Texas 75235.

"mild hypertension," the Hypertension Detection and Follow-up Program and the Australian Therapeutic Trial in Mild Hypertension. Taken together with the previous studies on hypertension, these new observations provide unequivocal evidence for the value of treatment of patients with diastolic blood pressures of 90 mm Hg or more.

II. MECHANISMS OF ESSENTIAL HYPERTENSION

Despite the accumulated work of several decades of intense investigations, the etiology of hypertension in most patients is unclear, and it is therefore termed "essential hypertension." Even though the precise etiology of hypertension remains elusive, significant advances have been made in our understanding of the basic physiological mechanisms that regulate the arterial blood pressure and the manner in which these mechanisms are altered in hypertension. It is well established that cardiac output and peripheral vascular resistance are the principal determinants of blood pressure. Thus, one can easily judge how the interplay of various factors affecting the cardiac output and peripheral vascular resistance can bring on changes in the level of blood pressure. Such factors include fluid volume, sympathetic tone, the renin–angiotensin system, prostaglandins, kinins, vascular elasticity, blood viscosity, and, perhaps, various local substances.

Although it is impossible to isolate one factor to the exclusion of others, a possible scheme can be constructed to explain the basis of essential hypertension. In the initial stages, the peripheral vascular resistance may be normal while the cardiac output is increased. This increased cardiac output could be caused by excessive fluid volume, perhaps because of abnormal renal retention of salt and water. Ultimately, however, as the hypertension becomes "established," the cardiac output is normal, and the peripheral resistance is high. This change in the hemodynamics is brought on by the process of autoregulation in which increases in the blood flow (cardiac output) lead to vasoconstriction which is maintained despite the subsequent restoration of normal cardiac output. Thus, elevated peripheral vascular resistance is the hemodynamic abnormality that is directly related to the degree of blood pressure elevation. The elevated peripheral resistance is related to an enhanced response to the vasoconstrictors norepinephrine and angiotensin and possibly to a defect in the vasodilatory prostaglandins. Additionally, Folkow has demonstrated that structural changes occur in the arterial walls that decrease elasticity and narrow the lumen, thus contributing to increased peripheral resistance.

The role of heredity in hypertension is important as a predisposing mechanism, but the precise mode of transmission has not been determined. In those genetically predisposed, high dietary sodium induces hypertension.

There are convincing epidemiological data showing a relationship between salt consumption and level of blood pressure.

III. MANAGEMENT OF ESSENTIAL HYPERTENSION

The goal of antihypertensive therapy is to prevent complications by sustaining blood pressure control for the remainder of the patient's life. Therefore, before embarking on a therapeutic program, the physician should perform a thorough physical examination after obtaining a detailed history. The physician should discuss the nature of the problem and the need for the patient's active participation in achieving the goal. Laboratory work-up should include complete blood count, urine analysis, and blood chemistries (SMA_{12}) in addition to cholesterol and triglycerides. Care must be taken to separate the blood cells from serum immediately after drawing to prevent potassium loss into the serum. Otherwise, the opportunity for diagnosing primary aldosteronism may be lost. An electrocardiogram and chest X-ray should be done. If renal artery stenosis is suspected because of abdominal bruit or severe hypertension, an arteriogram is necessary to evaluate the patient. A good rapport between the physician and the patient is integral to successful therapy.

A. Nonpharmacological Treatment

Although most patients with hypertension will require some form of drug therapy, there are certain nonpharmacological means that may be helpful in some patients. All hypertensive patients will benefit from restriction of dietary salt and reduction of excess body weight. An appropriate dynamic exercise program may also be helpful. Behavioral modification techniques aimed at reducing stress response reduce blood pressure temporarily in some mild hypertensives. However, there is no convincing evidence showing a prolonged antihypertensive effect from behavior modification. Thus, the therapeutic role of behavior modification is unsettled, and drug treatment remains the only established modality for long-term treatment of hypertension.

B. Dietary Restriction of Sodium

There is ample evidence linking high salt intake to hypertension in acculturated, industrialized societies. Modest restriction of salt intake (to 50–75 mEq/day) may cause reduction in blood pressure. Furthermore, restriction of salt enhances the antihypertensive effect of diuretic agents, permitting reduction of dosage and attenuating the degree of hypokalemia.

C. Antihypertensive Drugs

The initial drug in the treatment of hypertension is usually a diuretic. However, in several countries, β blockers are used as the step-1 agents. Other drugs should be added in sequence, and one should avoid using two different drugs belonging to the same class; the ineffective drug(s) should be withdrawn before adding other drug(s). The goal should be to control the hypertension with the minimal number of agents to assure patient compliance and to minimize the side effects and unfavorable drug interactions.

1. Diuretics

Although diuretics are extremely useful in lowering the blood pressure, the mechanism by which they do so is not fully understood. These agents increase urinary sodium excretion, resulting in reduced plasma volume, extracellular fluid volume, cardiac output, and blood pressure. After about 6–8 weeks, however, the cardiac output returns toward the control levels, and the lower blood pressure at this point is the result of a fall in peripheral vascular resistance, the mechanism of which is unknown.

a. Thiazides and Related Compounds

About 30–40% of patients with mild hypertension respond to thiazide therapy alone. The thiazide diuretics have a flat hypotensive dose response. Thus, larger doses than those listed in Table I produce little additional therapeutic effect but induce additional biochemical side effects.

The duration of diuresis caused by hydrochlorothiazide and other related benzothiadiazines is up to 12 hr. The effects of long-acting drugs such as methyclothiazide and polythiazide continue for 24 hr, with chlorathalidone even longer in duration. The thiazide group of diuretics inhibit the sodium absorption in the distal cortical diluting segment and cause excretion of as much as 10–15% of the filtered sodium. If the patient has normal renal function, ordinarily a thiazide diuretic should be the first choice. However, long-acting diuretics, metolazone and chlorthalidone, are equally effective, but the biochemical side effects accompanying their use are also prolonged.

The diuretics are particularly efficacious in the treatment of "volume-dependent" hypertension, examples of which include the so-called low-renin hypertension comprising 20–25% of all patients with essential hypertension, primary aldosteronism, and hypertension associated with chronic

Table I. Drugs Used in the Treatment of Hypertension

Drug	Total daily dose (mg)	Doses/day
Diuretics		
Thiazides		
Hydrochlorothiazide	50 to 100	1 to 2
Trichlormethiazide	2 to 4	1 to 2
Methyclothiazide	2.5 to 10	1
Metolazone[a]	2.5 to 10	1
Chlorthalidone	25 to 50	1
Furosemide[a]	40 to 240	2 to 4
Spironolactone	25 to 400	2 to 3
Triamterene	100 to 300	2
Amiloride	5 to 20	1 to 2
Adrenergic inhibitors		
Reserpine	0.10 to 0.25	1
Guanethidine	10 to 200	1
α-Methyldopa	500 to 3000	1 to 3
Clonidine	0.1 to 2.4	1 to 2
Prazosin	1 to 20	1 to 2
Propranolol	40 to 640	2 to 3
Metoprolol	50 to 400	2 to 3
Nadolol	40 to 640	1
Direct vasodilators		
Hydralazine	75 to 400	2 to 3
Minoxidil	5 to 100	1 to 2
Inhibitors of renin–angiotensin system		
Captopril	75 to 450	2 to 3

[a] Larger doses may be used in renal insufficiency.

renal disease. Some studies have shown that continued effectiveness of non-diuretic antihypertensive agents depends on the maintenance of a shrunken plasma volume, and, thus, the role of diuretics in the general treatment of hypertension is an important one. The patients should be advised to limit their salt intake, since ingestion of large quantities of salt may negate the therapeutic benefit of diuretics.

b. Loop Diuretics

The loop diuretics, furosemide and ethacrynic acid, are more potent than thiazides and inhibit the sodium chloride reabsorption from both the medullary and cortical segments of the ascending loop of Henle. It is important to note that the loop diuretics, although able to mobilize greater amounts of sodium than thiazides, are no more effective as antihypertensive agents, and some authors have found thiazides to be more useful than furosemide. The duration of action of loop diuretics is about 6 hr, and, therefore, multiple doses may be necessary to maintain the desired hemodynamic response. These drugs are effective in certain situations in which there is a need to mobilize large amounts of sodium and water, as in hypertension complicated by congestive heart failure and chronic renal disease. Thiazides decrease the glomerular filtration rate and are ineffective in some patients with chronic renal insufficiency; therefore, in these patients, furosemide may be the diuretic of choice. A disadvantage of furosemide is its short half-life, often necessitating administration of three or four doses daily to maintain smooth antihypertensive effectiveness. At the present time, the thiazide group of diuretics is usually preferred in the treatment of uncomplicated hypertension unless some contraindications exist. On the other hand, loop diuretics are preferred in patients with renal insufficiency and edematous states.

c. Potassium-Sparing Agents

Spironolactone, triamterene, and amiloride are classified as potassium-sparing diuretics because of their ability to conserve potassium during diuretic therapy. These agents inhibit sodium reabsorption at the sodium/potassium exchange site in the distal tubule and thus reduce the excretion of potassium. Spironolactone is a specific aldosterone antagonist, and its efficacy is directly related to the sodium-retaining and kaliuretic effects of aldosterone. Since the fraction of sodium reaching the exchange site in the distal tubule is relatively small, they cause a maximum excretion of less than 5% of filtered sodium. Therefore, they are ordinarily weak diuretic and antihypertensive agents but highly effective in excess aldosterone states. The potassium-sparing diuretics should ordinarily be used in combination with the thiazide or loop diuretics for the purpose of limiting the degree of hypokalemia.

Triamterene has more natriuretic activity than spironolactone, but, again, its primary use is to reduce potassium losses from other diuretics. Its activity is independent of aldosterone, although the locus of action in the nephron is thought to be the same as that of spironolactone. Amiloride is a relatively new (in the United States) potassium-sparing agent with slight natriuretic but profound potassium-sparing effect. The utility of amiloride appears to be in combination with other diuretics in order to enhance the natriuresis but attenuate the potassium losses. It should be emphasized that the use of any potassium-sparing agent requires balanced dosing to prevent hyperkalemia. These agents should be used with great caution or not at all in patients with renal insufficiency who are predisposed to develop hyperkalemia. It should be emphasized that concomitant administration of potassium supplements and potassium-sparing drugs enhances the risk for hyperkalemia, and thus, the combination should be limited to very select reliable patients while serum potassium is carefully monitored.

d. Side Effects of Diuretics

Most of the side effects of diuretics are directly associated with their pharmacological actions.

i. Hypokalemia. Hypokalemia is a common dose-related side effect of the diuretics, ranging from 0 to 40% in different studies. The diuretic-induced potassium losses are primarily a result of increased delivery of sodium to the distal tubule and of the degree of secondary hyperaldosteronism produced by the diuretic itself. Most subjects with mild hypokalemia are asymptomatic, but with prolonged or severe hypokalemia, symptoms such as muscle weakness and nocturia may appear. Patients with congestive heart failure, myocardial infarction, and diabetes mellitus may be quite sensitive to hypokalemia, and, therefore, adequate corrective measures must be undertaken. The degree of hypokalemia also depends on the type of diuretic used—it is more prominent with long-acting and potent diuretics. Therefore, a diuretic with intermediate duration of action such as hydrochlorothiazide is the best choice for uncomplicated hypertension.

There is no satisfactory answer to the question concerning the level of serum potassium that requires corrective steps. This should be individualized, and most patients with serum potassium less than 3.2 mEq/liter do need some form of supplementation or antikaliuretic agents. The hypokalemia can be corrected by restricting the salt intake, adjusting the dose of diuretic, and administering potassium chloride supplements or potassium-sparing agents, in that order.

ii. Hyperuricemia. Hyperuricemia, usually symptomless, also occurs as a function of diuretic dosage but ordinarily does not require specific therapy. Although diuretic-induced hyperuricemia rarely precipitates acute gout, close attention must be given to those with a history of this disorder. Some authorities recommend the use of a uricosuric agent, probenecid, if the serum uric acid is greater than 10 mg/dl. Although many physicians frequently use allopurinol, it can cause potentially lethal hematological problems and is not ordinarily used for asymptomatic diuretic-induced hyperuricemia.

iii. Hyperglycemia. The diuretics sometimes cause hyperglycemia and, rarely, frank diabetes. Part of the hyperglycemia can be ameliorated by restoring serum potassium. However, it can still occur with normal potassium. Although diabetes is not a contraindication for diuretic therapy, severe hyperglycemia may occasionally result, and the therapy for diabetes may have to be modified with the concomitant use of a diuretic. Alternatively, such patients should be carefully informed and motivated concerning substitution of a low sodium intake for the diuretic.

iv. Hyperlipidemia. Some workers have reported increases in serum cholesterol and triglycerides with diuretic therapy. The mechanism and clinical significance of this effect have not been determined.

v. Hypercalcemia. An insignificant rise in serum calcium level is frequently seen with effective diuretic therapy. In the evaluation of primary hyperparathyroidism, the diuretic should be discontinued for several weeks.

2. Adrenergic Suppressing Drugs

If the blood pressure is not adequately controlled, the next step is to administer an adrenergic blocking drug. The adrenergic inhibiting drugs were the first drugs shown to be effective in the treatment of hypertension. Over the past few years, significant advances have been made in the development of newer adrenolytic agents more specific in their action and causing fewer side effects. From a pathyphysiological view, the concept of adrenergic blockade is an important one. The adrenergic nervous system controls the circulatory system at various levels, and there is evidence to suggest abnormal sympathetic tone as one of the factors in the genesis or maintenance of hypertension. It is difficult to quantify the neural events taking place in the circulatory system, but suppression of adrenergic input is the goal of antihypertensive therapy for many patients.

The cardiovascular system is under the constant influence of the adrenergic nervous system, and certain afferent impulses originate from the cardiovascular system. These may come from volume receptors, pressure receptors, circulating catecholamines, state of sodium balance, etc. The brain provides a sophisticated network of "centers" that respond to these stimuli by transmitting necessary signals to the heart and blood vessels—impulses that result in changes of blood pressure. This sequence of adrenergic impulse transmission provides the basis for the application of adrenergic blocking drugs in the treatment of hypertension.

a. Methyldopa

Methyldopa is widely used in the treatment of hypertension. The major antihypertensive action of methyldopa is mediated by the α-adrenergic receptors in the brain, resulting in decreased sympathetic outflow and lowering of blood pressure. The blood pressure fall with methyldopa results mainly from a decrease in the peripheral resistance. Renal blood flow is preserved, and the drug is, therefore, widely used in patients with renal insufficiency. Although renin levels fall during methyldopa treatment, its antihypertensive effect is perhaps not related to changes in the activity of the renin–angiotensin system.

As with other drugs, the dose requirements of methyldopa vary from patient to patient. The beginning dose is 250 mg twice a day. The dose can be increased at biweekly intervals to a maximum daily dose of 3000 mg, the larger dose preferably taken at bedtime. In the treatment of mild hypertension, a single daily dose of methyldopa may be effective. As with other adrenergic inhibitors, methyldopa is best used in conjunction with a diuretic.

The most common side effects of methyldopa are sedation and drowsiness. The other side effects—such as depression, nightmares, and postural hypotension—are uncommon. Approximately 3% of patients develop dose-related abnormal liver function tests beginning with increased transaminases. However, this is rarely fatal, and discontinuing drug administration usually results in reversal of these abnormalities. A flu-like syndrome, which is caused by drug allergy, occurs in <2% of patients. About 20% of patients receiving methyldopa develop a positive antiglobulin (Coombs test) which is of significance only during typing and cross matching of blood for transfusions. Rarely, it may cause hemolytic anemia. The drug also has the potential of causing dose-related dry mouth, impotence, galactorrhea, and a withdrawal syndrome.

b. Clonidine

Clonidine has pharmacological properties nearly identical to those of methyldopa except that it rarely produces toxicity. It reduces the blood pressure by directly stimulating the central α receptors, which results in decreased peripheral sympathetic tone. Clonidine has little or no effect on renal blood flow or glomerular filtration rate but reduces the renal vascular resistance, a pattern similar to that observed with methyldopa. Although the bradycardia produced by clonidine could be caused by the diminished sympathetic tone, it may also be caused by activation of vagal centers. Clonidine also suppresses the plasma renin activity either directly or indirectly.

The starting dose of clonidine should be 0.1 mg given twice daily. The total daily dose should not exceed 1.8–2.4 mg and perhaps be even lower to minimize the sedative effects.

The most frequent side effects of clonidine are drowsiness and dry mouth which are more prominent during the initial stages of treatment and with high doses. A potentially serious side effect that may ensue following abrupt discontinuation of clonidine therapy is the rapid return of hypertension, sometimes associated with clinical and biochemical features of sympathetic overactivity. The exact incidence of this phenomenon is unknown, but it is more likely after abrupt discontinuation of large doses of the drug (greater than 1.2 mg/day). Blood pressure elevation during the clonidine withdrawal syndrome can be treated by administration of α and β blockers or readministration of clonidine. This withdrawal syndrome can be prevented in most patients by gradually decreasing dosage over a 5- to 7-day period.

c. Guanethidine

With the availability of more refined adrenergic blockers, the clinical role of guanethidine in the management of hypertension has declined. Guanethidine was used widely quite successfully until the availability of the new generation of adrenergic inhibitors. It produces its hypotensive effect by preventing norepinephrine release from peripheral sympathetic nerve endings. The predominant role of the sympathetic nervous system is to maintain increased cardiac output with upright posture and exercise, and since guanethidine blocks these mechanisms, it causes exercise intolerance, weakness, etc. However, it has no effect on catecholamine metabolism in the brain, and, therefore, sedation and other central nervous system side effects are not seen with guanethidine.

The antihypertensive response to guanethidine is highly variable among patients, so the maintenance dose ranges from 10 to 200 mg/day, and sometimes much higher doses are needed. It has a long half-life (>72 hr) and can be administered once a day with a diuretic. Other common side effects are diarrhea, failure of ejaculation, and impotence. Certain drugs such as ephedrine, amphetamines, and tricyclic antidepressants antagonize the effects of guanethidine.

3. α-Adrenergic Receptor-Blocking Drugs

The adrenergic neuron releases norepinephrine which interacts with receptors on the vascular smooth muscle to cause vasoconstriction. Adrenergic receptor-blocking drugs thus lower the peripheral vascular resistance and the blood pressure. The classical α blockers, phentolamine and phenoxybenzamine, are generally not used in the treatment of essential hypertension because of postural hypotension and other adverse effects. Prazosin is a selective α_1 (postsynaptic) adrenergic blocker. The side effects typical of classical α blockers are not seen with prazosin because it does not block the α_2 (presynaptic) receptors, and, therefore, feedback inhibition of norepinephrine release is maintained. Prazosin is used as a step-2 agent (after a diuretic) in the treatment of hypertension. Its effectiveness is clearly enhanced by concomitant administration of a diuretic. Since it also lowers the preload by causing venodilation, it has been employed in the treatment of refractory congestive heart failure. However, this effect on the veins is temporary, and tolerance may occur.

The most frequent side effects of prazosin are dizziness and postural hypotension, which particularly may occur with the first dose or with rapid increments in the doses. The "first-dose phenomenon" can be prevented by starting therapy with 1.0 mg taken at bedtime and increasing the dose gradually. The maintenance dose is variable between 3 and 40 mg/day.

4. β-Adrenergic Receptor-Blocking Drugs

These drugs are widely used in the treatment of hypertension, and this can be attributed to their effectiveness and relative freedom from troublesome side effects. The mechanism(s) by which these agents lower the blood pressure is not fully known. They do lower cardiac output and renin secretion and, with time, decrease peripheral vascular resistance. They can also stimulate the synthesis of vasodilatory prostaglandins; thus, more than one antihypertensive mechanism may be involved.

The β blockers are classified as cardioselective and noncardioselective depending on their ability to antagonize β receptors in various tissues. For example, metoprolol, acebutalol, and atenolol are more effective in inhibiting the effects of catecholamines on the heart (β_1 receptors) than on the bronchial tree (β_2 receptors). Propranolol, nadolol, oxprenolol, and pindolol are noncardioselective, thus blocking the β-receptor sites equally in all organs. The organ selectivity of β blockers is only possible at low doses. Thus, the clinical advantage of currently available cardioselective β blockers is linked to the dose administered. The pharmacological properties of various β blockers are shown in Table II.

In the United States, the β blockers have been recommended as step-2 agents. In some countries, β blockers are used as the initial therapy in the place of diuretics. Clearly, some patients respond to β blockers alone, so that the choice of initial therapy should be individualized. β-Adrenergic blockers may be the first choice for younger individuals, those with hyperkinetic circulatory states, and those with high-renin hypertension, whereas diuretics may be the initial drugs for older individuals, black patients, and patients with volume-dependent low-renin hypertension. Measurement of plasma renin activity may be helpful in making a choice about initial therapy, but it is not practical to do renin studies on each patient, as this test should be performed under standardized conditions.

a. Clinical Use

The β blockers are generally safe and well tolerated by most patients. They may be ineffective in low-renin hypertension and, in fact, have been reported to cause paradoxical hypertension, perhaps via a combination of fluid retention and unopposed α-receptor-mediated vasoconstriction. As

Table II. Pharmacological Properties of Some β Blockers

Drug	β-Blocking potency ratio (propranolol = 1)	Cardio-selectivity	Sympatho-mimetic agonist activity	Membrane-stabilizing activity
Acebutolol	0.3	+	+	+
Atenolol	1	+	0	0
Metoprolol	1	+	0	±
Nadolol	2 to 4	0	0	0
Oxprenolol	0.5 to 1.0	0	++	+
Pindolol	6	0	+++	+
Propranolol	1	0	0	++
Timolol	6	0	0	0

with other antihypertensive drugs, the effectiveness of β blockers is enhanced by a diuretic.

The antihypertensive efficacies of various β blockers are nearly identical. However, there are certain clinical situations in which one β blocker may be better than another. As a general rule, β blockers are contraindicated if bronchial asthma is present. But when their use is essential, a cardioselective drug may be used in low doses; higher doses may nullify the advantage of cardioselectivity. The recovery from insulin-induced hypoglycemia is more rapid in a patient receiving metoprolol than in one using propranolol. Nadolol, a nonselective β blocker, has the longest plasma half-life (>18 hr) of any known β blocker and therefore can be conveniently administered once daily. Thus, a physician should individualize the choice of a β blocker on the basis of the clinical situation.

The starting dose of propranolol is usually 40 mg twice daily which can be titrated until a therapeutic response is seen. Although doses up to 4000 mg a day have been used by some investigators, the dose response above 240–320 mg/day is extremely flat, and, consequently, megadoses are not justified. In conjunction with direct vasodilators (hydralazine, minoxidil), the dose of β blockers must be sufficient to block the reflex activation of sympathetic activity caused by direct vasodilators. The dosage of metoprolol is 100–400 mg daily, and nadolol doses are similar to those of propranolol. However, since nadolol is excreted unchanged by the kidney, the dosage interval should be adjusted for patients with renal insufficiency.

b. Adverse Effects

The adverse effects of β blockers are related to their known pharmacological actions. However, the number of adverse experiences can be minimized if patients with congestive heart failure, bronchial asthma, and peripheral vascular disease are excluded from the use of β blockers.

The β blockers, especially the nonselective ones, can aggravate or unmask bronchial asthma. Since the adrenergic nervous system plays an important role in supporting a failing myocardium, β blockers may precipitate or worsen congestive failure. Similarly, considerable caution must be exercised in using β blockers in patients with atrioventricular conduction block.

Aggravation of intermittent claudication or Raynaud's phenomenon can occur with β blockers. They may mask the features of hypoglycemia; on the other hand, worsening of diabetes has also been reported with certain β blockers. Cardioselective β blockers are safer than nonselective ones for diabetics. Various CNS effects—depression, insomnia, nightmares, etc.—have been reported with propranolol but are somewhat unusual and may occur only at high doses.

When propranolol is discontinued abruptly, symptoms of coronary artery disease may be aggravated, so the drug should be tapered off gradually. This phenomenon may be caused by a state of supersensitivity or an increase in the β-receptor pool as a result of the β blockade.

Despite some reports, patients with renal insufficiency can be safely treated with β blockers, but the dose of the long-acting β blocker nadolol may need adjustment.

Respiratory distress, bradycardia, and hypoglycemia have been observed in some fetuses when propranolol was administered during pregnancy. It is probably wise not to use this drug during gestation.

c. α- and β-Receptor-Blocking Agent

Labetolol is an adrenoreceptor blocking agent that is a competitive antagonist at both α- and β-receptor sites. It is not yet available in the United States, but it is widely used in some countries such as Great Britain. Although the β-blocking actions of labetolol closely resemble those of propranolol, its α-blocking activity is considerably less than that of the classical α blocker phenoxybenzamine. Labetolol has been found to be effective in the treatment of different degrees of hypertension. This drug has also proven successful in the management of hypertensive emergencies and hypertension associated with chronic renal disease.

5. Direct Vasodilators

If a diuretic and an adrenergic blocker do not control hypertension satisfactorily, a direct vasodilator should then be added to the regimen. Direct vasodilators, hydralazine and minoxidil, are very effective antihypertensive agents and have an important role in the management of moderate/severe or complicated forms of hypertension.

a. Hydralazine

Hydralazine was the only vasodilator available for long-term management of hypertension until the recent introduction of minoxidil. This drug directly relaxes the arterial smooth muscle. As a consequence, blood pressure falls, but this direct vasodilatation activates the sympathetic nervous system, and a number of unfavorable hemodynamic and subjective side effects are seen—namely, fluid retention and tachycardia. Therefore, to eliminate these effects and to retain the effectiveness of hydralazine, concomitant use of a diuretic and an adrenergic inhibitor, generally a β blocker, is necessary. The dose of the β blocker should be sufficient to attenuate the reflex tachycardia and should be adjusted accordingly. Hydralazine is an extremely useful agent in the treatment of moderate/severe hypertension, and its clinical applicability has vastly increased with the availability of β blockers which counteract the reflex tachycardia that this and other direct vasodilators cause.

Hydralazine, although it usually has been given four times a day, can be given on a twice-a-day schedule if it produces a satisfactory response. The maximum daily dosage should be kept below 400 mg to avoid a possible lupuslike syndrome. This reaction is very rare, can be reversed on discontinuation of the drug, and is more commonly induced in slow acetylators of the drug.

b. Minoxidil

This drug, a direct vasodilator, has recently been made available for general clinical use after many years of intense investigation. It works in a manner similar to hydralazine but is more potent and effective. Because of its potency, the use of this drug is usually limited to severe or complicated hypertension. In most clinical trials, minoxidil was used in patients not responding to multiple conventional antihypertensive drugs. Minoxidil, like other direct vasodilators, causes fluid retention and reflex tachycardia so that simultaneous administration of a diuretic and an adrenergic inhibitor is necessary. Fluid retention can sometimes be marked, and, hence, a potent diuretic such as furosemide should be administered. A side effect that is somewhat unique to minoxidil therapy is hair growth, and the facial hirsutism may be cosmetically unacceptable for women. Therefore, it is advisable to institute minoxidil therapy in women only when other conventional therapeutic modalities have absolutely failed. The treatment of hypertension associated with renal insufficiency has been made easier with the introduction of minoxidil, and this aspect is discussed in detail in Section IV.B. The previous reports of pulmonary hypertension caused by minoxidil have now been disproven.

The dosage of minoxidil should be begun with 5 mg/day and adjusted up to 60–100 mg/day as needed to produce desired effects. The drug can be given once a day, and the majority of patients can be managed successfully with doses less than 40 mg/day.

6. Inhibition of the Renin–Angiotensin System

Since the renin–angiotensin–aldosterone system may play a role in hypertension, compounds that inhibit this system have been thoroughly investigated. Saralasin, a competitive inhibitor of angiotensin II, has the disadvantage of inherent agonistic property in the volume-replete state and has to be given intravenously. It is therefore not suitable for routine clinical use.

Captopril is an orally effective antihypertensive drug that lowers the blood pressure by competitive inhibition of the enzyme responsible for the conversion of angiotensin I to the potent vasoconstrictor angiotensin II. However, this blood pressure-lowering effect is not limited to hypertensive states associated with high plasma renin activity. It also produces reductions of blood pressure in hypertensive states in which the plasma renin is low. Thus, although captopril appears to lower the blood pressure primarily through suppression of renin–angiotensin system, its complete mechanisms has not yet been fully delineated. Captopril has been shown to be effective in the treatment of all degrees of hypertension, including renal and renovascular hypertension.

The antihypertensive effect of captopril is associated with a fall in total peripheral resistance without significant change in cardiac output; renal blood flow is increased although glomerular filtration rate is unchanged. At the present time in the United States, the use of captopril is limited to severe or drug-resistant hypertension. Captopril is particularly effective in the treatment of hypertension associated with renal scleroderma. The usual starting dose of captopril is 75 mg/day which can be increased to a maximum of 450–500 mg/day. The bioavailability of captopril is reduced 30–40% by food; therefore, it should be taken 1 hr before or 3 hr after meals. The efficacy of captopril is enhanced by concomitant administration of a diuretic.

The side effects of captopril differ somewhat from those of other antihypertensive drugs. Neutropenia is reported in 0.3% of patients taking captopril; proteinuria has occurred in 1–2%. However, these adverse effects have occurred mostly in patients with complicated hypertension. Therefore, the significance of these side effects is not fully determined, but patients should be monitored closely, especially during the first 3–4 months of treatment. The other adverse effects are rash (10 per 100), taste impairment (6 to 7 per 100), and vague GI disturbances.

IV. SECONDARY FORMS OF HYPERTENSION

The important secondary causes of hypertension are shown in Table III. Together, these forms of hypertension constitute only a small fraction (<5%) of the hypertensive population. Although it is important to recognize secondary forms of hypertension, not every patient should undergo work-up for secondary hypertension, but the physician should be guided by certain clinical and biochemical parameters.

A. Oral Contraceptive Use

The use of oral contraceptive pills is probably the most common cause of secondary hypertension. The exact incidence of hypertension caused by oral contraceptive pills is debatable, and published reports suggest that anywhere from 0 to 18% of women on oral contraceptive pills develop hypertension. Data from the Royal College of General Practitioners indicate that the incidence of hypertension among pill users was 2.6 times greater than among nonusers. The incidence increases with the duration of oral contraceptive use and is likely to be greater in obese women and those over age 35.

The mechanism of hypertension caused by oral contraceptive pills has been the subject of several investigations. Although more than one mech-

Table III. Secondary Causes of Hypertension

Oral contraceptive use
Renal parenchymal disease
Renal artery stenosis
Primary aldosteronism
Pheochromocytoma
Miscellaneous causes:
    Coarctation of the aorta
    Cushing's syndrome
    Steroid use
    Licorice ingestion
    Hypercalcemia
    Hyper- and hypothyroidism
    Renal trauma
    Increased intracranial pressure
    Use of sympathomimetic drugs
    MAO inhibition/tyramine interaction

---

anism may play a role in the pathogenesis of this form of hypertension, present evidence strongly implicates the renin–angiotensin system as the major factor. The oral contraceptive pill or its components stimulate the production of renin substrate from the liver and, thereby, activate the renin–angiotensin–aldosterone axis, leading to sodium retention and hypertension. When the women with pill-induced hypertension are given the angiotensin antagonist saralasin, blood pressure falls in those who become normotensive on discontinuation of the pill.

The hypertension caused by oral contraceptives is usually mild, but sometimes it may be severe. Ideally, the oral contraceptive should be discontinued if hypertension is discovered, and alternate modes of contraception should be implemented. The blood pressure returns to normal levels in variable intervals in most after the discontinuation of the pill. In many patients, hypertension may abate within 3 months of discontinuation of the pill, but in some it may take up to 6 months. However, in some, the hypertension is maintained despite the discontinuation of the pill. Perhaps, in these patients, the pill might have uncovered the predisposition to develop essential hypertension.

If, for medical reasons, the pill cannot be discontinued, the hypertension should be treated by pharmacological means. Although the principles of antihypertensive therapy in general are the same as those for essential hypertension, pill-induced hypertension may respond better to the administration of the aldosterone antagonist spironolactone with or without concomitant use of thiazide diuretics. Additional drugs should be used as necessary to lower the blood pressure to the desired level. If the hypertension does not resolve within 3–6 months after discontinuation of the pill, appropriate work-up and therapy should be implemented. Practitioners are advised not to give more than a 6-month supply of oral contraceptives at a time so that patients' blood pressure can be monitored periodically.

B. Hypertension Associated with Renal Parenchymal Disease

Hypertension can be both a cause and a consequence of renal disease. The kidney is one of the target organs susceptible to damage by chronic untreated hypertension and by accelerated hypertension. On the other hand, hypertension is a common phenomenon in patients with any form of renal parenchymal disease in general and chronic glomerulonephritis in particular. Despite the availability of chronic hemodialysis, many patients succumb to the cardiovascular complications of renal failure—congestive heart failure, myocardial infarction, and stroke. Therefore, it is critical to control hypertension in all patients with chronic renal disease. As the renal disease progresses, hypertension becomes apparent and further accelerates renal dysfunction. Thus, to provide as long an interval as possible between the onset of renal disease and the need for dialysis or kidney transplantation, hypertension must be aggressively treated. This can be achieved with a wide spectrum of antihypertensive agents available today. Physicians caring for patients with renal disease should be familiar with the applied pharmacology of various antihypertensive drugs, since renal dysfunction alters the pharmacodynamics of some drugs.

1. Acute Glomerulonephritis

Although the typical syndrome of acute glomerulonephritis has become less common, it still occurs as an important cause of renal disease in childhood. It is now believed that this entity can be caused by a variety of agents other than type-specific Streptococcus. Usually, in the early phases, hypertension is present in association with edema and oliguria. Because the onset of hypertension is relatively rapid in acute glomerulonephritis, the patients are at risk of developing malignant hypertension and encephalopathy. Therefore, blood pressure should be adequately controlled. Although, for a long time, it has been thought that the elevation of blood pressure in acute glomerulonephritis results from fluid overload and high cardiac output, some recent observations suggest that peripheral resistance is also increased.

The hypertension should be treated by salt and water restriction and, in many cases, with a diuretic in a dose sufficient to produce gradual and steady diuresis. However, sometimes additional antihypertensive agents such as adrenergic blockers and vasodilators will be necessary. The classical disease is self-limited, but in some patients the disease may progress with inevitable chronic renal insufficiency.

2. Hypertension and Pyelonephritis

There is no convincing relationship between acute pyelonephritis and hypertension. However, hypertension can be a feature of chronic pyelonephritis. For many years, it has been claimed that patients with hypertension are susceptible to attacks of pyelonephritis, but this is unproven. The some-

times striking relationship between chronic pyelonephritis and hypertension probably results from the parenchymal destruction caused by pyelonephritis. Hypertension may be a result of vascular occlusion from scarring
and the resultant activation of renin release. High plasma renin activity can
be demonstrated in many, but not all, patients with pyelonephritis. Whatever
the underlying mechanism may be, the hypertension associated with pyelonephritis should be controlled in order to preserve renal function.

3. Diabetic Nephropathy and Hypertension

Hypertension is present in the majority of patients with diabetic nephropathy. The hypertension is the result of glomerular disease and also,
perhaps, arteriolar disease. Some patients affected by this disorder may have
hyporeninemic hypoaldosteronism which may predispose them to hyperkalemia, and, thus, potassium supplements or potassium-sparing agents
should be used with great caution or not at all. In formulating the antihypertensive regimen, one must give consideration to certain drugs (e.g., guanethidine) that can cause postural hypotension which is unwelcome, particularly in diabetics with autonomic insufficiency. One should also keep in
mind that certain diuretics (such as thiazides) may aggravate hyperglycemia,
necessitating close attention and possible adjustment in the insulin dose.

4. Polycystic Kidney Disease

Hypertension is frequently encountered in the adult form of polycystic
kidney disease. Cardiac and cerebrovascular events account for considerable
mortality and illustrate the significance of hypertension in this disease. The
mechanism of hypertension is not clear, but it could be the combination of
ischemia caused by the enlarging cysts and loss of vasodepressor (prostaglandins) function from the destruction of renal parenchyma. The hypertension, once detected, should be vigorously controlled.

5. Hydronephrosis

Hydronephrosis is not a common cause of secondary hypertension, but
there are reports of cure of hypertension following the correction of hydronephrosis. The mechanism of hypertension could be renal ischemia resulting
from compression of interlobular arteries or loss of prostaglandin-secreting
cells. It seems prudent to correct the hydronephrosis if possible in the hope
of alleviating the hypertension.

6. Scleroderma

When scleroderma affects the kidneys, hypertension appears very rapidly and causes a rapid decline in renal function, heralding an unfavorable
prognosis. The renal lesions seen in scleroderma are similar to those seen in

malignant hypertension. The fulminating course and the malignant hypertension suggest rapid renal ischemia from narrowing of the interlobular arteries. These patients have high levels of plasma renin activity. The blood pressure should be treated with potent antihypertensive agents, and, often, the patient should be hospitalized. The conventional agents are not uniformly effective in controlling the hypertension associated with renal scleroderma. There has been a revival of hope for these patients now with the availability of captopril, an inhibitor of angiotensin formation, following encouraging reports of improved survival of patients treated with captopril. The specific advantage of captopril in this situation is perhaps a reflection of the toxic role of the renin–angiotensin system in the scleroderma kidney, and captopril successfully antagonizes this pressor mechanism. The hypertension complicating scleroderma can also be treated with the potent vasodilator minoxidil. We hope that the availability of these new agents will change the otherwise grim outcome of this disorder.

7. Hypertension with Chronic Renal Disease

As alluded to earlier, hypertension can be both a cause and a result of renal disease. Since the kidney is a regulator of salt and water balance, the renin–angiotensin system, and vasodepressor substances (prostaglandins), it is easy to speculate how renal dysfunction can cause hypertension. On the other hand, chronic uncontrolled hypertension eventually causes nephrosclerosis with resultant renal insufficiency. With the availability of hemodialysis for the chronic care of patients with end-stage renal disease, hypertension has to be dealt with for long periods. Despite the introduction of potent antihypertensive drugs, hypertension is a significant problem and causes significant cardiovascular morbidity and mortality in patients with chronic renal failure. The blood pressure should be controlled in order to maintain the patient in good cardiovascular condition for possible kidney transplantation.

To treat hypertension in a patient with chronic renal disease, one should have insight into the possible mechanisms and the effects of various pharmacological agents on the kidney. On the basis of this knowledge, effective treatment can be implemented and maintained.

8. Mechanisms of Hypertension

There are two important factors that regulate the blood pressure in a patient with end-stage renal disease: salt and water balance and the vasopressor function of the kidney. In addition, the deficiency of vasodepressor substances (such as prostaglandins) may also be a factor, but data are lacking to support this view. The key abnormality that sets off the hypertension is, of course, the loss of functional nephrons.

Volume hypertension is an important, if not the only, mechanism. The patients with progressive renal insufficiency cannot excrete salt and water and, thus, stay in a "positive" balance. To some extent the renin–angiotensin system may also be involved, as the normal renin found in many patients with chronic renal disease may, in fact, be inappropriately high for the volume-expanded state. It was suggested that these patients may be divided into two groups—salt–water dependent and renin dependent—according to the blood pressure response to dialysis or bilateral nephrectomy. However, clinically, such a clear-cut separation is not possible, since in a given patient, both the fluid volume and renin may sustain the hypertension.

Initially, the hypertension in renal disease may start with increased cardiac output. With time, however, the cardiac output tends to decrease, whereas the peripheral vascular resistance increases. As the disease progresses, the cardiac output again increases, but the peripheral resistance fails to fall. The higher cardiac output in the patients with end-stage renal disease could also result in part from uremic anemia. In patients in whom the hypertension is mediated by high cardiac output, the pharmacological blockade of the renin–angiotensin system will have no effect on the blood pressure. However, once the volume factor is removed, the role of renin–angiotensin is uncovered.

9. Treatment of Hypertension in Chronic Renal Disease

In this category are patients who have not yet reached end-stage renal failure (i.e., the glomerular filtration rate may range between 10 and 30 ml/min) and who are not yet on dialysis. The renal insufficiency can be from any cause, and effective control of blood pressure delays or even arrests the progression of renal failure. The therapy of hypertension is important in protecting the failing kidney and the cardiovascular system. With proper control of blood pressure, even patients presenting with malignant hypertension survive for long periods of time.

10. Salt Restriction

Patients with impaired renal function are prone to salt and water retention, and, therefore, efforts should be made to limit the salt intake. However, a subgroup of patients with chronic renal disease may be "salt losers," and excessive salt restriction in these patients may result in salt and volume deficits. Therefore, the need for salt restriction should be assessed individually. It is necessary to restrict the sodium chloride to 2–4 g/day in most patients in order to control the blood pressure satisfactorily. Many patients cannot adhere to a salt-restricted diet and therefore need diuretics for proper regulation of salt and water balance.

11. Diuretics

As with essential hypertension, diuretics are the cornerstone of antihypertensive therapy in patients with renal insufficiency. Thiazide diuretics are not used because of their tendency to decrease the glomerular filtration rate and because of their ineffectiveness when the glomerular filtration rate is reduced below 20 ml/min. A loop diuretic (furosemide or ethacrynic acid) is usually the first agent to be used in the treatment of hypertension complicated by renal insufficiency. The daily dose of furosemide is quite variable and depends on the elevation of the blood pressure and the severity of renal impairment; the therapy may be begun with 40 mg twice a day and the dose adjusted as necessary. Some patients may require doses up to 480–600 mg/day. Potassium-sparing agents, spironolactone and triamterene, should be avoided when azotemia is present because of the risk of hyperkalemia. The risk is particularly present in those with diabetic nephropathy and hyporeninemic hypoaldosteronism. However, in individuals who develop hypokalemia with diuretics, a potassium-sparing agent may be added with due care and with periodic determinations of serum potassium levels. Some patients who are truly refractory to large doses of loop diuretics may respond after the addition of another diuretic, metolazone, but the combination of these diuretics should be used with great caution and under careful supervision because sometimes a brisk diuresis may ensue with attendant dangers.

12. Additional Therapy

If the blood pressure cannot be successfully controlled with diuretics, additional drugs will be needed. The second drug could be α-methyldopa or clonidine. Their pharmacological profiles and mechanisms of action are similar, and both preserve renal blood flow. The starting dose of clonidine is 0.1 mg given twice a day, and the dose should be titrated as necessary to a maximum of 1.8 to 2.4 mg/day. It is preferable to keep the daily dose below 1.2–1.6 mg/day because of sedation and other side effects with high doses. For α-methyldopa, the initial dose should be 250 mg twice a day and can be increased to a maximum daily dose of 3000 mg. The most common side effects of α-methyldopa and clonidine are drowsiness and dry mouth, particularly with high doses, and these effects may diminish with continued administration of the drugs. If the blood pressure is not controlled with a diuretic and methyldopa or clonidine, a direct vasodilator such as hydralazine or minoxidil should be used. If methyldopa or clonidine proves ineffective, it should be tapered off when alternate drug therapy is instituted. The direct vasodilators produce prompt response and are the most valuable agents for the control of hypertension associated with renal disease. Since the direct vasodilators usually produce reflex tachycardia and activation of the sympathetic nervous system, concomitant administration of an adrenergic blocker is mandatory. The dose of hydralazine is variable, and one can initiate the therapy with 25 mg twice a day, increasing it to a maximum of 300–400 mg/day.

An alternative to hydralazine is minoxidil, a potent vasodilator. Minoxidil has been found to be extremely useful in the treatment of severe hypertension not responding to conventional agents and hypertension associated with renal impairment. The availability of minoxidil has revolutionized the treatment of hypertension complicated by renal insufficiency. Until a few years ago, bilateral nephrectomy was performed in patients not responding to conventional antihypertensive agents, but now the need for such an irreversible procedure has been virtually eliminated by the use of minoxidil. There are reports showing significant improvement or stabilization of renal function during chronic therapy with minoxidil. A few patients were removed from hemodialysis after the recovery of renal function by aggressive control of hypertension with minoxidil. Therefore, minoxidil occupies an important therapeutic role in the management of hypertension in renal disease. The initial dose of minoxidil should be 5 mg/day depending on the response.

The reflex tachycardia accompanying the use of hydralazine and minoxidil can be blocked by the simultaneous administration of a β-adrenergic blocking agent such as propranolol, metoprolol, or nadolol. The dosage of β blocker should be assessed individually and be enough to attenuate the sympathetic response to vasodilators. Many patients appear to require upwards of 160 mg/day of propranolol to satisfactorily control the undesirable hemodynamic effects of vasodilators. Another side effect of vasodilators is fluid retention, particularly with minoxidil, and this should always be anticipated and treated with an appropriate dose of a loop diuretic. Thus, the maximum beneficial therapeutic effect of direct vasodilators can only be achieved with concomitant administration of a diuretic and a β blocker. If for some reason a β blocker cannot be used or is contraindicated, then one can use α-methyldopa or clonidine to block the activation of sympathetic tone.

Beta-blocking drugs alone are not too helpful in the management of hypertension complicated by renal dysfunction, but if the renal dysfunction is mild, they may be tried. The role of β blockers and their relationship to renal function have been controversial, as some earlier reports demonstrated deterioration in renal function with their use. But it is not clear whether these observations reflected direct drug effects or progression of the underlying renal disease. It is fair to say that β blockers are being used in large numbers of patients with renal disease without evidence of any toxic effect on the kidneys. Although effective blood pressure reduction in patients with chronic renal disease may sometimes be accompanied by rises in the BUN and serum creatinine levels, the physician should not get unduly alarmed by such observations, as the renal function will likely stabilize or improve with maintenance of blood pressure control.

13. Treatment of Hypertensive Patients with End-Stage Renal Disease

These patients have no meaningful excretory function and are on dialysis; therefore, their fluid volume and salt balance are critically important in maintaining the hypertension. In most patients in this stage, hypertension can be controlled by removal of sodium and water by ultrafiltration dialysis and by restriction of salt and fluid intake. If adequate blood pressure control cannot be maintained with regular dialysis and restriction of salt intake, additional antihypertensive measures are instituted similar to the guidelines outlined for patients who are not on dialysis. Appropriate doses of α-methyldopa or clonidine should be tried for several weeks, and, if response is less than optimal, these drugs should be replaced with the combination of hydralazine or minoxidil and β blockers. When minoxidil is administered in appropriate doses, many patients will show a response with rare exceptions. Of course, the accompanying reflex activation of sympathetic tone should be counteracted with a β blocker or methyldopa or clonidine.

If the patient's blood pressure cannot be controlled despite ultrafiltration dialysis, dietary restriction of salt and water, and use of antihypertensive drugs in the maximal doses that the patient can tolerate, then consideration should be given to bilateral nephrectomy, as the vasopressor function of the kidney may be responsible for severe hypertension. It should be reemphasized that with the availability of minoxidil, the need for bilateral nephrectomy is minimized. It has been suggested that the plasma renin activity may serve as a useful indicator of possible response to bilateral nephrectomy. However, because of overlapping values of plasma renin among patients with end-stage renal disease, and since many antihypertensive agents used in this situation affect the renins, it is not possible to recommend plasma renin activity as a predictive factor for response to bilateral nephrectomy. The decision is made as demanded by the patient's clinical condition after all available therapies have been given a sufficient trial.

Bilateral nephrectomy not only decreases the blood pressure; it also results in marked general improvement of the patient. The choice of antihypertensive drugs and the pharmacological principles for the anephric patient are the same as for those on maintenance dialysis.

C. Renovascular Hypertension

True renovascular hypertension should be defined as hypertension caused by occlusive disease of a renal artery, correction of which cures the hypertension. Renal artery stenosis may be present in the absence of hypertension. Therefore, there need not be a causal relationship between the observed stenosis and elevated blood pressure. The incidence figures for renovascular hypertension vary from 1% to 5% depending on the series studied. It is generally believed, on the basis of available data, that renal artery stenosis is present in 15% of the hypertensive population. Of this, one-third or 5% have renovascular hypertension. If 30 million Americans have hypertension, it means that about 1.5 million or so have renovascular hypertension which is potentially curable. Since the precise diagnosis of renovascular hypertension requires invasive procedures requiring hospitalization, considerable efforts have been made in recent years to identify the patients with this problem on the basis of clinical characteristics and outpatient procedures. Proper decision making is a difficult task because renal artery stenosis can result from multiple causes and may be associated with renal insufficiency and/or extrarenal vascular disease—factors that profoundly influence the ultimate prognosis. Since the evaluation of renovascular hypertension is not easy, and since hypertension can be treated medically with a wide variety of antihypertensive agents available, the physician is often faced with the dilemma about the degree of aggressiveness with which he should pursue this diagnosis.

1. Clinical Criteria

Although the National Cooperative Study of Renovascular Hypertension found a number of clinical criteria that distinguish the patients with renovascular hypertension from those with essential hypertension, there is considerable overlap between the two groups. Patients with renovascular hypertension were found to have a shorter duration of hypertension, less striking family history of hypertension, severe retinal findings, higher BUN, and greater frequency of proteinuria and urinary casts; each patient should be assessed on an individual basis.

The history, physical examination, and routine laboratory work-up are usually not helpful in identifying patients with renovascular hypertension. The presence of an epigastric or flank bruit—especially with both the systolic and diastolic components—may be a clinical clue, but the absence of an abdominal bruit does not rule out this condition. Careful auscultation of the abdomen should always be done in each hypertensive patient to detect abdominal bruits.

Renal artery stenosis, on an etiologic basis, can be broadly divided into two categories: atherosclerotic and resulting from fibromuscular dysplasia. Patients with atherosclerotic renal artery stenosis in general tend to be older (mean age 50 years) and have extrarenal vascular disease with greater target organ dysfunction. Fibromuscular hyperplasia is seen in the young (mean age 35 years), predominantly in females. There is a relationship between the operative mortality and the presence of coronary artery disease. Therefore, elderly patients should not be extensively evaluated for renovascular hypertension unless medical therapy has failed. Since renovascular hypertension is less prevalent in blacks, one should limit the work-up only to those presenting with severe or refractory hypertension.

Screening for renovascular hypertension should be restricted to the following groups:

1. Onset of hypertension before age 25 or after age 50.
2. Patients with severe elevation of blood pressure (diastolic greater than 120 mm Hg).
3. Patients presenting with accelerated or malignant hypertension.
4. Presence of an abdominal bruit, especially if high pitched and present during systolic plus diastolic phases.

5. Patients who cannot tolerate antihypertensive drugs.
6. Patients in whom a blood pressure cannot be properly controlled despite maximal drug therapy.

2. Diagnosis

The conclusive diagnosis of renovascular hypertension rests on the demonstration of renal artery stenosis and measurement of renal vein renins in order to assess the functional significance of the lesion. However, certain other less invasive tests can be performed prior to the renal arteriography. Only those patients who are candidates for possible surgery should be investigated.

a. Rapid Sequence Intravenous Pyelogram

This is a reasonable screening procedure and can provide useful information. The following are the major criteria used for diagnosing unilateral renal artery stenosis:

1. Delayed appearance of contrast media on the ischemic side.
2. Difference of more than 1.5 cm on one side from pole to pole.
3. An increased density and delayed disappearance of the dye on the ischemic side.

The intravenous pyelogram (IVP) is easily done and is a generally safe procedure. Although the published data are confusing, perhaps 15% of the IVPs are false positive or negative. Therefore, physicians should use the clinical impression regarding the pursuit of the diagnosis and not rely solely on the IVP.

b. Radioisotope Renography

Isotope renography utilizing labeled hippurate is sometimes used in the place of the IVP, but it gives fewer details than an IVP. Isotope detection probes are placed over each renal area to record the radioactivity within the kidneys which is plotted against time. As a screening procedure, the renogram has the advantage of using a very small amount of iodine as a tracer, and, therefore, the risk of an allergic reaction to iodine is virtually absent, but the procedure requires expensive equipment. Like the IVP, this test, too, suffers from the occurrence of false positive and negative responses.

c. Plasma Renin Activity

Although it has previously been believed that patients with renovascular hypertension have high plasma renin activity (PRA) in the peripheral blood, it is now accepted that a third of these patients have normal PRA. Thus, PRA level is not always a reliable indication of the presence of renovascular hypertension. But, if the PRA is indeed high when assayed under appropriate conditions, additional work-up for renovascular hypertension may be undertaken.

d. Angiotensin Blockade

Since renovascular hypertension is generally thought to be secondary to the increased activity of the renin–angiotensin system, the recent availability of specific inhibitors of the renin–angiotensin system has permitted a promising approach to the diagnosis of renovascular hypertension. Renin- and angiotensin-mediated hypertension may be identified by the demonstration of a decrease in the blood pressure following the administration of saralasin, a competitive antagonist of angiotensin. It has been demonstrated that intravenous infusion of this antagonist produces an immediate and sustained reduction of blood pressure in patients with renovascular hypertension. The results of saralasin infusion offer greater accuracy with prior sodium depletion, usually by furosemide. Saralasin is administered by a bolus injection or by continuous infusion starting with a dose of 0.1 μg/kg per min and gradually increased until a response occurs to a maximum dose of 10 μg/kg per min. False negative responses can occur if the subject is not adequately volume depleted. In low-renin patients, there is a potential for blood pressure elevation because of the agonist property of saralasin. At the present time, saralasin testing remains an experimental procedure restricted to research centers. When generally available, it may prove to be an additional tool in the work-up of hypertensive patients.

e. Confirmatory Tests

If there is a strong suspicion of the presence of renovascular hypertension, confirmation of the stenosis must be obtained by renal arteriography, the functional role of which must be, in turn, confirmed by renal vein renin estimation. We believe that renal arteriography must be performed first so that the need for renal vein renins can be eliminated if there is no demonstrable stenosis. The radiographer should pay particular attention to obtaining films showing the entire renal vasculature including oblique projections. By morphological appearance and location of the stenosis, one can judge whether it is a fibromuscular hyperplasia or an atherosclerotic lesion. The atherosclerotic lesion is usually annular and present in the proximal third of the renal artery, whereas in fibromuscular hyperplasia, the lesions have a "string of beads" pattern located in the middle third or distal portions of the renal artery.

Once the stenosis is seen on the arteriogram, its functional significance must be ascertained before its correction can be recommended. For this purpose, renal vein renin concentration from both the stenotic and nonstenotic sides must be estimated. It is advisable to discontinue drugs that inhibit renin (all the adrenergic blockers) at least 1 week prior to the renal vein renin sampling. If the stenosis is significant, the production of renin from the ischemic side will be much higher than that from the contralateral side. A positive test is a greater than 1.5 times difference between the stenotic and nonstenotic sides. If the difference in the ratio is less than 1.5, the chance of surgical cure will diminish.

3. Management

At the present time there are no data about the merits of surgical versus medical treatment of renovascular hypertension; no controlled study has ever been done. Therefore, the physician should take into account various factors before deciding on the therapeutic approach. Surgical repair should certainly be considered for patients with proven renovascular hypertension who are in good general health. Those with fibromuscular dysplasia in general show good results because these patients tend to be younger. The following factors should form the basis for considering medical or surgical approach:

1. The age of the patient. The older the patient, the greater will be the surgical risk because of associated extrarenal atherosclerotic disease. The best results are obtained in patients with a short duration of hypertension.
2. The stenosis itself. In general, the chances of surgical cure are better with fibromuscular dysplasia than with atherosclerotic disease, but there may be individual differences depending on the location of the obstruction, etc.
3. Renal function. If the stenosis is bilateral with significant loss of renal function, the surgical results are usually not good. Such cases must be assessed individually with respect to other factors involved.
4. Cardiovascular disease. Patients with coronary artery disease or cerebrovascular disease do not tolerate the surgery well and therefore should be considered for intensive medical therapy. However, special circumstances such as intolerance to drug therapy, progressive renal insufficiency because of a bilateral renal arterial obstruction, etc. may later change the decision towards surgery.

There are a number of surgical procedures for the relief of renal artery stenosis, and the details of the techniques are not within the purview of this chapter. Renal vascularization is the preferred procedure in most patients. However, nephrectomy is sometimes indicated in cases with an atrophic, nonfunctioning kidney or when revascularization is not technically feasible or has previously failed. Patients who are unwilling or unable to undergo general surgery may be considered for percutaneous transluminal dilation of the stenosis. The preliminary results with this procedure are encouraging, but the long-term results are not yet available.

Patients with renovascular hypertension can be successfully treated with drugs. The principles of drug administration and titration of doses are similar to those in essential hypertension, but since this form of hypertension is probably mediated by the renin–angiotensin system, the drugs that inhibit renin release such as the β blockers are particularly effective alone or in combination with other antihypertensive agents.

D. Primary Aldosteronism

Primary aldosteronism is a rare cause of secondary hypertension, accounting for less than 0.5% of all hypertensive disorders.

1. Pathophysiology

Aldosterone is the mineralocorticoid hormone synthesized and released from the glomerulosa cells of the adrenal cortex. It regulates the sodium and potassium balance, and under normal conditions aldosterone secretion is under the control of ACTH, angiotensin II, plasma sodium, and, perhaps, plasma potassium concentration. In primary aldosteronism, however, there is "autonomous" overproduction of aldosterone, resulting in various biochemical abnormalities and hypertension. Rarely, the syndrome has been reported in individuals with normal blood pressure or with normal plasma potassium level. The diagnosis is suspected in a hypertensive patient with unprovoked hypokalemia.

Although for many years it was believed that primary aldosteronism represented a classical example of "volume-dependent" hypertension, there is new evidence to implicate increased peripheral vascular resistance as an important mechanism. Since aldosterone plays a key role in sodium and water retention by the kidney, the result would be suppression of plasma renin activity, which is one of the diagnostic features of primary aldosteronism.

2. Diagnosis

The diagnosis of primary aldosteronism rests on demonstration in a hypertensive patient of (1) hypokalemia, (2) inappropriate urinary losses of potassium, (3) suppressed PRA, and (4) increased levels of aldosterone in the urine or plasma. Investigations for primary aldosteronism should not be undertaken if the patient does not have hypertension or until the diuretics have been discontinued for 3–4 weeks prior to the evaluation. Sometimes, but not always, patients may present with symptoms of potassium depletion—muscular weakness, paresthesia, visual disturbance, polyuria, and, very rarely, intermittent paralysis and tetany. Most often the diagnosis is considered because of persistent hypokalemia in a hypertensive patient.

Some patients are discovered only after challenge with diuretics, as the ensuing hypokalemia may be striking and prolonged.

The plasma potassium is often less than 3.5 mEq/liter. Twenty-four-hour urinary potassium must be quantitated while the patient is hypokalemic, on a normal sodium intake, and on no diuretics or potassium supplements. If the urinary potassium is more than 30 mEq/day, the diagnosis should be pursued, but if it is less than 30 mEq/day, primary aldosteronism is unlikely. The next step would be to determine PRA which is always low in patients with primary aldosteronism. The renin secretion should be stimulated by either a salt-restricted diet and 3–4 hr of upright posture or by administration of furosemide, to document renin suppression. An elevated PRA rules out primary aldosteronism and suggests secondary aldosteronism.

Finally, measurement of plasma or urinary aldosterone provides the confirmatory diagnosis of primary aldosteronism. Since plasma aldosterone level may fluctuate because of dynamic changes in its secretion, single values are not helpful; therefore, measurement of 24-hr excretion of aldosterone is a practical alternative. During the collection of urine, one should insure adequate intake of salt to be certain that high levels of aldosterone do not result from sodium restriction. Several techniques are used to further demonstrate inappropriate secretion and excretion of aldosterone, and these include oral administration of fludrocortisone, liberal intake of salt, and saline infusions. If aldosterone values remain high despite these maneuvers, primary aldosteronism is a likely diagnosis. Although clinical response to the aldosterone antagonist spironolactone has been advocated as a diagnostic test for primary aldosteronism, we do not recommend this test because many low-renin patients may also show a response.

3. Adenoma versus Hyperplasia

After making the diagnosis of primary aldosteronism by sequential tests outlined above, one should make the morphological distinction between adenoma and bilateral hyperplasia. Patients with hyperplasia do not respond even to bilateral adrenalectomy; therefore, preoperative distinction should be made. The majority of patients have adrenal adenomas, and only 15% or so have bilateral hyperplasia. However, in some instances, these entities may coexist. The clinical and biochemical manifestations are milder in patients with hyperplasia than in those with an adenoma. There are several procedures to distinguish adenoma from hyperplasia. The basal aldosterone levels are higher in the former; also, in the upright posture, plasma aldosterone level falls in a patient with adenoma, whereas it may rise in hyperplasia. Adrenal venography in experienced hands is of great value in localizing the tumor, and adrenal venous aldosterone measurements show unilateral increase in the case of an adenoma; in bilateral hyperplasia, bilateral increase is seen. Adrenal scintiscanning with [131I]cholesterol can distinguish an adenoma from hyperplasia, but this procedure is available only at a few centers at the present time. Computerized tomography has been successfully used to visualize aldosteronomas greater than 1.0 cm in diameter.

4. Management

Once the diagnosis is confirmed and the nature of primary aldosteronism is determined (adenoma or hyperplasia), the choice of therapy can be made. Adenoma should be resected if possible, whereas patients with hyperplasias should be treated medically with spironolactone with or without a thiazide-type diuretic. With appropriate doses, the clinical and biochemical features can be controlled indefinitely. The dose of spironolactone is quite variable. Some may require high doses up to 400 mg/day. If an operation is contemplated for the removal of an adenoma, the body stores of potassium must be restored in order to reduce the operative risk.

E. Pheochromocytoma

Pheochromocytoma is a neoplasm arising from chromaffin cells of the adrenal medulla or the sympathetic chain. It is estimated that it accounts for less than 0.5% of patients with newly diagnosed hypertension. Despite its rarity, much has been written about pheochromocytoma because of its spectacular clinical features. It is an important entity because it represents a curable form of hypertension and is potentially fatal if not diagnosed. Pheochromocytoma has been the subject of considerable research in recent years, and such endeavors have provided a better understanding of the pathophysiology of this disorder and insight into the applied pharmacology of the drugs capable of blocking the effects of catecholamines.

Most of the pheochromocytomas (perhaps 80%) arise from the adrenal medulla; 10% are bilateral, and 10% are malignant. Familial tumors show a pattern of autosomal dominance with frequent occurrence of bilateral tumors. Sipple's syndrome (multiple endocrine adenomata, type II) is comprised of medullary carcinoma of the thyroid, parathyroid hyperplasia, and bilateral pheochromocytoma.

1. Clinical Features

Pheochromocytoma may cause hypertension identical to essential hypertension, but usually other signs or symptoms secondary to increased levels of catecholamines may be present. Tumors producing only epinephrine are rare. Those from the adrenal medulla commonly secrete norepinephrine or a mixture of the catecholamines. The hypertension may be either sustained or paroxysmal. The paroxysms of hypertension are associated with headache, sweating, pallor, anxiety, tremor, nausea, and weakness. Some patients demonstrate marked fluctuations in the blood pressure. The attacks of hypertension may be precipitated by induction of anesthesia, smoking, changes in posture, and, with large tumors, by massage of the tumor.

Patients with pheochromocytoma are hypermetabolic, mimicking thyrotoxicosis; hyperglycemia is also common, particularly during the spells. The presence of hypermetabolism and hyperglycemia in a hypertensive patient is suggestive of pheochromocytoma. Postural hypotension is frequently encountered in pheochromocytoma. A few patients may present with congestive heart failure or cardiomegaly secondary to catecholamine cardiomyopathy. Intense vasoconstriction with necrosis has been reported in certain patients. Some patients will have evidence of neurocutaneous involvement with *café-au-lait* spots, axillary freckling, and neurofibromas. A patient with intermittent paroxysms may have a normal physical examination during the intervals.

2. Diagnosis

Since pheochromocytoma may present with diverse clinical features, it may be confused with various other entities. A pheochromocytoma should be suspected in any patient with persistent or paroxysmal hypertension accompanied by the clinical features described above.

The biochemical diagnosis of pheochromocytoma depends on the demonstration of high levels of catecholamines and their metabolites in the urine or plasma. Perhaps the best and most convenient procedure is a 24-hr urine for total metanephrines. This test is least affected by interfering substances, and the high levels of this metabolite generally parallel the levels of catecholamines. The vanillylmandelic acid (VMA) test is not specific and is subject to false results, but an increased VMA test in concert with other tests supports the diagnosis. If the metanephrines or VMA levels are high, further confirmation must be obtained by estimating 24-hr urine catecholamines. Plasma catecholamine assays are available in large centers and provide a distinction between essential hypertension and pheochromocytoma.

Pharmacological tests are no longer employed for the diagnosis of pheochromocytoma because of the occurrence of false responses and the risks involved. Once the diagnosis is confirmed biochemically, the tumor must be localized, keeping in mind that a majority of tumors are found in the abdomen, either in the adrenals or the sympathetic chain. A chest X-ray should be taken including the oblique views to rule out the rare tumor in the posterior mediastinum. Intravenous urography with tomograms can localize the tumor in 70% of the patients. Computerized axial tomography is an extremely valuable procedure and may localize the tumor correctly in many instances, especially if the tumor is over 1.0 cm in size. In a few research centers, pheochromocytomas were localized by scintigrams using a new radiopharmaceutical agent [131I]meta-iodobenzylguanidine. If the tumor cannot be localized by noninvasive means, selective arteriography is done after the patient has been treated sufficiently for several days with adrenergic blockers (see below).

3. Management

Once the tumor is localized, the definitive therapy is its resection. But it is important to treat the patient with α- and β-adrenergic blockers for at least 1–2 weeks prior to surgery to minimize the operative risk. Patients should be first treated with phenoxybenzamine, an α blocker, followed by the β blocker, propranolol. The doses of these drugs should be adjusted to control the sympathetic activity and clinical manifestations of the disease. Adrenergic blockade can also be achieved with α-methyl-*para*-tyrosine, a drug that inhibits the rate-limiting tyrosine hydroxylation step in the catecholamine synthesis. α-Methyl-*para*-tyrosine in the daily dose of 2–3 g can inhibit the catecholamine synthesis by 80–90%, thus providing a rational form of adrenergic blockade.

The surgery should be performed by an experienced surgeon who should explore all the other potential sites of the tumor after the resection of the obvious tumor. Sufficient quantities of phentolamine and nitroprusside should be available to manage possible hypertensive episodes during the operation.

For those with unresectable or malignant pheochromocytoma, chronic medical therapy with α and β blockers or with α-methyl-*para*-tyrosine proves quite successful in controlling the symptoms and signs of the disease. The serious nature of malignant pheochromocytoma is related to the possible cardiovascular complications and not to the "neoplastic" features; therefore, chronic medical therapy must be maintained.

F. Miscellaneous Causes

1. Coarctation of the Aorta

Usually detected in childhood, this is an uncommon form of secondary hypertension which is sometimes, but not always, reversible with appropriate surgical correction. Coarctation may occur independently or with other cardiac abnormalities. The cause of hypertension is unclear. Some believe that it results from mechanical obstruction, but others support the renal mechanism. Hypertension in the upper extremities with delay or absent femoral pulses is an important clue to the diagnosis of aortic coarctation. If it is detected, early opinion is recommended in order to avoid potentially fatal cardiac complications.

2. Cushing's Syndrome

Hypertension is an important feature of Cushing's syndrome. The diagnosis should be suspected on the basis of general clinical features and confirmed by hormone measurements.

3. Other Causes

Exogenous steroid administration for prolonged periods can cause hypertension, and this problem should be considered when treating chronic diseases that may need prolonged steroid use.

Licorice contains the mineralocorticoidlike substance glycyrrhizic acid which can cause retention of sodium and water and hypertension in persons who habitually take large amounts of licorice. A much greater frequency of hypertension is observed in patients with hypercalcemia both from hyperparathyroidism and other causes. The mechanism of hypertension is not understood, and the resolution of hypercalcemia does not always result in normotension. Both *hyperthyrodism* and *hypothyroidism* may be associated with hypertension. In the former, systolic with or without mild diastolic hypertension is seen, and after the restoration of euthyroid status, hypertension often improves. A large number of patients with untreated hypothyroidism have been reported to have hypertension, and many become normotensive with the treatment of hypothyroidism. In all of the above miscellaneous conditions, patients may have a coexistent essential hypertension; therefore, treatment of primary cause may not always relieve the hypertension.

Repeated use or abuse of any sympathomimetic drug in any form can elevate the arterial blood pressure. Patients who are on MAO inhibitors are at a risk of developing severe hypertension should they ingest foods with high tyramine content, but fortunately this is less of a problem now because of diminished use of MAO inhibitors in psychiatric medicine.

SUGGESTED READINGS

Alderman MM: Mild hypertension: New light on an old controversy. *Am J Med* 69:653–655, 1980.

Beechgaard P: A 40 years' follow-up study of 1000 untreated hypertensive patients. *Clin Sci Mol Med* 51:673s–675s, 1976.

Dahl LK: Salt and hypertension. *Am J Clin Nutr* 25:231–244, 1972.

Fries ED: Salt, volume and prevention of hypertension. *Circulation* 53:589–595, 1976.

Garay RP, Meyer P: A new test showing abnormal net Na^+ and K^+ in erythrocytes of essential hypertension patients. *Lancet* 1:349–353, 1979.

Gillum RF: Pathophysiology of hypertension in blacks and whites. *Hypertension* 1:468–475, 1979.

Guyton AC, Coleman TG, Cowley AW, et al: Arterial pressure regulation, over-riding dominance of the kidneys in long term regulation and in hypertension. *Am J Med* 52:584–594, 1972.

Hypertension Detection and Follow-up Program Cooperative Group: Five-year findings of the Hypertension Detection and Follow-up Program. I. Reduction of mortality of persons with high blood pressure, including mild hypertension. *JAMA* 242:2562–2571, 1979.

Joint National Committee on Detection, Evaluation and Treatment of High Blood Pressure: Report of the Joint National Committee on Detection, Evaluation and Treatment of High Blood Pressure. *Arch Intern Med* 140:1280–1285, 1980.

Kannel WB, Sorlie P: Hypertension in Framingham, Role of blood pressure in cardiovascular disease: The Framingham study. *Angiology* 26:1–14, 1975.

Kaplan NM: *Clinical Hypertension* (ed 3). Baltimore, Williams & Wilkins, 1982.

Kaplan NM: The Goldblatt Memorial Lecture: The role of kidney in hypertension. *Hypertension* 1:456, 1979.

The Management Committee: The Australian therapeutic trial in mild hypertension. *Lancet* 1:1261, 1980.

Melby JC, Dale SL: New mineralocorticoids and adrenocorticosteroids in hypertension. *Am J Cardiol* 38:805, 1976.

Perera GA: Hypertensive vascular disease, description and natural history. *J Chron Dis* 1:33, 1955.

Pickering G: Hypertension: Definitions, natural histories and consequences. *Am J Med* 52:570, 1972.

Relman AS: Mild hypertension: No more benign neglect, editorial. *N Engl J Med* 302:293, 1980.

Veterans Administration Cooperative Study Group on Antihypertensive Agents: Effects of treatment on morbidity in hypertension. Results in patients with diastolic blood pressure averaging 115 through 129 mm Hg. *JAMA* 292:1028, 1967.

Veterans Administration Cooperative Study Group on Antihypertensive Agents: Effect of treatment on morbidity in hypertension. II. Results in patients with diastolic blood pressure averaging 90 to 114 mm Hg. *JAMA* 213:1143, 1970.

Management of Essential Hypertension

Nonpharmacological Measures

Benson H, Rosner BA, Marzetta BR, et al: Decreased blood pressure in borderline hypertensive subjects who practice meditation. *J Chron Dis* 27:163, 1974.

Black HR: Nonpharmacologic therapy of hypertension. *Am J Med* 66:837, 1979.

Dustan HP: Obesity and hypertension, in Lauer RM, Skekelle RB (eds): *Childhood Prevention of Atherosclerosis and Hypertension.* New York, Raven Press, 1980, p 305.

Fries ED: Salt in hypertension and effects of diuretics. *Annu Rev Pharmacol Toxical* 19:13, 1979.

Ram, CVS, Garrett BN, Kaplan NM: Moderate sodium restriction and various diuretics in the treatment of hypertension: Effects on potassium wastage and blood pressure control. *Arch Intern Med* 141:1015, 1981.

Shapiro AP, Schwartz GE, Ferguson DCE, et al.: Behavioral methods in the treatment of hypertension: A review of their clinical status. *Ann Intern Med* 86:626, 1977.

Thiazides and Related Compounds

Beevers DG, Hamilton M, Harpur JD: The long term treatment of hypertension with thiazide diuretics. *Postgrad Med J* 47:639, 1971.

Bennett WM, McDonald WJ, Kuehnle E: Do diuretics have antihypertensive properties independent of natriuresis? *Clin Pharmacol Ther* 22:499, 1977.

Ram CVS, Reichgott MD: Treatment of loop-diuretic resistant edema by the addition of metolazone. *Curr Ther Res* 22:686, 1977.

Tarazi RC, Dustan HP, Frohligh ED: Long term thiazide therapy in essential hypertension. Evidence for persistent alteration in plasma volume and renin activity. *Circulation* 41:709, 1970.

Loop Diuretics and Potassium-Sparing Diuretics

Finnerty FA, Maxwell MM, Lunn J, et al: Long term effects of furosemide and hydrochlorothiazide in patients with essential hypertension: A two-year comparison of safety and efficacy. *Angiology* 28:125, 1977.

Kim KE, Onesti G, Moyer JH, et al: Ethacrynic acid and furosemide diuretic and hemodynamic effects and clinical use. *Am J Cardiol* 27:407–415, 1971.

Ram CVS, Holland OB, Kaplan NM: Attenuation of diuretic induced hypokalemia by amiloride, a new potassium sparing agent. *J Clin Pharmacol*, 21:484–487, 1981.

Adrenergic Suppressing Drugs

Achor RWO, Hanson NO, Gifford RW: Hypertension treated with rauwolfia serpentina (whole root) and with reserpine. *JAMA* 159:841–845, 1955.

Dollery CT, Harrington M: Methyldopa in hypertension: Clinical and pharmacological studies. *Lancet* 1:759–763, 1962.

Frohlich ED: Methyldopa—mechanisms and treatment 25 years later. *Arch Intern Med* 140: 954–959, 1980.

Onesti G, Schwartz AB, Kim KE, et al.: Antihypertensive effect of clonidine. *Circ Res* 28(Suppl II):53–69, 1971.

Pettinger WA: Drug therapy. Clonidine, a new antihypertensive drug. *N Engl J Med* 293:1179–1180, 1975.

α-Adrenergic Receptor-Blocking Drugs

Brogden RN, Heel RC, Speight TM, et al: Prazosin: A review of its pharmacological properties and therapeutic efficacy in hypertension. *Drugs* 14:163–197, 1977.

Ram CVS, Anderson RJ, Hart GR, et al: Alpha-adrenergic blockade by prazosin in the therapy of essential hypertension. *Clin Pharmacol Ther* 29:719–722, 1981.

β-Adrenergic Receptor-Blocking Drugs

Birkenhager WH, DeLeeuw PW, Wester A, et al: Therapeutic effects of β-adreno-receptor blocking agents in hypertension, *Ergeb Inn Med Kinderheilkd* 39:117–134, 1977.

Editorial: Adverse effects of beta-adrenergic blockade. *Br Med J* 2:3–4, 1974.

Laragh JH: Modern system for treating high blood pressure based on renin profiling and vasoconstriction–volume analysis: A primary role of beta-blocking drugs such as propranolol. *Am J Med* 61:797–810, 1976.

Ram CVS, Kaplan NM: Alpha- and beta-receptor blocking drugs in the treatment of hypertension, in: *Curr Probl Cardio* Vol 3 (Jan), 1979.

Direct Vasodilators

Chidsey CA III, Gottlieb TD. The pharmacological basis of antihypertensive therapy: The role of vasodilator drugs. *Prog Cardiovasc Dis* 17:99–113, 1974.

DuCharme DW, Freyburger WA, Graham BE, et al: Pharmacologic properties of minoxidil: A new hypotensive agent. *J Pharmacol Exp Ther* 184:622–670, 1973.

Koch-Weser J: Hydralazine. *N Engl J Med* 295:320–322, 1976.

Linus ST, Nies AS: Minoxidil. *Ann Intern Med* 94:61–65, 1981.

Perry HM: Late toxicity to hydralazine resembling systemic lupus erythematosus or rheumatoid arthritis. *Am J Med* 54:58–72, 1973.

Inhibitors of the Renin–Angiotensin System: Captopril

Captopril: Benefits and risks in severe hypertension, editorial. *Lancet* 2:129–130, 1980.

Hollenberg NK: Pharmacologic interruption of the renin–angiotensin system. *Annu Rev Pharmacol Toxicol* 19:559–582, 1979.

Ram CVS: Clinical application of therapeutic advances: Captopril. *Arch Intern Med* 142:914–916, 1982.

Secondary Forms of Hypertension

General

Berglund G, Anderson O, Wilhelmsen L: Prevalence of primary and secondary hypertension: Studies in a random population sample. *Br Med J* 2:544, 1976.

Garay RP, Elghozi J, Dagher G, et al: Laboratory distinction between essential and secondary hypertension by measurement of erythrocyte cation fluxes. *N Engl J Med* 302:769, 1980.

Gifford RW Jr: Evaluation of the hypertensive patient with emphasis on detecting curable hypertension. *Milbank Mem Fund Q* 47:179, 1969.

Grim CE, Weinberger MM, Higgins JT, et al: Diagnosis of secondary forms of hypertension. A comprehensive protocol. *JAMA* 237:1331, 1977.

Weinstein MC, Stason WB (eds): *Hypertension: A Policy Perspective.* Cambridge, Harvard University Press, 1976.

Oral Contraceptive Use

Beral V, Kay C: The pill and circulatory disease. *Am Heart J* 97:263, 1979.

Saruta T, Saade GA, Kaplan NM: A possible mechanism for hypertension induced by oral contraceptives. Diminished feedback suppression of renin release. *Arch Intern Med* 126: 621, 1970.

Weir RJ: When the pill causes a rise in blood pressure. *Drugs* 16:522, 1978.

Hypertension Associated with Renal Parenchymal Disease

Baldwin DS: Poststreptococcal glomerulonephritis. A progressive disease? *Am J Med* 62:1, 1977.

Brod J: Chronic renal parenchymal disease and hypertension. *Kidney Int* 8:S235, 1975.

Brown JJ, Dusterdieck GO, Fraser R, et al: Hypertension and chronic renal failure. *Br Med Bull* 27:128, 1971.

Brunner HR, Krishman D, Sealey JE, et al: Hypertension of renal origin: Evidence for two different mechanisms. *Science* 174:1344, 1971.

Hull AR, Long DL, Prati RC, et al: The control of hypertension in patients undergoing regular maintenance hemodialysis. *Kidney Int* 57:S184, 1975.

Kim KE, Onesti G, Schwartz AB, et al: Hemodynamics of hypertension in chronic end-stage renal disease. *Circulation* 46:456, 1972.

Kincaid-Smith P: Renal disease and hypertension. *Med Clin North Am* 61:611, 1977.

Kincaid-Smith P:, Fairley KF, Heale WF, et al: Pyelonephritis as a cause of hypertension in man, In: Onesti G, Kim KE, Moyer JH (eds): *Hypertension: Mechanisms and Management.* New York, Grune & Stratton, 1973, p 697.

Mitchell HG, Graham RM, Pettiger WA: Renal function during long term treatment of hypertension with minoxidil. Comparison of benign and malignant hypertension. *Ann Intern Med* 93:676, 1980.

Pettinger WA, Mitchell HC: Minoxidil—an alternative to nephrectomy for refractory hypertension. *N Engl J Med* 289:167, 1973.

Vertes V, Cangiano JL, Berman LB, et al: Hypertension in end-stage renal disease. *N Engl J Med* 280:978, 1969.

Weber MA, Drayer JI: Renal effects of beta-adrenoceptor blockade. *Kidney Int* 18:686, 1980.

Weidman P, Maxwell MH: The renin–angiotensin–aldosterone system in terminal renal failure. *Kidney Int* 8:S219, 1975.

Renovascular Hypertension

Baer L, Parra-Carrillo JZ, Radichevich J, et al: Detection or renovascular hypertension with angiotensin II blockade. *Ann Intern Med* 86:257, 1977.

Foster JH, Maxwell MH, Franklin SS, et al: Renovascular occlusive disease. Results of operative treatment. *JAMA* 231:1043, 1975.

Streeten DHP, Anderson GH Jr: Out-patient experience with saralasin. *Kidney Int* 15:S44, 1979.

Primary Aldosteronism

Conn JW: Primary aldosteronism, in Genest J, Koiw E, Kuchel O (eds): *Hypertension; Pathophysiology and Treatment.* New York, McGraw-Hill, 1977, p 768.

Ferriss JB, Beevers DG, Brown JJ, et al: The treatment of low-renin ("primary") hyperaldosteronism. *Am Heart J* 96:97–109 1978.

Horton R, Finck E: Diagnosis and localization of primary aldosteronism. *Ann Intern Med* 76: 885–890, 1972.

Weinberger MH, Grim CE, Hollifield JW, et al: Primary aldosteronism. *Ann Intern Med* 90: 386–395, 1979.

Pheochromocytoma

Amery A, Conway J: A critical review of diagnostic tests for pheochromocytoma. *Am Heart J* 73:129–133, 1967.

Bravo EL, Tarazi RW, Gifford RW Jr, et al: Circulating and urinary catecholamines in pheochromocytoma. *N Engl J Med* 301:682–686, 1979.

Manger WM, Gifford RW Jr: *Pheochromocytoma.* New York, Springer-Verlag, 1978.

Ram CVS, Engelman K: Pheochromocytoma: Pathophysiology, recognition and management, in: *Curr Probl Cardiol,* Vol. 4 Apr), 1979.

Management of Hypertension
Hypertensive Emergencies

C. VENKATA S. RAM

I. INTRODUCTION

Despite the large number of patients with chronic hypertension, hypertensive crisis constitutes a relatively rare medical emergency. However, marked and sudden elevation in blood pressure may represent an immediate threat to life. Prompt reduction of blood pressure in these situations is therefore essential and may be life saving.

In the majority of patients, hypertension progresses slowly and, if adequately controlled, seldom leads to a crisis. The consequences of severe elevation of blood pressure generally involve the brain, the cardiovascular system, and the kidneys. Therefore, rapid treatment of hypertension is necessary in order to prevent or reverse many of the morbid consequences. Any form of hypertension may lead to a crisis, the major determinant being the degree of blood pressure elevation rather than the etiology of the hypertensive state. Under certain circumstances, it is not only the degree of blood pressure elevation that determines the gravity of the clinical situation but also the rate of rise in blood pressure, as exemplified by eclampsia and acute glomerulonephritis in which hypertensive crisis can occur at blood pressures that are ordinarily tolerated by patients with chronic hypertension, e.g., blood pressures of 150–160/100.

Certain conditions qualify as hypertensive emergencies not so much because of the magnitude of blood pressure elevation but because of coexist-

C. VENKATA S. RAM • Department of Internal Medicine, Southwestern Medical School at the University of Texas Health Science Center at Dallas, Dallas, Texas 75235; and St. Paul Hospital, Dallas, Texas 75235.

ing complications that make even moderate hypertension dangerous. These include acute left ventricular failure, acute dissection of the aorta, and coronary artery disease. Hypertensive emergencies rarely develop in previously normotensive persons, and more commonly they occur in poorly controlled chronic hypertension. In previously normotensive individuals, acute elevations of blood pressure cause complications to a greater extent at any given level of blood pressure than in those with chronic hypertension. In the management of hypertensive emergencies, prompt therapy should take precedence over diagnostic procedures, and valuable time should not be wasted in the pursuit of an underlying etiology.

For practical purposes and therapeutic priorities, I am categorizing hypertensive crisis into *hypertensive emergencies* and *hypertensive urgencies*. Hypertensive emergencies (Table I) are conditions with dire prognosis in which delay of therapeutic intervention might potentially lead to irreversible sequelae. Hypertensive urgencies are conditions with less serious immediate prognosis but that may ultimately lead to complications if blood pressure is not aggressively treated. The examples of hypertensive urgencies are shown in Table II.

II. ACCELERATED AND MALIGNANT HYPERTENSION

The term malignant or accelerated hypertension is usually applied to the hypertensive state that is associated with rapidly deteriorating blood pressure control and grade-III or -IV Keith–Wagener retinopathy. No matter how severe the hypertension may be, it should not be classified as "malignant" unless papilledema is present. On the other hand, the term "accelerated" hypertension is characterized by the presence of hemorrhages or exudates in the retina. The funduscopic picture is also characterized by generalized arteriolar spasm.

A. Clinical Features

In malignant or accelerated hypertension, the sustained elevation of blood pressure is severe enough to cause damage to the vascular system. The

Table I. Hypertensive Emergencies

Hypertensive encephalopathy
Acute aortic dissection
Pulmonary edema
Pheochromocytoma crisis
MAO inhibitor + tyramine interaction
Intracranial hemorrhage
Eclampsia

Table II. Hypertensive Urgencies

Hypertension associated with coronary artery disease
Accelerated and malignant hypertension
Severe hypertension in the kidney transplant patient
Postoperative hypertension
Uncontrolled hypertension in the patient who requires emergency surgery

vascular damage is clinically manifested as neuroretinopathy or nephropathy. Malignant hypertension may develop during the course of essential hypertension or sometimes as a manifestation of a secondary form of hypertension, particularly renal artery stenosis. The clinical features of malignant or accelerated hypertension are shown in Table III.

More than 75% of patients with malignant hypertension have a previous history of blood pressure elevation, and in substantial numbers of these patients, there is also a strong positive family history of high blood pressure. The blood pressure in this condition is always high (usually greater than 200/130 mm Hg). The patient may be entirely without symptoms, the condition being discovered by accident, or the patient may present with clinical evidence of heart failure or renal insufficiency. Although some patients may be asymptomatic and free of complications, the majority of patients complain of headache that is most severe early in the morning. The consistent finding on physical examination of a patient with this condition is the presence of grade III or IV retinopathy (Keith–Wagener classification). The level of blood pressure itself, although important, is not a major criterion for the diagnosis. Except for hypertensive encephalopathy, which is described in detail in Section III, the symptoms of malignant hypertension are not distinctive. Gross hematuria, weight loss, visual disturbance, generalized malaise, and manifestations of secondary hyperaldosteronism (profound muscle weakness or paresthesias reflecting severe hypokalemia) are occasionally noted. The urinalysis usually reveals proteinuria or hematuria. There may be a certain degree of azotemia, which can sometimes be severe, and anemia. The peripheral blood smear may reflect the evidence of intravascular hemolysis which is presumably secondary to mechanical destruction of the RBCs.

The characteristic pathological lesion of accelerated or malignant hypertension is fibrinoid arteriolar necrosis predominantly occurring in the kidneys, brain, and retina.

Table III. Features of Accelerated or Malignant Hypertension

Marked elevation of diastolic BP
Malaise
Headache
Retinopathy
Renal failure (azotemia, proteinuria, hematuria, etc.)
Altered mental status

The prognosis of untreated malignant hypertension is extremely poor. Without adequate treatment, more than 80% of patients succumb within 12 months. The necrotizing arteriolitis of malignant hypertension is a rapidly progressive process that leads to irreversible renal failure if the process is uninterrupted, and therefore, the blood pressure should be urgently reduced to stop the necrotizing process and permit the damaged arterioles to heal. Modern antihypertensive therapy unquestionably has been shown to prolong life in patients with malignant hypertension.

B. Management

The patient with accelerated or malignant hypertension should be immediately hospitalized for intensive medical therapy (Table IV). If the patient has a normal mental status and is able to take oral medications, intensive medical therapy should be instituted. The most useful oral agents for rapid control of blood pressure are the diuretics and direct vasodilators such as hydralazine and the new agent minoxidil. Since the direct vasodilators almost always cause reflexive increases in the heart rate and cardiac output, simultaneous administration of an adrenergic blocking agent to counteract these adverse hemodynamic effects is advisable. The availability of minoxidil has favorably changed the prognostic outlook of these patients. If the patient's condition is severe, or if hydralazine is ineffective, minoxidil should be used. In some patients with malignant hypertension, administration of minoxidil not only preserves but also may improve the renal function. Captopril has been successfully employed in the management of hypertensive crisis and certainly is a good choice for those who do not show satisfactory response to other orally active agents. Patients with renal insufficiency receiving captopril should be closely monitored, since certain adverse effects of captopril (renal, hematological) have been reported mainly in this category of patients. In some institutions, guanethidine loading is used to rapidly reduce the blood pressure, but it is preferable to use a combination of a direct vasodilator and an adrenergic blocking agent. If the patient's condition is severe, or if he is not able to take oral medications, the blood pressure can be reduced to the desired level by using one of the potent parenteral antihypertensive agents such as diazoxide, sodium nitroprusside, or trimethaphan.

Table IV. Therapy of Accelerated and Malignant Hypertension

Bed rest
Diuretics, usually a loop diuretic
Hydralazine or minoxidil
Adrenergic blocking agents
Parenteral agents: diazoxide, nitroprusside, trimethaphan, or hydralazine

III. HYPERTENSIVE ENCEPHALOPATHY

Hypertensive encephalopathy is a medical emergency caused by abrupt and severe elevation of blood pressure; it is the most serious complication of accelerated hypertension. The present rarity of this syndrome reflects overall improved management of hypertension. It is important to diagnose hypertensive encephalopathy promptly, because rapid reduction of blood pressure results in the amelioration of the syndrome which is otherwise potentially fatal. Hypertensive encephalopathy occurs during the course of severe elevation of arterial blood pressure and is not limited to any specific etiologic type of hypertension, although the syndrome tends to occur more commonly as a complication of acute glomerulonephritis, toxemia of pregnancy, and renal artery stenosis. In hypertensive encephalopathy, the absolute level and the rapidity with which elevation of blood pressure occurs determine the development of symptoms. They may appear at relatively low levels of blood pressure when hypertension is of recent onset. Hypertensive encephalopathy occurs more frequently when hypertension is complicated by renal failure than when the kidney function is normal.

Normal cerebral blood flow (CBF) remains relatively constant despite the variations in systemic blood pressure. This constancy of CBF is maintained by the process of autoregulation. However, in hypertensive encephalopathy, the cerebral autoregulation is deranged.

A. Clinical Features

The clinical features of hypertensive encephalopathy are usually precipitated by a sudden increase in blood pressure from a previously stable hypertensive level or by abrupt appearance of hypertension in a previously normotensive patient (i.e., toxemia of pregnancy or acute glomerulonephritis). In those previously hypertensive, the manifestations of hypertensive encephalopathy usually do not occur until the blood pressure exceeds about 200–220/130 mm Hg. Hypertensive encephalopathy may occur at much lower levels of blood pressure when the onset of hypertension has been recent and abrupt. The onset of symptoms is usually subacute, and although the exact time period of evolution of the syndrome has not been documented, it often takes 24 to 48 hr to develop a full-blown encephalopathy. The symptoms are listed in Table V.

B. Management

Once the diagnosis of hypertensive encephalopathy seems likely on the basis of the constellation of clinical findings that have been discussed,

Table V. Salient Features of Hypertensive
Encephalopathy

Marked elevation of blood pressure
Headache
Nausea, vomiting
Papilledema
Visual complaints
Focal transient neurological deficits (seizures)
Altered mental status

the blood pressure should be lowered to near normal levels. The patient with encephalopathy should ideally be managed in an intensive care unit with constant monitoring of his vital signs. The most important aspect of therapy is to reduce the blood pressure rapidly to near normal levels. Although it has been warned that cerebral blood flow may be jeopardized by rapid lowering of blood pressure to normal levels in chronically hypertensive patients, one can avoid the hypotensive sequelae by reducing the blood pressure with an agent with a short duration of action so that unwanted reduction in the blood pressure can be reversed by discontinuing the drug. The presently available parenteral hypotensive drugs produce prompt and dramatic relief of symptoms of hypertensive encephalopathy.

Although it is sometimes difficult to distinguish hypertensive encephalopathy from other cerebral complications of severe hypertension (Table VI), the *sine qua non* of hypertensive encephalopathy is its prompt response to

Table VI. Features of Hypertensive Encephalopathy and Other Intracranial
Disorders

	Evolution	Headache	Consciousness	Signs
Hypertensive encephalopathy	Subacute (12–48 hr)	Severe, generalized, recent onset	Initially clear but progresses to coma	Nausea and vomiting, visual disturbance, seizures, transient neurological deficits
Cerebral infarction	Rapid (few min to 6 hr)	None or mild	Inattentive, coma very rare	Fixed neurological deficits
Cerebral embolus	Sudden	None or mild	Mild lethargy	Changing signs
Cerebral hemorrhage	Rapid	Sudden, severe, occipital	Rapid progression to coma	Dense deficits
Subarachnoid hemorrhage	Rapid	Sudden, severe, local to general	Normal or altered depending on the site and secondary involvement	Fever, stiff neck, aphasia, cranial nerve palsies

Table VII. Differential Diagnosis of
Hypertensive Encephalopathy

Acute cerebrovascular accidents
Uremic encephalopathy
Benign intracranial hypertension
Intracranial mass lesion
Seizure disorder
Drug overdose or interaction

antihypertensive therapy. Nitroprusside and diazoxide are the drugs of choice, whereas several untoward effects make trimethaphan a less desirable treatment choice. Because of their central actions, clonidine, methyldopa, and reserpine should not be used in this condition. If the patient's neurological syndrome does not improve or worsens with therapy, an alternate diagnosis should be sought (Table VII).

IV. SEVERE HYPERTENSION ASSOCIATED WITH CEREBROVASCULAR ACCIDENTS

Whereas there is good evidence that control of hypertension reduces the incidence of both intracranial hemorrhage and thrombotic strokes, a patient who presents with severe hypertension during an acute cerebrovascular accident presents a difficult problem. Many but not all physicians recommend reduction of blood pressure with parenteral administration of hypotensive drugs. With increased intracerebral pressure, the autoregulation curve or the relationship between the systemic blood pressure and the cerebral blood flow becomes unpredictable. The goal in the treatment of severe hypertension associated with cerebrovascular accidents is to lower the blood pressure without depressing mental functions. Therefore, agents with rapid onset but short duration of action are preferred.

In contrast to the intracerebral hemorrhage for which medical management is indicated, the treatment of intracerebellar hemorrhages is somewhat different. In this condition, surgical decompression of the cerebellar hematoma is indicated and in most cases is life saving. Thus, with the present state of our knowledge, no specific guidelines can be given about the management of hypertensive crisis occurring in patients with cerebrovascular accidents. However, based on the pathogenesis of these conditions, especially intracerebral hemorrhage and possibly subarachnoid hemorrhage, if the patient has severe hypertension, it is advisable to reduce the blood pressure gradually to 100–110 mm Hg diastolic or to a degree that will not compromise the cerebral function. Such a smooth desired level of blood pressure control is only achieved with either sodium nitroprusside or trimethaphan.

V. ACUTE AORTIC DISSECTION

The occurrence of dissecting aortic aneurysms in patients with hypertension and the frequent presence of hypertension in patients with dissecting aneurysm of the aorta are well established. Dissection of the aorta is the most common acute disease of the aorta and occurs at the rate of around five to ten cases per million population each year. In addition to being the most common catastrophe involving the aorta, the acute dissection is also the most lethal.

A. Clinical Features

The dissecting aortic aneurysms afflict men more frequently than women with a peak incidence around the sixth decade, although patients with types 1 and 2 (Table VIII, but compare Table IX) dissection are on the average somewhat younger. The usual patient with a dissection of the aorta, especially involving the ascending aorta, is an elderly male with a chronic history of hypertension who presents with severe and persistent chest pain. The symptoms of acute dissection are listed in Table X.

Of all the symptoms that are listed, severe pain is the most important manifestation of acute dissection. It is easily confused with the pain of acute myocadial infarction. There are, however, certain subtle qualitative differences between the pain of aortic dissection and myocardial infarction. The pain of dissection is abrupt in onset and is quite severe right from the onset, whereas patients with acute myocardial infarction rarely report that the pain began abruptly. The pain of myocardial infarction may wax and wane, whereas the aortic dissection pain occurs abruptly and persists. Although the patient's description of the pain may not indicate the site of dissection, it might sometimes reflect the extent of dissection. It is the quality of pain rather than its precise location that characterizes the patient with acute aortic dissection. Certain terms, such as tearing, lacerating, throbbin, ripping, excruciating, and burning, have been used by patients with acute dissections. The onset of pain is almost always sudden and is unremitting in most patients who fear that death is imminent. Frequently, the onset of pain is not preceded by any special activity, and many patients wake up with acute pain.

Table VIII. Debakey's Classification of Dissecting Aneurysms

Type 1 Begins in the ascending aorta and extends at least into the arch and possibly through the descending aorta.

Type 2 Dissection is localized to the ascending aorta only.

Type 3 Begins in the descending aorta. Sometimes a type 3 dissection may have a retrograde progression through the arch and may even dissect into the pericardium.

Table IX. The New ABC Therapeutic Classification

Class	Definition
A	Involves the ascending aorta
A1	With complications
A2	Without complications
B	Does not involve the ascending aorta
B1	With complications
B2	Without complications
C	Inoperable

Signs such as sudden pulselessness in an extremity or sudden appearance of a diastolic murmur together with appearance of such severe pain should alert the physician to the possibility of a dissection. Following the resolution of the initial attack, recurrence of pain may signify resumption of the dissection process.

B. Physical Findings

The physical findings of acute dissection are listed in Table XI.

Except for chest X-ray and angiography, the laboratory is of little help in making the diagnosis of dissecting aneurysm. The electrocardiogram is useful in a negative sense, to rule out the possibility of an acute myocardial infarction. Left ventricular hypertrophy is common, and the cardiac enzymes are usually normal, although sometimes the LDH may be elevated because of hemolysis within the false channel. Experience with echocardiography is limited but has been quite reliable in a few centers.

C. Initial Management

When acute aortic dissection is suspected, immediate measures should be instituted to stabilize the patient's condition before any additional studies

Table X. Clinical Features of Acute
Aortic Dissection

Severe pain in the chest, intrascapular
  region, neck, midback, sacral area
Syncope
Confusional state or headache
Blindness
Hemoptysis
Dyspnea
Nausea and vomiting
Melena or hematemesis
Oliguria, anuria, or hematuria
Paralysis

Table XI. Physical Findings of Acute Dissection

Hypertension
Tachycardia or bradycardia
Shocky appearance
Rales
Deficiency of pulses
Cardiac tamponade
Unilateral or bilateral jugular venous distension
Cardiomegaly
Hemothorax
Pericardial friction rub
Physical findings of aortic insufficiency
Hemiplegia, paraplegia
Facial paralysis
Paralytic ileus

are performed; intraarterial blood pressure should be closely monitored. If a previous chest X-ray is available for comparison, it would be helpful to see if there has been any enlargement of the mediastinal shadow. Once the diagnosis of acute aortic dissection is apparent (Table XII), the following steps should be undertaken.

If the patient is hypertensive, blood pressure should be reduced to near normal levels with an agent that causes the blood pressure to come down smoothly rather than drastically. The direct vasodilators which reflexly stimulate the heart should be avoided and, in fact, are contraindicated in acute aortic dissection. When instituting antihypertensive therapy, one should keep in mind that the force and velocity of ventricular contraction (dp/dt) and the pulsatile flow are important determinants of the shearing force acting on the aortic wall. Attempts should be made to decrease the dp/dt with a suitable agent; drugs that reflexly stimulate the heart such as diazoxide and Apresoline® should be avoided. The blood pressure should be reduced to near normal levels, and the ideal agent in this situation would be trimethaphan which has a smooth action and is rapidly effective. Since this drug is a ganglion-blocking agent, it decreases the neural transmission at the myocardial contractility sites, has a negative inotropic effect, and therefore decreases the pulsatile flow and also blunts the sharpness of the pulse wave generated by the heart. This mode of pharmacological approach to management has been shown to reduce mortality.

The alternative to trimethaphan is sodium nitroprusside in conjunction

Table XII. Differential Diagnosis
of Acute Aortic Dissection

Acute myocardial infarction
Acute pulmonary embolism
Cerebrovascular accident
Acute surgical abdomen
Rupture of the sinus of Valsalva

with the simultaneous administration of a β-adrenergic blocking agent such as propranolol (to reduce the rate of myocardial contractility and arrest the progression of the dissection). Sodium nitroprusside alone has been alleged to cause an increase in dp/dt, an effect that is harmful in these patients; the adverse effects of sodium nitroprusside occurred because of inadequate dosage of propranolol. When adequate doses of propranolol are given along with sodium nitroprusside, this is as effective and indeed is better tolerated than trimethaphan.

Only after the institution of measures aimed at restoring the vital signs should further work-up be undertaken. The goal of initial treatment is the elimination of pain and reduction of systolic blood pressure to 100–120 mm Hg or to the lowest level that is tolerated by the patient with adequate vital organ perfusion.

D. Angiography

The hazards of this technique are minimal with the proper precautions, and most patients tolerate this procedure fairly well if they have been stabilized. Retrograde angiogrphy allows accurate identification of the site of the origin of the dissection, a prerequisite if surgery is to be done.

E. Definitive Therapy

The choice between continuing medical therapy and surgical intervention depends on the different clinical behavior of proximal and distal dissections in the early phase of the disease. There has been considerable controversy in the literature regarding the surgical and medical therapy of aortic dissections. With the accumulation of a large quantity of data, prospective and retrospective in nature, certain generalities can be made. Surgery is the definitive treatment of choice for proximal dissection because of the potentially devastating consequences of the progression of the hematoma and frequent association of this type with pulse deficits, aortic regurgitation, pericardial tamponade, and neurological dysfunction. In a very small group of patients with proximal dissection (in patients who are unable or unwilling to undergo a surgical procedure), long-term medical therapy has been accomplished with variable results.

For the patients with uncomplicated distal dissection (type 3), continuation of chronic medical therapy offers a slight advantage over surgical therapy. The advantage of medical therapy is largely because patients with distal dissection tend to have advanced atherosclerotic or cardiac disease. Thus, in these patients, surgical morbidity and mortality are likely to be higher than in patients with proximal dissection. For a type 3 dissection, surgery should be undertaken if there is evidence of rupture or vital organ compromise or inability to contain the hematoma with appropriate medical therapy.

VI. ACUTE LEFT VENTRICULAR FAILURE

Acute left ventricular failure in a patient with moderate or severe hypertension is an indication for rapid lowering of the blood pressure. The lowering of the blood pressure in a patient with acute pulmonary edema decreases the work load of the failing myocardium, and, in fact, in many patients it is possible to restore adequate cardiac function with blood pressure lowering alone. The failing ventricle demonstrates an increased end-diastolic fiber length, an increased ventricular volume, and a reduced ejection fraction rate; these factors result in consumption of more oxygen in order to expel a smaller stroke volume. The essential effect that will be required then is an immediate reduction in the systemic vascular resistance in order to decrease the afterload on the failing myocardium and increase the cardiac output. The persistently elevated blood pressure is a costly burden on the failing myocardium, increasing its oxygen requirements. This could be particularly deleterious in patients who may have coexistent coronary artery disease.

Prompt reduction of blood pressure with a vasodilating agent such as sodium nitroprusside is indicated in this situation. Systemic vasodilators such as sodium nitroprusside, in addition to their hypotensive effect, dilate the capacitance vessels, decreasing the venous return to the heart. These actions therefore decrease the afterload and preload, both of which actions help to restore myocardial function and increase cardiac output. Drugs such as hydralazine and diazoxide should be avoided in treating this condition because they may cause reflex tachycardia. If nitroprusside cannot be infused for any reason, and the patient needs parenteral antihypertensive therapy, perhaps small doses of diazoxide can be given. The other alternative obviously would be trimethaphan which has a smooth onset of action, and blood pressure can be predictably lowered by adjusting the speed of infusion. Along with reduction in blood pressure, the conventional measures for managing pulmonary edema should be instituted.

VII. SEVERE HYPERTENSION ASSOCIATED WITH ISCHEMIC HEART DISEASE

Systemic hypertension increases the myocardial oxygen consumption by increasing the intraventricular pressure and, in some patients, by increasing the left ventricular diameter, both of which are known to increase the wall tension. Thus, theoretically, patients who have ischemic heart disease and have sustained high blood pressure should benefit from lowering of the blood pressure. Although it is logical to assume that severe hypertension occurring in a patient with ischemic heart disease should be treated, there are no definite data in the literature that uniformly suggest that treatment is beneficial. Despite the reported detrimental effects that hypertension may exert on patients with acute myocardial infarction, considerable controversy prevails on the pathophysiological significance of hypertension in patients with acute myocardial infarction. Reduction of blood pressure reduces the cardiac work, wall tension, and oxygen demand and may be a rational approach to decrease the frequency of angina and limit the necrosis in the early phase of infarction.

Some studies suggest that acute elevation of blood pressure in the setting of acute myocardial infarction is transient and does not seem to exert any adverse effect, but Fox *et al.* have assessed the prognostic significance of acute systolic hypertension in a larger series of patients and have concluded that the mortality rate and the incidence of cardiac failure were significantly greater in a group of patients who had systolic blood pressure greater than 170 mm Hg.

Shell and Sobel have indicated that reduction of systemic arterial pressure early in the course of acute myocardial infarction protects the myocardium as reflected by reduced release of CPK enzyme activity. In their series, the myocardial infarct size was decreased by 24% in hypertensive patients whose blood pressure was reduced with trimethaphan during the acute phase of myocardial infarction. It is reasonable to assume that hypertension would raise the ventricular afterload and thus may augment the myocardial oxygen demand and further compromise the coronary circulation.

Cautious treatment of hypertension in patients with acute myocardial infarction is likely to be beneficial. However, the reduction in the blood pressure should be carried on with adequate hemodynamic monitoring. Of the parenteral agents, sodium nitroprusside is widely used in this setting.

VIII. MISCELLANEOUS CAUSES

A. Pheochromocytoma Crisis

Pheochromocytoma crisis is extremely unusual but requires emergency control of the blood pressure. It presents with a constellation of striking clinical features. Typically, the blood pressure is markedly elevated (to as high as 300 mm Hg systolic), usually with a proportionate rise in the diastolic blood pressure and profound sweating. There is also marked tachycardia, pallor, especially on the face, and numbness, tingling, and coldness of the feet and hands. Many patients complain of pounding headache, nausea, vomiting, and epigastric discomfort. During the crisis, acute pulmonary edema and serious neurological deficits might result. A single attack will last from a few minutes to hours and may occur as often as several times a day to once a month or less. During the intervening periods, however, the patient is usually asymptomatic. Although severe hypertension is a notable finding, this is more so when the tumor is predominantly secreting norepinephrine. Epinephrine-producing tumors may not cause marked elevations in the blood pressure.

Once the diagnosis of pheochromocytoma crisis is apparent, an intravenous line should be established, and the patient given the α-adrenergic blocking drug phentolamine in a dose of 5 to 10 mg intravenously. The dosage of phentolamine may be repeated in a few minutes as warranted by the patient's clinical status. An alternative to phentolamine therapy would be sodium nitroprusside, but the former is more rational. There is no unanimity about the use of the β-blocking drug propranolol in managing pheochromocytoma crisis. The drug will certainly be useful if the patient has a concomitant cardiac arrhythmia. The administration of β-blocking agents should always be preceded by either phentolamine or phenoxybenzamine. If this is not done, the β-blocker can aggravate the unopposed peripheral vasoconstriction.

B. Clonidine Withdrawal Syndrome

A syndrome mimicking pheochromocytoma crisis has been reported following abrupt discontinuation of the antihypertensive drug clonidine. Clonidine exerts its antihypertensive effect by stimulating the α receptors in the brainstem and thus reducing the tone of peripheral sympathetic activity. When clonidine is abruptly discontinued or rapidly tapered, patients may experience nausea, palpitations, anxiety, sweating, nervousness, and headache with or without marked elevation of blood pressure. In some patients, overshoot in blood pressure has been reported following abrupt cessation of clonidine therapy. The so-called clonidine withdrawal syndrome is best explained by enhanced sympathetic activity on sudden discontinuation of drug therapy. In most of the published reports, the withdrawal syndrome has occurred in patients who had been receiving more than 1.2 mg/day of clonidine. Therefore, the withdrawal phenomenon is perhaps related to the total daily dose.

When a patient presents a syndrome of sympathetic overactivity and a history of therapy with clonidine, one should entertain the possibility of clonidine withdrawal syndrome and promptly institute appropriate therapy. The symptoms of clonidine withdrawal can be abated with reinstitution of clonidine alone if this can be done. If there is marked elevation of blood pressure and the patient is experiencing severe and annoying subjective side effects such as palpitations, chest discomfort, epigastric discomfort, etc., intravenous administration of phentolamine is recommended. The treatment of clonidine withdrawal syndrome does not differ significantly from that of pheochromocytoma. Clonidine withdrawal phenomenon, although rare, can be minimized by precautions to avoid abrupt discontinuation of the drug.

C. Hypertensive Crisis Associated with Drug and Food Interactions

Patients receiving monoamine oxidase (MAO) inhibitors are at risk of developing hypertensive crisis if they take drugs such as ephedrine or amphetamine or foods containing high quantities of tyramine (Table XIII). Monoamine oxidase inhibitors are sometimes used to treat depression, and examples of the drugs belong to this class are also listed in Table XIII.

Critical elevation of blood pressure has been reported following the interaction between these MAO inhibitors and certain foodstuffs. Fortunately, however, these reactions are rather uncommon because of the declining use of MAO inhibitors. The tyramine that is contained in these foodstuffs is an indirectly acting sympathetic amine and is ordinarily destroyed by MAO present in the liver and gastrointestinal mucosa. But in the presence of an inhibitor of MAO, tyramine escapes the oxidative degradation, enters the systemic circulation, and potentiates the actions of catecholamines. The diagnosis of a pressor reaction secondary to MAO inhibitors depends on the history of the usage of the drug and identification of the precipitating event such as a particular drug or foodstuff. The history of psychiatric depression is often a helpful clue in suggesting the diagnosis.

Intravenous injection of 5 to 10 mg of phentolamine will control the hypertension and can be repeated as necessary until the patient is stabilized or switched to an alternative medication such as sodium nitroprusside or infusion of phentolamine. Luckily, these pressor reactions are self-limited and are usually short-lived, but, nevertheless, proper recognition of the syndrome is essential in order to institute rational therapy.

D. Postoperative Hypertensive Crisis

Open heart operations and surgical manipulation of the carotid artery are sometimes followed by severe hypertension in the immediate postoperative period. Hypertension, even if it is of moderate degree, in the

Table XIII. Some MAO Inhibitors and Tyramine-Containing Substances

MAO inhibitors
  Pargyline (Eutonyl®)
  Nialamide (Niamid®)
  Furazulidone (Furoxone®)
  Phenelzine (Nardil®)
  Tranylcypromine (Parnate®)

Tyramine-containing foods
  Chianti wine
  Some beers
  Aged cheeses (cheddar, brie)
  Avocados
  Bananas
  Chocolate
  Chicken liver
  Fermented sausage
  Soy sauce
  Yeast extract

postoperative period may jeopardize the integrity of the vascular suture lines. Whatever the etiology for hypertension in the postoperative period may be, it should be managed promptly with parenteral agents. Sodium nitroprusside is usually the agent of choice because of the titratable dose. (Obviously, hypotension should be avoided in the postoperative period because of the danger of thrombosis around the vascular suture lines.) Trimethaphan should be avoided in the postoperative period because it may delay the return of bowel and bladder function.

E. Severe Hypertension Associated with Burns

Hypertensive crisis has been associated with extensive body burns, and the mechanism involved is not understood. The blood pressure may rise to critical levels and require the use of a promptly acting agent such as sodium nitroprusside or diazoxide.

F. Hypertensive Crisis in Quadriplegic Patients

Hypertensive crises have been reported in patients with high transverse lesions of the spinal cord, usually above the origins of the thoracolumbar sympathetic neurons. The mechanism appears to be one of autonomic overactivity. Any stimulation of dermatomes and muscles supplied by nerves below the injury evokes severe hypertension, profound headache, and bradycardia. The hypertension may be quite severe and may indeed cause cerebrovascular accidents and death. Given the current pathophysiological basis for such hypertensive reactions, critical blood pressure elevations can be prevented by avoiding the excessive stimulation of the susceptible portion of dermatomes. The hypertension should be treated with one of the parenteral antihypertensive drugs discussed.

IX. DRUGS USED IN THE TREATMENT OF HYPERTENSIVE CRISIS

The availability of potent antihypertensive drugs has revolutionized the therapeutic approach to hypertensive crises. The drugs that can be administered parenterally to reduce the blood pressure are nitroprusside, diazoxide, trimethaphan, and hydralazine.

Important considerations in treating patients with hypertensive emergencies are onset and duration of action of the drug. The other consideration should be the knowledge of possible hemodynamic effects of the drug on the patient. The patient's clinical, neurological, and hemodynamic status should be assessed before the beginning of antihypertensive therapy. The choice of the antihypertensive agent depends largely on the hemodynamic status of the patient. Before implementing the antihypertensive therapy, the physician should thoroughly ascertain the clinical status of the patient and possible diagnosis. It should be clearly emphasized that administration of these potent drugs has the potential of causing immediate circulatory compromise, and certainly, these are to be given only to patients with sustained hypertension with target organ dysfunction. It is better to withhold immediate therapy in patients demonstrating lability in blood pressure. Thus, individualization of therapy is of key importance.

A. Diazoxide

Diazoxide is a benzothiadizine derivative that closely resembles the thiazide diuretics but is different pharmacologically. When given intravenously, it has a direct relaxant effect on the vascular smooth muscle, causing a rapid fall in arterial blood pressure. The hypotensive effect of diazoxide is associated with striking increases in heart rate and cardiac output.

1. Clinical Use

Intravenous administration of diazoxide produces a rapid fall in blood pressure within 1 min, and the maximum effect is achieved within 2 to 5 min. The hypotensive effect of a single injection of diazoxide is maintained for 3 to 15 hr (Fig. 1), but if there is no effect from the first injection, an additional dose can be given within 30 min. Traditionally, the recommended dose of diazoxide is 300 mg or 5 mg/kg given as a rapid intravenous injection. To be maximally effective, the dose should be injected rapidly, between 10 and 30 sec; rapid injection is necessary to overcome the protein-binding effect of

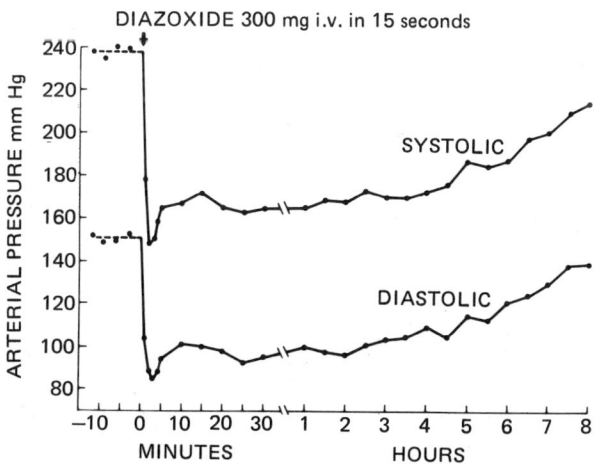

Figure 1. The usual response to 300 mg diazoxide. (From Koch-Weser J: Diazoxide. *N Engl J Med* 294:1271, 1976. Reproduced with permission.)

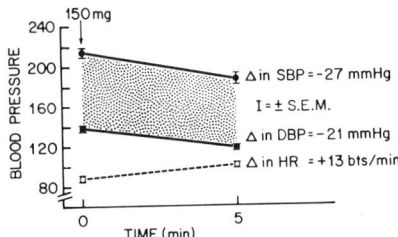

Figure 2. Blood pressure response to the initial injection of 150 mg diazoxide. Additional doses may be required every 5–10 min to reach the desired goal in some patients. (From Ram CVS, Kaplan, NM: Individual titration of diazoxide dosage in the treatment of severe hypertension. *Am J Cardiol* 43:627, 1979. Reproduced with permission.)

diazoxide. The injection should always be made into a stable intravenous line; since diazoxide is highly alkaline (pH 11.6), extravasation can cause severe local pain and cellulitis. Some recent studies indicate that diazoxide can be given by slow intravenous infusion, but further studies are needed before concluding that diazoxide infusions are effective. Injection of a relatively large single dose makes no allowance for variation in response and commits the physician to whatever degree of hypotensive effect may ensue. Severe hypotension with resultant myocardial ischemia and cerebrovascular insufficiency have been reported with the standard 300-mg dose of diazoxide.

We have evaluated the effectiveness of smaller dose bolus injections of diazoxide for the treatment of severe hypertension, reasoning that "minibolus" injections of diazoxide, if effective, would reduce the dangers of drastic and precipitous reduction in blood pressure. Diazoxide was administered in the small boluses of 150 mg every 5 min until the desired goal was reached. Such individual titration of the dose was highly effective (Fig. 2), and no major adverse effects were seen.

2. Disadvantages of Diazoxide

The most common side effects reported with diazoxide include nausea, vomiting, abdominal discomfort, sodium and water retention, and a sensation of warmth along the vein. More severe pain is noted when extravasation occurs. The other major side effect is an exaggerated hypotensive effect. The various side effects of diazoxide are listed in Table XIV. It is better to avoid diazoxide in patients who are or have recently been on other antihypertensive drugs.

B. Nitroprusside

Sodium nitroprusside is one of the most potent blood pressure-lowering drugs and possesses the property of rapid onset and offset of action. The fears of cyanide intoxication delayed its acceptance for clinical use.

The hypotensive response occurs within seconds after infusion is started and is dissipated almost as rapidly when the infusion is discontinued. The

Table XIV. Indications and Contraindications
for Diazoxide

Indications
    Accelerated or malignant hypertension
    Hypertensive encephalopathy
    Eclampsia (caution: inhibitory effect on labor)

Adverse effects
    Excessive response, hypertension
    Hyperglycemia with repeated injections
    Hyperuricemia
    Retention of sodium
    Elevated fatty acid levels
    Arrest of labor

Absolute contraindications
    Patients with acute myocardial infarction
    Acute dissection of the aorta

actions of nitroprusside are almost exclusively confined to the vascular smooth muscle, where it relaxes both the arteries and the veins. During nitroprusside administration, systemic arterial and venous pressures are reduced along with the systemic and pulmonary vascular resistance.

The immediate metabolic product of nitroprusside is cyanide which is probably liberated by the direct combination of nitroprusside with the sulfhydryl groups in the red cells and the tissues. The circulating cyanide is rapidly converted in the liver to thiocyanate (by the enzyme "rhodanase" or "transsulfarase"), which is removed almost exclusively by the kidney with a half-life of approximately 1 week.

1. Method of Administration

Sodium nitroprusside is supplied in 50-mg vials of dry powder and is usually reconstituted with 2 to 5 cc of 5% dextrose in water which yields an amber-colored solution. The 50 mg thus reconstituted is then added to 500 or 1000 cc of dextrose in water. A more concentrated solution can be made by adding 50 mg of nitroprusside to only 250 cc of dextrose of water for patients in whom fluid restriction is necessary. No diluent other than dextrose and water should be used, and no other drugs should be added to the nitroprusside solution. Since nitroprusside is light sensitive, the solution may acquire a darker tint if exposed to light. Because of its rapid onset of action and potency, nitroprusside infusion must be closely and accurately monitored, and whenever possible, this should be done by means of an infusion pump or a microdrop regulator. It is also strongly suggested that intraarterial blood pressure be monitored during nitroprusside infusion to safeguard the patient. To insure maximal benefit from nitroprusside, the drug should be titrated to effective doses as quickly as possible, but with due caution. Perhaps a safe initial dose is 0.5 μg/kg per min, and this can be increased every 5 min until the desired blood pressure level is obtained.

2. Advantages and Disadvantages

The major advantages of sodium nitroprusside are (1) rapid onset of action, (2) potency, (3) short duration of action, and (4) smooth regulation of blood pressure.

Hypotension can be rapidly reversed and, of course, can be prevented by careful monitoring and adjustments in the dosage. Thiocyanate toxicity (Table XV) is a potential problem in patients receiving nitroprusside for prolonged periods, especially in those with renal insufficiency. In such instances, plasma thiocyanate levels should be periodically monitored, and the treatment should be interrupted when the thiocyanate level is close to 10 mg/dl. The clinical manifestations of thiocyanate toxicity are anorexia, headache, disorientation, and sometimes psychotic behavior. Since cyanide is readily metabolized to thiocyanate, cyanide toxicity is not a significant problem with nitroprusside.

It has been shown that prophylactic infusion of hydroxycobalamin (vitamin B_{12}) decreases the RBC cyanide concentration during nitroprusside infusion. The rationale is that cyanide combines with hydroxycobalamin to form cyanocobalamin which is then excreted by the renal route. Whether this approach will find a useful role in the application of nitroprusside therapy remains to be seen.

C. Trimethaphan

Trimethaphan camsylate is a ganglion-blocking agent useful in the emergency treatment of hypertension. Trimethaphan competitively inhibits the action of acetylcholine in the postganglionic nerve terminals and prevents postsynaptic depolarization by stabilizing the membrane. The hypotensive effect of trimethaphan is accompanied by a reduction in the cardiac index, left ventricular ejection rate, and cardiac output. Trimethaphan should be administered as a continuous intravenous drip similarly to sodium nitroprusside. Constant monitoring is necessary, preferably in the intensive care unit. The usual starting dose of the drug should be about 1 mg/min and titrated to obtain the desired blood pressure level. The hypotensive effect is immediate and returns to pretreatment levels once the infusion is stopped

Table XV. Adverse Effects of Nitroprusside

Hypotension
Thiocyanate toxicity (mainly in renal failure)
Cyanide toxicity (extremely uncommon)

Table XVI. Advantages and Disadvantages of Trimethaphan

Advantages of trimethaphan
  Rapid onset and offset of action
  Smooth blood pressure control can be maintained with careful titration of the dose
  Brief duration of action
  Favorable effects on the myocardium: decrease in cardiac index and left ventricular
    ejection rate; this effect makes it an agent of choice in acute aortic dissection
    where the reduction in the rate of myocardial contractility and left ventricular
    wall tension are desirable in order to arrest the progression of the dissection

Disadvantages of trimethaphan
  Paralytic ileus
  Urinary retention
  Mydriasis
  ? Tachyphylaxis

(Table XVI). Prolonged infusion of trimethaphan causes tachyphylaxis because of intravascular volume expansion which can be partially overcome by effective diuretics. Table XVII compares the hemodynamic effects of trimethaphan with those of nitroprusside and diazoxide.

D. Phentolamine

Phentolamine, an α-receptor-blocking agent, is specifically indicated for treating hypertensive crises associated with increased circulating catecholamines, namely, pheochromocytoma crisis, certain cases of clonidine withdrawal syndrome, and crises resulting from MAO inhibitor and drug–food interaction. This drug is not effective in treating hypertensive crises from other causes. The hypotensive effect of a single intravenous bolus injection is short-lived and lasts less than 15 min. It is perhaps preferable to use sodium nitroprusside infusion instead of phentolamine infusion because the former drug is effective in treating any type of severe hypertension and is somewhat easier to handle than phentolamine.

All of the above agents have been successfully used in the treatment of hypertensive emergencies, and drugs such as minoxidil and captopril (Table

Table XVII. Hemodynamic Effects of Sodium Nitroprusside, Trimethaphan, and Diazoxide

	Sodium nitroprusside	Trimethaphan	Diazoxide
Mean arterial blood pressure	↓	↓	↓
Heart rate	↑	↑	↑
Cardiac index	↓	↓	↑
Total peripheral resistance	↓	↓	↓
Left ventricular ejection rate	↓	↓	↑

Table XVIII. Recent Advances
in the Treatment of Hypertensive
Emergencies

Captopril
Prazosin
Labetalol
Minoxidil
Oral clonidine loading

XVIII) are of special interest because of their potency and ease of administration. The details of using these agents are discussed in Chapter 13. Experience with these orally effective drugs is not extensive enough to give general guidelines, and interested readers should review pertinent publications.

E. Other Agents

Hydralazine hydrochloride has been successfully employed in the treatment of severe hypertension. Intramuscular or intravenous administration of hydralazine results in an unpredictable but definite fall in blood pressure. In the treatment of hypertensive emergencies, the initial dose should be 10 to 20 mg. The onset of the hypotensive effect occurs within 10 to 30 min and duration of action ranges from 3 to 9 hr. The dose and the frequency of administration necessary to control the blood pressure are highly variable. The delayed onset and unpredictable degree of hypotensive effect present difficulties in titration. Nevertheless, hydralazine has been, and continues to be, successfully employed in the treatment of severe hypertension, especially eclampsia. The sodium and water retention that occurs with the use of this direct vasodilator can be overcome by the use of a diuretic, and the reflex increases in the cardiac output and heart rate can be minimized by the administration of a β-adrenergic blocking agent.

F. Transition to Oral Therapy

Oral antihypertensive agents should be administered as soon as the patient is able to take them but only after the patient's presenting manifestations have either cleared or been stabilized. Institution of oral antihypertensive agents at the earliest possible time is necessary to avoid the inconvenience of parenteral injections after the hypertension has been controlled. In most patients, this is done by the administration of a diuretic and an adrenergic blocker with or without a vasodilator such as hydralazine. In patients recovering from acute cerebrovascular accident or hypertensive encephalopathy, one should not use centrally acting agents such as methyldopa or clonidine because of their sedative effects. One of the common errors in managing hypertensive crisis is to prematurely introduce the oral drugs, which should be given gradually rather than substituted abruptly for potent intravenous medications. Another common error is the failure to monitor the standing blood pressure in a convalescing patient who has been receiving potent antihypertensive agents in the supine position. This point should be emphasized, and whenever possible, standing blood pressure should also be taken during the transition to oral therapy so that supine normotension does not transform into postural hypotension.

X. GENERAL APPROACH TO THE MANAGEMENT AND CONCLUSIONS

The most important consideration in the treatment of hypertensive emergencies is to assess the patient's clinical state and ascertain whether the patient's condition truly warrants emergency management with parenteral agents or only further intensification of his previous therapy. Once the diagnosis of a hypertensive crisis is made, the management should ideally be carried out in an intensive care unit with continuous monitoring of the blood pressure, urine volume, and cardiac rhythm.

The level to which the blood pressure should be lowered varies with the type of hypertensive crisis and should be strictly individualized; there is no predestined arbitrary level that will be the goal of therapy. The complications of therapy, hypotension and ischemic brain damage, have occurred in patients who were given multiple potent antihypertensive drugs in large doses without adequate hemodynamic monitoring. Such catastrophes can and should be avoided by gentle lowering of blood pressure and individualization of therapy. Conditions such as hypertensive encephalopathy and acute aortic dissection warrant blood pressure reduction in a matter of "minutes to hours," whereas in accelerated and malignant hypertension, the blood pressure reduction is usually achieved in "days." While hypertensive emergencies are treated, cardiac, renal, and neurological status of the patient should be closely monitored in order to detect any possible effects of underperfusion to these vital organs. Although effective and rapid control of hypertension is sometimes accompanied by rises in BUN and creatinine, these are usually temporary, but careful reassessment is indicated.

The relatively asymptomatic patient who might present with severe hypertension, for example with a diastolic blood pressure of 130–140 mm Hg, should not be treated with parenteral drugs; these patients should be assessed on an individual basis, and the usual course would be to intensify or alter the previous antihypertensive therapy.

The therapy of hypertensive crisis does not end with the normalization of blood pressure, but the physician should probe into possible factor(s) that might have contributed to the precipitous elevation of the blood pressure, including:

1. Reasons for cessation of drug therapy.
2. Onset and/or progression of renal artery stenosis.
3. Inadequate antihypertensive therapy.

Physicians should inquire into the reasons for noncompliance with prior antihypertensive therapy and take steps to correct the precipitating event so that recurrence of the crisis can be avoided. For example, if an antihypertensive medication has caused significant side effects that have interfered with the patient's function, mental or physical, the choice of antihypertensive therapy should be one that will be more acceptable to the patient.

A recent study documents a high incidence of renal artery stenosis in patients presenting with severe hypertension. Thus, it seems prudent that in patients who present with acute onset of hypertension and rapid deterioration of blood pressure control, apart from treating the hypertensive crisis, one should look into the possibility of an underlying etiology.

True hypertensive crises are uncommon, and we should not overreact to elevated blood pressures that do not constitute emergencies. The conditions described here comprise complex clinical problems. The term "hypertensive crisis" implies an elevation of blood pressure severe enough to cause dysfunction of vital organs if the blood pressure is not reduced immediately. In some cases, it is not the absolute level of the blood pressure but the rapidity of rise in blood pressure that determines the gravity of the situation. There are some conditions that are categorized as hypertensive emergencies not because of the height of the blood pressure but because coexisting complications make even moderate hypertension dangerous.

Potent antihypertensive drugs are available for rapid reduction of blood pressure. Before using these drugs, the physician should assess the neurological and hemodynamic status of the patient as well as the possible hemodynamic effects of the drugs on the patient. Basic understanding of the mechanism of action and the possible adverse effects is vital to the proper application of parenteral antihypertensive agents. Familiarity with the natural history, prognosis, pathophysiology, and hemodynamic determinants of hypertensive emergencies is invaluable in the rational approach to hypertensive crises.

SUGGESTED READINGS

AMA Committee on Hypertension: The treatment of malignant hypertension and hypertensive emergencies. *JAMA* 228:1673–1679, 1974.

Bhatia SK, Frohlich ED: Hemodynamic comparison of agents useful in hypertensive emergencies. *Am Heart J* 85:367–373, 1973.

Bohle A, Grund KE, Helmchen U, et al: Primary malignant nephrosclerosis. *Clin Sci Mol Med* 51:23S–25S, 1976.

Byrom FB: The evolution of acute hypertensive arterial disease. *Prog Cardiovasc Dis* 17:31–37, 1974.

Cohn JN, Burke LP: Nitroprusside. *Ann Intern Med* 91:752–757, 1979.

Davidov ME, Mroczek WJ, Gavrilovich L, et al: Long-term follow-up of aggressive medical therapy of accelerated hypertension with azotemia. *Angiology* 26:396–407, 1975.

Davis BA, Crook JE, Vestal RE, et al: Prevalence of renovascular hypertension in patients with grade III or IV hypertensive retinopathy. *N Engl J Med* 301:1273–1276, 1979.

Fox KM, Tomlinson IW, Portal RW, et al: Prognostic significance of systolic hypertension after acute myocardial infarction. *Br Med J* 3:128–130, 1974.

Goldby FS, Beilin LJ: How an acute rise in arterial pressure damages arterioles. Electron microscopic changes during angiotensin infusion. *Cardiovasc Res* 6:569–584, 1972.

Jellinek EM, Pointer M, Prineas J, et al: Hypertensive encephalopathy with cortical disorders of vision. *Q J Med* 33:239–256, 1967.

Keith NM, Wagner HP, Barker MW: Some different types of essential hypertension. Their course and prognosis. *Am J Med Sci* 197:332–343, 1939.

Keith TA III: Hypertension crisis; recognition and management. *JAMA* 237:1570–1577, 1977.

Koch-Weser J: Hypertensive emergencies. *N Engl J Med* 290:211, 1974.

Kanada SA, et al: Angina-like syndrome with diazoxide therapy for hypertensive crisis. *Ann Intern Med* 84:696, 1976.

Luft FC, Bloch R, Szwed JJ, et al: Minoxidil treatment of malignant hypertension: Recovery of renal function. *JAMA* 240:1985, 1978.

McDonald WJ, et al: Intravenous diazoxide therapy in hypertensive crisis. *Am J Cardiol* 40:409, 1977.

Meyer JS, Bauer RB: Medical treatment of spontaneous intracerebral hemorrhage by the use of hypotensive agents. *Neurology* 12:36, 1962.

Mills SE, Teja K, Crosby IK, et al: Aortic dissection: Surgical and nonsurgical treatments compared. *Am J Surg* 137:240, 1979.

Mohler ER, Fries ED: 5-Year survival of patients with malignant hypertension treated with antihypertensive agents. *Am Heart J* 60:329, 1960.

Palmer RF, Lasseter KC: Sodium nitroprusside. *N Engl J Med* 292:294, 1975.

Palmer RF, Lasseter KC: Nitroprusside and aortic dissecting aneurysms. *N Engl J Med* 294:1403, 1976.

Ram CVS: Hypertensive encephalopathy—recognition and management. *Arch Intern Med* 138:1851, 1978.

Ram CVS, Kaplan NM: Individual titration of diazoxide dosage in the treatment of severe hypertension. *Am J Cardiol* 43:627, 1979.

Shell WE, Sobel BE: Protection of jeopardized ischemic myocardium by reduction of ventricular afterload. *N Engl J Med* 291:481, 1974.

Slater E, DeSanchs RW: Dissection of the aorta. *Med Clin North Am* 63:151, 1979.

Wheat MW: Treatment of dissecting aneurysms of the aorta: Current status. *Prog Cardiovasc Dis* 16:87, 1973.

Whisnant JP: Medical therapy for intracerebral hemorrhage, in Toole JF, Siekert RG, Whisnant JP, et al (eds): *Cerebral Vascular Diseases.* New York, Grune & Stratton, 1968, p 167–178.

Wood BC, Sharma BN, Crouch TT: Oral minoxidil in the treatment of hypertensive crisis. *JAMA* 241:163, 1979.

15

Hypertension and Renal Disease during Pregnancy

LINDA L. FRANCISCO and THOMAS F. FERRIS

I. PHYSIOLOGICAL CHANGES IN PREGNANCY

The systemic hemodynamic and renal vascular changes that occur in pregnancy lead to striking alterations in function of the kidneys during gestation. It is necessary to understand these normal physiological alterations before an attempt is made to interpret data from pregnant patients with known or suspected hypertension and/or renal disease.

A. Blood Volume and Arterial Pressure

Pregnancy is associated with an approximately 50% increase in blood volume, with a rise in both plasma volume and red cell mass, beginning in the first trimester. The greater increase in plasma volume is responsible for the hemodilution and physiological anemia of pregnancy. Cardiac output also increases in the first trimester and reaches a maximum of 30–50% above the nonpregnant level at approximately the 24th week of gestation. This increase in cardiac output occurs without a rise in arterial blood pressure, and actually, blood pressure falls during pregnancy (approximately 10–15 mm Hg), so that a striking reduction in total peripheral resistance occurs.

LINDA L. FRANCISCO and THOMAS F. FERRIS • Department of Internal Medicine, University of Minnesota, Minneapolis, Minnesota 55455.

B. Humoral Alterations

Accompanying the blood volume expansion in pregnancy is an extraordinary increase in renin and aldosterone secretion. This increase in plasma renin and aldosterone occurs in the first trimester. In response to the rise in plasma renin, plasma angiotensin II reaches 78 ± 24 pg/ml compared with the 5 to 35 pg/ml found in nonpregnant women. It has been found that, at least in the pregnant rabbit, the elevated plasma angiotensin is physiologically important in maintaining arterial blood pressure, since angiotensin blockade results in hypotension. It appears that vasodilatation and reduced peripheral vascular resistance are the most likely causes for the increase in renin secretion during pregnancy. The cause of the vasodilation, on the other hand, is not certain. It is interesting in this regard, however, that pregnant women have elevated plasma prostaglandin E_2 (PGE_2) and 6-keto-$PGF_{1\alpha}$ (the breakdown product of PGI_2) concentrations. These vasodilators may be contributing to the systemic vasodilatation and fall in peripheral vascular resistance that is observed in pregnancy. In addition to alterations in the renin–angiotensin–aldosterone and prostaglandin systems, urinary kallirein has also been found to be elevated in pregnancy. Like renin, it increases in the first trimester of pregnancy and remains elevated throughout gestation. Since urinary kallikrein is increased both by intrarenal angiotensin and prostaglandin E infusions, the elevated excretion might be caused by the increased plasma concentration of both in pregnancy.

C. Renal Blood Flow

The 30–50% increase in renal blood flow during pregnancy is in part caused by the increased cardiac output and blood volume. However, blood flow to all organs does not uniformly increase; for example, no increase in cerebral or hepatic flow has been detected in pregnancy. Since blood pressure is unchanged, there must be a selective decrease in renal vascular resistance to account for this marked rise in blood flow. The etiology of this fall in renal vascular resistance is not clear, but it is known that PGE_2 and PGI_2 are potent renal vasodilators, and with the high levels that exist in pregnancy, renal synthesis of both could lead to the fall in resistance in the renal vascular bed. It is also known that human growth hormone increases renal blood flow by extracellular fluid volume expansion and decreased renal resistance. Although growth hormone levels are normal during pregnancy, human somatomammotropin, which is immunologically and chemically similar to human growth hormone, is present as early as the sixth week of gestation. Whether or not somatomammotropin has effects similar to those of growth hormone in causing renal vasodilatation and increased renal blood flow is unknown, but increases in somatomammotropin seen with hydatidiform mole and choriocarcinoma have not been reported to result in increased renal blood flow.

D. Glomerular Filtration Rate

An increase in glomerular filtration rate (GFR) occurs as early as the second month of pregnancy, accompanying the increase in renal blood flow. This increase is reflected in the mean blood urea nitrogen (BUN) (8.7 ± 1.5 mg/dl) and serum creatinine (0.46 ± 0.6 mg/dl) found in pregnancy. The increases in GFR and renal plasma flow remain proportional until late in pregnancy, when a disproportionate increase in glomerular filtration occurs. In late pregnancy, arterial blood pressure and angiotensin sensitivity increase slightly, and thus, efferent arteriolar resistance may increase. There is also a fall in plasma oncotic pressure in late pregnancy which could increase glomerular filtration rate and filtration fraction.

E. Renal Tubular Function

1. Sodium Reabsorption

In spite of an extraordinary increase in filtered sodium during pregnancy, there is no evidence that pregnant women do not retain sodium normally. Sodium balance is attained in third-trimester pregnant women on a 10-mEq sodium intake as readily as in nonpregnant women. Plasma aldosterone, although higher in pregnant women, is probably not the major factor in this capacity to reabsorb sodium, since pregnant women with Addison's disease also maintain sodium balance without increasing mineralocorticoid dose. There are undoubtedly other factors, hormonal or physiological, that occur in the pregnant woman to maintain sodium balance.

2. Glucose and Amino Acid Transport

Glomerular tubular balance, so effective in preventing sodium loss during pregnancy, is not as efficient in glucose and amino acid resorption. Pregnancy is frequently (in 5 to 40%) associated with glucosuria which results in part from the inability of the proximal tubules to increase glucose resorption in parallel with filtration. In addition to glucosuria, aminoaciduria develops during pregnancy with corresponding reductions in the plasma amino acid levels. In the case of histidine, the percentage of filtered amino acid reabsorbed is decreased. This increased excretion of the nutrients also makes the gravid urine more susceptible to infection.

3. Urate Clearance

There is an increase in urate clearance in normal pregnancy resulting in a mean serum urate level of 3.0 ± 0.17 mg/dl in contrast to values in nonpregnant women of 4.2 ± 1.2 mg/dl. The increase in urate clearance may reflect the rise in renal plasma flow, increasing delivery of urate to its secretory site.

F. Acid–Base Balance in Pregnancy

Pregnancy is associated with a compensated respiratory alkalosis. The alkalosis is thought to result from the effect of elevated progesterone on centrally mediated hyperventilation so that the arterial P_{CO_2} decreases from a normal of 40 mm Hg in nonpregnant women to 30 mm Hg during gestation. Pregnant women are therefore more prone to develop severe acidosis because of the lowered bicarbonate induced by the respiratory alkalosis. Mean plasma bicarbonate in pregnancy is approximately 18 to 20 mEq/liter.

Ammonium chloride loading in a pregnant woman has demonstrated normal excretion of both titratable acid and ammonium following an acid load.

G. Urinary Concentration and Dilution in Pregnancy

Pregnant women are capable of attaining normal, maximal, and minimal urinary osmolality.

H. Serum Tonicity during Pregnancy

Serum sodium falls approximately 5 mEq/liter during late pregnancy with a fall in serum tonicity of approximately 10 mOsm/kg of water. It is suggested that part of the explanation for this fall in serum tonicity is an increase in ADH release and a resetting of the osmostat. In addition, there is increased secretion of the renin–angiotensin system in pregnancy, and stimulation by angiotensin of the thirst center could lead to a subsequent increase in water intake and dilution of the serum sodium in the face of a reset osmostat.

II. ANATOMIC CHANGES OF THE URINARY TRACT

There are multiple anatomic changes of the urinary tract that occur during pregnancy that need to be understood in order to interpret normal versus abnormal anatomic configuration during pregnancy.

From early pregnancy through the puerperium, the renal collecting structures are dilated and produce the so-called physiological hydronephrosis of pregnancy. The etiology of the anatomic changes is hormonal, since they have been reproduced in both nonpregnant animals and men following estrogen and progesterone therapy. This dilatation of the renal collecting system during pregnancy clears within 2 weeks of delivery in 60% of patients and within 12 weeks after delivery in essentially all patients. The right ureter tends to dilate more than the left with pregnancy and may indicate some element of obstruction from the fetus.

Hypomotility of the ureters with a decrease in frequency and amplitude of peristaltic waves has been reported. The volume of urine contained in the renal pelvis and ureters is greatly increased and may also be a factor in the frequency of urinary tract infections during pregnancy.

In comparisons of pyelographic studies done in the immediate pre-parium, kidney size is more than 1 cm larger than those repeated 6 months post-partum. This enlargement is undoubtedly related to the increase in renal vascular volume and blood flow occurring with pregnancy.

Vesicoureteral reflux has been reported in approximately 3% of pregnant women. There did not, however, appear to be an increased incidence of infection, prematurity, or preeclampsia in women with reflux. This usually resolved within 6 months after delivery.

III. RENAL DISEASE AND PREGNANCY

A. Acute Renal Diseases

1. Acute Glomerulonephritis

Acute glomerulonephritis (AGN) is a rare complication during pregnancy. Case reports of 20 patients have appeared in the literature, and the calculated incidence of the disease is approximately one in 40,000 pregnancies. Fetal loss occurs in most pregnant patients with acute glomerulonephritis, although successful pregnancies have been reported. When spontaneous abortion does not occur with AGN, therapeutic abortion has been advocated. This, however, may not be necessary since there is no evidence that AGN improves in the mother after termination of the pregnancy, and when blood pressure and fluid balance are controlled during pregnancy, a viable fetus can be delivered. At delivery, there is no evidence of renal disease in the babies, possibly indicating that the soluble antigen–antibody complexes causing the glomerulonephritis are too large to cross the placental circulation or that fetal glomeruli do not react similarly to immune complexes.

If superimposed preeclampsia occurs, delivery of the fetus is indicated. This diagnosis is a difficult clinical differentiation in the face of AGN and may only be suspected if hypertension and renal disease rapidly worsen. This is one circumstance in which a renal biopsy in pregnancy is possibly justified therapeutically to differentiate between the two conditions. Each situation must be evaluated individually, with attention directed to the clinical status of the patient, the risk of the abortion, and the patient's own attitude concerning the pregnancy. If AGN occurs early in pregnancy, the attack may resolve and the remainder of the pregnancy be uneventful.

In those women with a previous history of acute glomerulonephritis with complete resolution of the event documented by a negative urinalysis, there is no increased risk associated with pregnancy. Since, however, a normal urine after acute glomerulonephritis has been described in patients in whom renal biopsy had demonstrated persistent activity of the disease, patients with a history of glomerulonephritis should be followed closely during pregnancy so that any change in blood pressure or the appearance of proteinuria is quickly detected.

Focal glomerulonephritis, or Berger's disease, represents a relatively common cause of hematuria and minimal proteinuria in young adults. Pregnancy in women with focal glomerulonephritis does not increase the incidence of preeclampsia.

2. Acute Pyelonephritis

Acute pyelonephritis develops in 20–40% of pregnant women with bacteriuria. Treatment of the bacteriuria becomes of vital importance since it lowers the subsequent incidence of pyelonephritis by about 90%. Therefore, it is important to screen all pregnant women for the presence of asymptomatic bacteriuria and to treat those with significant bacteriuria and/or positive cultures.

There is some disagreement about the treatment of urinary tract infections in the gravida. Some authors believe that the pregnant woman has a hign relapse rate and therefore recommend continuous antibiotic treatment until after delivery. However, approximately 50% of patients have bladder involvement only, and most appear to respond to a simple 8- to 12-day course of therapy. No one therapeutic agent has any advantage over another; sulfonamides are inexpensive; sulfisoxazole, 0.5 g four times a day, will eradicate the bacteriuria in 70–80% of women treated. Follow-up cultures should be obtained, and if there is persistence of bacteriuria, retreatment with another agent is recommended. In the small percentage of women whose bacteriuria is not eradicated with two courses of treatment, underlying renal disease is frequently present. These women should have continuous treatment throughout pregnancy.

If acute pyelonephritis does occur in pregnancy, it requires hospitalization with intravenous hydration and antibiotics appropriate for the organism.

3. Acute Renal Failure

Acute renal failure is one of the most serious complications of pregnancy. Those with acute renal failure can be divided into two groups: (1) those in whom acute renal failure occurs early in pregnancy as a result of septic abortion and (2) those who develop acute renal failure in the last trimester of pregnancy in association with toxemia or an obstetric complication.

In women in whom acute renal failure develops early in pregnancy, infection of the uterus is the most common cause. The incidence of acute renal failure during the first trimester, however, has extraordinarily decreased since the liberalization of abortion laws. *Clostridium welchie* and *Streptococcus pyogenes* are the usual offending organisms when a septic abortion does occur. With clostridial uterine infection, mortality approaches 30%. Emptying the uterus of infected and necrotic debris is essential, and hysterectomy is occasionally necessary. Irreversible renal failure in this group is unusual, and with adequate therapy for renal failure, recovery of function can be expected.

Development of acute renal failure late in pregnancy is usually related to an obstetric complication. The great danger of acute renal failure in late pregnancy is the high incidence of cortical necrosis. This is a rare complication, in the nonpregnant patient, and its occurrence in pregnancy is related to the increased incidence of intravascular coagulation during pregnancy. The diagnosis of cortical necrosis should be considered when oliguria lasts more than 14 to 21 days. A renal biopsy is helpful in establishing the diagnosis.

4. Postpartum Renal Failure

The disease consists of rapid development of renal failure 2 to 10 weeks post-partum, with findings of malignant nephrosclerosis at autopsy. The disease has been termed postpartum hemolytic uremic syndrome, malignant nephrosclerosis in women post-partum, postpartum renal failure with microangiopathic hemolytic anemia, and postpartum hemolytic uremic syndrome. The pathological changes in the kidneys are fibrin deposits in glomeruli and afferent arterioles as well as marked intimal hyperplasia attributed to organization of fibrin deposits in the arcuate and interlobular arteries. Unlike children with hemolytic uremic syndrome in whom a good prognosis is usually assumed, 75% of these adults die or must be placed on long-term hemodialysis because of irreversible renal failure.

Symptoms before the onset of acute renal failure include vomiting, diarrhea, or an influenzalike illness. This is followed by oliguria, hematuria, proteinuria, and severe microangiopathic hemolytic anemia with anisocytosis and schizocytosis. Frequent findings are indirect bilirubinemia, plasma hemoglobinemia, reticulocytosis, and severe thrombocytopenia.

Treatment has not been uniformly helpful in reversing the disease and has consisted of anticoagulation.

Characteristic pathological lesions are thickening of the glomerular capillary wall as a result of endothelial cell swelling and the appearance of a widened, lucent subendothelial space containing mucinous material. Capillary thrombi are seen, and vascular changes in arterioles are consistent with involvement of the intralobular arteries in this syndrome more frequently than in childhood hemolytic uremia.

Other diseases with multisystem involvement occurring during or immediately after pregnancy that might have a common basis, e.g., intravascular coagulation, are acute fatty liver of pregnancy, postpartum myocardiopathy, and postpartum necrosis of the anterior pituitary.

B. Chronic Renal Diseases

The prognosis in pregnant women with chronic renal disease is dependent on whether hypertension or reduction in GFR sufficient to lead to azotemia (BUN > 20 mg/dl) precedes the pregnancy. Since two or more of the usual features of preeclampsia, i.e., proteinuria, hypertension, and edema, are present before pregnancy, the patient must be carefully observed during gestation for changes in blood pressure, BUN, and plasma creatinine and uric acid concentration. Women with renal disease should be seen frequently during pregnancy, and any rise in blood pressure or rapid weight gain must be considered significant. Treatment during pregnancy consists of maintaining normal blood pressure with antihypertensive agents. Diuretics should be used throughout pregnancy in the hypertensive patient. The potential slight extracellular fluid depletion from chronic diuretic therapy poses less risk to fetal and maternal survival than hypertension. Hypertensive women on chronic diuretic therapy retain the sodium necessary for normal fetal growth. There is no evidence that chronic diuretic therapy increases fetal mortality.

1. Chronic Glomerulonephritis

The risk of pregnancy in a woman with chronic glomerulonephritis is primarily the increased incidence of superimposed toxemia. Not only is the incidence higher, but the occurrence of toxemia is earlier, often before the 28th week of gestation. Indeed, the onset of preeclampsia before the 28th week of gestation suggests preexisting renal disease. In addition, if preexisting azotemia is present, the likelihood of a successful pregnancy is further reduced. Therefore, the physician should advise women with azotemia against pregnancy except under exceptional circumstances.

2. Nephrotic Syndrome

In women with the nephrotic syndrome, the risk of pregnancy is similar to that in chronic glomerulonephritis without nephrosis. Birth weight correlates best with serum albumin levels, and severe hypoproteinemia often results in prematurity. Whether nephrotic syndrome is caused by minimal change disease or membranous or membranoproliferative glomerulonephritis, the majority of patients will have a successful outcome of the pregnancy. If, however, the nephrotic syndrome is accompanied by azotemia or hypertension, the chance for a successful pregnancy is less likely. In women with nephrotic syndrome, infection, particularly of the urinary tract, is a frequent problem during pregnancy because of associated hypogammaglobulinemia and, in certain cases, steroid therapy.

A rare form of nephrosis is the "nephrotic syndrome of pregnancy" in which proteinuria develops during pregnancy, disappears after delivery, and recurs with subsequent pregnancies. The possibility of a sensitizing antigen, either a fetal or placental protein, resulting in immune-complex deposits in glomeruli has been postulated, but no immunofluorescent studies of glomeruli in this rare disease have been described.

3. Chronic Interstitial Nephritis

Chronic interstitial nephritis, regardless of the cause, may be associated with hypertension, and the clinical course of pregnancy seems to correlate best with the hypertension and preexisting azotemia.

C. Renal Diseases Associated with Systemic Disease

1. Systemic Lupus Erythematosus

In patients without renal involvement, systemic lupus erythematosus (SLE) can run a variable course during pregnancy. Some SLE patients note an improvement during pregnancy and a postpartum exacerbation of symptoms similar to that reported by patients with rheumatoid arthritis. Diffuse lupus glomerulonephritis has a variable course in pregnancy, but in women whose disease has been quiescent for 6 months prior to conception, the risk of pregnancy worsening the activity of the lupus is approximately one in three. Most women with SLE have live babies, and the prematurity rate is not greatly different from that in a normal population. When worsening of the lupus nephropathy occurs during the pregnancy, it is usually transient, with reversal post-partum. When clinical activity of SLE is present in the 6-month period before pregnancy, clinical manifestations remain unchanged in about half and worsen during pregnancy in the other half. There is little evidence, however, that the lupus nephropathy is permanently worsened by pregnancy. Patients requiring steroids for suppression of the disease activity should be maintained on them throughout pregnancy. There is no evidence of SLE in infants of mothers with exacerbation of their disease during pregnancy; however, transmission of the LE phenomenon can occur.

2. Diabetes Mellitus

The course of diabetic nephropathy during pregnancy is similar to that of other renal diseases, with little or no evidence that the renal disease is worsened specifically by the pregnancy. Although therapeutic abortion has been advocated when diabetic nephropathy precedes pregnancy, studies at the Joslin Clinic have demonstrated that diabetic women can have normal pregnancies with a good chance of fetal survival and no evidence of accelerated deterioration of renal function. However, preeclampsia is approximately three times as frequent in a diabetic population than in a normal population. The cause of this increase is probably related to the underlying vascular disease, renal and uteroplacental, as well as the propensity of the diabetic women to have large babies. The chances for a successful pregnancy appear to diminish with the extent of the diabetic complications. Renal involvement *per se* does not appear to be the factor deciding the outcome of the pregnancy but rather the more global complications of diabetes in an individual patient.

D. Hereditary Renal Diseases

1. Polycystic Renal Disease

Since 41 years of age is the average age for onset of symptoms and signs of polycystic renal disease, women with undiagnosed or asymptomatic polycystic kidney disease are usually past childbearing age when clinical manifestations of the disease appear. In large retrospective studies, no risk posed by pregnancy was demonstrable in women with polycystic kidney disease without hypertension or azotemia. As with other renal diseases, however, when hypertension or azotemia precedes the pregnancy, the incidence of preeclampsia and perinatal mortality are increased. Since polycystic kidney disease is transmitted as an autosomal dominant trait with high penetrance, the incidence of the disease in large families is 50%. Thus, couples may wish to limit family size or to adopt children when they are aware of the presence of the disease in their families. Approximately 20% of patients with polycystic kidney disease have intracranial aneurysms. Conceivably, these might burst during pregnancy and delivery.

E. Renal Calculi

Although ureteral and pelvic dilatation predisposes to stasis and infection, renal calculi are relatively rare during pregnancy. The incidence of nephrolithiasis in pregnancy is approximately one in 1150 women, which is about the same as in nonpregnant women. Although calculi are uncommon, they represent a frequent cause of pain requiring hospitalization for diagnosis and treatment during pregnancy. In one series of women with symptomatic stones, two-thirds required surgical intervention during pregnancy.

The diagnosis of the stone is sometimes difficult during pregnancy. It seems reasonable to perform an intravenous pyelogram on all pregnant women with a history suggestive of stone disease, acute symptoms of infection, and a previous history of a renal calculus or recurrent urinary tract infection during pregnancy. The danger to the fetus is minimal if shielding and image intensification procedures are followed.

F. Hemodialysis during Pregnancy

There have now been several reports of hemodialysis in pregnant women with chronic or acute renal failure. Hypotension and vaginal bleeding have been reported in these women, but other complications appear to be minimal. With the decrease in peripheral vascular resistance, filtration rates need to be carefully monitored in the pregnant woman to prevent severe hypotension. Pregnant women are more prone to develop hypoglycemia, so glucose-containing dialysates have been recommended. Bleeding problems have been avoided with the use of low-dose heparinization with maintenance of the activated clotting time to less than 2 min. The compensated respiratory alkalosis that occurs with pregnancy makes the fall in serum bicarbonate that is seen early in hemodialysis with an acetate dialysate bath more accentuated then in the nonpregnant women. Thus, bicarbonate-containing dialysates should probably be used in pregnancy. One report has noted the removal of progesterone by hemodialysis and questioned whether the presence of premature contractions of labor may be more apt to occur in dialyzed patients because of this progesterone depletion. It has been suggested to administer parenteral progesterone in the pregnant woman on hemodialysis until the onset of labor is desired.

G. Pregnancy following Renal Transplantation

As more renal transplants are being performed, pregnancy in women who have received renal allografts is becoming more common. As with other aspects of transplantation, the outcome of the pregnancy seems to be better when the transplanted kidney comes from a living donor. The majority of the pregnancies succeed, but there are significant maternal and fetal risks, for the most part because of the immunosuppression, e.g., steroid-induced hyperglycemia, hypertension, septicemia, intrauterine growth retardation, congenital anomalies, and prematurity. There are criteria that have been established for recommendation of pregnancy in transplant recipients.

1. Stable renal function for 18–24 months following transplantation.
2. The absence of hypertension and proteinuria.
3. The absence of azotemia.
4. Drug therapy: prednisone $\leq$ 15 mg/day and azathioprine $\leq$ 3 mg/kg per day.
5. No evidence of pelvocalyceal distension on IVP prior to gestation.

IV. DIAGNOSIS OF RENAL DISORDERS DURING PREGNANCY

The diagnosis of renal disease can usually be made by the physician on the basis of the clinical history, physical examination, and urinalysis. Examination of the urine is the single most valuable procedure in the recognition and differential diagnosis of renal disease. It is necessary that the urine be a concentrated, usually first-voided specimen for optimal resolution of proteinuria, cylinduria, hematuria, and pyuria.

A. Proteinuria

Proteinuria is an important sign of renal disease, and significant proteinuria points to changes in glomerular basement membrane permeability to plasma proteins. Protein excretion is abnormal when the total excretion exceeds 150–250 mg/day. The use of paper strips for detection of protein coupled with sulfosalicylic acid tests should detect both albuminuria and other proteinuria. If these are both positive, a 24-hr quantitation should be obtained.

Heavy proteinuria, more than 2 g/day, is caused by renal diseases that primarily affect the glomerulus. These diseases include acute and chronic glomerulonephritis, intercapillary glomerulonephritis, systemic lupus erythematosus, membranous glumerulonephritis, lipoid nephrosis, and renal venous congestion. Moderate proteinuria between 150 mg and 2 g daily is more apt to be present with chronic interstitial nephritis, nephrocalcinosis, and hypercalcemic and hypokalemic nephropathy.

B. Hematuria

Hematuria is so frequently caused by extrarenal bleeding from the genitourinary tract that one must determine if red blood cell casts are present or not. This finding indicates inflammation of and injury to the glomerulus. The causes of hematuria run the gamut of the glomerulonephritides and will not distinguish any of them. It is important that preeclampsia, in which a definite lesion of the glomerulus has been demonstrated, results in proteinuria but no hematuria. If hematuria exists, it usually is indicative of underlying renal disease.

C. Pyuria

Pyuria may be seen in any renal disease but when found in great numbers usually indicates the presence of infection. White blood cells, casts, and pyuria can, however, be present in the absence of documented bacterial infection in response to inflammation of either the glomerulus or interstitium of the kidney. Thus, it is not unusual in acute glomerulonephritis to find leukocytes and leukocyte casts because of the polymorphonuclear inflammation in the glomeruli. If pyuria is present, however, a quantitative urine culture demonstrating greater than 100,000 organisms/ml is necessary to document the presence of infection in cases suspected of having pyelonephritis.

D. Renal Biopsy

There is an increased risk of complication if renal biopsy is performed during pregnancy, particularly in the hypertensive patient. The increased risk is probably related to technical difficulties in performing a biopsy in a pregnant patient, the increase in renal blood flow, and the hypertension which is usually present in the pregnant woman undergoing renal biopsy. Because of these risks, renal biopsy should not be carried out during pregnancy unless the potential gain to the patient's care warrants the risk.

E. Other Laboratory Studies

After a careful urinalysis, base-line studies of renal function in patients with possible renal disease should include a serum creatinine, BUN, and uric acid. In patients with heavy proteinuria, a serum protein and cholesterol should be obtained. The BUN and creatinine must be interpreted in light of the knowledge that it is only after a 60 to 70% reduction in GFR that these levels rise above the "normal" values. When renal disease exists without elevations in BUN or serum creatinine, a 24-hr creatinine clearance is needed to determine GFR. A base-line serum urate determination is important in early pregnancy, since a rise in serum urate points to the development of preeclampsia.

V. HYPERTENSION DURING PREGNANCY

Hypertension occurring during pregnancy can be the result of the pregnancy or simply an indication that blood pressure is often taken for the first time during pregnancy. Although hypertension was previously felt to be an ominous sign regarding the outcome of the pregnancy, the prognosis for a successful pregnancy in a woman with hypertension is virtually similar to that in normotensive women if the blood pressure is maintained normal throughout pregnancy.

A. Essential Hypertension

Essential hypertension accounts for approximately one-third of all cases of hypertension during pregnancy. The history frequently reveals hypertension, diabetes mellitus, and obesity in other family members. Women in whom hypertension develops in the second half of pregnancy but who show no other evidence of toxemia (i.e., edema, proteinuria, hyperuricemia) can be regarded as having latent essential hypertension unmasked by pregnancy, and a high proportion of them remain permanently hypertensive after pregnancy. An intensive work-up of hypertension during pregnancy is unnecessary. Auscultation of the abdomen to determine if a murmur, suggestive of renal artery stenosis, is present and palpation of the femoral arteries to exclude coarctation are indicated.

The retina should be examined for evidence of longstanding hypertension, i.e., increased light reflex, arteriolar narrowing, and arteriovenous nicking. An electrocardiogram to determine the presence of left ventricular hypertrophy may also be used as a guide to the chronicity of the hypertension. The presence of retinal hemorrhages and exudates indicates accelerated hypertension and warrants immediate hospitalization. Base-line serum urate should be obtained, and in hypertensive women without toxemia, it is usually 4 mg/100 ml or less.

1. Complications

Although the prognosis for a successful pregnancy in a woman with essential hypertension is excellent, hypertension increases the risk of obstetric complications such as premature separation of the placenta and abruptio placenta. It also predisposes to the development of toxemia and myocardial infarction. The likelihood of developing toxemia is increased two- to sevenfold if there is underlying essential hypertension, but essential hypertension generally is associated with an uneventful pregnancy if blood pressure is controlled. In studies prior to the availability of antihypertensive medications, it was noted that if blood pressure is below 160/100 mm Hg, the spontaneous abortion rate is no greater than that in normotensive women. Higher values of blood pressure increased fetal mortality. With available antihypertensive therapy, there is no reason for blood pressures higher than 160/100 mm Hg during pregnancy. Pregnant women with hypertension should therefore be treated exactly as they would be if they were not pregnant, maintaining blood pressure as close to normal as possible with the use of antihypertensive agents.

2. Treatment

Because of the proven efficacy of antihypertensive therapy in preventing complications of hypertension, more women on antihypertensive drugs are being followed through pregnancy. Patients with essential hypertension should have their blood pressure maintained below 140/90 with whatever antihypertensive regimen is best suited to them. Table I depicts the antihypertensive drugs that have been used in pregnant women with essential hypertension. Most patients on long-term therapy for essential hypertension

Table I. Antihypertensive Medications in Pregnancy

Chronic essential hypertension	Toxemia
Diuretics	
Thiazide, 1–2 tab q.d.	Thiazide, 1–2 tab q.d. Furosemide (Lasix®), 40 mg PO or IV
Central adrenergic blockers	
Methyldopa (Aldomet®), 0.5–3 g q.d. Clonidine (Catapres®), 0.2–2 mg q.d.	Methyldopa, 0.5–2 g PO q.d. or 0.5 g IV q6h
α-Adrenergic blocker	
Prazosin (Minipres®), 2–20 mg q.d.	Not used
β-Adrenergic blockers	
Propranolol (Inderal®), 20–80 mg b.i.d. Metoprolol (Lopressor®), 100–200 mg b.i.d. Nadolol (Corgard®), 80–300 mg q.d.	Encouraging preliminary studies
Arteriolar dilators	
Hydralazine (Apresoline®), 25–50 mg q.i.d. Minoxidil (Loniten®), 5–40 mg q.d. Nitroprusside, IV	Hydralazine, 25–50 mg q6h PO or 10–40 mg IV q3h Diazoxide, 300 mg IV

will be on a combination of methyldopa and a diuretic or a combination of propranolol, hydralazine, and a diuretic. The drugs should be continued throughout the pregnancy. In some women reduction of the dose and, in a few, elimination of medications may be necessary during the pregnancy because of a reduction in pressure. However, this should be done only with careful monitoring, and the blood pressure should be maintained normal throughout the pregnancy. Diuretics should be continued through the pregnancy, since significant volume depletion does not occur with chronic diuretic administration, and their antihypertensive effect is independent of sustained volume depletion. It has been demonstrated that women on chronic diuretic therapy retain the normal 900 mg of sodium required during pregnancy without difficulty.

Patients with essential hypertension should be seen every 2 to 3 weeks during pregnancy and weekly after the 32nd week. The development of proteinuria or a rise in blood pressure is indication for immediate hospitalization. Although there is no evidence that antihypertensive medication increases urinary estriol excretion, there is evidence it increases perinatal survival. Birth weights in women treated with antihypertensive drugs were similar to controls, and there was no evidence for altered fetal growth in the treated group. The condition of the neonates at birth was also similar. In hypertensive women developing toxemia before the 32nd week, delivery is indicated if urinary estriols are low, since the chance for further fetal growth seems slim. In patients with essential hypertension, ergot preparations are contraindicated; oxytocin, which has little pressor activity, should be used to induce labor.

3. Mortality

The incidence of mortality in pregnant women wth essential hypertension is under 1%. When death occurs, it is usually a result of a sudden rise in blood pressure with consequent cerebral hemorrhage, acute left ventricular failure, or malignant encephalopathy. These complications can now be prevented with antihypertensive agents, and mortality should be virtually eliminated. A woman with hypertension who develops toxemia does not necessarily develop toxemia with subsequent pregnancies. If the toxemia occurred early in pregnancy, subsequent pregnancies are more apt to be associated with toxemia.

Malignant hypertension associated with retinal hemorrhages, exudates, or papilledema developing during the course of pregnancy was an indication for delivery in the past. There was no hope for fetal survival in the era prior to the availability of antihypertensive therapy with malignant hypertension; this may not now be the case.

B. Primary Aldosteronism (Conn's Syndrome)

Women with primary aldosteronism have been followed during a pregnancy, and the hypokalemia, but not hypertension, disappeared during pregnancy, presumably because of the antagonistic effect of the elevated progesterone of pregnancy on the action of aldosterone. Thus, the hypokalemia of primary aldosteronism may be relieved during pregnancy, but hypertension persists.

C. Renal Artery Stenosis

Women with proven renal artery stenosis have undergone pregnancy, and most develop toxemia. Although there is evidence in animals that hypertension induced by renal artery constriction improves during pregnancy, hypertension has been induced in pregnant animals with constriction of the renal artery in late pregnancy. The appropriate course of management would be to maintain blood pressure normal with antihypertensive drugs and evaluate and possibly operate on the patient post-partum. Hypertension caused by renal artery stenosis can be treated medically as readily as other forms of hypertension. Although the angiotensin I-converting enzyme inhibitors are useful in the treatment of renal vascular hypertension, they would seem to be contraindicated in pregnancy because of adverse effects on uterine PGE_2 synthesis and fetal mortality in pregnant rabbits.

D. Coarctation of the Aorta

Coarctation of the aorta is a rare hypertensive complication of pregnancy but may be associated with toxemia. Of ten patients requiring surgical repair of their coarctation during pregnancy, nine had uncomplicated deliveries of living infants. One patient died in her seventh month of pregnancy from an aneurysm of the aorta at the anastomotic site. The major danger to the pregnant woman with an aortic coarctation is rupture of the cystic medial necrosis often present in the aortic wall. Causes for the rupture could include the increase in cardiac output of pregnancy, increase in blood pressure during toxemia, or the strain of labor.

E. Pheochromocytoma

Pheochromocytoma is a potentially lethal form of secondary hypertension. It is an extremely rare cause of hypertension during pregnancy, with only 93 pheochromocytomas during pregnancy having been reported in the English literature. Symptoms of severe headache, profuse sweating, palpitations, nausea and vomiting, blurred vision, vertigo, tremulousness, seizures, and general weakness are frequently present. Physical findings suggestive of hyperthyroidism—tachycardia, lid lag, and fine tremor—should alert the obstetrician to the possibility of a pheochromocytoma. In pregnant women with pheochromocytomas, maternal mortality rate is approximately 50%. The cause of death is usually pulmonary edema, cerebral hemorrhage, and cardiovascular collapse. Once the diagnosis has been established, the tumor should be removed surgically. Concern about the dangers of x-ray in localizing the tumor is inappropriate with this potentially lethal condition.

VI. ANTIHYPERTENSIVE DRUGS

The Food and Drug Administration has developed a system for evaluating the risk to the fetus for all drugs. This will help to resolve the problem that most drugs have received inadequate testing in pregnant animals and that consequently all drugs are stated to be contraindicated in pregnancy in the package insert or in the Physician's Desk Reference. The categories to be used in the future are the following:

1. Category A. Control studies in women of drugs that fail to demonstrate a risk to the fetus in the first trimester (and there is no evidence of a risk in later trimesters), and the possibility of fetal harm appears remote.
2. Category B. Either animal reproduction studies have not demonstrated a fetal risk but there are no controlled studies in pregnant

women, or animal reproduction studies have shown an adverse effect (other than a decrease in fertility) that was not confirmed in controlled studies in women in the first trimester (and there is no evidence of a risk in later trimesters).

3. Category C. Either studies in animals have revealed adverse effects on the fetus (teratogenic or embryocidal effects or others) and there are no controlled studies in women, or studies in women and animals are not available. Drugs should be given only if the potential benefit justifies the potential risk to the fetus.

4. Category D. There is positive evidence of human fetal risk, but the benefits from use in pregnant women may be acceptable despite the risk (e.g., if the drug is needed in a life-threatening situation or for a serious disease for which safer drugs cannot be used or are ineffective). There will be an appropriate statement in the "warnings" section of the labeling.

5. Category X. Studies in animals or human beings have demonstrated fetal abnormalities, or there is evidence of fetal risk based on human experience, or both, and the risk of the use of the drug in pregnant women clearly outweighs any possible benefit. The drug is contraindicated in women who are or may become pregnant. There will be an appropriate statement in the "contraindications" section of the labeling.

Although evaluations have not yet been provided for antihypertensive drugs, it would seem from the information available that most will be in the B–C category. As with the use of any drug, a risk–benefit analysis must be made that, in the case of antihypertensive drugs, is clearly in favor of their use in the pregnant woman.

A. Diuretics

Table I depicts the various pharmacological categories of drugs that are used in the treatment of hypertension during pregnancy. Some have been used in the acute hypertension of toxemia whereas others have been used primarily in the pregnant woman with chronic essential hypertension. All have had wide experience in nonpregnant subjects. There are a large number of thiazide preparations, all with essentially the same potency per tablet. They are the first step in the treatment of all hypertensive patients. They not only have intrinsic antihypertensive properties but prevent the refractoriness that develops with the use of other antihypertensive drugs which usually cause salt retention.

Approximately 10% of patients receiving one thiazide daily develop serum potassium below 3.5 mEq/liter, but since the potassium wasting with diuretic therapy is dependent on aldosterone secretion, hypokalemia below 3.5 mEq/liter will usually suppress aldosterone secretion, and the potassium wasting ceases. Chlorthalidone (Hygroton®) is a long-acting thiazide preparation that causes hypokalemia more often than shorter acting preparations such as chlorothiazide (Diuril®) or hydrochlorothiazide (Hydrodiuril®). Cardiac arrhythmias in the fetus have been described with maternal hypokalemia, but potassium depletion in pregnancy can be prevented by either the administration of 40 to 60 mEq KCl daily or by adding a potassium-sparing diuretic, i.e., triamterene, to the thiazide. Diazide®, the most commonly used diuretic in the treatment of hypertension, represents such a combination of a thiazide and triamterene.

Diuretics have been used throughout pregnancy in patients with essential hypertension, and there is no evidence that they increase fetal mortality, whereas there is an abundance of evidence that uncontrolled hypertension results in increased fetal and maternal mortality.

With acute toxemia, thiazides can be given intravenously, but the more potent diuretic furosemide should be used when an intravenous use of a diuretic is needed. Furosemide in a dose of 40 mg intravenously every 4 hr can be given for treatment of severe toxemia, particularly when a vasodilating agent is also used. Vasodilators cause salt retention, and their antihypertensive effects are potentiated by concomitant use of a diuretic, Furosemide has been demonstrated to reduce left ventricular filling pressure prior to the natriuresis by increasing venous capacitance and diminishing venous return. This effect makes the drug particularly helpful in toxemic patients with congestive heart failure. Although cardiac output and extracellular volume fall with initiation of diuretic therapy, both return to normal during chronic diuretic administration, but a sustained reduction in peripheral resistance occurs. The mechanism of the reduction in peripheral resistance with diuretic therapy is not understood. It has been suggested that the dilatation of arterioles occurs as a result of altered concentration of sodium and calcium in vessel walls. The fact that diazoxide, chemically similar to the thiazides, is a potent peripheral vasodilator but not a diuretic suggests a similar action for thiazides independent of natriuresis.

A disadvantage in the use of a diuretic in pregnancy is that an elevation in uric acid may occur and obscure the best chemical marker of the development of toxemia. However, urate seldom rises above 6.5 mg/100 ml with diuretics alone, and higher levels usually indicate toxemia. Serial determination of plasma urate throughout pregnancy in hypertensive women taking a diuretic throughout pregnancy will usually show a rise if toxemia supervenes.

B. Adrenergic Blocking Drugs

Although the sympathetic depleting agents reserpine and guanethidine were used in the past for the treatment of essential hypertension, they have been replaced by drugs with fewer side effects. Two major drugs that act as adrenergic blockers in the central nervous system are methyldopa

(Aldomet®) and clonidine (Catapres®). Methyldopa acts primarily by the buildup within the central nervous system of a false neurotransmitter, α-methylnorepinephrine. Its antihypertensive effect is caused by a decrease in peripheral resistance with little change in cardiac output or pulse. Clonidine stimulates central α-adrenergic receptors, thereby decreasing sympathetic outflow from the CNS and reducing peripheral resistance.

Methyldopa may be utilized to lower blood pressure acutely: 500 mg is given intravenously, and repeated at 6-hr intervals. Hypertension usually responds within 6 to 8 hr, and after 24–48 hr of parenteral therapy, oral methyldopa in equivalent doses may be substituted. Methyldopa depletes the brain of biogenic amines which accounts for the somnolence and depression that occur in some patients. The incidence of a positive Coomb's test in patients on methyldopa averages between 10 and 20%, but only rarely does a hemolytic anemia occur. This reaction is not of concern when methyldopa is used for the acute treatment of toxemia. Occasionally, fever associated with eosinophilia occurs during initiation of therapy, and abnormalities of liver function such as elevated alkaline phosphatase, SGOT, and SGPT have been reported. The dose varies from 250 mg to 1 g t.i.d. Fluid retention occurs as with most antihypertensive agents.

The most common side effects of clonidine are sedation and a dry mouth, as well as severe hypertension which may follow abrupt withdrawal of the drug. Clonidine reduces cardiac output and pulse with a decrease in peripheral resistance. It is also used with a diuretic to prevent fluid retention. Both drugs have been used in pregnancy, and follow-up studies in the children born of mothers taking methyldopa revealed normal mental and physical development. Interestingly and perhaps coincidentally, the children born of mothers taking methyldopa throughout pregnancy scored consistently higher than untreated controls on five main indices of intellectual and motor development.

C. α- and β-Adrenergic Blockers

Prazosin (Minipres®) acts as a postsynapatic α-adrenergic blocking agent. Its hemodynamic effects cause a fall in peripheral resistance with no change in cardiac output. The drug is equally potent to methyldopa, and it can be combined with a β-adrenergic blocking drug such as propranolol to provide a further reduction in blood pressure by lowering cardiac output. The drug can cause severe postural hypotension after the first dose, but this effect is usually a transient phenomenon. No studies of this drug during pregnancy have been reported, but in a woman with well-controlled hypertension on prazosin, there would appear to be no theoretical reason to stop the drug.

Propranolol is a β-adrenergic blocking drug that lowers blood pressure primarily by blocking cardiac β receptors with a consequent fall in cardiac output and pulse rate. Other actions that might play a role in its antihypertensive effect include inhibition of renin release from the kidney and blockade of β-adrenergic receptors in the central nervous system with production of bradycardia and peripheral vasodilatation. Although peripheral β-adrenergic blockade theoretically could cause peripheral vasoconstriction with Raynaud's phenomenon by unopposed α-receptor activity, this effect is not usually seen because of the sparcity of peripheral β-adrenergic receptors. The drug is always combined with a diuretic and usually with a vasodilator. All β blockers are contraindicated in the face of asthma or obstructive lung disease, but significant side effects have proven to be less of a problem than those of the central adrenergic blockers. Fatigue, depression, cold extremities, and insomnia rarely occur.

The use of β-adrenergic blocking agents during pregnancy is controversial. Adverse effects on the fetus such as intrauterine growth retardation, neonatal bradycardia, and hypoglycemia, have been reported. Since β blockers cross the placenta and reduce fetal heart rate and cardiac output in the pregnant ewe, there has been fear that the β-adrenergic blockage in the fetus would mask signs of fetal distress. Also since β-adrenergic drugs such as isoproteronol suppress myometrial activity, and β-adrenergic blockade enhances uterine activity in experimental animals, premature labor could be a theoretical complication of a β-adrenergic blocker. However, studies utilizing β-adrenergic blocking drugs in pregnant women with essential hypertension have not demonstrated an increase in premature delivery.

The adverse effects of these drugs have been for the most part isolated case reports. In the largest series of pregnant women treated throughout pregnancy for essential hypertension with β-adrenergic blocking drugs, hydralazine, and diuretics, the perinatal mortality was 1.9%. At the present time, a reasonable approach would be that pregnant women with essential hypertension who are adequately controlled on a β blocker be kept on the drug throughout pregnancy. Further experience should be developed in the use of β-adrenergic blockers for the treatment of acute toxemia, but initial studies from Europe are very encouraging.

D. Arteriolar Dilators

There are several drugs that lower blood pressure by a direct vasodilating effect on arterioles; the most commonly used are hydralazine and diazoxide. Oral hydralazine is not a potent antihypertensive agent when used alone. By contrast, the combination of hydralazine, a diuretic, and a β blocker, which prevents the reflex tachycardia that occurs with a vasodilator, is an effective regimen in the treatment of essential hypertension. It controls moderately severe hypertension without side effects.

The arteriolar dilator diazoxide (Hyperstat®) is a most potent antihypertensive agent when given intravenously. It acts by directly altering reactivity of arteriole smooth muscle with a decrease in peripheral vascular resistance. Like all vasodilators, it causes sodium retention and must be used in conjunction with a diuretic. There is an increase in heart rate and cardiac output following diazoxide because of a compensatory response of the carotid baroreceptors to the fall in pressure. There is no reduction in renal blood flow or glomerular filtration. The drug acts within 10 to 15 sec with a maximum effect achieved within 3 to 40 min. The usual dose is 300 mg either given rapidly (10 to 15 sec) or in boluses of 50 mg/min. If a satisfactory fall in pressure does not occur within 5 to 10 min, a second dose of 300 mg is given. The effect of the drug usually lasts 3 to 8 hr after injection. It has been used in severe toxemia and is the agent of choice when acute hypertensive emergencies develop during the course of toxemia. Diazoxide induces hyperglycemia when given chronically and is not useful for the treatment of chronic hypertension. It frequently causes cessation of labor, but this effect can be overcome by an oxytocic agent.

Hydralazine is the most commonly used vasodilator in pregnancy. Its mode of action is not clear, but it may act by inhibiting movement of calcium into the smooth muscle cell. It causes peripheral vasodilation with a greater effect on resistance than capacitance vessels. Accompanying the vasodilation, heart rate and cardiac output increase. These compensatory reflexes cause tolerance to hydralszine to develop, but when it is combined with either a β-adrenergic blocker such as propranolol or a central adrenergic blocker such as methyldopa or clonidine, hydralazine becomes quite effective as an antihypertensive agent. No adverse effects have been described in pregnant women given hydralazine, and in studies of pregnant animals hydralazine has been noted to cause an increase in uterine blood flow.

Minoxidil (Loniten®) is a potent arteriolar dilator which is not used except in severe hypertension refractory to other medications. There is no report of its use during pregnancy.

Nitroprusside, another potent vasodilator, is quite effective in controlling hypertensive emergencies, but it has not gained favor in severe toxemia since studies in pregnant ewes demonstrated thiocyanate and cyanide accumulation in the fetus.

The angiotensin-blocking agents captopril and saralasin have not been used in pregnancy, but experiments in pregnant rabbits demonstrate a striking increase in fetal mortality with captopril. This drug was found to decrease uterine PGE_2 synthesis, indicating that uterine PGE_2 synthesis in the rabbit is dependent on angiotensin II generation, and this may be the mechanism of its detrimental effect on fetal viability.

SUGGESTED READINGS

Ferris TF: Hypertension and toxemia in pregnancy, in Burrow GN, Ferris TF (eds): *Medical Complications of Pregnancy* (ed 2). Philadelphia, WB Saunders, 1982, pp. 1–35.
Lindheimer MD, Katz AI (eds): The kidney in pregnancy. *Kidney Int* 18:147–278, 1980.

16

Nutrition in Renal Disease

WILLIAM E. MITCH

I. INTRODUCTION

A nutrient can be defined as something eaten (or infused) that promotes growth and/or acts to repair the consequences of excessive catabolism of body tissues. Therefore, nutritional management of renal insufficiency should be directed not only toward promoting growth (in children) or maintaining weight and muscle mass (in adults) but also towards correcting abnormalities that lead to net catabolism of muscles, bones, and to loss of residual kidney function. Success in achieving these goals is possible because certain consequences of renal failure (bone disease, acidosis, etc.) and many uremic symptoms are closely linked to the quantity of accumulated waste products derived from food eaten by the patient.

Accumulation of unexcreted waste products is a predictable consequence of the reduced renal clearance. When dietary intake of a waste product (or its precursor) is constant, the amount of a waste product that must be excreted each day, $U_x V$, for the patient to maintain a steady state can be eliminated only if the plasma concentration, P_x, of that waste product increases to balance the lower clearance, C_x. This follows from rearrangement of the clearance formula $C_x = U_x V / P_x$ to $(C_x)(P_x) = U_x V$.

In renal insufficiency, the consequence of the reduction in clearance can be compensated for, at least partially, by nutritional therapy. Nutritional therapy attempts to decrease the quantity of accumulated waste products and, hence, the plasma level of the product by reducing the intake of precursors of toxic products. Simply stated, if intake of the product is lowered, less

WILLIAM E. MITCH • Department of Medicine, Harvard Medical School; and Brigham and Women's Hospital, Boston, Massachusetts 02115.

of the product must be excreted each day, and the plasma level will fall. At the same time, sufficient amounts of essential nutrients must be provided to maintain lean body mass and to combat any tendency for wasting. Thus, it is critical that sufficient dietary protein be prescribed to prevent wasting of body protein, but at the same time, excessive protein intake must be avoided since almost all of the accumulated nitrogenous waste products are derived directly from dietary protein. Not only do nitrogenous waste products arise during catabolism of dietary or endogenous (e.g., muscle) protein but also the daily amount of inorganic ions [phosphate, sulfate, hydrogen, potassium, and sodium (Fig. 1)] that must be excreted increases during protein degradation. Reducing dietary protein, therefore, reduces the accumulation of these inorganic ions as well.

II. DIETARY PROTEIN

A. Minimum Requirements

The minimum daily protein requirement of adults with normal renal function is approximately 0.5–0.6 g/kg (35–40 g/day). This amount is necessary to replenish protein lost during the normal daily process of protein turnover. Although early studies suggested that patients with chronic renal failure (CRF) needed only 20 g/day (about 0.3 g/kg per day), this was subsequently found to be incorrect, and it is now clear that patients with CRF need

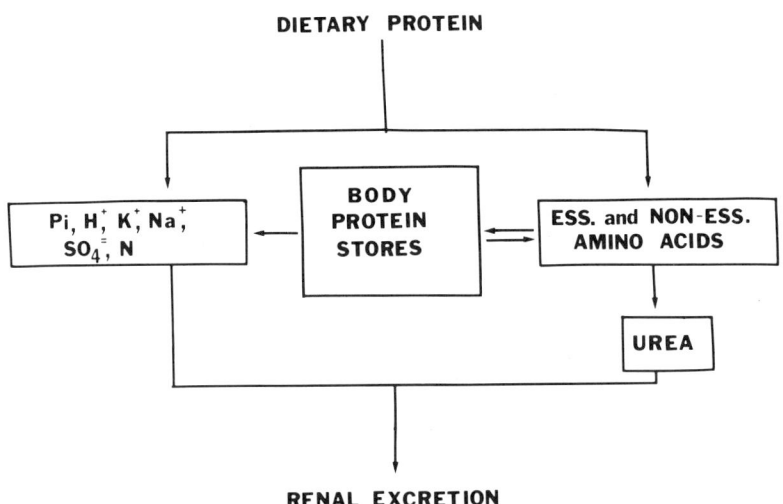

Figure 1. Breakdown of dietary protein enlarges the pool of essential and nonessential amino acids which can be used to synthesize body protein. The amino acids also are used to produce urea which must be excreted. Besides nitrogenous waste products, dietary protein catabolism yields inorganic ions that must be excreted.

about the same amount of protein as do normal subjects. In addition to a minimum quantity, there also is a restriction regarding protein quality. Patients with renal insufficiency eating the minimal amount of 40 g/day of protein must select foods with "high-quality" protein (eggs, milk, etc.). These foods contain a high proportion of the essential amino acids (leucine, isoleucine, valine, threonine, tryptophan, lysine, methionine, phenylalanine, and histidine). Since these amino acids cannot be synthesized by the body, they must be provided in the diet, or the body cannot synthesize new protein. Thus, protein quality is as important as quantity, and diets with less than 40 g/day of high-quality protein can lead to net catabolism of endogenous protein and ultimately to muscle wasting.

B. Deviations from Minimal Requirements

Patients with the nephrotic syndrome require an additional intake of high-quality protein that is at least as great as the amount of protein lost in the urine. If inadequate amounts of protein or low-quality protein is eaten by these patients, severe protein wasting can occur.

Hemodialysis patients require at least 0.8–1 g/kg per day of protein to prevent protein catabolism and muscle wasting. Their increased protein requirement results in part from the loss of nutrients during dialysis; the dialysis membrane is nonselective and removes amino acids, vitamins, and other nutrients as well as urea and other waste products.

When protein intake is restricted to less than 40 g/day to control symptoms, then a supplement of essential amino acids must be provided either as the essential amino acids themselves or as their nitrogen-free analogues. With such supplements, dietary protein can be restricted to 20–25 g/day, and it is no longer necessary to specify that dietary protein consist only of "high-quality" protein. since protein quality need not be restricted, the greater variety of foods that can be eaten may improve patient compliance even though the allotment of dietary protein is lower.

In any patient, protein wasting must be detected early and treated appropriately. There are three ways to detect net protein catabolism: first, nitrogen balance (see Section III.A) will become negative; secondly, the urea appearance rate (see Section III.C) will increase; and thirdly, the serum concentrations of albumin and transferrin will decrease if dietary protein is inadequate for prolonged periods.

III. NITROGEN METABOLISM

A. Nitrogen Balance

Digestion of dietary protein or degradation of endogenous protein releases amino acids into the body's pool of amino acids. Amino acids in this pool have two fates; they can be used to synthesize protein, to replenish protein degraded during daily protein turnover, or they may be degraded to nitrogen, carbon dioxide, and water (Fig. 1). The nitrogen is converted almost exclusively to urea. Nutritional therapy must maintain the balance between body protein synthesis and endogenous protein degradation so that protein wasting does not occur. The most simple way to determine if this has been accomplished is to measure nitrogen balance, B_N. A positive B_N indicates that protein synthesis exceeds degradation; a negative B_N indicates the opposite. Normal adults are in neutral B_N.

In normal subjects, B_N is measured as the difference between dietary nitrogen and nitrogen excreted in urine and feces. Since urea is the major nitrogen-containing product of endogenous and exogenous protein catabolism, an increase in urine urea excretion when dietary nitrogen is constant suggests that B_N is negative; a decrease, that B_N is positive. Unfortunately, in patients with renal insufficiency, urea excretion usually does not change rapidly following a change in B_N or a change in dietary nitrogen. In fact, when urea clearance is low, the half-life of an increase or decrease in the size of the urea pool is measured in days (in normal subjects, the half-life is in hours). Thus, in patients with CRF, a change in dietary protein or nitrogen balance cannot be detected unless both urea excretion and changes in the urea nitrogen pool are measured. Therefore, B_N for a patient with renal failure must be calculated as intake minus output (in urine and feces) of nitrogen minus the change in the size of the urea nitrogen pool. For example, if an anuric patient receives an infusion of urea nitrogen, total nitrogen intake increases, but urine nitrogen will be constant. If the enlarged urea pool is not included in the calculation of B_N, nitrogen balance will appear to become positive. In fact, it may not have changed. Theoretically, all nonprotein nitrogenous compounds should be measured in this way, but the total nitrogen contained in all of these compounds is so small in comparison to urea, they may be ignored.

B. Urea

From these considerations, it is obvious that one of the most important waste products is urea. In dialysis patients, an excessively high serum urea concentration (SUN > 150 mg/dl) has been found to be associated with headache, nausea, vomiting, and lethargy, i.e., the symptoms of uremia. Thus, urea itself may be toxic. Moreover, urea levels also correlate well with uremic symptoms because the nitrogen in protein is ultimately converted to urea. Therefore, the amount of urea produced each day directly reflects the amount of dietary (or endogenous) protein degraded each day. Since protein degradation not only leads to urea production but also to production of other nitrogen waste products, the amount of urea produced each day must be parallel to the amount of all nitrogen-containing waste products produced each day. Consequently, treatment programs that reduce the rate of urea production reduce the rate of production of other nitrogenous waste products and *vice versa*. For example, the rate of production of "middle molecules," etc. increase when dietary protein rises, and the change will be mirrored by an increase in urea accumulation; when dietary protein is lowered, waste nitrogen production decreases, and any toxicity caused by these putative uremic toxins must be diminished.

Urea that is produced has two possible fates; a portion is degraded by gastrointestinal bacteria to form ammonia and carbon dioxide which are recirculated to the liver, and the remaining urea is either excreted by the kidney or accumulates in body water. This latter quantity (excretion plus accumulation) is termed urea appearance and is the most important physiological and nutritional index of nitrogen equilibrium. Moreover, it is a major determinant of nitrogen balance.

C. Urea Appearance Rate

Fortunately, the size of the urea pool can be estimated easily because urea has the same concentration throughout body water. In a patient without edema, water is approximately 60% of body weight, and the size of the urea nitrogen pool can be calculated as the product of body water and SUN (Table I). The size of the urea pool can be measured more accurately by isotope dilution techniques, but for clinical purposes, this is rarely necessary. The rate of urea appearance is calculated as the sum of the rate of accumulation of urea nitrogen (which can be either positive or negative) plus the average daily rate of urinary excretion of urea nitrogen (determined over the same period) (Table I). Obviously, when weight and SUN are constant, urea appearance is equal to urea excretion.

D. Urea Appearance and Nitrogen Balance

A clinically useful estimate of B_N can be calculated from dietary protein (I_N) and the urea appearance rate (U). This is possible because the total

Table I. Representative Calculation of Urea Nitrogen Appearance Rate[a]

	Day 1	Day 5
Weight (kg)	80	90
Body water (liter)	48	54
SUN (mg/dl)	50	41
Urea nitrogen pool (g N)	24	22.1

[a] Body water is calculated as 60% weight, and the urea nitrogen pool as body water (liter) $\times$ SUN (g/liter). Urinary urea nitrogen averages 6.4 g N/day. Urea nitrogen accumulation = (urea nitrogen pool$_1$ − urea nitrogen pool$_2$) ÷ 5 = −0.4 g N/day. Urea nitrogen appearance rate = average urea nitrogen excretion plus urea nitrogen accumulation or U = 6.4 g N/day − 0.4 g N/day = 6.0 g N/day.

nonurea nitrogen excretion (NUN) including fecal nitrogen, the nitrogen in urinary creatinine, uric acid, protein, etc., and skin losses is relatively constant, averaging about 2.5 g N/day. Thus, $B_N = I_N - U - 2.5$ g N/day. In addition, the urea appearance rate can be used to estimate dietary compliance if urea clearance is known and balance is assumed to be neutral ($B_N = 0$). This is possible because the quantity of urea nitrogen that must be excreted each day (UV) equals nitrogen intake, I_N, minus NUN (or 2.5 g N/day), and the steady-state SUN expected for the diet can be calculated.

E. Steady-State SUN

Rearrangement of the urea clearance formula to ($I_N - 2.5$ g N/day) ÷ urea clearance (in liters/day) yields the steady-state SUN (in mg/liter) that must occur considering the patient's urea clearance and protein intake (Table II). The steady-state SUN calculation helps to determine the cause of an unexpected change in the SUN. For example, the SUN could increase when too much protein is eaten or when gastrointestinal bleeding or a catabolic illness is present. The relationship between the predicted steady-state SUN and the prescribed protein intake can help to sort out these possibilities. If the predicted SUN value is considerably lower than the measured value, then the patient either has not been following the prescribed diet or there may be gastrointestinal bleeding. It should be emphasized that gastrointestinal bleeding need not be massive to cause an increase in the SUN of a patient with renal insufficiency. This is because the time for a patient with a low urea clearance to excrete the urea nitrogen arising from catabolism of the absorbed protein following gastrointestinal bleeding is prolonged and because there is as much as 4 g of potential urea nitrogen in 100 ml blood. A catabolic illness or treatment with corticosteroids can also increase the SUN since endogenous protein is degraded to form urea. In the case of a wasting disease, the diagnosis frequently will be obvious.

F. Urea Degradation

The portion of urea produced each day that is degraded to ammonia and carbon dioxide by the bacteria of the gastrointestinal tract is an endogenous, nonprotein nitrogen source supplied directly to the liver. It was proposed that this ammonia could be used for synthesis of amino acids and ultimately protein and therefore that the ammonia would allow dietary protein to be restricted to a very low level in patients with CRF even though nitrogen balance was maintained. However, it has been shown that less than 3% of albumin nitrogen is derived from urea breakdown in patients with CRF. Moreover, when urea degradation by gut bacteria was suppressed in patients with CRF, it was found that their nitrogen balance improved, and urea appearance did not change. If nitrogen derived from urea degradation were

Table II. Effect of Protein Intake on Steady-State SUN in Patients with CRF[a]

Clearance			UV		SUN	
Creatinine (ml/min)	Urea		40-g-protein diet (g N/day)	80-g-protein diet (g N/day)	40-g-protein diet (mg/dl)	80-g-protein diet (mg/dl)
	ml/min	liter/day				
20	12	17.3	3.9	10.3	23	60
10	6	8.6	3.9	10.3	45	120
5	3	4.3	3.9	10.3	91	239

[a] Urea clearance is assumed to be 60% of creatinine clearance. Since 16% of protein is nitrogen, the daily steady-state excretion of urea nitrogen equals nitrogen intake minus nonurea nitrogen excretion (averaging 2.5 g N/day). Rearrangement of the urea clearance formula to $SUN = UV \div C_u$ permits calculation of the steady-state SUN resulting from a defined protein intake. (UV is the daily urinary excretion of urea nitrogen, and SUN is the serum urea nitrogen concentration.)

being used to synthesize amino acids, the amount of urea nitrogen appearing in urine and body fluids should increase when urea degradation was suppressed. On the other hand, if nitrogen from urea were being used simply to resynthesize urea, then the quantity of urea appearing in urine and body fluids should remain constant. It was found that urea appearance did not change in these studies, and it was concluded that urea nitrogen is not nutritionally important for patients with CRF.

IV. METABOLISM OF CREATINE AND CREATININE

A. Creatine Conversion to Creatinine

Creatine arises from endogenous synthesis and from preformed dietary creatine, and it is contained primarily in muscle. Each day, 1.7% of the creatine pool is dehydrated nonenzymatically to form creatinine. Since the size of the creatine pool is proportional to muscle mass, and since a constant amount of creatine is converted to creatinine each day, the amount of creatinine produced is proportional to the muscle mass. Because muscle mass remains fairly constant, daily creatinine excretion is often considered to be almost constant. In fact, it varies by 10–20% even when 24-hr urine specimens are collected carefully. Because such a small fraction of the creatine pool is converted to creatinine each day, the day-to-day variation in creatinine excretion is almost certainly not caused by variation in muscle mass or in the amount of meat eaten (and hence creatine intake). This follows from the following example:

> A 28-year-old male has about 128 g of creatine and excretes about 1.85 g/day of creatinine. A change in his creatinine excretion of 10% would mean that his creatine pool would have changed by 10–11 g.

Since the creatine content of meat is approximately 4.2 mg/g wet weight, a 10% change in creatinine excretion would require a 2.5-kg per day change in meat intake or a change in muscle mass of 2.5 kg. Such a day-to-day variation in diet or muscle mass is highly unlikely. A more likely explanation for the variability in creatinine excretion is that the diet causes a change in the smaller creatinine pool. In fact, creatine in meat is converted to creatinine by cooking; eating an additional 10 oz of cooked ground beef could increase urinary creatinine by as much as 900 mg. In addition, creatinine clearance might change slightly.

B. Other Determinants of Creatinine Production

Age and sex are also important determinants of creatinine excretion. Creatinine excretion decreases 2½-fold between the ages of 20 and 90 years, apparently because the creatine pool (and therefore muscle mass) diminishes with age. Women excrete less creatinine than men of the same age because muscle mass is a smaller fraction of their body weight. Clearly, determination of the values for "normal" rates of creatinine excretion and clearance should take diet, age, and sex into account.

C. Chronic Renal Failure

In CRF, steady-state creatinine excretion is reduced compared to normal subjects of the same age, sex, and weight. This occurs because creatinine is degraded to noncreatinine products. In fact, in patients with severe renal insufficiency, creatinine degradation can account for as much as 50% of the total amount of creatinine removed from the body each day. The rate of creatinine degradation can be expressed in terms of an "extrarenal clearance" which equals the quantity degraded each day divided by the serum creatinine concentration. Because this extrarenal clearance is relatively constant, the amount of creatinine degraded each day increases as serum creatinine rises.

D. Daily Creatinine Production

The amount of creatinine produced each day can be calculated because it (like urea) has three fates: it can be degraded, it can be excreted in the urine, or it can accumulate in body fluid. The fact that extrarenal clearance is fairly constant can be used to estimate the amount degraded; the amount that is excreted and accumulated in body fluids can be measured. An estimate of creatinine production is useful since creatinine production is proportional to muscle mass and, therefore, can be used to compare the muscle mass of a patient with CRF to that of normal subjects of the same age, sex, and weight. Thus, in the steady state, when weight and serum creatinine are constant, creatinine production (P) equals the rate of creatinine excretion (U_cV) plus the rate of creatinine degradation (M_c). The creatinine degradation rate is equal to the product of extrarenal clearance (0.04 liter/kg per day) and serum creatinine (S) expressed in mg/liter. Thus:

$$P\text{(mg/kg per day)} = U_cV\text{(mg/kg per day)} + 0.04\text{ (liter/kg per day)} \times S\text{(mg/liter)}$$

Estimated values for P may be compared to the creatinine production rates of normal subjects to determine in individual patients whether marked changes in creatinine production and hence muscle mass have occurred.

Normal men: $P\text{(mg/kg per day)} = 28 - 0.2 \times \text{age}$
Normal women: $P\text{(mg/kg per day)} = 23.8 - 0.17 \times \text{age}$

V. OTHER NITROGEN WASTE PRODUCTS

A. Ammonia

Besides urea and creatinine, other nitrogenous compounds that might affect nitrogen balance or cause symptoms in patients with CRF are ammonia, uric acid, urine protein, and fecal nitrogen. Ammonia arises from two sources: from catabolism of glutamine by the liver, kidney, and gut and from bacterial degradation of urea. Ammonia produced is detoxified by conversion to urea. In patients with CRF, there does not appear to be any abnormality of hepatic ammonia detoxification or abnormal ammonia accumulation.

B. Uric Acid

Serum uric acid rises in patients with CRF because uric acid clearance by the kidney is reduced. Usually, the increase is small because the dietary content of uric acid falls when protein and hence purine intake is restricted. In addition, uric acid, like urea, is degraded by gastrointestinal bacteria. The increase in serum uric acid rarely causes clinical problems and should not be treated unless the patient has a history of gout or unless it is above 13 mg/dl in men or 10 mg/dl in women. Above these levels, uric acid might cause further loss of residual renal function.

C. Proteinuria

Large losses of protein in the urine will lead to endogenous protein catabolism unless the losses are replaced. As indicated in the section on protein requirements, dietary protein should be increased by 1 g for each gram of proteinuria. As renal insufficiency progresses, protein clearance decreases, and protein intake should be lowered accordingly.

D. Intestinal Nitrogen Losses

Fecal nitrogen losses of patients with CRF may be greater than those of normal subjects because occasional patients will have "low-grade" gastrointestinal bleeding, especially in severe uremia. When there is no bleeding, the daily quantity of fecal nitrogen is remarkably constant. Presumably this is because fecal nitrogen does not arise from dietary protein (except in malabsorption) but arises from gastrointestinal bacteria and from protein that is secreted into the intestine.

E. Nonurea Nitrogen

When the nitrogen contained in urinary creatinine, uric acid, etc. and feces is combined, it is termed "nonurea nitrogen" to distinguish it from urea nitrogen. As pointed out earlier, the excreted quantity of nitrogen contained in all of these compounds varies only slightly from day to day. For this reason, an average value of 2.5 g N/day may be used in calculating the nitrogen balance and steady-state SUN of patients with CRF (Section III.D).

VI. IMPORTANCE OF CALORIES

A. Consequence of Anorexia

The requirement for energy is directly proportional to the subjects' level of activity whether or not they have renal disease. Unfortunately, patients with renal failure tend to eat fewer calories than they require for their level of activity. This can lead to catabolism of body fat and muscle to provide energy, producing a decrease in lean body mass. Furthermore, there is suggestive evidence that an inadequate energy intake by these patients leads to poor utilization of dietary protein. When protein intake is restricted to minimal levels, poor utilization of dietary protein to synthesize body protein makes it even more likely that endogenous protein catabolism will occur. It is not surprising, therefore, that patients eating an inadequate amount of foods providing energy will lose weight and have reduced fat stores, a reduction in total body potassium, and low values for serum albumin and transferrin concentrations. These are all indications of prolonged negative nitrogen balance.

B. Energy Requirements

To meet energy requirements, it is recommended that adults with renal insufficiency receive 30–50 kcal/kg per day. Children with renal failure need even more calories (about 50–100 kcal/kg per day) to meet their requirements for growth as well as for daily activity. The importance of supplying adequate amounts of energy precursors cannot be overemphasized, but because of anorexia and because the variety of foods may be limited, it may be difficult to maintain an adequate energy intake. For this reason, it is advisable to periodically have the patient list all foods eaten over a 3-day period and analyze calorie intake.

VII. METABOLIC AND ENDOCRINE ABNORMALITIES

A. Glucose Intolerance

Glucose intolerance is frequently present in uremic patients but rarely requires treatment. The fasting blood sugar is almost always less than 150 mg/dl, and postprandial blood sugar is usually less than 200 mg/dl. Furthermore, ketoacidosis does not occur. Glucose intolerance is caused by a reduced uptake of glucose by peripheral tissues, especially muscle, because of a relative insensitivity to the hypoglycemic action of insulin. Besides insensitivity to insulin, glucose intolerance is aggravated by the high carbohydrate intake given to increase calorie intake to desired levels. The higher blood glucose levels stimulate insulin release, leading to an increase in plasma insulin levels until defective glucose uptake is overcome and glucose uptake balances glucose production. In this new steady state, hyperglycemia and hyperinsulinemia are present.

B. Insulin Metabolism

In addition to the stimulus for insulin secretion, there is defective degradation of insulin. Catabolism of insulin in muscle and kidney (and possibly other organs) is diminished in uremia, and a consequence of this that has practical importance is that the insulin requirement of diabetic patients with renal insufficiency may decrease dramatically as renal failure advances. Occasionally, well-managed diabetic patients begin to have hypoglycemic attacks without a change in their insulin dose because advancing kidney disease results in less degradation of insulin and, hence, in excessive levels of insulin and hypoglycemia.

C. Hypertriglyceridemia

Hypertriglyceridemia is commonly present in patients with CRF just as it is in patients with diabetes mellitus who have normal renal function. It has been suggested that hypertriglyceridemia contributes to the accelerated atherosclerosis that frequently occurs in dialysis patients, although this is not established. Regarding the pathogenesis of this disorder, the major defect appears to be decreased removal of VLDL triglycerides from plasma. Impaired removal of triglycerides has been linked to reduced activity of the enzymes that degrade triglycerides, i.e., adipose tissue triglyceride lipase and plasma lipoprotein lipase.

D. Treatment of Hypertriglyceridemia

There are at least three methods of lowering triglycerides in patients with CRF: initiation of an exercise program, dietary alteration, and drug therapy. These patients, like other patients with chronic illness, often become depressed and adopt a sedentary existence.

1. Exercise

Increased exercise and improvement in exercise tolerance not only tend to lower blood lipid levels and improve the overall mental and physical condition of the patient, they also counteract glucose intolerance (as they do in patients with diabetes). For example, it has been shown that increasing the exercise tolerance of dialysis patients led to an improvement in glucose tolerance, to lower plasma insulin and triglyceride levels, and to an increase in plasma HDL cholesterol (a higher HDL cholesterol level is associated with a lower risk of coronary artery disease). Also, there was less difficulty in controlling hypertension in these same patients. Considering these potential benefits, a program of increased exercise should be planned for each patient, but care should be taken to avoid abrupt, excessive exercise because of the tendency of patients with CRF to have coronary atherosclerosis. The exercise program should be initiated gradually and will require enthusiasm and encouragement from the physician to achieve compliance. Debilitated patients should begin with short walks and increase the distance gradually. Guidelines for exercise programs for patients with coronary disease are quite suitable for patients with CRF.

2. Dietary Alteration

Changing the diet of patients with CRF can improve both glucose intolerance and hypertriglyceridemia whether or not they are being treated by dialysis. As noted above (Section VII.A), a high carbohydrate intake (which is often prescribed in order to increase caloric intake) coupled with reduced glucose uptake by peripheral tissues even in the presence of insulin results in mild hyperglycemia and exacerbates the tendency towards abnormal plasma lipids.

When the distribution of foods in the diet is changed so that the content of carbohydrates is lower, and the content of unsaturated fat is raised, and saturated fat is lowered, the fasting plasma triglyceride concentration will decrease. Furthermore, the increase in plasma triglycerides after meals will be lower than observed previously. This occurs in dialysis and nondialysis patients as well as in normal subjects. Not only are triglycerides lowered when the ratio of polyunsaturated to saturated fat is increased in the diet but also serum cholesterol and free fatty acids remain stable in spite of an increase in dietary fat. Interestingly, glucose and insulin levels do not change although fasting plasma insulin does not rise as sharply after meals.

3. Drugs

In addition to exercise and alteration in diet, administration of clofibrate will increase plasma triglycerides in patients with renal insufficiency. Presumably this occurs through enhancement of lipase activity; clofibrate has been shown to increase the activity of adipose tissue lipase and total plasma (hepatic triglyceride and lipoprotein) lipase of dialysis patients. In one study, the increase in lipase activity was accompanied by lower plasma triglyceride and VLDL triglyceride concentrations. Because the consequences of isolated hypertriglyceridemia are unclear, and because the effects of long-term administration of clofibrate to patients with renal insufficiency are unknown, the drug should be used with caution, especially since there are reports of clofibrate-induced myositis.

VIII. MINERALS AND ELECTROLYTES

In patients with CRF, important changes in mineral and electrolyte metabolism occur that must be considered in designing nutritional therapy. Metabolism of sodium, potassium, and calcium and phosphorus are discussed in detail in other chapters, so only those problems specifically related to nutritional therapy will be reviewed here.

A. Body Fluid Volumes

Body fluid volumes are surprisingly well maintained in patients with CRF, supporting the contention that steady-state regulation of salt excretion is adequate. For example, total body water is usually normal unless the patient is malnourished. Measurements of extracellular volume are often increased, but in many patients, this may not be a true expansion of the extracellular fluid (ECV) but falsely high because of the method used to measure ECV. However, in patients with hypertension and in dialysis patients who are functionally anephric, the ECV may be expanded and require dietary salt restriction.

B. Sodium

Frequently, the salt intake of patients with CRF is restricted because it is assumed that their capacity to excrete sodium is severely limited. In fact, the capacity of patients with CRF to regulate sodium excretion in the steady state is well preserved. Their problem lies more in inability to change the rate of sodium excretion rapidly in response to abrupt changes in dietary salt. Even when creatinine clearance is as low as 10 ml/min, dietary salt rarely needs to be limited below 6 g/day or 102 mEq/day of sodium (1 g salt contains 17 mEq sodium), since such patients can readily excrete this amount of sodium. However, if dietary salt is withdrawn abruptly, such patients cannot lower their sodium excretion in response to the reduced intake for several days (normal subjects eating 10 mEq/day can lower sodium excretion to this level within 2 days). This inability to decrease sodium loss results in loss of extracellular fluid and a further decline in GFR. Even when CRF is less severe, the renal adjustment to changes in salt intake remains sluggish. It is clear that unwarranted salt deprivation can have unfortunate consequences including a fall in blood pressure and further loss of renal function.

C. Dietary Salt

The importance of these considerations to nutritional therapy leads to the following conclusions. First, even in patients with severe CRF, dietary salt does not have to be greatly restricted unless there is poorly controlled hypertension (see Chapter 13). Secondly, dietary salt must not be restricted abruptly, or salt depletion will occur and cause further renal impairment. The amount of salt that can be permitted in the diet can be determined easily if the patient is in the steady state (when weight and renal function are constant, then the amount of sodium being excreted is constant). One method of determining the dietary salt allowance is to subtract the sodium contained in the amount of sodium bicarbonate required to treat acidosis from the average daily sodium excretion. Another method is to gradually increase dietary salt until pedal edema can just be detected at the end of the day but is absent in the morning. This slight edema indicates that an adequate extracellular volume and renal perfusion are present. Regardless of which method is used, once an amount of dietary salt is prescribed, the patient should maintain a daily record of body weight so that adjustments can be made as required. If weight increases, furosemide can be used to reduce weight to the desired level. If weight decreases, dietary salt must be increased to prevent further loss of ECV and a decline in renal function. Canned soup is a simple, palatable means of increasing dietary salt and can be added to the diet until the patient's weight increases to the desired level.

D. Potassium

Although the serum potassium concentration of patients with CRF is usually normal or slightly high, there is considerable evidence that body stores of potassium are low, especially in malnourished or severely ill patients. Body potassium stores are usually normal in well-dialyzed patients, although serum potassium is high. These findings indicate that there is an abnormal distribution of potassium across cell membranes. In spite of the abnormal cellular distribution of potassium in patients with CRF, the ability of the kidney to excrete potassium adapts so that it is unusual to have to restrict dietary potassium until creatinine clearance falls below 5–7 ml/min. Even at this level of renal function, specific instructions regarding potassium are required only rarely because usually the diet is restricted in protein content and consequently also will be restricted in potassium (Fig. 1). In contrast, dialysis patients not only have lost the capacity for renal potassium excretion, they also eat a higher protein (and hence potassium) diet (see above). Almost always, they must avoid foods with a high potassium content such as citrus fruits. An important factor raising the serum potassium is the acid–base status, since acidosis causes a shift of potassium from cells to the extracellular fluid. In fact, a high serum potassium often may be lowered simply by using sodium bicarbonate to correct acidosis.

E. Divalent Ions

Abnormalities of mineral metabolism in patients with CRF are discussed in Chapters 3–5. In CRF, the development of secondary hyperparathyroidism is linked closely to the retention of dietary phosphorus. The retention of phosphorus and the development of hyperparathyroidism not only affect bone, they also may lead to deposition of calcium and phosphorus in soft tissues, including the damaged kidney. Moreover, there is evidence from animals with experimentally induced CRF that the deposition of calcium and phosphorus in the kidney can contribute to progressive loss of residual renal function. To prevent progressive bone disease and soft-tissue calcification and possibly to prevent further deterioration in renal function, serum phosphorus must be maintained in the normal range.

1. Phosphate

Control of serum phosphorus begins with control of dietary phosphorus. A diet that is restricted in protein is also restricted in phosphorus content (Fig. 1), but often certain foods that are especially high in phosphorus (milk products, including ice cream and cheese) must be eliminated when serum phosphorus cannot be maintained in the normal range. In patients with advanced CRF, even dietary phosphorus restriction may not be adequate to maintain a normal serum phosphorus, and aluminum hydroxide "phosphate binders" become necessary.

2. Calcium

In patients with renal insufficiency, serum calcium is often low. A low serum calcium may be caused by resistance to the action of parathyroid hormone, the high serum phosphorus, or low vitamin D (Chapter 3). A low total serum calcium also may be related to a low serum albumin even though ionized calcium (the physiologically important fraction) is normal. A formula that corrects for a low serum albumin is:

$$\text{``True'' calcium} = \text{measured calcium} - \text{serum albumin} + 4$$

If the calculated "true" calcium is within the normal range, then the low serum albumin probably accounts for the lower total serum calcium. To correct this, emphasis should be placed on improving the patient's nutrition.

Another nutritionally important fact to consider when the serum calcium is low is the adequacy of dietary calcium. Because gastrointestinal absorption of calcium is abnormally low in patients with CRF, calcium intake must be at least 1.5 g/day to achieve calcium balance. Unfortunately, when dietary protein is restricted, calcium intake falls, and it may be necessary to prescribe calcium supplements. It should be reemphasized, however, that a high serum phosphorus will tend to lower serum calcium. Thus, serum phosphorus must be brought into the normal range before calcium supplements are prescribed.

IX. VITAMINS AND TRACE METALS

A. Folic Acid and Vitamin C

Patients with uremia frequently have low serum folate levels, and they also may have circulating inhibitors of folate. To combat these problems and possibly to improve the patient's anemia, a folic acid supplement of 1 mg/day usually is prescribed. There is less evidence for deficiencies of other water-soluble vitamins including vitamin C because patients with renal insufficiency usually eat adequate amounts of fruits and vegetables.

B. Pyridoxine and B Vitamins

Pyridoxine deficiency has been reported in patients with CRF, especially in dialysis patients. Because pyridoxine is a cofactor for certain enzymes responsible for amino acid metabolism, a deficiency of this vitamin might impair overall amino acid metabolism. For this reason, pyridoxine supplements of 10–25 mg/day are usually prescribed when dietary protein is restricted, especially when essential amino acid or ketoacid supplements are given. Dialysis patients require a supplement of water-soluble B and C vitamins because they are partially removed during a dialysis treatment.

C. Vitamin A

The plasma level of vitamin A is increased in uremic patients, and there is ample evidence that their vitamin A stores are increased also. In fact, certain of the abnormalities of calcium metabolism, bone mineralization, and fat metabolism that occur in chronic renal failure have been linked to vitamin A excess, but the association is not proven. Regardless, there is no evidence for vitamin A deficiency, and multivitamin preparations containing vitamin A should not be given.

D. Iron

Iron deficiency may occur in patients with renal insufficiency for three reasons. First, many of these patients have intermittent gastrointestinal bleeding which can deplete iron stores. For this reason, repeated stool guaiac tests should be performed whenever bleeding is suspected, for example, when the degree of anemia is out of proportion to the degree of renal impairment or when an unexplained increase in the urea appearance rate occurs (see Section III.E). Secondly, iron is dialyzable, and when iron stores or intake are limited, dialysis can cause iron deficiency. Thirdly, the iron restriction that accompanies a protein-restricted diet can lead to iron deficiency. In addition, the patient with uremia may have a lower hemoglobin than normal subjects with the same iron stores because of impaired erythrocytosis associated with uremia. Iron deficiency is often difficult to recognize in patients with renal insufficiency because a chronic disease (such as CRF) will lower serum iron concentration even when iron stores are adequate. In addition, serum transferrin becomes less valuable as a diagnostic aid because it is affected by the nutritional state of the patient, being depressed in malnourished subjects. However, when serum iron is less than 40 μg/dl or when serum transferrin is less than 16% saturated, iron supplements should be prescribed. Iron should be taken for a minimum of 6 months, since it takes this length of time to replenish iron stores.

E. Zinc and Copper

It also has been suggested that patients with CRF (and especially dialysis patients) develop zinc and/or copper deficiency. In fact, the anorexia and decreased ability to taste that occur in uremia have been ascribed to zinc deficiency, although this has not been proven. Low levels of copper in serum, muscle, and other tissues of undialyzed uremic children have been reported, but their pathophysiological significance is not clear. At present, recommendations for zinc or copper supplementation are not established, and it would seem prudent to avoid prescribing supplements of trace metals unless there is a clear indication of a deficiency state. Such practice will avoid potential toxicity occurring from excessive intake of these metals.

X. DESIGN OF THE DIET

From the foregoing discussion, it is clear that there are many abnormalities in renal insufficiency that are related to excesses in or affected by deficiencies of the diet. These include accumulation of nitrogen waste products, changes in mineral and electrolyte metabolism, and possibly a relationship between excessive dietary phosphorus and progressive loss of renal function. Thus, the goals of nutritional therapy for patients with renal insufficiency (Table III) are directed to combat these problems.

A. Protein Restriction

When should dietary protein restriction begin? There is no clear-cut answer to this question, but when the patient is symptomatically uremic, protein restriction will almost always lead to an improvement in fatigue, nausea, irritability, and other symptoms. Besides the presence of symptoms, protein restriction should be instituted when serum phosphorus is poorly controlled or when the SUN exceeds 80 mg/dl. When serum urea nitrogen is above this level, patients frequently will develop fatigue or other symptoms of uremia, and these can be detected by taking a careful history. Since degradation of dietary protein leads to the accumulation of toxic waste products, and since the rate of urea appearance (and hence the rate of urea nitrogen accumulation) is directly proportional to protein intake, a lower SUN following reduction of dietary protein can be used as an indication that the rate of accumulation of all nitrogenous products as well as inorganic ions (Fig. 1) is lower. The choice of 80 mg/dl as the SUN level at which nutritional therapy should be started should not be considered absolute and is chosen only because most patients will be at least mildly symptomatic at this level. The best guide is the presence of symptoms attributable to uremia, however mild.

Table III. Goals of Nutritional Therapy for
Patients with Renal Insufficiency

To maintain the serum urea nitrogen concentration
  below a level that causes symptoms
To maintain protein nutrition
To minimize electrolyte disturbances
To slow the rate of loss of residual function

B. Representative Diet

A diet for patients with CRF is presented in Table IV. This diet is designed to provide 40 g/day of high-quality protein and is suitable for patients with advanced CRF. When renal function is less severely impaired, a more liberal diet can be prescribed. Increasing dietary protein can be accomplished most easily by increasing the amount of meat in the diet. For example, if the lunch described in Table IV contained 2 oz of turkey rather than 1 oz, and the fish included in the supper was increased to 4 oz, the total protein intake would be 61 g/day. Obviously, this increase in dietary protein means that in the steady state an additional 3.2 g of urea nitrogen (Table II) and about 200 mg of phosphorus must be excreted.

Table IV. Sample Diet for Patients with Chronic
Renal Failure[a]

Breakfast
   ½ cup orange juice or half grapefruit
   1 cup corn flakes with ½ cup skim milk or 1 egg
   Sugar, 2 tsp
   1 slice toast
   2 tsp margarine
   1 tbsp jelly
   Coffee, tea, 2 tsp sugar, and nondairy creamer

Lunch
   1 oz turkey
   2 slices white bread
   1 tbsp mayonnaise
   Salad (lettuce and tomato), oil and vinegar dressing
   Apple or other fruit
   12-oz can soft drink

Supper
   2 oz fish, broiled in margarine
   1 medium baked potato
   ½ cup green beans
   1 small dinner roll
   5 tsp margarine (for potato, beans, roll)
   ½ cup canned fruit cocktail
   Coffee, tea, 2 tsp sugar, and nondairy creamer

Snacks
   2 cups apple juice
   Hard candy (Lifesavers[®], 1 roll)

Totals
   Protein   40 g
   Calories   2250–2300
   Fat   72 g (with egg, 78 g)
   Phosphorus   550–600 mg

[a] This diet was designed by Cheryl Mistrick, R.D.

The sample diet must be adjusted to provide an adequate salt and calcium intake. Methods for establishing the salt requirement are discussed in Section VIII, as is the need for a higher calcium intake for patients with CRF. In this same section, it was pointed out that excessive phosphorus intake might be related to further deterioration of renal function. This possibility is the basis for the fourth goal of nutritional therapy (Table III), to delay the progressive loss of residual renal function.

XI. PROGRESSION OF RENAL INSUFFICIENCY

During evaluation of a patient with CRF, it is important to obtain an accurate estimate of the rate of loss of residual renal function. This rate traditionally has been calculated for a group of patients with advanced disease of several causes or for a group of patients all with the same disease. Unfortunately, such a method of prognosis has a large variation which limits its clinical usefulness. For example, the average time for patients to progress from a serum creatinine of 5 mg/dl to initiation of dialysis has been estimated to be 10.8 months, but in individual patients, the time varied from 1 month to more than 2 years. Clearly, 10.8 months cannot be the prognosis for all patients. Likewise, this rate could not be used to study the effect of therapy on the rate of loss of renal function of an individual patient.

A. Serum Urea Nitrogen Concentration

The serum concentration of urea nitrogen is not useful as a measure of the rate of loss of renal function because it does not rise or fall solely with changes in renal function; it is also affected by protein intake. In addition, subjects with nephrosclerosis may have a marked depression of their urea clearance which is out of proportion to the loss of other indices of renal function, e.g., creatinine clearance; such a patient will have an excessively high SUN.

B. Serum Creatinine Concentration

The rate of creatinine production is much less influenced by protein intake, and, therefore, it would seem more appropriate to use the serum creatinine to estimate the loss of GFR or the loss of creatinine clearance. In fact, there are nomograms and formulas available for estimating creatinine clearance from serum creatinine concentration, but, unfortunately, they were derived from data taken from patients with normal kidneys or with mild renal impairment and may not be applicable to patients with CRF. Moreover, they do not take into account the degradation of creatinine that occurs in patients with CRF. In addition, the change in serum creatinine concentration that occurs as GFR falls is difficult to describe mathematically and therefore is poorly suited for assessing changes in real function.

C. Creatinine Clearance

When GFR is below 20 ml/min, creatinine clearance can be 20–30% higher than GFR. The difference is related in part to excretion of noncreatinine chromagen and in part to the fact that creatinine secretion becomes increasingly important in total renal creatinine clearance at low levels of renal function. This leads to an overestimate of GFR. A more accurate estimate of the GFR of patients with CRF is the average of their creatinine and urea clearances, but repeated collections of 24-hr urine aliquots is prohibitively cumbersome and expensive when patients are followed for prolonged periods.

D. Reciprocal of the Serum Creatinine Concentration

The rate of loss of renal function of most patients with CRF can be calculated by a relatively simple method using the reciprocal of serum creatinine (Fig. 2). In a study of 34 patients, sequential values of the reciprocal of serum creatinine concentration were plotted against time for each patient,

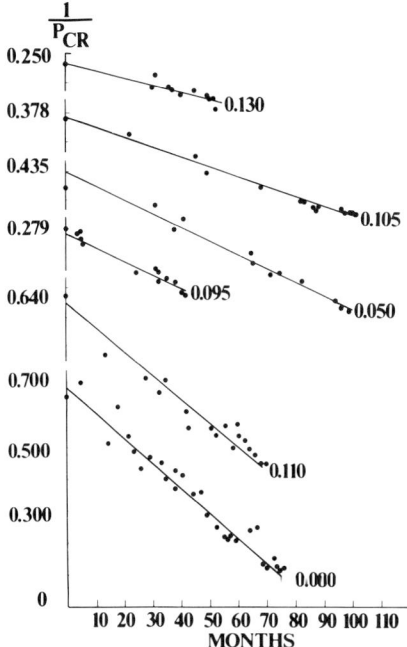

Figure 2. Rate of loss of renal function measured as the linear change in the reciprocal of serum creatinine concentration with time. Data from six patients are shown—two with glomerulonephritis, two with interstital nephritis, and two with medullary cystic disease.

and it was found that the reciprocal declined linearly with time for more than 90% of the subjects; for three patients, the relationship was nonlinear. The slope of the line is an estimate of the rate of loss of renal function and can be used to determine the effect of therapy on the rate of loss of residual renal function. Besides the change in the reciprocal of serum creatinine, it has also been proposed that the logarithm of serum creatinine increases linearly with time in some patients with CRF. However, the slope of sequential values of the log of serum creatinine increased abruptly and unexpectedly in some patients, making this method less valuable as a means of determining whether a certain therapy caused a change in renal function. Obviously, a linear change in both the reciprocal and the logarithm cannot be correct mathematically or physiologically, since a decrease in the reciprocal transformation is consistent with a constant rate of loss of function, whereas an increase in the logarithm suggests that a constant fraction of residual function is being lost with time. It seems advisable to use the logarithm method if the reciprocal method is not found to be linear. When a linear relationship of the change in renal function is established, then the slope of the line (rate of loss of renal function) and its error can be calculated by linear regression analysis to determine the effects of therapy on the course of disease. Furthermore, an estimate of prognosis can be made.

XII. NUTRITIONAL THERAPY AND PROGRESSION OF CHRONIC RENAL FAILURE

A technique for assessing the rate of loss of residual renal function permitted study of the effects of nutritional therapy on the rate of loss of residual renal function. The study was begun because it seemed possible that nutritional therapy might slow the rate of loss of renal function. A likely mechanism by which nutritional therapy might affect this rate is by correcting hyperphosphatemia. As suggested previously, calcium and phosphorus deposition in the kidney might be an important factor in the usually inexorable loss of residual renal function. For example, it has been reported that animals with CRF fed a phosphorus-restricted diet do not develop progressive loss of renal function.

To study the effect of nutritional therapy prospectively, dietary phosphorus was reduced for four patients with a serum creatinine of 10 mg/dl who had an established linear decline in the reciprocal of their serum creatinine concentration. They also received sufficient aluminum hydroxide to maintain their serum phosphorus concentration between 3 and 4 mg/dl. The rate of loss of renal function during the treatment period was then compared with the rate of loss that had occurred before institution of this program. Progression of renal insufficiency was arrested for more than a year in two patients, one with rapidly progressive glomerulonephritis (Fig. 3) and one with interstitial nephritis. Two other patients (one with diabetic nephrop-

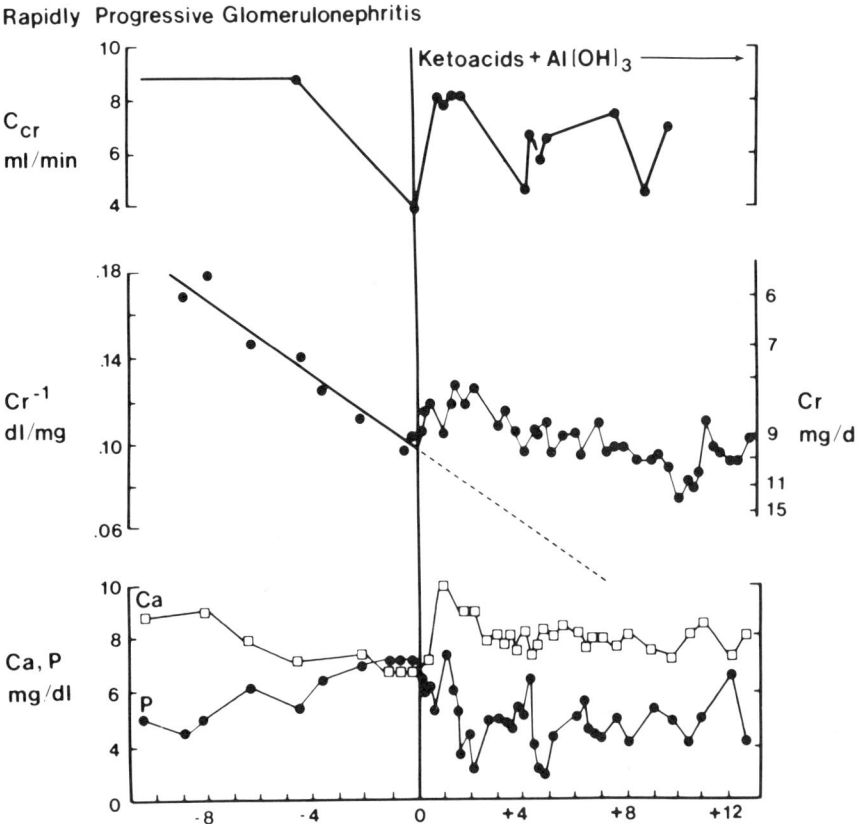

A.P.
Rapidly Progressive Glomerulonephritis

Figure 3. Effects of controlling serum phosphorus on changes in renal function. At a serum creatinine of 10 mg/dl, the constant loss of renal function (indicated by the linear decline of the reciprocal of serum creatinine) was stopped for more than 12 months by use of a phosphate-restricted diet and phosphorus-binding gel. Serial measurements of creatinine clearance confirmed that renal function was stabilized by this regimen.

athy and one with interstitial nephritis and chronic renal infection) had transient slowing of their progressive loss of renal function lasting several months, but subsequently the rate of loss of residual function returned to its previous value. How frequently this might occur if larger numbers of patients were managed similarly is not known. It is possible, however, that an even larger impact might be made on the course of the disease in patients with lower initial serum creatinines. These data clearly indicate the importance of a careful assessment of the rate of progression and raise the possibility that the course of CRF need not always be one of inexorable progression to end-stage renal disease.

ACKNOWLEDGMENT. This work was supported in part by a Research Career Development Award AM 00750 from The National Institutes of Health.

SUGGESTED READINGS

Bricker NS, Fine LG: The pathophysiology of chronic renal failure, in Maxwell MH, Kleeman CR (eds): *Clinical Disorders of Fluid and Electrolyte Metabolism*, ed 3. New York, McGraw-Hill, 1980, pp 799–825.

DeFronzo RA, Andres R, Edgar P, et al: Carbohydrate metabolism in uremia: A review. *Medicine* 52:469–481, 1973.

Dossetor JB: Creatinemia versus uremia. The relative significance of blood urea nitrogen and serum creatinine concentrations in azotemia. *Ann Intern Med* 65:1287–1299, 1966.

Fessel WJ: Renal outcomes of gout and hyperuricemia. *Am J Med* 67:74–84, 1979.

Goldberg AP, Hagberg JM, Delmez JA, et al: Metabolic effects of exercise training in hemodialysis patients. *Kidney Int* 18:754–761, 1980.

Holliday MA, McHenry-Richardson K, Portale A: Nutritional management of chronic renal disease. *Med Clin North Am* 63:945–950, 1979.

Ibels LS, Alfrey AC, Haut AL, et al: Preservation of function in experimental renal disease by dietary restriction of phosphate. *N Engl J Med* 298:122–126, 1978.

Kopple JD, Coburn JW: Metabolic studies of low protein diets in uremia. I. Nitrogen and potassium. *Medicine* 52:583–595, 1973.

Kopple JD, Coburn JW: Metabolic studies of low protein diets in uremia. II. Calcium, phosphorus and magnesium. *Medicine* 52:597–607, 1973.

Kopple JD, Swendseid ME: Vitamin nutrition in patients undergoing maintenance hemodialysis. *Kidney Int* 7:S79–S85, 1975.

Mitch WE: Nutrition in renal disease, in Klahr S, Massry S (eds): *Contemporary Nephrology*, vol 1. New York, Plenum Press, 1981, pp 551–577.

Mitch WE: Conservative management of chronic renal failure, in Brenner BM, Stein JH (eds): *Contemporary Issues in Nephrology*, vol 7: *Chronic Renal Failure*. Edinburgh, Churchill Livingstone, 1981, pp 116–152.

Mitch WE, Buffington G, Lemann J Jr, et al: Progression of chronic renal failure: A simple method of estimation. *Lancet* 2:1326–1328, 1976.

Mitch WE, Collier VU, Walser M: Creatinine metabolism in chronic renal failure. *Clin Sci* 58:327–335, 1980.

Mitch WE, Wilcox CS: Disorders of body fluids, sodium and potassium in chronic renal failure. *Am J Med*, 72:536–550, 1982.

Walser M: Determinants of ureagenesis, with particular reference to renal failure. *Kidney Int* 17:999–1007, 1980.

Walser M: Keto acid therapy in chronic renal failure. *Nephron* 21:57–74, 1978.

Walser M, Mitch WE, Collier VU: Essential amino acids and their nitrogen-free analogues in the treatment of chronic renal failure, in Schreiner G (ed): *Controversies in Nephrology*, Washington, D.C., National Kidney Foundation, 1979, pp 404.

Diagnosis and Therapy of Nephrolithiasis

CHARLES Y. C. PAK

I. INTRODUCTION

Nephrolithiasis is a common disorder affecting 0.1–0.5% of the population in the Western World. It is associated with considerable morbidity by causing obstruction, hematuria, or infection.

Although the ultimate symptomatic presentation may be the same, it is clear that nephrolithiasis is heterogeneous with respect to chemical composition and pathogenetic origin. Renal stones typically contain calcium (calcareous calculi); they are less commonly composed of cystine, struvite, or uric acid (noncalcareous calculi). Specific physicochemical and physiological disturbances have been identified. Thus, the urinary environment of patients with stones has been shown to be supersaturated with respect to stone-forming salts and to possess reduced inhibitor activity (against crystallization) and possibly enhanced promoter activity. Many patients with stones have been found to suffer from a variety of physiological (metabolic) disturbances including hypercalciuria, hyperoxaluria, and hyperuricosuria.

The above recognition has led to the refined classification and treatment of nephrolithiasis. Thus, it has been possible to formulate reliable diagnostic criteria for nephrolithiasis on the basis of underlying metabolic derangements in patients with nephrolithiasis. Moreover, treatments could be spe-

CHARLES Y. C. PAK • Department of Internal Medicine, Section of Mineral Metabolism, Southwestern Medical School at the University of Texas Health Science Center at Dallas, Dallas, Texas 75235.

cifically selected for their ability to "reverse" the particular underlying physicochemical and physiological disturbances.

This selective approach argues for a thorough diagnostic differentiation of various causes of nephrolithiasis and emphasizes the need for a careful selection of treatment program for each cause of nephrolithiasis. Its feasibility and practicality are considered in detail here.

II. DIAGNOSTIC CONSIDERATIONS

A. Heterogeneity of Chemical Composition of Calculi

Calcareous renal calculi comprise more than 75% of stones. They are usually composed of calcium oxalate as the predominant phase with calcium phosphate as a minor constituent. Stones of pure calcium oxalate or calcium phosphate (hydroxyapatite or brushite) are less common. Noncalcareous calculi include stones of uric acid (5%), cystine (1%), struvite (<20%), and rarely xanthine and 2,8-dihydroxyadenine.

The exact chemical nature of stones may have an intrinsic diagnostic value and may sometimes yield pathophysiological clues. Presence of cystine stones is diagnostic of cystinuria, and that of struvite (magnesium ammonium phosphate) implicates infection of the urinary tract with ureasplitting organisms. Uric acid lithiasis suggests gouty diathesis or chronic diarrheal syndromes. However, the occurrence of calcium-containing stones may have a limited diagnostic value (other than exclusion of causes of noncalcareous stones), since it may be associated with numerous metabolic disturbances.

B. Metabolic Classification of Nephrolithiasis

A simple and logical method of diagnostic differentiation of nephrolithiasis is categorization on the basis of underlying physiological abnormalities (Table I). This classification assumes that physiological disturbances are pathogenetically important in stone formation. Although complete validation is lacking, it is generally agreed that excessive renal excretion of calcium, uric acid, oxalate, or cystine may contribute to stone formation by rendering the urinary environment supersaturated with respect to stone-forming salts. This classification is based on major or principal physiological abnormalities. It is recognized that several disturbances may coexist in a given disorder.

Table I. Classification of Nephrolithiasis

Calcareous renal calculi
  Hypercalciuria (40–75%)[a]
    Resorptive
    Absorptive
    Renal
  Hyperuricosuria (~10% pure; 30–50% mixed)
  Hyperoxaluria (<5%)
    Primary
    Secondary
  Inhibitor deficiency/promoter excess (~5% pure; ~50% mixed)
  No metabolic abnormality (5–10%)

Noncalcareous renal calculi
  Uric acid stones (5%)
    Hyperuricosuria
    Low urinary pH
  Cystine stones (1%)
    Cystinuria
  Infection stones (<20%)
    Infection with urea-splitting organisms

---

[a] All values in parentheses refer to the total stone population.

III. PATHOGENESIS OF DIFFERENT CAUSES OF NEPHROLITHIASIS

A. Hypercalciuria

Three major causes of hypercalciuria, each associated with calcium nephrolithiasis, have been recognized.

In *resorptive* hypercalciuria, characterized by primary hyperparathyroidism, the initial event is the excessive resorption of bone from the hypersecretion of parathyroid hormone. The intestinal absorption of calcium is often elevated consequent to the parathyroid hormone-dependent stimulation of the renal synthesis of 1,25-dihydroxyvitamin D. These effects increase the serum concentration and the renal filtered load of calcium. Hypercalciuria often develops because of increased filtration of calcium and the suppressive effect of hypercalcemia on calcium reabsorption despite augmentation of calcium absorption by parathyroid hormone.

Hypercalciuria of primary hyperparathyroidism therefore originates from increased skeletal resorption and/or high calcium absorption. Only some patients with primary hyperparathyroidism present with hypercalciuria or nephrolithiasis. In stone-forming patients with this condition, hypercalciuria and urinary supersaturation with respect to calcium oxalate and brushite are usually found. Following successful parathyroidectomy, urinary calcium and saturation decline toward normal commensurate with a cessation or reduction in the rate of stone formation. However, many patients with primary hyperparathyroidism are free of renal stones despite persistent hypercalciuria and supersaturation of urine with respect to calcium salts. Reduced renal excretion of urinary inhibitors and/or increased urinary activity of promoters that facilitate crystallization have been proposed in stone-forming patients. Thus, nephrolithiasis may be the result of the combined influence of urinary supersaturation and reduced inhibitor and/or increased promoter activity.

The basic abnormality in *absorptive* hypercalciuria is the intestinal hyperabsorption of calcium. The consequent increase in the circulating concentration of calcium augments the renal filtered load of calcium and suppresses parathyroid function. Hypercalciuria results from the exaggerated renal filtered load of calcium and reduced renal tubular reabsorption of calcium consequent to parathyroid suppression. The excessive renal loss of calcium compensates for the high calcium absorption and maintains serum calcium concentration in the normal range.

The exact cause for the increased calcium absorption in absorptive hypercalciuria is not known. Several lines of evidence suggest the operation of a vitamin D-independent process. Intestinal calcium absorption remains elevated during treatment with adrenocorticosteroids, orthophosphate, or thiazide, agents that have been shown to alter vitamin D metabolism and urinary calcium excretion. The fractional (intestinal) calcium absorption bears no direct relationship with the serum concentration of 1,25-dihydroxyvitamin D. Finally, intestinal perfusion studies have disclosed high calcium absorption in jejunum but not in ileum and normal magnesium absorption. This selective jejunal hyperabsorption of calcium indicates a lack of an important pathogenetic role for vitamin D, since classic effects of vitamin D (or its metabolites) include enhancement of absorption of both calcium and magnesium in both intestinal segments.

However, that the increased calcium absorption may be vitamin D dependent is suggested by the finding of an elevated serum concentration of 1,25-dihydroxyvitamin D in approximately one-third of patients with absorptive hypercalciuria. To explain this rise, a scheme implicating an important role of hypophosphatemia has been proposed. It has been assumed that certain patients with absorptive hypercalciuria may have a primary "renal leak" of phosphate. The ensuing hypophosphatemia would then stimulate the renal synthesis of 1,25-dihydroxyvitamin D and increase calcium absorption. Although feasible, this scheme probably does not apply to the whole group. Hypophosphatemia and reduced renal threshold concentration for phosphorus are found in only a minority of patients with absorptive hypercalciuria when evaluated under the same dietary regimen and study setting as control subjects. Serum concentration of 1,25-dihydroxyvitamin D is not correlated with serum phosphorus or renal threshold concentration for phosphorus in patients with absorptive hypercalciuria. Finally, orthophosphate therapy does not reduce intestinal calcium absorption even though it lowers the serum concentration of 1,25-dihydroxyvitamin D.

In *renal* hypercalciuria, the primary abnormality is the impairment in the renal tubular reabsorption (renal leak) of calcium. The consequent reduction in serum calcium concentration stimulates parathyroid function. There may be an excessive resorption of bone from secondary hyperparathyroidism. Although clinical bone disease is rare, a significant reduction in bone density has been shown by ^{125}I photon absorptiometry. The intestinal calcium absorption may be increased in some patients. As in primary hyperparathyroidism, this increase is believed to result from the parathyroid hormone-dependent stimulation of the renal synthesis of 1,25-dihydroxyvitamin D. The serum concentration of 1,25-dihydroxyvitamin D is positively correlated with fractional calcium absorption. The correction of renal leak of calcium by thiazide restores normal calcium absorption commensurate with a fall in serum parathyroid hormone and 1,25-dihydroxyvitamin D.

The cause for the renal leak of calcium is not known. Complete renal tubular acidosis is not a part of the syndrome. Serum concentrations of sodium, potassium, chloride, and carbon dioxide are typically normal, and urinary pH is not different from that of control subjects. However, an inadequate renal handling of exogenous acid load, indicative of incomplete renal tubular acidosis, may be found in some patients. An exaggerated calciuric response to carbohydrate ingestion and enhanced natriuresis to hydrochlorothiazide have been reported, findings suggesting that abnormalities in tubular function may be present.

In all three forms of hypercalciuria, the urinary environment is characteristically supersaturated with respect to calcium oxalate and brushite, principally because of the high urinary concentration of calcium. Moreover, the formation product ratio (limit of metastability) of both calcium salts is often decreased. These effects combine to enhance the propensity for the spontaneous nucleation (or heterogeneous nucleation by naturally occurring nuclei) of calcium salts. In addition to the reduced metastable limit, the crystal growth and aggregation may sometimes be exaggerated, a finding indicating the operation of low inhibitor activity and/or high promoter activity. The above physicochemical profile is not unique to any one form of hypercalciuria, although the reduced limit of metastability is more commonly encountered in primary hyperparathyroidism.

B. Hyperuricosuria

Hyperuricosuria may be the only recognizable physiological abnormality in some patients with calcium nephrolithiasis. Such an abnormality (hyperuricosuric calcium oxalate nephrolithiasis) is found in 9–15% of calcium stone formers. The hyperuricosuria is usually the result of dietary overindulgence with purine-rich foods and sometimes is the sequela of a primary overproduction of uric acid. The urinary pH is typically greater than the pK_a for the first proton of uric acid (5.47), although it is reported to be lower than in non-stone-forming subjects in some series. Clinical gout is rare. Hyperuricosuria may coexist with all three forms of hypercalciuria.

The essential finding in hyperuricosuric calcium oxalate nephrolithiasis is the urinary supersaturation of monosodium urate which results from a high urinary content of uric acid and a favorable pH range (>5.5) in which this urate phase is stable. Although not yet proven conclusively, it has been suggested that either a colloidal or crystalline monosodium urate forms from such a supersaturated environment and initiates formation of calcium stones by (1) a direct induction of heterogeneous nucleation of calcium oxalate or (2) adsorption of certain mucopolysaccharides (which are inhibitors of crystal aggregation or spontaneous nucleation of calcium oxalate).

C. Hyperoxaluria

Although primary hyperoxaluria is a rare cause of calcium nephrolithiasis, enteric hyperoxaluria, associated with an inflammatory disease of the small bowel or with intestinal bypass surgery, may account for 1–5% of calcium nephrolithiasis. An increased intestinal absorption of oxalate is present and accounts for the hyperoxaluria. Two influences probably combine to cause the intestinal hyperabsorption of oxalate. The intestinal transport of oxalate may be primarily increased by the action of bile salts on the permeability of intestinal mucosa to oxalate. The total amount of oxalate absorbed may also be increased because of an enlarged intraluminal pool of oxalate available for absorption. The intestinal fat malabsorption characteristic of ileal disease may exaggerate soap formation with divalent cations, limit the amount of "free" divalent cations to complex oxalate, and thereby raise the available oxalate pool. The intestinal absorption and renal excretion of calcium are often decreased in enteric hyperoxaluria. Urine output may be substantially reduced consequent to excessive fluid loss from the intestinal tract. Urinary citrate and magnesium are usually reduced.

In calcium oxalate nephrolithiasis associated with enteric hyperoxaluria, there is an increased saturation of urine with respect to calcium oxalate because of the high oxalate concentration even though urinary calcium is low. Low urine volume exaggerates urinary supersaturation. Moreover, inhibitor activity against crystallization of calcium salts is reduced because of low renal excretion of citrate and magnesium.

D. Inhibitor Deficiency

There is some evidence that renal excretion of certain substances that retard crystallization of calcium salts may be deficient in some patients with nephrolithiasis. It is well known that the renal excretion of citrate is impaired in renal tubular acidosis and in enteric hyperoxaluria. Urinary citrate is also reduced in approximately 50% of patients with other causes of calcium nephrolithiasis. Low urinary pyrophosphate has been found in male patients with nephrolithiasis. Although unconfirmed, reports have appeared suggesting that urinary glycosaminoglycans, other organic inhibitors, and magnesium are reduced in nephrolithiasis.

There is some evidence that certain stone-forming urinary environments may contain substances that enhance crystallization of calcium salts. However, there are limited data concerning identification and characterization of such promoter substances.

E. Uric Acid Stones

The pK for the first proton of uric acid is 5.47. Thus, below this pH, uric acid, and not its salt, is the stable phase. Uric acid is sparingly soluble in this acid environment. The formation of uric acid stones is typically associated with the persistent passage of urine of low pH (<5.5) and/or hyperuricosuria. The conditions are therefore favorable to the formation of uric acid stones, because of the stability of uric acid, and since the urinary environment is usually supersaturated with respect to this phase.

F. Cystine Stones

Cystinuria is a disease of inborn error of metabolism characterized by a disturbance in renal and/or intestinal handling of dicarboxylic acids, including cystine.

Some patients with cystinuria may develop cystine stones. Stone formation is probably the result of an excessive renal excretion of cystine and the low solubility of this dicarboxylic acid in the normal acid pH of urine. Cystine solubility is pH dependent; at pH 5, only 200–300 mg cystine may be dissolved per liter of urine, whereas at pH 7.5, as much as 500 mg cystine may go into solution. Some patients with cystinuria often excrete more than 300 mg of cystine per day. In the normal acid environment, their urine may be supersaturated with respect to cystine, a condition favoring the formation of cystine stones.

G. Infection Stones

Urinary tract infection sometimes accompanies nephrolithiasis. When it results from non-urea-splitting organisms, the stone typically contains constituents other than struvite (magnesium ammonium phosphate). It is not known whether infection caused the stone or developed as a complication of the stone. When urea-splitting organisms (*Proteus*, certain species of *Staphy-*

lococcus, Pseudomonas, Klebsiella) are responsible for infection, stones typically contain struvite with varying amounts of apatite.

In some patients, struvite stones may have formed *de novo* as a consequence solely of infection. In others, specific metabolic disorders associated with the formation of other types of renal stones could be identified, such as hypercalciuria. Struvite stone formation in the latter instance probably results as follows: metabolic disorder → formation of nonstruvite stone → urinary tract infection with urea-splitting organisms → formation of struvite stone.

The physicochemical basis for struvite lithiasis is probably the same whether such stones form primarily or secondarily. The initial event is the formation of ammonia in urine on enzymatic degradation of urea by bacterial urease. The ammonia undergoes hydrolysis to form ammonium and hydroxyl ions. The resulting alkalinity of urine stimulates the dissociation of phosphate to form more trivalent phosphate ions and lowers the solubility of struvite. The activity product or the state of saturation of urine with respect to struvite ($MgNH_4PO_4 \cdot 6H_2O$) is therefore increased. Stone formation ensues when sufficient oversaturation is reached.

H. No Metabolic Abnormality

In fewer than 10% of patients with renal calculi, none of the above derangements may be present. Some of them may have formed stones from an acquired defect, since they give a history of low fluid ingestion and present with low urine output. Stones probably develop from the passage of concentrated urine which exaggerates supersaturation with respect to stone-forming salt. In the remaining patients, a disturbance in renal excretion of heretofore unidentified inhibitors or promoters best explains stone formation.

IV. DIAGNOSIS OF DIFFERENT CAUSES OF NEPHROLITHIASIS

A. History and Physical Examination

A positive family history of stones suggests absorptive hypercalciuria, cystinuria, or primary hyperoxaluria. A history of peptic ulcer disease and pathological skeletal fracture warrants a search for primary hyperparathyroidism. Patients with gout may form stones of either uric acid or calcium oxalate. A history of chronic diarrhea, ileal disease, or intestinal surgery should arouse the suspicion of uric acid stones or calcium oxalate stones (enteric hyperoxaluria). Absorptive hypercalciuria should be suspected in middle-aged Caucasian men with a history of recurrent passage of calcium stones, with no history of bone disease, and who have a positive family history of renal stones. Renal hypercalciuria may be present in patients with a history of recurrent urinary tract infection, especially if the infection preceded the onset of stone disease. Women are more commonly affected in primary hyperparathyroidism, whereas men outnumber women in absorptive hypercalciuria and hyperuricosuric calcium oxalate nephrolithiasis. The two sexes are equally affected in renal hypercalciuria.

A detailed history of dietary habits and drug ingestion should be taken. A high-calcium diet, as from an ingestion of an excessive amount of dairy products, may aggravate the stone disease in those patients with an intestinal hyperabsorption of calcium. A high-purine diet may cause hyperuricosuria and contribute to calcium stone formation (hyperuricosuric calcium oxalate nephrolithiasis). Adrenocorticosteroids, nonabsorbable antacids that bind phosphate, and vitamin D (in pharmacological amounts) may cause hypercalciuria. Vitamin D and ingestion of oxalate-rich foods (e.g., spinach) in excessive amounts may increase renal oxalate excretion. Acetazolamide may impair renal acidification and cause calcium phosphate nephrolithiasis.

The physical examination rarely yields any specific diagnostic clues, although the disclosure of band keratopathy or tophi would suggest the presence of hypercalcemia or hyperuricemia, respectively.

B. Stone Analysis and Roentgenologic Examination

Stone composition, if available or known to the patient, may provide the diagnosis or suggest the area needing a more thorough evaluation. The presence of struvite or carbonate apatite indicates infection with urea-splitting organisms. Cystine stones are pathognomonic of cystinuria. Uric acid stones suggest a disturbance in uric acid metabolism. Stones of calcium oxalate or calcium phosphate or both may indicate disorders of oxalate, urate, or calcium metabolism. Stone analysis may be obtained from several commercial laboratories, including Urolithiasis Laboratory, P.O. Box 25375, Houston, Texas, and Louis C. Herring and Co., P.O. Box 2171, Orlando, Florida.

The roentgenologic appearance of stones may be useful in diagnosis. Uric acid and xanthine stones are radiolucent. Struvite and calcium-containing stones are radioopaque. Cystine stones are opaque, though less so than calcium stones. Staghorn calculi may be seen with urinary tract infection with urea-splitting organisms, cystinuria, or with primary hyperparathyroidism. Nephrocalcinosis may be seen with renal tubular acidosis and primary hyperparathyroidism; it should be distinguished from medullary sponge disease which may be associated with stones and which may coexist with the metabolic derangements previously enumerated such as hypercalciuria.

C. Description of Ambulatory Diagnostic Protocol

Any medications that could affect the metabolism of calcium, uric acid, or oxalate should be discontinued prior to and throughout the period of evaluation. These medications would include vitamin D, aspirin, ascorbic acid, acetazolamide, as well as those that may have constituted the stone treatment program such as thiazide, phosphate, or magnesium.

Several approaches have been introduced for the diagnosis of different causes of nephrolithiasis, involving both inpatient and outpatient evaluation. Unfortunately, many of the diagnostic procedures have been developed in research centers, utilizing sophisticated procedures and a constant dietary regimen and involving trained nursing, dietary, and technical personnel. They may therefore be impractical or not applicable for evaluation in an ambulatory setting.

We have thus developed a reliable diagnostic protocol which could be performed in an ambulatory setting without the use of sophisticated instrumentation. It requires three outpatient visits and may be completed within a month. This evaluation depends largely on procedures that should be available in a routine clinical laboratory. Certain specialized procedures may be obtained commercially. An outline of our protocol for ambulatory patients with a summary of the laboratory tests obtained is shown in Table II.

Briefly, three 24-hr urine samples are collected. Two (random samples) are obtained while patients adhere to a random diet and reflect customary food intake. The third (restricted) sample is collected after a week of calcium and sodium restriction in order to standardize diagnostic tests. The week on a restricted diet is also a necessary preparation for the "fast and calcium load" study which is performed on the third visit. Blood samples are obtained on each visit.

On the first visit, the stone should be analyzed if it is available. A urological roentgenogram should be obtained if it has not been performed previously. Blood studies (on fasting venous blood) comprise complete peripheral blood cell count (CBC); a multichannel screen (SMA) including

Table II. Laboratory Tests in Protocol for Ambulatory Patients[a]

	Blood			Urine								Qualitative cystine
	CBC	SMA	PTH	Ca	UA	Cr	Na	pH	TV	Ox	cAMP	analysis
Visit 1	X	X	X	X	X	X	X	X	X			X
Visit 2		X		X	X	X	X	X	X			
Visit 3		X		X	X	X	X	X	X	X	X	
Fast				X		X					X	
Load				X		X					X	

[a] On visit 1, history is taken, physical examination is performed, and a 24-hr urine sample taken (random diet). On visit 2, another 24-hr urine sample is taken (random diet), and the patient is given a restricted (400 mg Ca, 100 mEq Na per day) diet to follow for at least 1 week. On visit 3, a restricted-diet 24-hr urine sample is collected, and fast and load tests are performed.

serum calcium, phosphorus, total proteins, albumin, alkaline phosphatase, sodium, potassium, carbon dioxide, chloride, creatinine, and uric acid; and serum immunoreactive PTH (PTH). Urine tests include spot sample for urinalysis, culture, and qualitative cystine, and 24-hr sample collected on a random diet for calcium (Ca), uric acid (UA), creatinine (Cr), sodium (Na), pH, and total volume (TV). Serum PTH may be obtained commercially (e.g., from Mayo Medical Laboratories, Rochester, Minnesota, or the Nichols Institute, San Pedro, California).

On the second visit, another 24-hr urine sample collected on a random diet is analyzed for calcium, uric acid, creatinine, sodium, pH, and total volume. Another blood sample is drawn for SMA. A diet history is taken, and the patient is given a diet of approximately 400 mg calcium and 100 mEq sodium per day to be maintained until the third visit (at least 1 week).

On the third visit, the 24-hr urine sample collected on the restricted diet is assayed for calcium, uric acid, creatinine, sodium, pH, total volume, oxalate (Ox), and cyclic AMP (cAMP) (the latter two tests may be obtained commercially, e.g., Bio-Science Laboratories, Van Nuys, California). Fasting venous blood is analyzed again for SMA. Following the collection of this restricted urine sample, the study of "fast and calcium load" is performed. It entails collection of a fasting 2-hr urine sample after an overnight fast and a 4-hr sample following an ingestion of 1 g calcium by adding appropriate amounts of NeoCalglucon® (Dorsey Laboratories, Lincoln, Nebraska) to a synthetic meal (Calcitest®, Doyle Pharmaceutical Co., Minneapolis, Minnesota) or milk. The samples are analyzed for calcium, creatinine, and cyclic AMP.

A high renal excretion of calcium during the fasting state is believed to denote either that there is an excessive mobilization of calcium from bone or that an impaired renal tubular reabsorption (renal leak) of calcium is present. The fasting urinary cyclic AMP may provide a measure of parathyroid function. The extent of renal calcium excretion following an oral load of calcium provides an indirect assessment of intestinal calcium absorption. These suppositions provide the basis for a simple test useful in the differentiation of the two major forms of idiopathic hypercalciuria. Fasting urinary calcium and cyclic AMP are increased in renal hypercalciuria because of the renal leak of calcium and secondary hyperparathyroidism. In absorptive hypercalciuria, these values are within the normal range, but there is an exaggerated urinary calcium excretion following an oral calcium load, reflecting the enhanced intestinal calcium absorption. It should be emphasized that the value of fasting urinary calcium depends on the preparation of patients on a low-calcium, low-sodium diet prior to the test. In patients with intestinal hyperabsorption of calcium, "abnormally" high values of fasting urinary calcium may be found if they are not so prepared.

As already stated, urinary cyclic AMP may be used as an indirect measure of parathyroid function. Urinary cyclic AMP is partly filtered from the general circulation, but much of this substance is produced within the renal tubules and "secreted" into the urine in response to parathyroid hormone.

The measurement of urinary cyclic AMP may be expressed in mmoles per milligram creatinine or, after multiplying this term by the serum creatinine (in mg per 100 ml), as nmoles per 100 ml glomerular filtrate (GF). The latter term is preferred because it not only adjusts the urinary cyclic AMP excretion for variations in body size but also for differences in renal function. Although urinary cyclic AMP measurements have proven to be a very reliable index of parathyroid function in many laboratories, other laboratories have not found this test to be useful. If a reliable PTH assay is available, measurement of urinary cyclic AMP may be deleted.

D. Diagnostic Criteria

Table III lists the normal values for pertinent serum and urinary data as determined in our laboratory. Although they should generally apply to different laboratory settings, these normal ranges should be validated for each laboratory. From comparison with these normal values, diagnostic criteria for each cause of nephrolithiasis may be formulated.

Absorptive hypercalciuria, type I is characterized by normocalcemia, normal fasting urinary calcium (<0.11 mg/100 ml GF), exaggerated urinary calcium following an oral calcium load (>0.2 mg/mg creatinine), normal or suppressed parathyroid function (serum PTH <36 μl Eq/ml using Isotex®

Table III. Normal Values for Serum and Urinary Data

Serum	
Ca (mg/dl)	<10.5
P (mg/dl)	>2.5
Uric acid (mg/dl)	Male <9.0, female <7.7
Bicarbonate (mEq/liter)	22–32
Chloride (mEq/liter)	97–108
24-hr urine	
Volume (ml/day)	>2000
pH	5.5–6.7
Ca	Random <4 mg/kg per day, restricted <200 mg/day
Na (mEq/day)	75–200
Uric acid (mg/day)	<600
Oxalate (mg/day)	<44
Cyclic AMP (nmole/100 ml GF)	<5.40
Qualitative urinary cystine	Negative
Fast	
Ca (mg/100 ml GF)	<0.11
Cyclic AMP (nmole/100 ml GF)	<6.85
Load	
Ca (mg/mg Gr)	<0.20
Cyclic AMP (nmole/100 ml GF)	<4.60

antiserum and 24-hr urine cyclic AMP in a restricted sample <5.4 nmole/100 ml GF), and urinary calcium on a restricted diet (400 mg calcium and 100 mEq sodium/day) of greater than 200 mg/day. These values reflect increased intestinal calcium absorption, resultant parathyroid suppression, and hypercalciuria.

Absorptive hypercalciuria, type II is characterized by the same biochemical features as type I except for normocalciuria (<200 mg/day) on a restricted diet. Apparently, intestinal calcium absorption from a low calcium intake is normal, whereas that from a high calcium intake is elevated. Indeed, if these patients are placed on a diet of 1000 mg calcium and 100 mEq sodium/day, urinary calcium exceeds 4 mg/kg per day or 250 mg/day. Absorptive hypercalciuria associated with hypophosphatemia has been termed hypophosphatemic absorptive hypercalciuria or *absorptive hypercalciuria, type III.*

Renal hypercalciuria is manifested by normocalcemia, high fasting urinary calcium (>0.11 mg/100 ml GF), and parathyroid stimulation (serum iPTH >36 μl Eq/ml using Isotex® antiserum and/or 24-hr urinary cyclic AMP on a restricted sample >5.4 nmole/100 ml GF). These results are indicative of a renal leak of calcium with compensatory parathyroid stimulation. It should be noted that either the serum PTH or urinary cyclic AMP (on the restricted 24-hr sample) must be elevated to diagnose renal hypercalciuria. In most patients, the urinary cyclic AMP, which is high in the fasting state, decreases to the normal range following an oral calcium load, a finding indicative of the suppressibility of parathyroid stimulation. Bone density may be decreased in patients with renal hypercalciuria, and in some cases osteopenia may occur.

Primary hyperparathyroidism may be recognized by the presence of hypercalcemia, hypophosphatemia, hypercalciuria, and increased or inappropriately high serum PTH and/or urinary cAMP. The fasting urinary cyclic AMP tends to be high and is not restored to normal following an oral calcium load, a result suggesting relative nonsuppressibility of PTH secretion. Hypercalcemic symptoms, peptic ulcer, or bone disease (osteitis, pathological fractures, osteoporosis) may be present.

Hyperuricosuric calcium oxalate nephrolithiasis is characterized by hyperuricosuria (urinary uric acid >600 mg/day on mean of three samples and on at least two samples), normocalcemia, normal fast and calcium load response, normal urinary calcium (<200 mg/day on a restricted diet) and oxalate (<44 mg/day), and calcium nephrolithiasis. Hyperuricosuria, defined functionally here by the upper normal limit of 600 mg/day, has been found to correlate well with the urinary supersaturation with respect to monosodium urate and with the propensity for calcium stone formation. (Other laboratories employ a higher upper limit for urinary uric acid, e.g., 750 mg/day for women and 800 mg/day for men.) Urinary pH is typically greater than 5.5. Hyperuricosuria may be the only abnormality present in patients with calcium stones, or it may coexist with various forms of hypercalciuria.

Hyperoxaluria, defined as urinary oxalate >44 mg/day, is associated with calcium oxalate stones. If urinary oxalate is >80 mg/day, primary or enteric hyperoxaluria is probably present. In primary hyperoxaluria, urinary glycolate or glycerate may be increased in addition to oxalate. Moreover, oxalosis (tissue deposition of calcium oxalate), anemia, and renal failure are common in primary hyperoxaluria. In eneteric hyperoxaluria, there is a history of small bowel disease, ileal bypass, or resection. Urinary calcium is typically low (<100 mg/day). Serum calcium and magnesium may be low or low normal, and parathyroid function may be stimulated. Serum bicarbonate and urinary citrate may be reduced. Even in the absence of intestinal disease, a mild to moderate hyperoxaluria (urinary oxalate 44–80 mg/day) may occur with vitamin D therapy, overindulgence with oxalate-rich foods (particularly spinach), or severe dietary calcium deprivation. Mild hyperoxaluria may also be seen in patients with increased calcium absorption, such as absorptive hypercalciuria.

One of the causes of *inhibitor deficiency* is renal tubular acidosis. *Renal tubular acidosis* is characterized by systemic hyperchloremic metabolic acidosis and high urinary pH (>6.8) in the absence of infection. Hypokalemia may also be present. Nephrocalcinosis is more common than nephrolithiasis, but calcium stones may occur. There is also an incomplete form of renal tubular acidosis characterized by normal serum pH and bicarbonate but an impaired ability to acidify the urine following ammonium chloride load. A high fasting urinary pH (>6) provides a clue to its existence. Both complete and incomplete forms may be associated with hypercalciuria and low urinary citrate (<400 mg/day).

Urinary citrate may be reduced in some patients with calcium nephrolithiasis independently of a defect in acidification.

Uric acid lithiasis is disclosed by the finding of uric acid on stone analysis. Typically, urinary pH is unusually low (<5.5), and serum uric acid high. Urinary uric acid may be normal or high. A microscopic examination of urinary sediment may show the presence of uric acid crystals.

In *cystinuria,* the cyanide–nitroprusside test provides a qualitative measure of the cystine content of urine. If positive, a quantitative test should be performed. In patients with cystine stones, urinary cystine is increased (>400 mg/day).

Infection lithiasis is disclosed by the presence of magnesium ammonium phosphate on stone analysis. Such struvite stones are often associated with pyuria, positive urine culture for urea-splitting organisms (*Proteus,* certain species of *Staphylococcus, Pseudomonas,* and *Klebsiella*), and high urinary pH (>7.0). Struvite stones are radioopaque and sometimes may attain a large (staghorn) size.

Rarely, patients with renal lithiasis may be found on intravenous pyelogram to have ectopic kidney, polycystic disease, or horseshoe kidney. Stones are typically radioopaque and usually consist of apatite or struvite. It is generally believed that these stones form secondarily to urinary tract infection.

Medullary sponge kidney is often associated with renal stones containing calcium oxalate and/or calcium phosphate. The same spectrum of metabolic abnormalities underlies this condition as in the overall population of stone formers.

Features of *no metabolic abnormality* are normal renal structure on pyelogram, normocalcemia, normal fast and calcium load response, normal serum PTH, normal values for urinary cyclic AMP, calcium, uric acid, and oxalate, and calcium nephrolithiasis. Urine volume is often less than 1 liter/day.

Diagnostic criteria for some of the major causes of nephrolithiasis are summarized in Table IV.

V. THERAPEUTIC CONSIDERATIONS

Improved elucidation of pathophysiology and formulation of diagnostic criteria for different causes of nephrolithiasis have made feasible the adoption of a selective or optimum treatment program. Such a program should (1) reverse the underlying physicochemical and physiological derangements, (2) inhibit new stone formation, (3) overcome nonrenal complications of the disease process, and (4) not cause serious side effects.

Table IV. Diagnostic Criteria[a]

	PHPT	AH-I	AH-II	AH-III	RH	HUCN
Serum Ca	↑	N	N	N	N	N
Serum P	↓/N	N	N	↓	N	N
Urinary Ca	↑/N	↑	N	↑/N	↑	N
Serum PTH	↑	N/↓	N/↓	N/↓	↑	N
Urinary cyclic AMP	↑	N/↓	N/↓	N/↓	↑	N
Urinary cyclic AMP (fasting)	↑	N	N	N	↑	N
Urinary cyclic AMP (1-g Ca load)	↑	N	N	N	N	N
α	↑/N	↑	↑/N	↑/N	↑/N	N
Urinary Ca (1-g Ca load)	↑/N	↑	↑	↑	↑/N	N
Urinary Ca (fasting)	↑/N	N	N	N	↑	N
Bone density	N/↓	N	N	N	N/↓	N
Urinary uric acid	N/↑	N/↑	N/↑	N/↑	N/↑	↑

[a] Fasting samples represent 2-hr urine collections obtained in the morning following an overnight fast. One-gram Ca load samples were obtained over a 4-hr period subsequent to oral ingestion of 1 g Ca. Fractional Ca absorption (α) was obtained from fecal recovery of radioactivity following oral administration of radiocalcium with 100 mg Ca. Bone density was obtained in the distal third of the radius by photon absorptiometry. PTH, immunoreactive parathyroid hormone; ↑, high; ↓, low; N, normal; PHPT, primary hyperparathyroidism; AH-I, absorptive hypercalciuria type I; AH-II, absorptive hypercalciuria type II; AH-III, hypophosphatemic absorptive hypercalciuria; RH, renal hypercalciuria; HUCN, hyperuricosuric oxalate nephrolithiasis.

The rationale for the selection of a treatment program according to its ability to reverse physicochemical and physiological abnormalities as outlined previously is the assumption that the particular physicochemical and physiological aberrations identified with the given disorder are etiologically important in the formation of renal stones and that the correction of these disturbances would prevent stone formation. Moreover, it is assumed that such a selected treatment program would be more effective and safe than a "random" treatment. Despite a lack of conclusive experiment verification, these hypotheses appear reasonable and logical.

A. Mechanism of Action of Therapeutic Modalities

For many treatment programs recommended for nephrolithiasis, sufficient information is now available to characterize their physicochemical and physiological actions. Tables V and VI summarize available data concerning the mode of action of some of the common therapeutic modalities for nephrolithiasis. Based on these actions, it may be possible to suggest optimal indications.

B. Selective Treatment Programs

1. Primary Hyperparathyroidism

Parathyroidectomy is the optimum treatment for nephrolithiasis of primary hyperparathyroidism. Following removal of abnormal parathyroid tissue, urinary calcium is restored to normal commensurate with a decline in

Table V. Physicochemical Actions of Therapeutic Modalities[a]

	PTX	SCP	PO₄	DiP	TZ	Allop	Mg	H₂O
Urine Ca	↓↓	↓↓↓	↓	—	↓↓	—	↑	—
Urine P	—	↑	↑↑↑	—	↑/—	—	↓	—
Urine Ox	—/↓	↑↑↑	↑/—	↑/—	↑/↓	—	↓	—
Urine Citr	↓	—	↑	—	↓	—	—	—
Urine P₂O₇	↓	—	↑↑	—	↑	↑/—	—	—
Brushite APR	↓	↓↓	↑	—	↓	—	↑	↓↓
FPR	↑	—	↑	↑	↑	↑/—	—	—
CG	↓	—	↓/—	↓	—	—	—	?
CaOx APR	↓	↓/—	↓	—	↓	—	—	↓↓
FPR	↑	—	↑	↑	↑	↑	—	↑
CG	↓	—	↑/—	↓	—	↓	—	?
Aggr	?	?	↓	↓	?	?	?	?

[a] Abbreviations: ↓, decrease; —, no change; ↑, increase; PTX, parathyroidectomy; SCP, sodium cellulose phosphate; PO₄, orthophosphate; DiP, diphosphonate; TZ, thiazide; Allop, allopurinol; Ox, oxalate; Citr, citrate; P₂O₇, pyrophosphate; APR, activity product ratio or state of saturation; FPR, formation product ratio or limit of metastability; CG, crystal growth; Aggr, aggregation.

Table VI. Physiological Actions of Therapeutic Modalities

	Primary action	Secondary action
PTX[a]	↓PTH	↓Serum Ca, Ca absorption, urinary Ca
SCP	↓Intestinal Ca absorption	↓Urinary Ca
PO_4	?	↓Urinary Ca, ↑citrate and P_2O_7
DiP	↑Urinary DiP	
TZ	↓Urinary Ca	↓Ca absorption in renal hypercalciuria, not in absorptive hypercalciuria
Allop	↓Uric acid synthesis	↓Urinary uric acid
Mg	↑Urinary Mg, ↓oxalate absorption	
H_2O	↑Urine output	↓Urinary concentration of stone-forming substances

[a] Abbreviations as in Table V.

serum concentration of calcium and in intestinal calcium absorption. The urinary environment becomes less saturated with respect to calcium oxalate and brushite, and its limit of metastability (formation product ratio) of these calcium salts increases. There is typically a reduced new stone formation rate unless urinary tract infection is present. Parathyroidectomy is contraindicated in secondary hyperparathyroidism of renal hypercalciuria and in absorptive hypercalciuria.

There is no established medical treatment for the nephrolithiasis of primary hyperparathyroidism. Although orthophosphates have been recommended for disease of mild to moderate severity, their safety or efficacy has not yet been proven. They should be used only when parathyroid surgery cannot be undertaken.

2. Absorptive Hypercalciuria

There is currently no treatment program that is capable of correcting the basic abnormality of absorptive hypercalciuria, although several drugs are available that have been shown to restore normal calcium excretion. *Sodium cellulose phosphate* best meets the criteria for optimum therapy. When given orally, this nonabsorbable ion-exchange resin binds calcium and inhibits calcium absorption. However, this inhibition is caused by limiting the amount of intraluminal calcium available for absorption and not by correcting the basic disturbance in calcium transport.

The above mode of action accounts for the two potential complications of sodium cellulose phosphate. First, the treatment may cause magnesium depletion by binding dietary magnesium as well. Second, sodium cellulose phosphate may produce secondary hyperoxaluria by binding divalent cations in the intestinal tract, reducing divalent cation–oxalate complexation, and making more oxalate available for absorption. These complications may be overcome by oral magnesium supplementation (1.0–1.5 g magnesium gluconate twice a day separately from sodium cellulose phophate) and mod-

erate dietary restriction of oxalate. Under such circumstances, sodium cellulose phosphate at a dosage of 10–15 g/day (given with meals) has been
shown to lower urinary calcium without significantly altering urinary
oxalate or magnesium, to reduce urinary saturation of calcium salts, and
to retard new stone formation. This drug therapy is contraindicated in
other forms of hypercalciuria because it may further stimulate parathyroid
function.

Thiazide exerts the same hypocalciuric action and physicochemical effects in absorptive hypercalciuria as in renal hypercalciuria (see treatment of
renal hypercalciuria). Unfortunately, the intestinal hyperabsorption of calcium is not corrected by this treatment in absorptive hypercalciuria, unlike
the case of renal hypercalciuria. The fate of retained calcium, reflected by the
reduced calcium excretion in the face of high calcium absorption, is not
known. Despite this uncertainty, thiazide has received a wide usage for
absorptive hypercalciuria, type I, since sodium cellulose phosphate is currently unavailable in the United States.

In *absorptive hypercalciuria, type II,* no specific drug treatment may be
necessary. Normal urinary calcium may be obtained by a moderate dietary
calcium restriction. Because urinary output is often low, a high fluid intake
sufficient to produce a urinary volume of at least 2 liters per day should be
encouraged.

Oral administration of *orthophosphate* (neutral or alkaline salt of sodium and/or potassium, 0.5 g phosphorus three or four times a day) has been
shown to lower serum concentration of 1,25-dihydroxyvitamin D. However,
it does not restore normal calcium absorption in absorptive hypercalciuria.
The treatment reduces urinary calcium, probably by directly impairing renal
tubular reabsorption of calcium. Urinary phosphorus is markedly increased
during therapy, a finding reflecting the absorbability of soluble phosphate.
Physicochemically, orthophosphate reduces urinary saturation of calcium
oxalate but increases that of brushite. Moreover, the urinary inhibitor activity
is increased, probably because of stimulated renal excretion of pyrophosphate and citrate. Although controversial, this treatment program has been
reported to cause soft tissue calcification and parathyroid stimulation. It
may be particularly indicated in *absorptive hypercalciuria, type III.* It is
contraindicated in nephrolithiasis complicated by urinary tract infection.

3. Renal Hypercalciuria

Thiazide is ideally indicated for the treatment of renal hypercalciuria.
This form of diuretic has been shown to correct the renal leak of calcium by
augmenting calcium reabsorption in the distal tubule and by causing extracellular volume depletion and stimulating proximal tubular reabsorption of
calcium. The ensuing correction of secondary hyperparathyroidism restores
normal serum 1,25-dihydroxyvitamin D and intestinal calcium absorption.
Physicochemically, the urinary environment becomes less saturated with
respect to calcium oxalate and brushite during thiazide treatment, largely

because of the reduced calcium excretion. Moreover, urinary inhibitor activity, as reflected in the limit of metastability, is increased by a heretofore undisclosed mechanism. These effects are shared by hydrochlorothiazide 50 mg twice a day, chlorthalidone 50 mg/day, or trichlormethiazide 4 mg/day. Potassium supplementation (40–60 mEq/day) may sometimes be required to prevent hypokalemia and attendant hypocitraturia. Concurrent use of triamterene, a potassium-sparing agent, should be undertaken with caution because of recent reports of triameterene stone formation. Thiazide is contraindicated in primary hyperparathyroidism because of potential aggravation of hypercalcemia.

4. Hyperuricosuric Calcium Oxalate Nephrolithiasis

Allopurinol (100 mg three times a day) is the physiologically meaningful drug of choice in hyperuricosuric calcium oxalate nephrolithiasis resulting from uric acid overproduction because of its ability to reduce uric acid synthesis and lower urinary uric acid. Its use in hyperuricosuria associated with dietary purine overindulgence is also reasonable, since dietary purine restriction is impractical. Physicochemical changes ensuing from restoration of normal urinary uric acid include a reduction in urinary saturation of monosodium urate and a commensurate increase in the urinary limit of metastability of calcium oxalate. Thus, the spontaneous nucleation of calcium oxalate is retarded by treatment, probably via inhibition of monosodium urate-induced stimulation of calcium oxalate crystallization.

5. Enteric Hyperoxaluria

Oral administration of large amounts of *calcium* (0.25–1.0 g four times a day) or magnesium has been recommended for the control of calcium nephrolithiasis of ileal disease. Although urinary oxalate may decrease (probably by binding of oxalate by divalent cations), the concurrent rise in urinary calcium may obviate the beneficial effect of this therapy, at least in some patients. Cholestyramine does not cause a sustained reduction in oxalate excretion. A limitation of dietary oxalate intake and partial replacement of dietary fat with medium-chain triglycerides may be helpful.

Treatment with potassium *citrate* or bicarbonate (60–120 mEq/day) may correct the hypokalemia and metabolic acidosis and restore urinary citrate toward normal. A high fluid intake is recommended to assure adequate urine volume.

6. Inhibitor Deficiency

Soluble *alkali* (sodium or potassium salt of bicarbonate or citrate, 20–30 mEq three or four times a day) may be effective in correcting acidosis, reducing urinary calcium, and increasing urinary citrate in *renal tubular acidosis*. The potassium alkali is probably superior to the sodium alkali with respect to the latter two actions. However, care should be taken in patients with renal insufficiency. Soluble alkali may also be effective in incomplete renal tubular acidosis in reducing urinary calcium and augmenting citrate excretion. The role of alkali therapy in promoting citrate excretion in other hypocitraturic states has not been clarified.

In patients with presumed deficiency in urinary inhibitors, therapy may be directed at stimulating the renal excretion of endogenous inhibitors or at providing exogenous inhibitors that would appear in urine. Treatment with *thiazide* (for example, hydrochlorothiazide 50 mg twice a day) may promote renal excretion of pyrophosphate and zinc, whereas that with *orthophosphate* (500 mg P three or four times a day) may augment excretion of pyrophosphate, citrate, and phosphocitrate.

Alternatively, an inhibitor such as *diphosphonate* may be given exogenously. Diphosphonate is a synthetic analogue of pyrophosphate. Unlike pyrophosphate, it is hydrolyzed *in vivo*. Approximately 5% of the oral dose of diphosphonate is absorbed. After saturation of bone, the absorbed diphosphonate eventually appears in urine in an unaltered form. A sufficient amount of diphosphonate may be excreted to inhibit the crystallization process and retard stone formation. Unfortunately, the usefulness of the commercially available diphosphonate (disodium etidronate) for the control of calcium nephrolithiasis is limited because of the potential for the induction of osteomalacia.

7. Uric Acid Stones

Oral administration of soluble salts of *bicarbonate* or *citrate* may increase urinary pH and create an environment in which uric acid is unstable. Unfortunately, an overaggressive alkali therapy may be complicated by calcium stone formation. Moderate amounts of alkali (~20 mEq three times a day) sufficient to increase urinary pH to a range of 6–6.5 may be helpful in the management of uric acid lithiasis without producing a significant risk for calcium stone formation. Potassium alkali is probably preferable to the sodium alkali.

Allopurinol may be used to control hyperuricosuria; a dose of 300 mg/day in three divided doses is generally sufficient to restore normal urinary uric acid. Dietary purine restriction is seldom practical. Probenecid is contraindicated because of its uricosuric action.

8. Cystine Stones

The object of treatment is to reduce the urinary concentration of cystine to below its solubility limit (200–300 mg/day). The initial treatment program includes a high fluid intake to promote an adequate urine flow and oral administration of soluble alkali (bicarbonate or citrate, 60–120 mEq/day) at a dose sufficient to raise urinary pH above 7. If this program is ineffective,

d-penicillamine (2 g/day in divided doses) may be used. Vitamin B_6 (50 mg/day) should be added to avoid pyridoxine deficiency. Potential side effects include nephrotic syndrome, dermatitis, and pancytopenia.

9. Infection Stones

If longstanding effective control of infection with urea-splitting organisms can be achieved, there is some evidence that new stone formation can be averted, or some dissolution of existing stones may be achieved. Unfortunately, such control is difficult to obtain with antibiotic therapy. If there is an existing struvite stone, it is difficult to completely clear the infection because the stone often harbors the organisms within its interstices. Even if "sterilization" of urine can be achieved by antibiotic therapy, reinfection could occur by harbored organism. For these reasons, it has been customary to recommend surgical removal of the struvite stones.

In recent clinical trials, acetohydroxamic acid, a urease inhibitor, has been shown to reduce urinary saturation of struvite and to retard stone formation.

10. No Metabolic Abnormality

Although they may have no physiological derangements, some of the patients with no metabolic abnormality present with low urine output, probably because of reduced fluid intake. A high *fluid* intake in amounts sufficient to achieve a minimum urine output of 2 liters/day may be efficacious. It has been shown to reduce urinary saturation of calcium oxalate, brushite, and monosodium urate and to inhibit spontaneous nucleation of calcium oxalate.

C. General Treatment Measures

In additional to the above specific measures, the following general measures may be imposed. A moderate oxalate restriction is instituted by discouraging ingestion of spinach, rhubarb, and chocolate. Ascorbic acid supplementation is denied because of potential metabolism of vitamin C to oxalate. A high sodium intake is discouraged by advising avoidance of "salty" food and salt shakers in an attempt to achieve an intake of less than 150 mEq/day. Patients are encouraged to drink at least 3 liters of fluids per day so as to achieve a minimum urine output of 2 liters per day. No attempt is made to control purine intake in an effort to alter uric acid excretion.

ACKNOWLEDGMENTS. This work has supported in part by USPHS grants P50-AM20543, M01-RR-00633, and R01-AM16061.

SUGGESTED READINGS

Coe FL: *Nephrolithiasis: Pathogenesis and Treatment.* Chicago, Year Book Medical Publishers, 1978.

Pak CYC: *Calcium Urolithiasis: Pathogenesis, Diagnosis, and Management.* New York, Plenum Medical Book Company, 1978.

Pak CYC (ed): Symposium on urolithiasis. *Kidney Int* (special issue), vol 13, 1978.

Pak CYC, Britton F, Peterson R, et al: Ambulatory evaluation of nephrolithiasis: Classification, clinical presentation and diagnostic criteria. *Am J Med* 69:19, 1980.

Thomas WC Jr: *Renal Calculi.* Springfield, Illinois, Charles C Thomas, 1976.

18

Bone and Mineral Disturbances in Renal Insufficiency

EDUARDO SLATOPOLSKY and JACK W. COBURN

I. INTRODUCTION

The kidney plays a key role in the metabolism of parathyroid hormone and vitamin D, the two main hormonal systems responsible for the regulation of calcium and phosphate balance. The homeostasis of calcium, phosphate, and magnesium in the body involves precise mechanisms that regulate the function of the skeleton, kidney, and gastrointestinal tract. In patients with chronic renal insufficiency, these intricate and complex feedback mechanisms are disrupted. Thus, alterations in bone and mineral metabolism become apparent. The aim of this chapter is to describe recent advances in the therapeutics of the alterations in bone and mineral metabolism observed in patients with chronic renal failure.

II. PATHOGENESIS OF RENAL OSTEODYSTROPHY

As the number of nephrons decreases and the glomerular filtration rate (GFR) approaches 60–70 ml/min, a series of disturbances in bone and mineral metabolism becomes apparent. Some of these manifestations are detected

EDUARDO SLATOPOLSKY • Department of Medicine, Washington University School of Medicine; Renal Division, Barnes Hospital; and Chromalloy American Kidney Center, St. Louis, Missouri 63110.   JACK W. COBURN • Research and Training Program in Nephrology, Veterans Administration Wadsworth Medical Center; and Department of Medicine, UCLA School of Medicine, Los Angeles, California 90024.

only if special analytical procedures are performed, i.e., determination of parathyroid hormone by radioimmunoassay. As the disease progresses and the degree of renal insufficiency becomes more marked (GFR < 25 ml/min), other abnormalities become apparent, and patients may develop symptomatic manifestations. If bone biopsies are performed in patients with advanced renal failure, histological abnormalities consistent with osteitis fibrosa and osteomalacia are present in the majority of patients. Osteosclerosis and osteoporosis are also present in some patients with advanced renal insufficiency.

A. Secondary Hyperparathyroidism

Secondary hyperparathyroidism is a universal complication of chronic renal disease. Chief cell hyperplasia of the parathyroid glands and high levels of radioimmunoassayable parathyroid hormone (iPTH) are among the earliest findings affecting mineral metabolism in patients with chronic renal failure. Mild elevations in iPTH in serum have been reported in patients with only slightly abnormal renal function (GFR 60–80 ml/min). Although many factors are responsible for the regulation and secretion of parathyroid hormone, it seems that in patients with renal insufficiency the most important cause for the development of secondary hyperparathyroidism is a reduced serum ionized calcium. The factors that may contribute to the development of secondary hyperparathyroidism in renal insufficiency include (1) phosphate retention, (2) altered vitamind D metabolism, (3) a skeletal resistance to the calcemic action of PTH, (4) impaired degradation of parathyroid hormone, and (5) altered feedback relationships between ionized calcium and the secretion of parathyroid hormone (Fig. 1).

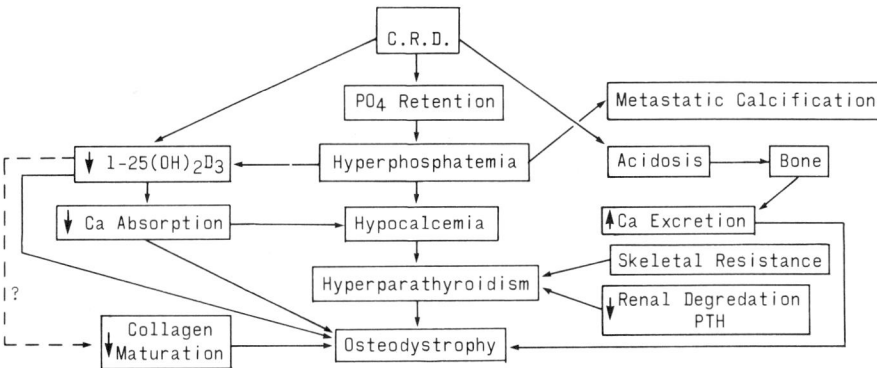

Figure 1. Diagrammatic representation of the pathogenetic factors responsible for the development of renal osteodystrophy. (From Slatopolsky E: *Kidney Int* S-253, 1975. Reprinted with permission.)

B. Phosphate Retention

Considerable evidence supports an important role of phosphate retention in producing secondary hyperparathyroidism. Reiss and collaborators demonstrated that a load of phosphorus that provided 1 g of elemental phosphorus led to an increase in serum phosphorus, a fall in ionized calcium levels, and an increase in serum iPTH in normal subjects. Other investigators have shown that the long-term feeding of a diet high in phosphate to animals with normal renal function can produce secondary hyperparathyroidism. Studies in experiemental renal failure in the dog have shown that the restriction of dietary phosphate could prevent the development of secondary hyperparathyroidism in azotemic dogs followed for 2 months, and subsequent studies showed a substantial reduction in serum iPTH levels in animals with renal failure treated with proportional reduction of phosphate for 2 years. Llach and collaborators demonstrated that a reduction in dietary phosphate intake in proportion to the decrease in GFR over a 2-month period in humans with a creatinine clearance of 50–90 ml/min was associated with a decrease iPTH to normal. Other studies have shown that serum iPTH levels correlate positively with the degree of hyperphosphatemia in patients undergoing dialysis. This observation provides support for a role of hyperphosphatemia in causing parathyroid hyperplasia in patients with advanced uremia.

The action of phosphate in through its effect of lowering ionized calcium concentration. Phosphate *per se* does not affect the release of parathyroid hormone. Although high concentrations of serum phosphate (7–9 mg/100 ml) increase the precipitation of calcium in soft tissue, the mechanism by which mild hyperphosphatemia affects the concentration of ionized calcium in serum is not known. Potentially, it may decrease the release of calcium by bone. More studies are necessary to precisely define the mechanism by which mild hyperphosphatemia affects the concentration of ionized calcium in serum. It is important to emphasize that in patients with far advanced renal failure (GFR less than 20 ml/min), correction of hyperphosphatemia alone will not reverse secondary hyperparathyroidism, since many other factors are responsible for the increased parathyroid hormone levels in blood.

C. Alterations in Vitamin D Metabolism

The kidney is the organ responsible for the conversion of vitamin D_3 to its active form, 1,25–dihydroxycholecalciferol [$1,25(OH)_2D_3$]. Thus, certain clinical disorders such as renal osteodystrophy may arise in part because of defective renal production in the active form of vitamin D in advanced renal failure. The liver hydroxylates vitamin D_3 to 25-hydroxycholecalciferol [$25(OH)D_3$], the predominant form of vitamin D_3 present in plasma. High plasma levels of 25 $(OH)D_3$ are observed after the ingestion of pharmacological doses of vitamin D. On the other hand, the renal conversion of 25 $(OH)D_3$ to $1,25(OH)_2D_3$ is closely regulated. The responsible enzyme, 25-hydroxycholecalciferol-1-hydroxylase, is localized in the mitochondrial fraction of the proximal tubular cells. Parathyroid hormone plays a key role in the stimulation of the 1-hydroxylase. This enzyme is also activated by diets low in phosphate. On the other hand, lack of parathyroid hormone or hyperphosphatemia decreases the action of the 1-hydroxylase and stimulates the activity of the 24-hydroxylase. Thus, the kidney is also geared to produce in those circumstances a different metabolite: 24,25-dihydroxychole-calciferol $[24,25(OH)_2D_3]$ (Fig. 2). Since one of the main actions of vitamin D is to stimulate intestinal transport of calcium, it is easy to understand that in patients with far-advanced renal insufficiency and low levels of $1,25(OH)_2D_3$, the absorption of calcium in the intestine is decreased.

The evidence that altered vitamin D metabolism contributes to abnormal calcium metabolism in advanced renal failure is considerable. Metabolic balance studies usually show that fecal calcium losses are equal to or greater than dietary calcium intake in patients with advanced renal insufficiency, and radioisotopic techniques also show reduced intestinal absorption of calcium in most patients with far-advanced renal failure. What is not known at the present time is at what level of renal insufficiency vitamin D metabolism becomes abnormal. This question is of considerable importance in considering the pathogenesis of secondary hyperparathyroidism of uremia.

Recently, Slatopolsky and collaborators have compared the levels of $1,25(OH)_2D_3$ and iPTH in a group of patients with normal renal function, patients with mild decrease in GFR (GFR between 40 and 60 ml/min), patients with advanced renal failure (GFR between 5 and 20 ml/min), and patients on dialysis. Of interest is that the plasma level of $1,25(OH)_2D_3$ is normal or even slightly elevated in patients with creatinine clearance greater than 40 ml/min. As expected, patients with severe renal insufficiency had low levels of $1,25(OH)_2D_3$, and dialysis patients had extremely low levels or undetectable levels of $1,25(OH)_2D_3$. If one assumes that a patient with a GFR of 50 ml/min has lost roughly one-half of the renal mass although the levels of $1,25(OH)_2D_3$ are normal, one has to conclude that the production of $1,25(OH)_2D_3$ per unit of renal mass is greatly increased. This could be a result of secondary hyperparathyroidism which is usually present in patients with mild renal insufficiency. Moreover, patients with a mild degree of renal insufficiency do not have calcium malabsorption.

Coburn and collaborators measured intestinal calcium absorption utilizing [47]Ca istopic techniques in patients with different degrees of renal insufficiency. They found that patients with mild renal failure and serum creatinine less than 2.5 mg/100 ml have calcium absorption values no different from those observed in normal volunteers. Another study of a large group of patients has indicated that as GFR decreases, there is a concomitant decrease in the absorption of calcium. However, this abnormality became evident only at GFR values below 30 ml/min. The results obtained in patients with GFRs

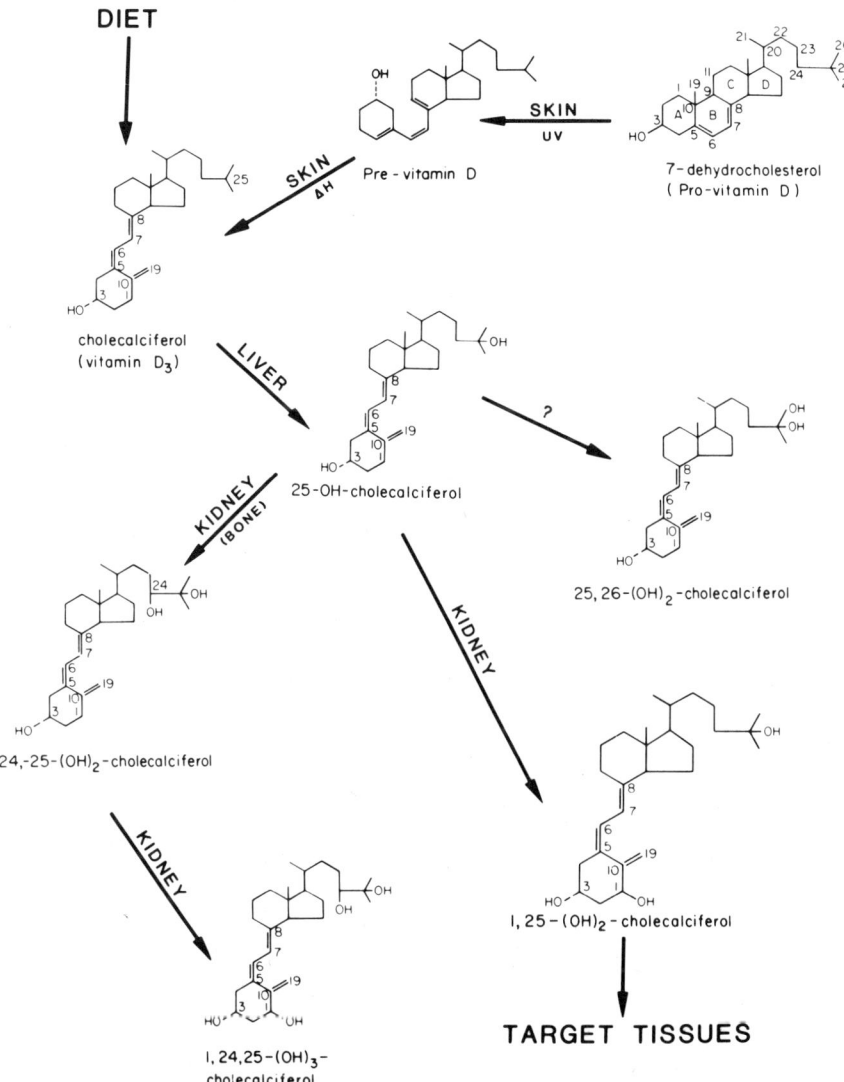

Figure 2. Schematic illustration of the bioactivation of vitamin D, which may arise either from the skin, via 7-dihydrocholesterol, or from the diet. UV, ultraviolet light; H, increased temperature. (From Coburn JW, Slatopolsky E: in Brenner B, Rector F (eds): *The Kidney*, ed 2. Philadelphia, WB Saunders, 1981. Reprinted with permission.)

greater than 60 ml/min were not different from those obtained in patients with normal renal function. Thus, there is no good evidence from the published data to support the concept that there is calcium malabsorption or low serum levels of 1,25(OH)$_2$D$_3$ in patients with early renal insufficiency.

Although the levels of $1,25(OH)_2D_3$ in most patients with advanced renal failure (GFR less than 20 ml/min) are low, many patients lack features of vitamin D deficiency. Thus, the reduced generation of $1,25(OH)_2D_3$ may not be the only factor responsible for the development of osteomalacia in this group of patients. Moreover, the lesions of osteomalacia occur in only a fraction of patients with advanced renal failure, and bone biopsies may fail to show histological evidence of vitamin D deficiency even in some anephric patients. It is possible that in some of these patients the occurrence of normal or elevated serum phosphorus levels may protect uremic patients from osteomalacia. The role of an abnomal generation of other vitamin D sterols and in particular of 24,25-dihydroxy D_3 in the pathogenesis of renal osteodystrophy remains uncertain. The kidney is the major organ responsible for the formation of $24,25(OH)_2D_3$, but there is evidence that this metabolite may also be produced in the intestine and bone. However, most of the recent information tends to indicate that patients with advanced renal insufficiency have low levels of $24,25(OH)_2D_3$.

D. Skeletal Resistance to the Action of Parathyroid Hormone

Skeletal resistance to the calcemic action of PTH may also play a role in the development of hypocalcemia seen in patients with renal insufficiency. In other words, higher circulating levels of PTH may be needed for the maintenance of a normal serum calcium in patients with renal failure. This is based on the observations of a delayed recovery from induced hypocalcemia in patients with mild renal insufficiency compared to results in normal subjects. Dietary phosphate restriction improves the calcemic response to the standardized infusion of parathyroid extract in patients with renal insufficiency.

That skeletal resistance to parathyroid hormone is an important factor in the development of secondary hyperparathyroidism has recently been challenged. A low-phosphate diet prevents the development of secondary hyperparathyroidism in experimental animals. However, those animals with renal failure developed skeletal resistance to the calcemic action of PTH. Thus, despite the presence of skeletal resistance to PTH, the dogs did not develop secondary hyperparathyroidism. Moreover, recent studies demonstrated that uremic dogs that received the intact PTH[1-84] molecule had an abnormal calcemic response. On the other hand, when the same animals received the biologically active amino-terminal fragment PTH[1-34], the calcemic response was normal. Abnormal metabolism of intact parathyroid hormone by the liver has been demonstrated in renal insufficiency. Thus, it is possible that the response to the administration of PTH[1-84], which has been used in the majority of studies in uremic animals, may not truly represent a state of skeletal resistance to parathyroid hormone. This particular issue requires further investigation.

E. Impaired Degradation of PTH
Secondary to Reduced Renal Function

Parathyroid hormone, a single-chain polypeptide containing 84 amino acids, is synthesized within the parathyroid glands from a biosynthetic precursor, a prohormone known as pro-PTH which has six additional amino acids attached to the amino terminal of the PTH$^{1-84}$ molecule. Pro-PTH is converted to PTH by proteolytic cleavage in the Golgi apparatus. Parathyroid hormone is secreted and rapidly metabolized by the liver and the kidney. Although PTH fragments also can be directly secreted by the parathyroid glands, the majority of fragments that circulate in blood are a product of peripheral metabolism of parathyroid hormone. The half-life of the intact molecule of PTH is rather short, less than 4 min, and the appearance of fragments in the periphery arises in part from the metabolism of PTH by the liver and kidney.

The uptake of iPTH by the liver is selective for intact hormone, indicating that the liver does not remove either amino-terminal or carboxy-terminal fragments from the circulation. The liver is a source of the carboxy-terminal and, presumably, the amino-terminal iPTH fragments found in the circulation. The kidney, on the other hand, removes from the circulation both intact PTH and amino- and carboxy-terminal PTH fragments. The biologically active forms of PTH (both intact and amino-terminal fragments) are removed by both peritubular uptake and glomerular filtration, whereas the biologically inactive carboxy-terminal fragments of iPTH depend exclusively on glomerular filtration and tubular reabsorption for their catabolism. Since the kidney is the only organ responsible for the removal of carboxy-terminal fragments, there is a marked accumulation of these fragments in peripheral plasma in patients with chronic renal failure, as predicted from the dependence of these fragments on glomerular filtration for the removal from the circulation. Thus, in patients with chronic renal insufficiency, the high levels of circulating immunoreactive parathyroid hormone result in part from increased secretion because of chief cell hyperplasia but also from a decreased catabolism secondary to the decreased number of nephrons and the effect of uremia on liver metabolism.

F. Altered Feedback Regulation between
Ionized Calcium and the Secretion of Parathyroid Hormone

It seems that the fine control whereby ionized calcium regulates the secretion of parathyroid hormone may be blunted in patients with chronic renal insufficiency. Hyperplastic parathyroid glands display less sensitivity to calcium than does normal tissue. This suggests that a mechanism for increased parathyroid hormone levels may be the shift in the set point for calcium as well as the increased tissue mass.

The set point is defined as the amount of calcium necessary to suppress the secretion of parathyroid hormone by 50%. The shift in the set point for calcium to inhibit hormone secretion is also manifested as an increase in the calcium concentration that inhibits the adenylatecyclase activity of membranes prepared from hyperplastic parathyroid glands obtained from patients with chronic renal insufficiency. Thus, normal concentrations of serum calcium may not be sufficient to suppress hyperplastic glands, and serum calcium may have to be increased to or even above the upper limits of normal to control the release of PTH in patients with secondary hyperparathyroidism.

G. Osteomalacia

Osteomalacia is another important feature of the skeletal disease seen in patients with advanced renal failure. Osteomalacia is defined as an increase in the osteoid seam width accompanied by a decrease in the mineralization front. The pathogenesis of impaired skeletal mineralization in patients with chronic renal failure is not clear, and although alterations in vitamin D metabolism undoubtedly play an important role, other factors may also potentially intervene in the pathogenesis of this disorder.

The mechanism whereby altered vitamin D metabolism leads to impaired demineralization of bone is poorly understood. Whether vitamin D or 1,25-dihydroxy D_3 can directly stimulate bone mineralization or whether they lead to mineralization by increasing the levels of calcium and phosphate in the extracellular fluid surrounding bone remains a matter of controversy. Although the plasma levels of 1,25-dihydroxy D_3 are reduced in patients with far-advanced renal insufficiency, overt osteomalacia is found in only a small fraction of patients with end-stage uremia. Moreover, osteomalacia may be absent even in anephric patients. Thus, other factors could also participate in the pathogenesis of osteomalacia in uremia patients.

The role of 24,25$(OH)_2D_3$ in the pathogenesis of osteomalacia has not been clarified up to this point. Another factor that may influence the development of osteomalacia is the plasma level of phosphorus. Hypophosphatemia per se can produce severe osteomalacia, even in patients with normal renal function. Alterations in collagen synthesis and maturation also may play an important role in the development of osteomalacia. Experimental studies in uremic rats have shown a preponderance of immature soluble collagen that fails to mineralize normally. Treatment of such uremic animals with 25-hydroxy D_3 can restore the collagen maturation toward normal.

Bone crystal maturation is also affected in patients with renal insufficiency. Immature bone contains large quantities of amorphous calcium phosphate. Other alterations in bone include an increase in magnesium, elevated levels in pyrophosphate, and diminished carbonate content. The combination of these factors may play a role in the maturation of the bone and potentially contribute to the development of osteomalacia. Acidosis may also contribute to a skeletal disease. In chronic renal insufficiency, the skeleton plays an important role buffering the excess of hydrogen entering the body. Administration of bicarbonate and correction of the acidosis in azotemic patients can reduce the urinary fecal calcium. Acidosis also may affect the metabolism of vitamin D and in this manner affect the mineralization of bone. Finally, retention of trace element and water contaminants such as aluminum may play an important role in the development of osteomalacia. In many patients with high concentrations of aluminum in serum, the major source of aluminum is believed to be that present in the dialysate. In certain locations with high aluminum content in the water, the incidence of osteomalacia appears to decrease with deionization of the water. There may be sporadic cases in which the aluminum may arise, in large part, from phosphate-binding antacids. In these patients, phosphate restriction in the diet is mandatory to allow a decrease in the amount of phosphate binders ingested. Finally, recent evidence suggests that the lack of parathyroid hormone, as has been seen in patients after total parathyroidectomy, may have precipitated in the development of osteomalacia.

H. Clinical and Biochemical Features of Altered Divalent Ion Metabolism

Most symptoms related to altered divalent ion metabolism appear only when renal failure is advanced. On the other hand, certain biochemical alterations appear early in the course of renal insufficiency. Knowledge of the presence of these alterations may help the physician to introduce treatment early in the course of renal insufficiency and aid in the prevention of severe complications in bone and mineral metabolism.

In addition to bone pain and fractures, numerous signs and symptoms can occur in association with altered divalent ion metabolism in uremia. Bone pain can develop and progress slowly to a point at which the patient is bedridden; moreover, this can occur independently of whether the skeletal pathology is osteitis fibrosa or osteomalacia. The bone pain is generally vague and commonly located in the lower back, hips, knees, and legs. Low back pain may arise from a collapse of a vertebral body, and sharp chest pain may be the indication of a spontaneous rib fracture. Physical findings are frequently lacking.

Muscular weakness, when present, is usually proximal and appears slowly and progresses as time goes by. Plasma levels of muscle enzymes, creatinine phosphokinase and transaminase, are usually normal and the electromyographic changes are nonspecific. The pathogenesis of such muscle weakness is uncertain. In patients with myopathy, electron micrography has revealed localized disorganization of the myofibrils and dispersion of Z-band, material changes that revert to normal following 25-hydroxy D_3. The muscular weakness has also been attributed to secondary hyperparathyroidism on a neuropathic basis.

Pruritus is a common symptom in uremic patients: it is common in patients with severe secondary hyperparathyroidism. The levels of calcium in the skin may be elevated in such patients. Pruritus also can develop in uremic patients receiving pharmacological doses of vitamin D and during the infusion of calcium. *Peripheral ischemic necrosis* and *vascular calcification* have been reported in rare patients. The lesions may involve the tips of the toes and fingers, and the skin becomes violaceous. Ulcerations and scar formation may occur with clear demarcation of the lesions from the surrounding skin. Most of the patients with these alterations have concomitant severe secondary hyperparathyroidism, and some of these patients have benefited from subtotal parathyroidectomy.

Acute pain and swelling around one or more joints may develop in uremic patients. The syndrome of *calcified periarthritis,* which may be caused by the deposition of hydroxyapatite crystals, is accompanied by marked hyperphosphatemia. Spontaneous rupture of the tendon can occur in uremic patients. Abnormality of collagen metabolism, as is thought to exist in uremic bone, may occur in tendons and predispose to this disorder.

Skeletal deformities are common in azotemic children who are growing. Bowing of the tibia and femur and deformities from slipped epiphyses are not uncommon. Children with renal trickets sometimes exhibit typical radiographic findings of vitamin D deficiency. In adults with renal failure, particularly those with osteomalacia, marked skeletal deformities with lumbar scoliosis, thoracic kyphosis, and deformities of the thoracic cage may be observed. *Growth retardation* is usually seen in young children both before and during maintenance hemodialysis. Several factors such as malnutrition, chronic acidosis, and severe osteomalacia may contribute to the retarded growth. Caloric supplementation, correction of acidosis, and addition of 1,25-dihydroxy D_3 may improve the growth retardation.

From the biochemical point of view, one of the early changes in patients with renal insufficiency (GFR between 60 and 80 ml/min) is the presence of elevated levels of circulating iPTH. As the disease progresses (GFR less than 30 ml/min) *hypocalcemia* may be present in a number of patients. Alterations in ionized calcium are seen earlier than changes in total serum calcium. This is because of an increase in the complexed fraction of calcium. In patients with advanced renal insufficiency, the serum calcium may remain close to normal, and values below 7.5 mg per 100 ml are infrequent. Usually, hypocalcemia is more marked in those patients who have severe osteomalacia and in those with profound metabolic acidosis. Occasionally, *hypercalcemia* may be observed in uremic patients, particularly those undergoing long-term dialysis. This can arise from severe secondary hyperparathyroidism or the ingestion of large amounts of calcium or vitamin D or occur from unrelated diseases such as sarcoidosis or malignancy or with a "pure" mineralizing defect.

Hyperphosphatemia is usually common in patients with GFR less than 25 ml/min. The degree of hyperphosphatemia depends on the amount of phosphate ingested in the diet, the fraction absorbed in the intestine, and that excreted into the urine. Obviously, if the patient ingests phosphate binders, the serum phosphorus may remain normal despite advanced renal insufficiency. Other factors such as parathyroid hormone also influence the concentration of phosphate in serum. Although parathyroid hormone decreases the reabsorption of phosphorus in the renal tubule, it also mobilizes phosphate from bone. Thus, patients with severe hyperparathyroidism and advanced renal insufficiency usually have higher concentrations of serum phosphate in plasma.

Hypermagnesemia occurs in patients with renal insufficiency when the GFR falls below 15 ml/min. The intake of magnesium-containing antacids by patients with severe renal failure can lead to abrupt and marked hypermagnesemia. The increase in serum magnesium levels is usually associated with an increased content of magnesium in bone, a factor that may affect crystal formation. In patients receiving chronic hemodialysis, the dialysate often contains a magnesium concentration of 1.5 mEq/liter, and blood levels of 2.5 and 3.5 mEq/liter are commonly seen with this dialysate concentration of magnesium.

Total serum alkaline phosphatase levels are commonly increased in uremic patients with osteitis fibrosa, osteomalacia, and mixed lesions. Alkaline phosphatase is comprised of isozymes arising from the intestine, liver, kidney, and bone, Despite the heterogeneity of the enzyme, alkaline phosphatase measurements can provide an indication for increased osteoblastic activity. In dialysis patients, the serum alkaline phosphatase can correlate with the osteoid surface covered with osteoblasts, resorbing surfaces, the number of osteoclasts, and the percentage of osteoid seams that take up tetracycline. Coexistent liver disease should be excluded as a cause of elevated alkaline phosphatase.

I. Bone Histology

Bone biopsies are critical in the diagnosis and management of patients with renal osteodystrophy. The most common finding in bone histology is osteitis fibrosa secondary to high levels of parathyroid hormone. In these patients, the histology usually reveals increased numbers of osteoclasts, increased woven osteoid, increased bone resorption surface, and many Howslip's lacunae. These patients also show increased quantities of woven osteoid which differ from the usual laminar osteoid in that the former exhibits a haphazard arrangement of collagen fibers. Woven osteoid can become mineralized in the absence of vitamin D. However, the calcium may be deposited as amorphous calcium phosphate rather than as hydroxyapatite. The excess deposition of calcium phosphate in the woven osteoid may explain the presence of osteosclerosis in some patients. The presence of an increased quantity of osteoid *per se* does not indicate the presence of osteomalacia or defective mineralization. The amount of osteoid present in bone depends on the rate of apposition of osteoid by osteoblasts, the rate of its calcification, and the extent of the bone surface involved in apposition and mineralization. Thus, the diagnosis of osteomalacia depends on the presence of osteoid and an abnormal mineralization front.

The extent of the bone surface undergoing calcification can be measured by staining with toluene blue *in vitro* or by tetracycline labeling *in vivo*. A decrease in the calcification front has been taken to be evidence for osteomalacia. The use of double tetracycline labeling in conjunction with quantitative histomorphometric techniques can provide the best method for identification of defective mineralization. Patients showing a preponderance of osteomalacia may have a tendency towards hypocalcemia with a low calcium–phosphate product in serum. Bone turnover rate measured with double tetracycline labeling is normal or increased above normal in patients with osteitis fibrosa, whereas it is below normal in patients with osteomalacia.

Another subgroup of dialysis patients with pure osteomalacia or mineralizing defect with little or no evidence of secondary hyperparathyroidism has been identified. This group of patients has failed to improve following treatment with 1-α-hydroxy D_3 or $1,25(OH)_2D_3$.

J. X-Ray Features of Secondary Hyperparathyroidism

Standard techniques as applied in clinical practice are often inconsistent in identifying the progression of renal osteodystrophy. Techniques to increase the sensitivity of X-rays which are particularly useful in views of the hands include the use of fine-grain film (i.e., Kodak M industrial film or mammography film), the use of manual rather than automatic film developing methods, the omission of grid or screen techniques, and magnification techniques. The main feature of secondary hyperparathyroidism is an increase in bone resorption more commonly seen on the subperiosteal surfaces of bone. Erosions that occur in conjunction with formation of new bone may appear as cysts or osteoclastomas (Brown tumors). The presence of subperiosteal erosions correlates with serum iPTH and histomorphometric features of osteitis fibrosa on biopsy.

Subperiosteal resorption of the phalanges detected by fine-grain hand radiographs may be the most sensitive radiographic sign of secondary hyperparathyroidism. The tuft of the terminal phalanx or the second or third digit commonly shows resorption. With severe tuft erosions, there may be a collapse of the soft tissue and a change in the contour of the tuft so that the finger appears to show clubbing. Bone erosions may also occur at the upper end of the tibia, the neck of the femur or the humerus, and the lower surface of the medial end of the clavicle. In the skull, resorption leads to a mottled and granular appearance commonly associated with altering areas of osteosclerosis. The lamina dura often shows erosions in primary hyperparapthyroidism but is uncommonly affected by secondary hyperparathyroidism. Increased endosteal resorption, manifested by scalloping of the endosteal surface or widening of the central canal of long bones, may also occur as part of secondary hyperparathyroidism. Osteosclerosis is thought to be another feature of osteitis fibrosa arising from an increase in the thickness and number of trabeculae in spongy bone. Osteosclerosis can lead to a typical "rugger jersey" appearance of the spine.

K. Radiographic Features of Osteomalacia

The X-ray features of osteomalacia are far less distinctive than those of secondary hyperparathyroidism. The Looser zone or pseudofracture are the only pathognomonic findings of osteomalacia in the adult. The typical X-ray features of rickets, i.e., widening of the epiphyseal growth plate, cannot develop after epiphyseal closure and hence are limited to children. With mechanical stress of severe prolonged vitamin D deficiency, a Looser zone may extend across the full width of the bone and produce a true fracture with displacement of fragments. Features such as increased haziness of indistinctiveness of the trabecula, biconcavity of the vertical bodies, particularly in association with normal body density, and bending deformities of long bones are said to be typical of osteomalacia, but these findings are uncommon and may not be easily recognized. Uremic patients with osteomalacia commonly have secondary hyperparathyroidism with concomitant X-ray features of the latter. Thus, a diagnosis of osteomalacia rests on histological examination, and one can only be certain of this diagnosis from bone biopsy.

L. Extraskeletal Calcifications

The factors that predispose to the appearance of soft-tissue calcification include an increase in the calcium–phosphate product in plasma, the degree of secondary hyperparathyroidism, the magnitude of alkalosis, and local tissue injury. Three major varieties include (1) calcification of medium-sized arteries, (2) articular or tumoral calcifications, and (3) visceral calcifications affecting the heart, lung, and kidney. Arterial calcification often involves the media of the vessel. These calcifications are diffuse and continuous along the vessels, and their appearance contrasts to the regular discrete appearance of calcified intimal plaques. Such medial calcifications of the vessels may be first seen in the dorsalis pedis artery where it appears as a ring or tube as it descends between the first and second metatarsal. Other sites commonly involved are the ankles, abdominal aorta, feet, pelvis, hands, and wrists.

M. Miscellaneous Determinations of Bone Mineral Content

Several methods have been used to measure the content of bone mineral for the purpose of quantitating bone mass. These include photon absorptiometry and neutron activiation. Although these methods can provide a quantitation of bone mass or mineral content, they offer no information regarding the cause of the abnormality or change. Photon absorptiometry provides a noninvasive method for the serial measure of bone mass. Measurements are conventionally taken over the phalanges, radius, and ulna. With this methodology, the mineral content of the midradius and ulna has been found to be lower in dialysis patients than in age-matched controls. Moreover, a progressive bone loss may occur with the duration of dialysis therapy. Neutron activation may provide an accurate method for measuring total bone mineral calcium in the whole body or in isolated parts of the skeleton. This technique has been useful in research studies of bone mineral content, particularly when the serial measurements are followed to evaluate the response to a specific treatment method.

III. PREVENTION AND TREATMENT

The objectives of the treatment of abnormal mineral metabolism and bone disease in patients with chronic renal insufficiency are (1) to return the blood levels of calcium and phosphorus to normal, (2) to suppress secondary hyperparathyroidism, (3) to reverse the histological abnormalities in the skeleton, and (4) to prevent and reverse extraskeletal deposits of calcium and phosphate. Different therapeutic regimens to be considered in the management of renal osteodystrophy are outlined below and summarized in Table I.

A. Control of Phosphate

Hyperphosphatemia is a major factor leading to the development and maintenance of secondary hyperparathyroidism in chronic renal failure. Phosphate retention also aggravates renal osteodystrophy by decreasing the activity of the 1-hydroxylase, therefore reducing the conversion of 25-hydroxy D_3 to 1,25-dihydroxy D_3. Moreover, high serum phosphorus levels contribute to the development of soft tissue calcification. Thus, the restriction of dietary phosphorus intake and the prevention of hyperphosphatemia are critical in the management of renal bone disease.

The usual phosphorus intake by normal adults in the United States is 1 to 1.5 g per day. One can lower the dietary intake of phosphate in proportion to the decrease in GFR in patients with mild renal insufficiency. Thus, dietary phosphate intake can be reduced to 600–800 mg, or approximately 60% of normal, by restricting the ingestion of dairy products and with rigid adherence to a low-protein diet. However, there will be great difficulty in lowering phosphorus intake in proportion to the reduction in GFR in patients with advanced renal failure; thus, aluminum-containing compounds that reduce the intestinal absorption of phosphorus must be given.

Table I. Guidelines for Management of Renal Osteodystrophy

Early treatment
  GFR 30 to 40 ml/min

Control of serum phosphorus (P) (3.5–5.0 mg/dl)
  Restrict phosphorus intake in diet to 600 to 800 mg/day
  Phosphate-binding antacids: aluminum carbonate or hydroxide; individualize dosage:
    Basalgel®, Dialume®, Alucap®, Amphogel®, 1–4 cap. with each meal
  Hypophosphatemia should be avoided
  Predialysis phosphorus: 4.5–5.5 mg/dl

Adequate calcium intake
  Oral calcium supplements providing 1–2 g/day when serum P is controlled: Os-Cal®,
    Titralac®
  Dialysate Ca, 6.5–6.8 mg/dl (3.25–3.40 mEq/liter)

Use of vitamin D sterols
  Indications for treatment: adequate control of serum P and
    Hypocalcemia
    Overt 2° hyperparathroidism (high iPTH and bone erosions) with serum Ca < 11.0 mg/dl
    Osteomalacia (with 2° hyperparathyroidism)
    Children with chronic renal failure
    Concomitant anticonvulsant therapy
    Proximal myopathy
    ? Prophylaxis
  Types and approximate daily doses
    Vitamin D_2 or D_3, 50,000 to 250,000 IU (1.25 to 6.25)
    Dihydrotachysterol, 0.25–2.0 mg/day
    25-hydroxyvitamin D_3 (calcifidiol), 25–100 μg/day (Calderol®)
    1,25-dihydroxyvitamin D_3 (calcitriol), 0.25–1.0 μg/day (Rocaltrol®)
    1-hydroxyvitamin D_3, 0.5–2.0 μg/day

Parathyroidectomy: Indications are evidence of severe secondary hyperparathyroidism (bone
    erosions and increased iPTH) plus any of the following:
  Persistent hypercalcemia (serum Ca > 11.5–12.0 mg/dl)
  Progressive or symptomatic extraskeletal calcification
  Persistently elevated serum calcium × phosphorus product
  Pruritus not responsive to medical treatment
  Calciphylaxis (ischemic ulcers and necrosis)
  Symptomatic hypercalcemia after renal transplantation

Other management considerations
  Appropriate dialysate magnesium 0.6–1.0 mg/dl (0.5–0.7 mEq/liter)
  Water treatment for dialysate preparation: remove fluoride, aluminum, calcium, and
    magnesium
  Avoid unnecessary treatment with barbiturates, phenytoin, or glutethemide
  Normalize acid–base status

Table II illustrates the calcium and phosphorus content of commonly consumed foods in the American diet. The goal with the use of phosphate binders is to reduce serum phosphorus to near normal. Thus, predialysis serum phorphorus should be maintained at 4.5 to 5.5 mg/ml to prevent the development of hypophosphatemia at the end of the dialysis (Fig. 3). When a patient's creatinine clearance is 5–10 ml/min, the administration of a diet

Table II. Comparative Calcium and Phosphorus Content of Commonly Consumed Foods in the American Diet[a]

Food	Ca (mg)	P (mg)	Food	Ca (mg)	P (mg)	Food	Ca (mg)	P (mg)
Cottage cheese, large curd, 1 cup	212	342	Frankfurter	4	76	Chili con carne with beans, canned, 1 cup	82	321
Saltines, 10	6	26	Cheddar cheese (prepackaged slices), 1 slice	158	100	Chicken chow mein without noodles, home cooked, 1 cup	58	293
Fried egg, 1 large	28	102	Lettuce raw, shredded, 1 cup	19	14			
Flounder fillet baked with butter	23	344	White bread, enriched, 1 slice	24	27	Coffee, instant, 1 cup	4	7
Lamb chops, loin, broiled, 6 (9 oz ea) [yield from 1 lb chops with bone)	24	429	Tomatoes, ripe tomato, approx. 7 oz	24	49	Chocolate chip cookies, homemade, 4 cookies	14	40
			Spinach, canned, drained, 1 cup	242	53	Corn-on-the-cob, cooked, 1 ear	2	69
Shrimp, french fried, 1 oz	20	54	Broccoli (frozen), boiled, drained, 1 cup	100	104	Beef liver, fried, 1 slice	9	405
Beef noodle soup, canned, prepared with water, 1 cup	7	48	Cauliflower (frozen), boiled, drained, 1 cup	31	68	Lobster Newburg, 1 cup	218	480
						Oatmeal, cooked, 1 cup	22	137
Chicken noodle soup, canned, prepared with water, 1 cup	10	36	Beans, green canned, 1 cup	81	50	Orange juice, frozen, 6-oz glass	19	32
			Ice cream (plain), hard, 1 cup	194	153	Peanut butter, 1 tbsp	9	61
Minestrone soup, canned, prepared with water, 1 cup	37	59				Peas (frozen), boiled, 1 cup	30	138
			Bacon, cooked, 2 thin slices	1	22	Apple pie, average slice	9	26

Food		
Tomato soup, canned, prepared with water, 1 cup	15	34
Vegetable beef soup, canned, prepared with water, 1 cup	12	49
Spaghetti, home cooked with tomato sauce and meatballs, topped with Parmesan cheese, 1 cup	124	236
Winter squash, baked, mashed, 1 cup	57	98
Tuna, canned, drained, 1 cup	13	374
Pumpkin pie, average slice	58	79
Puffed rice cereal	3	14
Danish pastry (plain), 1 piece	21	46
Hard roll	24	46
Rye bread, 1 slice	19	37
Bologna	1	17
Pork and beans, canned, 1 cup	138	235
T-bone steak, cooked (yield from 1 lb raw)	24	490
Ground beef, cooked, 3-oz patty	10	196
Beef and vegetable stew, home-cooked, 1 cup	29	
Biscuit mix made with milk, 1 biscuit	19	65
Bran flakes with raisins, 1 cup	28	146
Chocolate devil's food cake, without icing, 1 cupcake	24	45
Peanuts, roasted, salted	21	114
Cheese, American, pasteurized processed pre-packaged slices, 1 slice	188	208
Chicken, fried, 1 drumstick	6	89
Cherry pie, average slice	17	30
Popcorn, with oil and salt added, 1 cup	1	19
Ham, baked, 3 oz	9	201
Pork chops, broiled, 8 (2 oz ea; yield from 1 lb raw chops with bone)	28	624
French fries, 10 strips	12	87
Mashed potatoes, milk added, 1 cup	50	103
Potato chips, 10	8	28
Pretzels (3-ring), 10	7	39
Rice, white, long-grain, cooked, 1 cup	21	57
Milk, whole, 1 cup	288	227
Sesame seeds, dry, hulled, 1 tbsp	9	47
Ice cream, plain, soft-serve, 1 cup	253	199

a Adams CF: Nutritive Value of American Foods in Common Units. Handbook No. 456, Agricultural Research Service, United States Department of Agriculture, 1975.

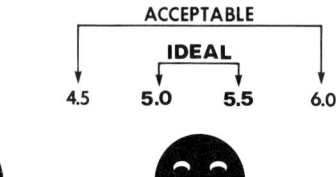

Figure 3. Diagrammatic representation of the ideal predialytic serum phosphate.

restricted in phosphorus, in the range of 600–700 mg/day, and the administration of two to four capsules of aluminum carbonate or aluminum hydroxide gel with each meal will usually maintain serum phosphorus within the normal range. If the patients are not yet on dialysis, the serum phosphorus should be maintained between 3.5 and 4.5 mg/100 ml. If the serum phosphorus decreases below 3.5/100 ml or remains above the desired range, the number of capsules should be decreased or increased, respectively, by one or two capsules with each meal. Antacids containing magnesium should be avoided because of the risk of hypermagnesemia. Several phosphate binders are available in the market (Table III) in liquid, tablet, or capsule form. The

Table III. Phosphate Binders[a]

Aluminum carbonate gel

  Basaljel®
    Tablets or capsules
      Equivalent to 608 mg dried aluminum hydroxide gel

    Suspension
      One teaspoonful (5 ml) equivalent to 500 mg aluminum hydroxide

    Extra strength suspension
      One teaspoonful (5 ml) equivalent to 1000 mg aluminum hydroxide

Aluminum hydroxide gel

  Amphogel®
    Tablets
      0.3 g (300 mg) aluminum hydorxide
      0.6 g (600 mg) aluminum hydroxide

    Suspension
      One teaspoonful (5 ml) contains 320 mg aluminum hydroxide

  Dialume®
    Capsules
      500 mg aluminum hydroxide powder

  Alu-Cap®
    475 mg dried aluminum hydroxide

  Alu-Tab®
    600 mg dried aluminum hydroxide

[a] These commercial preparations containing magnesium should not be prescribed to uremic patients: Aludrox®, Camalox®, Creamalin®, Gelusil®, Gaviscon®, Maalox®, Mylanta®, Riopan®, Silain-gel®, Tricreamalate®, and Wingel®.

tablets and capsules are less effective than liquid gels in binding phosphorus, but a patient's compliance is easier to achieve with the use of capsules and tablets than with liquid forms. If a patient develops hypophosphatemia, this is easily corrected by temporarily discontinuing the medication. However, if severe hypophosphatemia persists, drugs that will rapidly correct the hypophosphatemia are available (Table IV).

One of the obstacles to the use of aluminum-containing gels is the potential development of aluminum accumulation. There is substantial evidence that the administration of a large quantity of aluminum may be fatal to rats if it is given orally as poorly soluble aluminum gels or parenterally as a soluble aluminum salt. The possibility of aluminum accumulation in humans as a consequence of antiacid ingestion has been raised. Of the two main sources whereby aluminum may enter the body—the ingestion of aluminum-containing drugs described above and aluminum contamination of dialysate—the latter source of aluminum entrance into the body is the most signficant. Presently, no means are available for controlling the inevitable hyperphosphatemia in uremia other than by the use of aluminum-containing compounds: thus, weighing the known hazards of hyperphosphatemia against the theoretical risk of aluminum toxicity, one is left with no choice other than recommending the use of these compounds to control serum phosphorus levels.

B. Control of Calcium

Because of restriction in dairy products, the majority of patients treated with maintenance hemodialysis ingest diets containing only 400 to 700 mg of calcium per 24 hr. Several balance studies have demonstrated that the majority of patients with GFR lower than 20 ml/min have a significant degree of calcium malabsorption. Thus, patients with far-advanced renal insufficiency or those maintained on hemodialysis are in constant negative calcium balance unless their diets are supplemented. Positive calcium balance can be achieved in uremic patients with calcium carbonate, citrate, or lactate if the total intake of calcium is increased to 1.5 to 2 g of elemental calcium per day.

Calcium carbonate is the first choice as a source of supplemental calcium as it contains a high fraction of calcium and is inexpensive, tasteless,

Table IV. Phosphorus Preparations

Oral	
Whole cow's milk	100 ml = 90.0 mg phosphorus
Neutra-Phos®	1 capsule = 250 mg phosphorus
Fleet Phospho-Soda®	1 ml = 120 mg phosphorus
Parenteral	
Na-Phosphate Abbott®	(15-ml vial to be diluted)
	1 ml = 99 mg phosphorus

and relatively well tolerated. Moreover, calcium carbonate can bind phosphorus in the intestine and aid in the control of hyperphosphatemia. Also, because of the carbonate, this form of calcium helps to control the metabolic acidosis. Calcium carbonate contains 40% elemental calcium compared to only 12% for calcium lactate and 9% for calcium gluconate. To maximize calcium absorption, the quantity of calcium should be divided into several small doses taken throughout the day rather than as one or two large doses.

One should not attempt to correct hypocalcemia until the serum phosphorus is under good control. If the patient has hyperphosphatemia and ingests large amounts of calcium, the increments of their concentrations in blood can produce metastatic calcification. If possible, the serum calcium should be maintained at the upper limits of normal. This is because a higher concentration of calcium is required to suppress the release of PTH by hyperplastic parathyroid glands compared to normal glands. There are several commercially available calcium preparations (Table V).

Treatment with oral calcium supplements is not without risk. Patients with advanced renal failure who are given dietary supplements of calcium may be more likely to develop hypercalcemia than are normal individuals, since patients with renal failure lack the mechanism for increasing the urinary excretion of calcium if calcium absorption increases more than expected. Hypercalcemia may be more prone to develop in patients whose serum phosphorus levels are rapidly lowered to below 3 mg per 100 ml. Supplemental calcium administration should be discontinued if the serum calcium increases above 11.5 mg/100 ml.

The concentration of calcium in dialysate can clearly affect serum calcium levels in patients treated with maintenance hemodialysis. Predialysis iPTH levels have been found to vary indirectly with plasma calcium levels in dialysis patients using a dialysate calcium level below 6 mg/100 ml for more than 6 months. On the other hand, plasma iPTH levels often decrease with the use of dialysate levels of 6.5 to 7 mg/100 ml and when the serum phosphorus is maintained between 4.5 and 5.5 mg/100 ml. The ideal calcium concentration in the dialysate is between 6.25 and 6.75 mg/100 ml. Concentrations above 7 mg/100 ml should not be used because of the high incidence of pruritus and increased deposition of calcium in the skin.

C. Use of Vitamin D

Despite dietary control of phosphorus, the use of phosphate binders, the adequate intake of calcium in the diet, and appropriate levels of calcium in the dialysate, a significant number of uremic patients still develop skeletal disease. Vitamin D and its metabolites are important and effective agents in the treatment of renal osteodystrophy. The prevention of renal osteodystrophy may be favored with treatment with an active vitamin D sterol early in the course of renal insufficiency. However, no conclusive data are available regarding the efficacy or safety of such therapy in humans.

Table V. Calcium Preparations

Oral	
Os-Cal®	1 tablet = 250 mg calcium
Os-Cal® 500	1 tablet = 500 mg calcium
Titralac®	1 tablet = 168 mg calcium
Parenteral	
Calcium Chloride Bristol®	1 g in 10 ml (10% calcium)
Calcium Gluceptate Abbott®	1 ampule = 90 mg calcium

1. Principles of Usage, Effectiveness and Chemistry

Vitamin D and its metabolite, 25-hydroxycholecalciferol and 1,25-dihydroxycholecalciferol, are effective in the treatment of altered divalent ion metabolism in patients with chronic renal insufficiency. Humans normally acquire vitamin D either from the diet or through ultraviolet irradiation of the provitamin, 7-dehydrocholesterol, a compound present in the skin. The quantity of vitamin D_3 produced endogenously depends on the geographical latitude, the season, and the degree of exposure to sunlight and may average 2.5 to 10 μg/day (100–400 IU), values near the minimum daily requirement. Vitamin D can also be ingested as D_3 (cholecalciferol) or D_2 (ergocalciferol), a compound produced synthetically by the ultraviolet irradiation of a plant sterol (ergosterol); the latter is added to dairy products and bread in the United States. Vitamin D is absorbed in the proximal small bowel, carried in plasma bound to a specific vitamin D-binding protein, molecular weight 59,000, and transported to the liver and other tissues. The liver hydroxylates vitamin D to $25(OH)D_3$, the predominant form of vitamin D_3 present in plasma.

There is a seasonal increase in plasma $25(OH)D_3$ levels late in the summer; marked increases in plasma level of $25(OH)D_3$ occur after ingestion of pharmacological doses of vitamin D_3. 1,25-Dihydroxyvitamin D_3 is approximately 100 times more potent than $25(OH)D_3$ in increasing calcium absorption in the gastrointestinal tract.

2. Side Effects

The most common and important side effect of vitamin D administration is the development of hypercalcemia. Patients with mild hypercalcemia may be totally asymptomatic. However, as serum calcium increases to above 12.0 mg/100 ml, numerous symptoms may be present, and numerous organs of the body may be effected. The most common symptoms are nausea, vomiting, polyuria, polydipsia, lack of concentration, fatigue, somnolence, mental confusion, and even death (see Table VI and Chapter 3). Hypercalcemia also may cause both acute and reversible decrement in GFR or chronic nephropathy. In addition, acute hypercalcemia may produce natriuresis and ECF vol-

Table VI. Clinical Manifestations of Hypercalcemia

General
  Apathy, lethargy, weakness

Cardiovascular
  Cardiac arrhythmias, hypertension, vascular calcification

Renal
  Polyuria, hypercalciuria, stones, nephrocalcinosis, impaired concentration of urine, renal
    insufficiency

Gastrointestinal
  Anorexia, nausea, vomiting, polydypsia, constipation, abdominal pain, gastric ulcer,
    pancreatitis

Neuropsychiatric and muscular
  Headache, impaired concentration, loss of memory, confusion, hallucination, coma, myalgia,
    muscle weakness and arthralgia

Metastatic calcification
  Band keratopathy, conjunctival irritation, vascular calcification, periarticular calcification

---

ume contraction. In chronic hypercalcemic nephropathy, there is a fall in GFR and a decrease in the maximum concentrating capacity.

Calcium has an inotropic effect on the cardiovascular system. An increase in peripheral resistance and hypertension occur in 20–30% of patients with chronic hypercalcemia. The positive inotropic effect of digitalis is enhanced by calcium, so that digitalis toxicity may be aggravated by hypercalcemia. Occasionally, abdominal pain, distension and ileus may be present. Calcium increases the release of gastrin and hydrochloric acid in the stomach. Moreover, the incidence of pancreatitis is also increased. Patients with chronic hypercalcemia also may develop band keratopathy, which is the appearance of a corneal calcification; these corneal changes are usually permanent.

Another less frequent side effect of vitamin D is the development of hyperphosphatemia. A rise in serum phosphate has been observed in uremic patients receiving metabolites of vitamin D. Most of the clinical effects of hyperphosphatemia are related to secondary changes in calcium metabolism. Besides hypocalcemia, ectopic calcification is an important complication of hyperphosphatemia. It seems that when the calcium-phosphate product exceeds 70, the chances for precipitation are greatly increased. In addition to the effect of a high calcium–phosphate product, local tissue factors may favor calcium precipitation. For example, local alkalosis may favor calcification of the cornea and lungs. When vitamin D metabolites are used in patients with reduced GFR, increased concentrations of calcium and phosphate in blood and the deposition of calcium in the kidney may lead to further deterioration of renal function.

3. Kinetics

Vitamin D and its metabolites are well absorbed from the gastrointestinal tract. 25-Hydroxyvitamin D_3 (calcifidiol), when administered orally like vitamin D, is absorbed via the lacteals with bile salts playing an obligatory role. Studies performed in healthy volunteers indicate that 62 to 77% of an oral dose is absorbed over a dose range between 1 and 10 μg/kg. Peak responses were observed at 4–8 hr. A specific carrier has been shown to bind 25-hydroxy D_3 mole for mole with a K_d of 6.4 $\times$ 10^{-8} M. Both vitamin D_3 and $1,25(OH)_2D_3$ are also bound by this protein, but they are bound with a lower affinity constant. Both vitamin D and 25(OH)D_3 are widely distributed to many tissues. Skeletal muscle is an important site for the accumulation of 25-huydroxy D_3. 25-Hydroxyvitamin D_3 is the main circulating form of vitamin D, with a normal plasma level of 20–40 ng/ml. The disappearance of vitamin D from the circulation occurs with a plasma half-life of about 20–30 hr; in contrast, 25(OH)D_3 has a plasma half life of 12–23 days following its oral administration. The principal route of excretion of 25(OH)D_3 appears to be via the bile, and there is evidence for enterohepatic recirculation.

1,25-Dihydroxyvitamin D_3, (calcitriol) has a half life of 14–18 hr when radioacitve calcitriol is administered. A single oral dose of calcitriol results in maximum serum levels in approximately 3–4 hr independently of the doses employed from 1 to 5 μg. The half-life was calculated to be 5–6 hr, and the daily turnover rate was calculated to be approximately 0.5 μg/day. Compartmental analysis indicated that the renal rate of synthesis is approximately 0.3–1 μg/day, and the daily turnover rate in adults is approximately 0.5 μg/day. Calcitriol stimulates intestinal phosphate transport by a mechanism that appears to be independent of calcium. The intestine and the skeleton are the two most important target organs for the action of calcitriol.

There are at least two important pathways of inactivation of calcitriol. The first pathway is characterized by the side-chain oxidative cleavage of calcitriol. The second is the conversion to 1-α-24R,25-trihydroxyvitamin D_3 which occurs in the intestine and kidney and which is about one-third as active as 1,25-dihydroxy D_3.

4. Preparation and Dosage

Vitamin D is formulated in capsules containing 50,000 IU (1 mg is equal to 40,000 IU). The recommended dose is 50,000 to 250,000 IU per day.

25-Hydroxyvitamin D_3 or calcifidiol (Calderol®) is available in soft gelatin capsules containing the drug in two strengths, 50 μg (orange opaque) or 20 μg (white opaque). Each strength is available in bottles of 60 capsules. The recommended dose is 50 to 100 μg per day.

1,25-Dihydroxyvitamin D_3 or calcitriol (Rocatrol®) is available in gelatin capsules in two strengths, 0.25 μg (light orange) and 0.5 μg (dark orange). Each strength is available in bottles of 30 and 100 capsules, and the recommended dose is 0.25 to 1 μg per day.

1α-Hydroxyvitamin D_3, 1-Alpha®, is produced by Leo Pharmaceutical in Europe and Alpha-D_3® by Teva in Israel; the recommended dose is 0.5 to 2 μg per day.

Dihydrotachysterol (DHT), a synthetic sterol, is produced by Winthrop Laboratories with the trade name of Hytachyrol® and by Philips Roxane with the name of Dihydrotachysterol® tablets. Hytachyrol® is available in capsules of 0.5 mg and in oil in volumes of 15 ml containing 0.25 mg/ml of active drug. Dihydrotachysterol® tablets are supplied as white tablets in two strengths: 0.125 mg and 0.4 mg. A 0.2-mg strength is available as a pink tablet. The recommended dose for dihydrotachysterol is 0.25 to 2 mg per day. Dihydrotachysterol is biologically active without the necessity for 1α-hydroxylation by the kidney. The hydroxyl group responsible for biological activity is in the position of carbon atom 3, but the A ring is rotated to give a "pseudo-1α-hydroxy" group that is equivalent to carbon atom 1 of $1,25(OH)_2D_3$. Dihydrotachsteral and 1α-hydroxy D_3 undergo hepatic hydroxylatin, and 25-hydroxy DHT and 1,25-dihydroxy D_3 are the major circulating forms for these agents.

Presently $24,25(OH)_2D_3$ is still an experimental drug and it is not available for general use. The results obtained in several research facilities are too preliminary to draw strong conclusions about the drug's effects or usefulness.

5. Clinical Applications

As described previously, the two main components of renal osteodystrophy are osteitis fibrosa and osteomalacia. Excellent results have been obtained in patients with secondary hyperparathyroidism in whom the serum calcium was returned to normal after previous correction of their hyperphosphatemia. Regardless of the pathogenetic mechanisms responsible for the development of secondary hyperparathyroidism, hypocalcemia is the main factor responsible for the continuous increased secretion of parathyroid hormone in uremic patients. Thus, achievement of positive calcium balance in patients with chronic renal failure would represent a conservative, noninvasive therapeutic approach to correcting secondary hyperparathydoidism.

However, in some circumstances, the addition of calcium to the diet may not be sufficient to induce positive calcium balance. Numerous papers have clearly indicated the beneficial effects of vitamin D metabolites in the treatment of overt secondary hyperparathyroidism. Thus, appropriate doses of vitamin D, dihydrotachysterol, $25(OH)D_3$, $1-(OH)D_3$, and $1,25(OH)_2D_3$ can improve symptoms, bone disease as determined from X-rays, and skeletal histology. These compounds will also lower the serum levels of alkaline phosphatase and immunoassayable parathyroid hormone. If the main abnormality in patients with chronic renal failure is the presence of severe hypocalcemia, $1,25(OH)_2D_3$ is the drug of choice. Since $1,25(OH)_2D_3$ is extremely effective in the gastrointestinal tract, addition of supplemental calcium to the diet will easily correct the hypcalcemia. Moreover, because of the short half life of calcitriol, if hypercalcemia results, it will subside within 3–4 days.

Unfortunately, the results obtained in the treatment of osteomalacia are more controversial and less rewarding. Although nutritional osteomalacia in patients with normal renal function is secondary to a deficiency in vitamin D ingestion, the osteomalacia seen in uremic patients may arise from factors not related to vitamin D. Only a fraction of patients with renal osteomalacia have shown improved bone histology after $1,25(OH)_2D_3$. This may be in part related to the small dose of $1,25(OH)_2D_3$ given to these patients. Because of the great gastrointestinal response to $1,25(OH)_2D_3$, enhanced calcium reabsorption may lead to hypercalcemia. On the other hand, the gastrointestinal effect of $25(OH)D_3$ is 100 times less potent than that of $1,25(OH)_2D_3$. Doses in the range of 50–100 μg/day can be used in the majority of patients. Moreover, investigators have shown that some patients with nutritional osteomalacia show improvement after the use of $25(OH)D_3$ but not after $1,25(OH)_2D_3$. Thus, if the main bone histological lesion is osteomalacia, it seems advisable to start with a drug such as $25(OH)D_3$ (calcifidiol) which is less likely to produce hypercalcemia. Unfortunately, a study comparing the actions of vitamin D metabolites on bone disease in uremic patients does not exist at present.

D. Subtotal Parathyroidectomy

The treatment modalities outlined above can lead to improved homeostatis of calcium and phosphorus, a reversal of symptoms of bone disease, and suppression of parathyroid hypersecretion. However, such measures may be unsuccessful, and certain features of secondary hyperparathyroidism may dictate the need for parathyroid surgery. Indications for parathyroid surgery include (1) persistent hypercalcemia, particularly when symptomatic, (2) intractable pruritus which does not respond to dialysis or other medical treatment and is associated with high levels of parathyroid hormone, (3) progressive skeletal calcification in conjuction with a calcium–phosphorus product that is consistently above 75–80 despite appropriate phosphate restriction, (4) severe progressive skeletal pain and pathological fractures associated with high levels of parathyroid hormone, and (5) the appearance of calciphylaxis with ischemic lesions of the soft tissues and skin, vascular calcifications, and high levels of parathyroid hormone.

Because of lack of compliance, many patients are unable to control their serum phosphorus levels; in these cases, neither calcium supplementation nor vitamin D or its metabolites can be recommended safely. Moreover, this is the type of patient that usually develops severe secondary hyperparathyroidism, and surgical parathroidectomy may be the treatment of choice. Parathyroid surgery can lead to a transient lowering of blood phosphorus and the resolution of ectopic calcification. However, secondary hyperparathyroidism with all its manifestations will recur if the patient does not follow the prescribed treatment of phosphorus restriction. Postoperative hypocalcemia may pose a problem if the remaining parathyroid tissue is inadequate. The chances for development of hypocalcemia are enhanced if marked skeletal erosions are present preoperatively. Preoperative treatment of such patients with $1,25(OH)_2D_3$ (calcitriol) may obviate such problems.

Tetany and even seizures can occur during the postoperative period, and the intravenous infusion of calcium gluconate or other calcium supplements may be needed. Serum levels of phosphorus and magnesium sometimes decrease after parathyroid surgery, and aluminum-containing phosphate binders should be withheld if the serum phosphate falls below 2.5 mg/100 ml. However, the serum phosphorus should not be allowed to increase above 4.0 mg/100 ml, as this may aggravate the hypocalcemia. Rapid remineralization of the skeleton occurs during this period, and once the "hungry bones" have been mineralized, serum calcium will rise. A fall in the elevated plasma alkaline phosphatase toward normal may be a clue that rapid skeletal remineralization is nearly completed and indicate that calcium supplements and vitamin D dosage may be reduced or discontinued.

Although in the past the removal of 3½ glands was the procedure of choice, surgeons have gained experience with total parathyroidectomy followed by autotransplantation of parathyroid tissue into the patient's forearm. The tissue that is transplanted to the forearm is more accessible for subsequent surgical removal if necessary. Another risk of parathyroid surgery is the development of hypoparathyroidism. To avoid this, parathyroid tissue may be frozen and stored to be implanted later should hypocalcemia be persistent. Total parathyroidectomy may have little place in the management of renal bone disease, as this may predispose to the development of isolated mineralizing defect or osteomalacia in uremic patients.

E. Other Treatment Considerations

We strongly recommend that the water used in the dialysis procedure be treated for removal of all trace elements, including aluminum and fluoride, since the presence of the aluminum, as noted above, may predispose to the development of osteomalacia. Treatment of uremic patients with calcitonin has failed to lead to clear-cut improvement. Experimental studies with isolated parathyroid cells indicate that the blockade of β-adrenergic receptors can decrease the secretion of parathyroid hormone. Nevertheless, the long-term use of propranolol alone to suppress secondary hyperparathyroidism may not be practical. Moreover, ionized calcium would continue to be the most important factor regulating the secretion of parathyroid hormone.

Cimetidine has been reported to suppress secondary hyperparathyroidism in patients on chronic hemodialysis and in dogs with experimentally induced renal insufficiency. Administration of this drug for a prolonged period, however, is associated with an "escape" from its effects, and high levels of PTH reoccur. Recent studies have failed to demonstrate that cimetidine suppresses the release of parathyroid hormone in patients with chronic renal failure. Thus, its use in the treatment of secondary hyperparathyroidism remains speculative at this time.

ACKNOWLEDGMENTS. This work was supported by USPHS NIAMDD grants AM-09976, AM-07126, AM-14750, and RR-00036 and by Veterans Administration research support funds.

The secretarial assistance of Mrs. Pat Verplancke in the preparation of this manuscript is gratefully acknowledged.

SUGGESTED READINGS

Bourgoignie J, Jacob A, Gavellas G, et al: Effects of cimetidine on parathyroid hormone in chronic uremia, in Massry SG, Ritz E, Jahn H (eds): *Phosphate and Minerals in Health and Disease.* New York, Plenum Press, 1979, pp 505–514.

Brown EM: Set point for calcium: Its role in normal and abnormal parathyroid secretion, in Cohn DV, Talmage RV, Matthews JL (eds): *Hormonal Control of Calcium Metabolism.* Amsterdam, Excerpta Medica, 1981, pp 35–43.

Coburn JW, Koppel MH, Brickman AS, et al: Study of intestinal absorption of calcium in patients with renal failure. *Kidney Int* 3:264, 1973.

Coburn JW, Brickman AS, Sherrard DJ, et al: Defective skeletal mineralization in uremia without relation to vitamin D, serum Ca or P. *Kidney Int* 12:455, 1977.

Flueck JA, DiBella FP, Edis AJ, et al: Immunoheterogeneity of parathyroid hormone in venous effluent serum of hyperfunctioning parathyroid glands. *J Clin Invest* 60:1367, 1977.

Goldsmith RS, Johnson WJ: Role of phosphate depletion and high dialysate calcium in controlling dialytic renal osteodystrophy. *Kidney Int* 4:154, 1973.

Jacob AI, Canterbury JM, Gavellas G, et al: Reversal of secondary hyperparathroidisim by cimetidine in chronically uremic dogs. *J Clin Invest* 67:1753–1760, 1981.

Kopple JD, Coburn JW: Metabolic studies of low potein diets in uremia. II. Calcium, phosphorus and magnesium. *Medicine* 52:597, 1973.

Llach F, Massry SG, Singer FR, et al: Skeletal resistance of endogenous parathyroid hormone in patients with early renal failure: A possible cause for secondary hyperparathyroidism. *J Clin Endocrinol Metab* 41:338, 1975.

Llach F, Massry SG, Koffler A, et al: Secondary hyperparathryroidism in early renal failure: Role of phosphate retention. *Kidney Int* 12:459, 1977.

Martin KJ, Hruska KA, Lewis J, et al: The renal handling of parathyroid hormone. Role of peritubular uptake and glomerular filtration. *J Clin Invest* 60:808, 1977.

Mirahmade KS, Duffy BS, Shinaberger JH, et al: A controlled evalution of clinical and metabolic effects of dialysis. *Trans Am Soc Artif Intern Organs* 17:118, 1971.

Omsahl JL, Allen RC, Eaton RP: Computer modeling of vitamin D metabolism, in Norman AW, (ed): *Vitamin D Basic Research and its Clinical Application.* Berlin, W deGruyter, 1979, pp 515–521.

Parfitt AM: Soft tissue calcification in uremia. *Arch Intern Med* 124:544, 1969.

Reiss E, Canterbury JM, Bilinsky RT: Measurement of serum parathyroid hormone in renal insufficiency. *Trans Assoc Am Physicians* 81:104, 1968.

Schoenfeld PJ, Martin JA, Barnes B, et al: Amelioration of myopathy with 25-dihydroxyvitamin D$_3$ therapy (25(OH)D$_3$) in patients on chronic hemodialysis, in: *Abstract Book, Third Workshop on Vitamin D, Asilomar, California.* Berlin, Walter deGryer, 1977, p 160.

Slatopolsky E, Cricker NS: The role of phosphorus restriction in the prevention of secondary hyperparathroidism in chronic renal disease. *Kidney Int* 4:141, 1973.

Slatopolsky E, Gray R, Adams N, et al: The pathogenesis of secondary hyperparathyroidism in early renal failure, in Norman AW (ed): *Vitamin D Basic Research and Its Clinical Application.* Berlin, Walter deGruyer, 1979, p. 1209.

Therapy of the Acute Renal Failure Syndrome

GARABED EKNOYAN

I. INTRODUCTION

Acute renal failure (ARF) is a clinical syndrome of diverse etiologies in which a sudden deterioration in renal excretory function results in the inability of the kidneys to regulate normal homeostasis in general and solute and water balance in particular. It may occur in the face of a reduced, normal, or high urine flow, although in the majority (two-thirds), the urine volume is reduced. Its importance stems from the abruptness and severity of the clinical manifestations with which patients with ARF usually present and the potential for reversibility of the condition with proper therapeutic and supportive management.

Unfortunately, despite the fact that ARF is a self-limited condition and one instance of reversible organ failure for which replacement (dialytic) therapy is available, its mortality rate remains high. One major cause of death is the development of complications of renal failure, the therapy of which is the subject of this chapter. Another more important cause of death is the underlying primary illness of the patient. Although this aspect of the management will not be discussed in this chapter, under no circumstances should the attention focused on the dramatic events and complications that develop in ARF be allowed to relegate the management of the primary underlying disease to a secondary status.

The hallmarks of ARF are rapidly progressive azotemia and oliguria. With the onset of ARF, the urea load normally excreted by the kidney is

GARABED EKNOYAN • Department of Medicine, Renal Section, Baylor College of Medicine, Houston, Texas 77030.

reduced, and azotemia ensues. The magnitude of the azotemia that develops depends on the degree of reduction in filtration rate (GFR) and the rate of production of urea. With near complete cessation of filtration, the azotemia is progressive, with the BUN concentration rising in increments of about 10 mg/dl per day in uncomplicated cases of ARF, whereas in hypercatabolic cases, considerably more dramatic increments of 30 to 100 mg/dl per day are not unusual. Oliguria is said to be present if the daily urine volume is lower than the volume necessary to excrete the body's waste products. The daily urine excretion necessary to maintain normal homeostasis is about 400 to 500 ml in an individual on a normal diet, with normal renal function, and who is concentrating the urine maximally. The following set of principles is important to the understanding of this basic concept:

1. To maintain balance, the amount of solute to be excreted daily by a normal adult is 450–600 mOsm, with urea constituting 40–50% of the solute load and sodium or potassium salts the bulk of the balance. The normal human kidney is able to maximally concentrate urine to 1100 to 1200 mOsm/kg of water. It therefore follows that the maximally concentrating kidney would be able to excrete the "obligatory solute load" in about 400 to 500 ml of urine per day.

2. The normal daily urine output of 1000–1500 ml reflects the intake of water in excess of the amount necessary to maintain homeostasis. This obviously results in the excretion of a less concentrated urine. Thus, the daily urine is determined by the obligatory excretion of water and solute necessary to maintain balance.

3. Oliguria should not be equated with ARF. In an individual on a low dietary intake of protein or in a patient unable to break down protein to urea (as in cirrhosis of the liver), the amount of urea to be excreted is diminished. Since urea constitutes half the normal solute load to be excreted, the urine output necessary to maintain balance in these individuals is more in the range of 300 ml/day, as the amount of water obligated to excrete urea is reduced. Conversely, in a hypercatabolic state (as in burned patients), when urea production is increased, a proportionately larger volume of urine would be necessary to excrete the now larger solute load.

4. In individuals on restricted salt intake or in a patient whose kidneys are in a sodium retention state (as in heart failure, nephrotic syndrome, or cirrhosis of the liver), the urine output necessary to excrete the solute load is also reduced to the extent that the amount of sodium to be excreted and, therefore, the amount of water obligated to it are reduced.

5. If the kidneys are unable to concentrate maximally, a larger urine volume would be needed to excrete the daily load of solutes. Thus, if the kidneys were able to concentrate the urine up to only 600 mOsm/kg water, 1000 ml of urine would have to be excreted to maintain homeostasis, whereas if it could concentrate urine up to only 300 mOsm/kg water, 2000 ml of urine would have to be excreted. It is the acute development of such a concentrating defect (resulting from

Table I. Range of Daily Urine Composition

	Normal	Prerenal failure	Acute renal failure	
			Oliguric	Nonoliguric
Volume (ml/24 hr)	800–1500	<400	<400	>1500
Urea (g/24 hr)	20	15	5	10
(mmole/24 hr)	350	250	85	170
	(250–400)			
Creatinine (g/24 hr)	1–1.5	>1.0	<1.0	<1.0
Sodium (mEq/24 hr)	100	5	25	100
(mEq/liter)	50–70	10	>50	>50

tubular cell damage) coupled with a modest reduction in glomerular filtration rate that results in the "nonoliguric acute renal failure" that currently accounts for 10–25% of the cases of ARF.

6. It is evident then that an acute reduction in the kidneys' regulatory function or ARF may occur in the face of a reduced, normal, or high urine flow (Table I).

Acute renal failure does not necessarily imply renal parenchymal damage (renal failure). It may occur in the presence of essentially normal kidneys if the renal blood flow or perfusion pressure are sufficiently reduced in response to extrarenal stimuli (prerenal failure) or if the urine outflow is obstructed (postrenal failure). As a guide to therapy, it is useful to classify ARF into these three general categories (Table II). The prompt recognition and appropriate treatment of prerenal and postrenal failure are vitally important not only for the correct management of the underlying derangements but also to prevent the renal failure that is bound to ensue if prolonged underperfusion or obstruction are allowed to persist.

Table II. Major Causes of Acute Renal Failure

Prerenal failure
  Salt depletion
    Gastrointestinal losses
      Vomiting
      Diarrhea
    Fluid sequestration
      Burns
      Gastrointestinal: pancreatitis, peritonitis
      Trauma: crush injury
      Surgical: venous ligation
    Renal losses
      Diuretics
      Diabetic ketoacidosis
  Blood loss
  Cardiac shock, circulatory insufficiency
    Congestive heart failure
    Myocardial infarction
    Tachyarrhythmias
    CNS injury

(continued)

Table II. Major Causes of Acute Renal Failure (*Continued*)

Prerenal failure (continued)
   Septicemia, endotoxic shock
   Anoxia (requires salt depletion)

Postrenal failure
   Prostatic hypertrophy (benign or malignant)
   Bladder, pelvic, or retroperitoneal tumors
   Renal calculi
   Blood clots
   Ureteral edema (infection or surgical manipulation)
   Retroperitoneal fibrosis
   Inadvertent ureteral ligation
   Papillary necrosis

Renal
   Primary damage to tubular epithelium—acute tubular necrosis
   "Ischemic." Consequent to prerenal causes if sufficiently severe and prolonged. Also
       caused by renal embolization, clamping of renal artery, transplanted kidney, open heart
       surgery. Most common cause of acute tubular necrosis. Also referred to as "lower nephron
       nephrosis," "shock kidney," and "crush syndrome."
   "Nephrotoxic"
       Drugs: aminoglycosides, methoxyfluorane, cytolytic agents, phenytoin, *cis*-platinum, bis-
           muth, rifampin
       Radiopaque contrast agents
       Respiratory pigments
           Hemoglobin: transfusion reactions, cold agglutinins
           Myoglobin: muscle injury
       Poisons
           Heavy metals: mercury, arsenic, lead, gold
           Carbon tetrachloride
           Animal toxins
       Intratubular precipitation
           Uric acid
           Myeloma proteins
           Mucoprotein
           Sulfas
           Calcium
           Xanthine
           Oxalate
   Primary damage to glomeruli and small renal vasculature
       Acute glomerulonephritis. Rapidly progressive glomerulonephritis.
       Collagen vascular disease: lupus nephritis, Goodpasture syndrome, periarteritis nodosa
       Malignant hypertension
       Serum sickness
       Thrombotic thrombocytopenia purpura, hemolytic uremic syndrome
   Parenchymal necrosis
       Cortical
       Papillary
   Major renal vessel lesions
       Renal artery thrombosis
       Renal artery embolization
       Renal arterial atheroembolism
       Renal vein thrombosis: sudden, total

II. PRERENAL FAILURE

Prerenal failure results from the renal response to a variety of renal and extrarenal signals indicating contraction of the circulating blood volume. The latter may reflect an actual reduction in circulating volume (as in salt depletion because of gastrointestinal or renal losses or blood loss through hemorrhage) or a decrease in effective circulating volume (as in circulatory insufficiency resulting from myocardial insufficiency or endotoxic shock) (Table II). It is important to appreciate that an abrupt and rather drastic reduction in renal perfusion may develop even in the absence of overt shock.

In their attempt to preserve the true or effective circulating blood volume, the kidneys sustain acute functional changes without any demonstrable organic or structural damage. The most important of these changes is severe but reversible renal vasoconstriction with preferential renal cortical underperfusion. The resultant reduction in renal blood flow (RBF), if severe, may be associated with a reduction in glomerular filtration and thus a decrease in the filtration of solutes, although a drop in GFR need not always be present. Under all circumstances, the reduction of RBF is greater than that of GFR, such that the filtration fraction (GFR/RBF) is increased. This, coupled with other volume-stimulated factors, results in the tubular absorption of a greater fraction of the glomerular filtrate (urea, water, sodium). Additionally, there usually is a simultaneous stimulation of antidiuretic hormone and aldosterone secretion in response to the volume depletion. Thus, the oliguria that results is associated with a urine that is characteristically very highly concentrated and low in sodium content (Table III, Fig. 1).

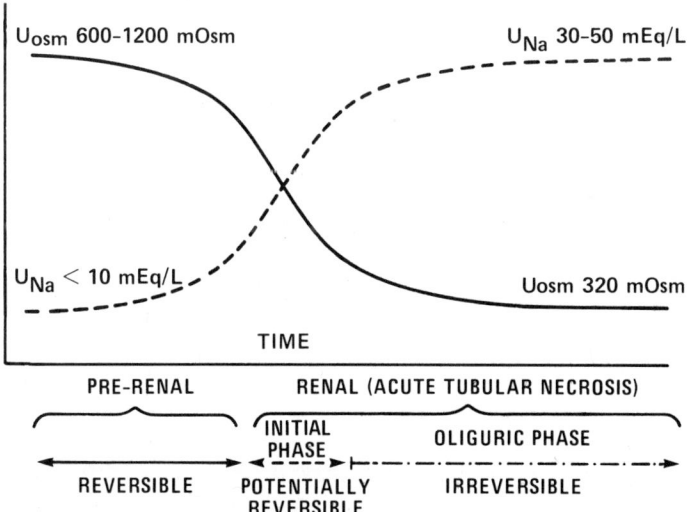

Figure 1. Changes in the urine concentration (U_{osm}) and sodium content (U_{Na}) during the progression from the prerenal type of ARF to the renal category.

Table III. Differential Urinary Findings in Prerenal and Renal Failure[a]

	Prerenal	Renal
Urine sediment	Few hyaline and granular casts	Numerous tubular cells, tubular cell casts, coarse broad granular casts
Urine specific gravity	>1.015	<1.010
Urine osmolality (mOsm/kg H_2O)	>500	<350
Ratio of urine osmolality to plasma osmalality	>1.5	<1.2
Urine Na^+ concentration (mEq/liter)	<20, usually <10	>20, usually >40
Ratio of urine to plasma urea concentration	>15 : 1	<10 : 1
Ratio of urine to plasma creatinine concentration	>15 : 1	<10 : 1
Fractional sodium excretion $\left(\dfrac{U_{Na}}{P_{Na}} \Big/ \dfrac{U_{cr}}{P_{cr}}\right) \times 100$	<1.0	>3.0

[a] In acute tubular necrosis that occurs against a background of severe volume depletion, the urine sodium concentration may continue to be <20 mEq/liter, whereas the urine in prerenal azotemia associated with diabetic ketoacidosis may be marked by an elevated urinary sodium concentration. This is true of other conditions associated with an osmotic diuresis (bicarbonate, mannitol, contrast dye). Furthermore, the presence of underlying chronic renal disease or the prior administration of a diuretic may make the interpretation of an isolated urine sodium concentration impossible.

The azotemia that may be present is in great part the result of increased reabsorption of the filtered urea and may develop in the absence of a drop in glomerular filtration rate. When renal circulation is restored, these patients will respond with a prompt diuresis and therefore a correction of the azotemia and oliguria.

Although this category of ARF may be identified by the usually accompanying signs of peripheral circulatory failure (orthostatic hypotension and tachycardia), the composition of the urine is the main clue to its diagnosis (Table III). The urine is characteristically low in sodium content (<10 mEq/liter) and high in concentration ($U_{osm} > 500$ mOsm/kg H_2O), and the sediment is essentially negative, containing only occasional granular or hyaline casts and few, if any, cellular elements.

An important aspect of prerenal ARF is that it represents an earlier and reversible change in the renal circulation which, if left uncorrected, may ultimately result in organic renal cell damage. If the cause of prerenal ischemia is corrected before this critical point is reached, the kidneys can recover, and normal function is restored. On the other hand, if uncorrected, it can evolve into the renal category of "ischemic" acute tubular necrosis which accounts for a significant number of ARF cases (Fig. 1). The critical period of ischemia before cell damage occurs is variable, depending on the severity of the ischemia and the underlying condition of the patient (with age, anoxia, and nephrotoxins being detrimental factors). To prevent the evolution of this potentially reversible form of ARF, prompt and appropriate remedial measures must be instituted to correct the circulating volume.

A. Evaluation

The history (GI losses, diuresis) and physical examination (orthostatic hypotension and tachycardia, poor skin turgor) can be invaluable in determining the nature and magnitude of the volume losses sustained in the majority of cases. In some cases, when one is confronted with hypotension of unknown etiology and when one cannot establish the adequacy of cardiac function, it is extremely useful to be guided during volume replacement by central venous and systemic arterial pressures. This is one situation in which central venous pressure (CVP) line placement is particularly useful. When the CVP is very low (less than 2 cm H_2O) in association with arterial hypotension, it denotes absolute or effective volume depletion. In these situations, the central venous line provides the additional advantage of easy access for fluid replacement.

With the CVP reading and the use of fluid challenge, one can "titrate" the patient's right ventricular Starling curve. One recommended technique is as follows:

1. Decide on a volume of fluid and infuse over 10 min. The choice of fluid depends on the clinical situation (a rough rule of thumb: if the CVP is less than 10, give 200 cc; if the CVP is greater than 10, give 100 cc of isotonic saline).
2. If the rise is greater than 5 cm of H_2O from the base-line value, stop the fluid challenge and observe the patient.
3. If the CVP rises greater than 2 but less than 5 cm H_2O above the base line during the 10-min infusion period, slow the infusion and wait 10 min. If the CVP then drops to within 2 cm of H_2O of the base line, resume the fluid challenge.
4. If the CVP does not rise greater than 2 cm of H_2O during the 10-min infusion period, give another fluid load over 10 min.
5. Do not open the intravenous line and come back a half-hour later to see what happened; fluid challenges must be monitored closely and carefully.

The interpretation of the data obtained from this type of dynamic situation is much more reliable and useful than the absolute CVP value alone, particularly when it is interpreted in the context of the clinical evaluation, i.e., improvement in mental status, increase in urine output, increase in the blood pressure, change in the orthostatic pressure drop, pulse rate, respiratory rate, and appearance of the skin of the extremities.

B. Diagnostic Challenge

In addition to volume expansion, a diagnostic challenge with mannitol or loop diuretics may be employed to rule out prerenal ARF as a cause of the oliguria and azotemia (Fig. 2). These should be undertaken cautiously (see cautions listed below) and only after correction of the volume status (as outlined above), determination of baseline parameters (urine flow), and under close monitoring.

1. Obtain a spot sample of urine to be used in the diagnostic work-up (Table III).
2. Inject a bolus of 12.5 g of mannitol (one 50-ml ampule of 25% mannitol) intravenously over 5 min.
3. An increase in urine output to over 30 ml/hr over the next 2 hr is considered a positive response.
4. If the response is positive, follow by an infusion of 10% mannitol (100 g mannitol in 1 liter of 5% D/W) over the next 24 hr to maintain the same rate of urine output.
5. If no response to mannitol occurs after the first 2 hr, repeat the same dose of mannitol (12.5 g over 5 min) together with a single intravenous dose of 240 mg furosemide.
6. If no response is obtained within the next hour, an additional dose of 480 mg furosemide may be administered intravenously (see cautions listed below).
7. If no response is obtained following the final dose of furosemide, the patient is considered to have sustained tubular cell necrosis and to have progressed to ischemic acute tubular necrosis.

Several cautions must be observed in the use of mannitol and diuretics.

1. Careful monitoring of the central venous pressure and of serum electrolytes is essential for the proper use of hypertonic mannitol. Mannitol as an extracellular solute will raise extracellular osmolarity and lead to intracellular water shifts, resulting in hyponatremia and plasma volume expansion (about 1–3 ml per kilogram body weight for every 5 g of mannitol). Consequently, if oliguria persists, and the mannitol is not excreted, the intravascular volume overload may result in pulmonary edema in the patient with a compromised circulatory system. On the other hand, if mannitol results in a significant diuresis, hypernatremia might result because of the loss of water in excess of salt in the urine. An increase in serum potassium might also result from the administration of hypertonic mannitol.
2. Furosemide may produce tinnitus and deafness, although these are usually reversible. The dose of furosemide should not exceed 1 g per 24 hr.

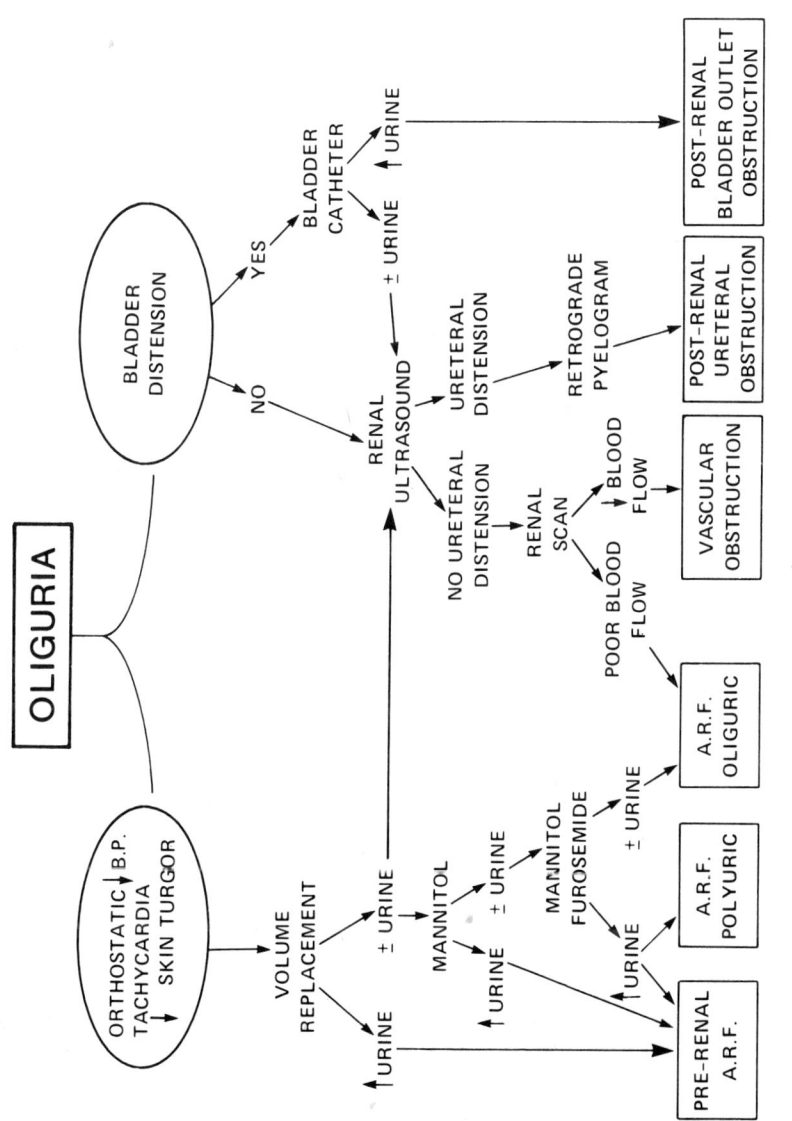

Figure 2. Work-up of the patient with oliguria.

3. The diuresis that might result may be marked, and it is essential that urine output be monitored closely for the adequate replacement of fluid losses. Hypotension is a potential side effect of the diuresis that might be induced with mannitol or furosemide, even in the apparently well-hydrated patient. Whenever this occurs, discontinue diuretics and replace fluid.

III. POSTRENAL FAILURE

This category includes all causes resulting in mechanical obstruction of the urine flow distal to the renal parenchyma proper. It is particularly important because it is immediately remediable by early relief of the obstruction. Normal function can be restored if the cause for the obstruction is removed quickly. On the other hand, chronic obstruction can result in irreversible damage.

A feature of postrenal ARF that may be of diagnostic value is anuria (<50 to 75 ml/day) which at times is succeeded by massive polyuria only to be followed by recurrence of the anuria. Other differentiating features are a history of renal colic or flank pain, absence of or minimal proteinuria, and a serum urea nitrogen level higher than expected for the accompanying creatinine value (the BUN : creatinine ratio is usually >20 : 1). The latter is partly the result of reabsorption of urea by the urinary tract mucosa from the stagnated urine.

The initial step in the evaluation of obstruction is to exclude prostatic or some other form of bladder outlet disease (Fig. 2). If the outlet is patent, a renal ultrasound is the screening method of choice to identify an obstructive nephropathy. A flat plate of the abdomen (KUB) can be useful in identifying calculi. Retrograde studies may become necessary if extrarenal obstruction is still not excluded. Unilateral ureteral catheterization is usually sufficient to rule out this possibility. Although bilateral ureteral obstruction is rare, it does occur and must be kept in mind. Obviously, the obstruction may occur in a unilateral kidney, which occurs with sufficient frequency (1 : 800 persons have a single kidney) to warrant consideration. A high-dose intravenous pyelogram with tomography and late films at 6 and 24 hr can be useful if extrarenal obstruction remains a possibility.

The management of these cases is in general surgical, and a urological consultation must be obtained as soon as the diagnosis of obstruction as a cause of ARF is entertained.

IV. RENAL FAILURE

Although in its broadest terms this category of ARF includes among other such diverse entities as acute glomerulonephritis, cortical necrosis, and papillary necrosis (Table II), acute renal failure commonly denotes those forms of renal failure caused by ischemia, nephrotoxic agents, or a combination of both, which together account for the vast majority (75–80%) of the cases of ARF. These two major causes of ARF have been variously termed "crush kidneys," "lower nephron nephrosis," "acute vasomotor nephropathy," "hemoglobinuric nephrosis," "oliguric acute renal failure," and "acute tubular necrosis." Both in the experimental model and in man, the damage is most evident in the tubular cells, and the preferred terminology which will be used here is that of acute tubular necrosis (ATN).

Renal ischemia is the most common cause of ATN. Although any of the disorders associated with prerenal ARF can result in ATN, it most commonly occurs in patients with hypotension, particularly in settings of sepsis and surgery. The surgical procedures associated with the highest risk are abdominal aortic, open heart, and gallbladder surgery. In general, most cases of ATN are related to surgery (40–45%), although about 25% are caused by medical causes (septicemia, volume depletion from renal or gastrointestinal losses), and at least in the older literature 10% are obstetric in origin, with a significant reduction in the incidence of ATN in obstetric cases in the more recent past. Another 10% each result from trauma and nephrotoxins. There appears to be an increased incidence (>20%) in nephrotoxin-related ATN since the introduction of aminoglycoside antibiotics. The cause of ATN is of considerable prognostic significance, as the mortality rate, which ranges from 50 to 70% in surgical and traumatic cases, is about 30 to 35% in medical cases and less than 10% in obstetric cases. An important variable that affects the prognosis favorably in all instances of ATN, independent of etiology, is the development of the nonoliguric type of ATN.

The diagnosis of ARF is primarily one of exclusion. Examination of the urine is extremely valuable for the diagnosis of ATN and its differentiation from prerenal ARF (Table III). A careful examination of the urine sediment is essential. Tubular epithelial cells with epithelial cell and broad granular casts suggest tubular injury, most commonly caused by ATN. Eosinophiluria, demonstrated by Wright stain preparation of a freshly voided urine sediment, is strongly suggestive of a drug-induced interstitial nephritis. The presence of red blood cells and red blood cell casts coupled with heavy proteinuria is almost always caused by glomerular disease or vasculitis. A renal biopsy can be useful to rule out glomerular disease. However, its value is questionable in the early stages of ARF in the absence of specific findings suggestive of glomerular disease. If the oliguric phase lasts for 3 weeks or longer, renal biopsy is indicated.

In cases that first present to the hospital in renal failure, if the onset of the renal failure cannot be documented, chronic renal failure must be ruled out. Small kidney size measured by ultrasound, cardiomegaly, hypertension, anemia, edema, and a pale itchy skin all denote chronic renal failure.

The clinical course of ATN can be divided into four phases: (1) initiating phase, (2) oliguric phase, (3) diuretic phase, and (4) recovery phase. Treatment of each varies and will be considered individually.

A. Initiating Phase

This is the period of ischemia or exposure to the nephrotoxic agent and continues until cell injury develops. Obviously, it overlaps with prerenal failure. The importance of identifying this phase is that it represents a reversible stage (Fig. 1). The length of this phase varies depending on the causative mechanism, being shorter (hours) in ischemic ATN and longer (days) in antibiotic-induced nephrotoxicity. In general, with the nephrotoxic agents, any decrease in glomerular filtration rate is preceded by several days of an abnormal sediment, tubular proteinuria, β_2 microglobinuria, lysozymuria, and a renal concentrating defect. Hence the importance of monitoring these variables and discontinuing the nephrotoxic agent.

Evidence exits that prostaglandins exert a protective effect in renal autoregulation during vasoconstrictive insults. It is important then to remember that the use of inhibitors of prostaglandin synthesis may subject the kidney to more severe ischemia and precipitate ATN. Aspirin, indomethacin, and other nonsteroidal analgesics all exert an inhibitory effect on prostaglandin synthesis, and their use should be strictly avoided in these patients.

B. Oliguric Phase

Oliguria will be present in 70 to 80% of cases of ATN, and another 20 to 30% will have nonoliguric renal failure. First reported in burn patients, nonoliguric ARF is beginning to be encountered with increasing frequency, particularly in antibiotic-induced nephrotoxicity. Since the glomerular filtration may be reduced to similar degrees in oliguric and nonoliguric ATN, the variability in urine volume must reflect differences in tubular damage and reabsorption. In general, in nonoliguric ATN, tubular damage occurs without an accompanying severe reduction of filtration. The kidney is, therefore, unable to concentrate the filtrate sufficiently to excrete the daily solute load and can respond only by increasing the urine output. It is important to distinguish between the nonoliguric state from the outset of the acute renal failure episode and that induced by diuretics (see above). In the former, the GFR is higher, and the prognosis better. With the nonoliguric state induced by mannitol or high-dose diuretics, the GFR remains low, and the mortality does not seem to be favorably affected, although fluid management becomes easier.

The average duration of the oliguric phase is 1 to 2 weeks. Anuria (urine output <50 to 75 ml/day) is uncommon in ATN. If oliguria continues for longer than 4 weeks, other possibilities (cortical necrosis, glomerulonephritis, vasculitis) must be considered and a renal biopsy performed. The duration of oliguria is of some prognostic significance, with the longer duration carrying a greater risk of complications and, therefore, a fatal outcome.

Despite considerable experimental work over the past decade, no single pathogenetic sequence of events appears to account for the development of oliguria. Currently, the balance of evidence favors the view that tubular obstruction is important. Changes in glomerular permeability and filtration rate and excessive "back leak" of the filtrate across the damaged tubular epithelium also appear to be contributing mechanisms (Fig. 3). The degree of involvement of any of these potential pathogenetic factors in the causation of oliguria will vary depending on the nature, severity, and duration of the initial insult.

The availability of dialysis has greatly simplified the management of patients with ATN. Nevertheless, despite dialysis, the mortality rate in ATN remains high, and certain principles governing water and electrolyte balance must be adhered to. The basic goals of management are maintenance of fluid and electrolyte balance, adequate nutrition, and, if present, the treatment of infection and uremic symptoms.

1. Water

In the oliguric patient, unless water intake is curtailed, dangerous volume expansion will occur. Water intake must be restricted to a volume equivalent to urine output plus extrarenal losses. Insensible losses (800 ml/day) must be restored. Because of the endogenous water production (combustion of carbohydrate and fat) of 350–400 ml/day, only 400–450 ml of water is needed to replace insensible losses. Thus, in the alert patient, daily water intake equals 400 ml plus the previous day's urine volume and extrarenal losses. Insensible losses must be increased with high ambient temperature, fever, and low relative humidity. If the patient is eating, the water content of food (500 to 700 ml) must be taken into consideration. A practical approach to accomplish water balance is:

1. Monitor daily intake and output. A bladder catheter for the measurement of urine output is usually not necessary. Once the diagnosis of ATN is established, the bladder catheter used in the initial patient

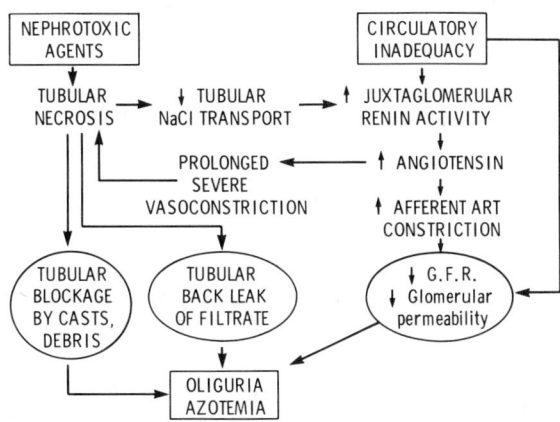

Figure 3. Postulated pathogenetic sequence of events in the development of acute tubular necrosis.

evaluation should be discontinued except in cases of bladder outlet obstruction. An indwelling catheter will result in an increased incidence of urinary tract infection. In male patients, an external drain catheter is usually sufficient to monitor daily urine output. In the comatose patient, catheterization once daily, under strict aseptic conditions, is sufficient to document daily urine volumes.

2. Weigh patient at the same time each day. Since ATN is a catabolic state, the patient should lose about 0.2 to 0.3 kg (½–¾ lb) per day. Any weight gain can only represent excess fluid administration.

3. Measure serum sodium. The sodium concentration should remain between 135 and 145 mEq/liter. A rise in the serum sodium level would indicate inadequate water replacement, whereas a drop would reflect excessive water replacement. As in normal individuals, hyponatremia reflects water excess and should be treated with water restriction and ultrafiltration. Always rule out causes of pseudohyponatremia (hyperglycemia, hyperlipemia, and hyperproteinemia) prior to instituting corrective measures.

2. Sodium Chloride

Sodium chloride usually is not required after the initial replacement during the prerenal phase when the patient first presents in vascular collapse or compromise. The guiding principles of sodium chloride replacement are:

1. Body weight losses in excess of 300 mg/day with a continued normal serum sodium level should prompt replacement (milliliter per gram) with isotonic saline.

2. Gastrointestinal losses must be replaced with salt. Gastric fluid should be replaced with half-normal saline. Pancreatic biliary and small intestinal losses should be replaced with isotonic saline. Diarrheal losses from the large intestine should be restored with 5% dextrose in water to which sodium bicarbonate (45 mEq/liter) has been added.

3. If the patient is alert and able to eat, limit salt intake to 2 g (88 mEq) per day.

3. Potassium

Potassium intake must be restricted. Small deficits should not be replaced. Hidden sources of potassium must be kept in mind (stored blood, salt substitutes, potassium salts of drugs). Hypolakemia, unless severe (<3 mEq/liter), should not be corrected. In patients without serious complications, plasma potassium increases about 0.5 mEq/liter per day. In severe catabolic states, increments of 1 mEq/liter every few hours may occur. Internal imbalance of potassium particularly in catabolic states, remains a threat to life even if external potassium is restricted. In the alert patient, limit potassium intake to 2 g (70 mEq) per day.

Hyperkalemia, formerly a common cause of death, continues to be one of the most serious problems confronting the patient with ATN. Serum potassium must be closely monitored in all patients, particularly in those with ATN following surgery and trauma. The electrocardiogram (ECG), although a poor correlate of serum potassium concentration, remains a reliable source of information on the electrophysiological state of the myocardium and must be closely monitored. Hyperkalemia may be treated by one or more of the following:

1. Correct the acidosis which is a usual coexisting and aggravating factor of the hyperkalemia. One ampule of sodium bicarbonate (50 mEq) may be injected over 5 min while the ECG is monitored. If cardiac conduction abnormalities persist, repeat in 15 min. Remember that sodium bicarbonate represents a sodium load and may produce hypernatremia and hyperosmolality. Additionally, the alkalosis induced by sodium bicarbonate may provoke hypocalcemic tetany.

2. Infuse 200 ml of 20% dextrose in water over 30 min together with the administration of 10 units of regular insulin. The volume of fluid may be reduced by using 50 ml of 50% dextrose in water infused over 10 min.

3. Inject one 10-ml ampule of 10% calcium gluconate over 5 min cautiously while monitoring the ECG. In the digitalized patient, calcium injection may result in an abnormal rhythm and is best avoided.

4. Use a cation-exchange resin such as sodium polysterene sulfonate (Kayexalate®) to remove potassium from the body. This may be given orally, 15–30 g Kayexalate® with 50 ml of 20% or sorbitol administered two to four times daily, or by retention enema, 50 g Kayexalate® in 200 ml of 20% sorbitol. The enema must be retained for 30–60 min to be effective and can be repeated every 4 to 6 hr. Each gram of Kayexalate® removes 1 mEq of potassium in exchange for its sodium. The rectal route is by far the more rapid of the two to reduce potassium.

5. Hyperkalemia is always an indication to consider dialysis as early as possible.

4. Acid–Base

With the loss of the kidneys' ability to excrete the hydrogen ions of fixed acids, metabolic acidosis will develop. Serum bicarbonate concentration will decrease by 1 to 2 mEq per day. If serum bicarbonate is less than 15 mEq/liter, it should be corrected by oral intake of bicarbonate salts or Shohl's solution (sodium citrate). If the patient is being dialyzed, discontinue the alkalizing agents to avoid the severe alkalosis that is bound to ensue considering the high citrate or acetate content of the dialysis fluid. Remember that bicarbonate salts represent a sodium load and may precipitate heart failure. Also, sudden and zealous correction of acidosis can precipitate tetany.

5. Divalent Ions

Hypermagnesemia may be caused by the use of magnesium-containing antacids. Signs of toxicity will develop with levels exceeding 5 mEq/liter. Magnesium-containing antacids and laxatives should be avoided. Hyperalimentation usually lowers serum magnesium, and supplementation is required. Aminoglycoside nephrotoxicity may also cause hypomagnesemia. Hypomagnesemia can be corrected with 10% magnesium sulfate in a dose of 1 to 2 g given IV over 15 to 30 min. Alternatively, 1 g of magnesium sulfate can be given intramuscularly every 6 hr.

Hypocalcemia develops early in ATN. In cases of trauma and rhabdomyolysis, the hypocalcemia can be a prominent feature. It usually results from the deposition of calcium in necrotic muscle and from low levels of circulating $25(OH)D_3$. Hypercalcemia will appear during the recovery phase of the ATN. Theses are self-limited processes that require no treatment except in the presence of hypocalcemic symptoms (tetany). The calcium may be replaced as the gluconate (4 mEq of Ca^{2+} per ampule) or chloride (14 mEq of Ca^{2+} per ampule). The former form of calcium is preferred to avoid the acidosis caused by the chloride ion of the latter form.

Phosphate levels are high in ATN and may be corrected by the oral administration of aluminum hydroxide gels. Phosphate levels will be low with hyperalimentation and would require supplementation as potassium phosphate.

6. Anemia

With the loss of renal function, the production of erythropoietin will be reduced. This coupled with reduction of red blood cell life-span will invariably result in some degree of anemia in most patients with ATN. Blood losses sustained prior to the onset of ATN or during its course will aggravate the anemia that accompanies the developing uremic state. The anemia of uremia may persist during the diuretic and recovery phases of ATN. In most patients, spontaneous correction of the anemia may be anticipated. Transfusion should be given as needed to maintain the hematocrit between 25 to 30%.

1. Prior to considering any replacement therapy, rule out the relative anemia of volume overload and dilution.
2. In the hypovolemic patient, transfusions may be given as whole blood.
3. In the absence of hypovolemia, packed red blood cells should be given, preferably during dialysis, to avoid intravascular volume overload.
4. Stored blood bank is a source of potassium (10–20 mEq/liter), and the serum potassium should be monitored.

7. Gastrointestinal Complications

Gastrointestinal complications are frequent. Nausea and vomiting are best treated by limiting oral intake. Should they persist, they can be effectively controlled with prochlorperazine (Compazine®) in a dose of 10 mg every 8–12 hr. Avoid overdosage which might result in orthostatic hypotension and extrapyramidal signs of toxicity. More serious is the development of gastrointestinal bleeding which is a significant cause of death in some series. Frequent dialysis diminishes the incidence of bleeding. The use of an H_2-receptor antagonist (cimetidine) has been shown to be effective in stress ulcers and may be used in a dose of 300 mg intravenously every 12 hr. Neutropenia has been reported as a side effect of cimetidine, particularly in patients with renal failure, and leukocyte count should be monitored in these individuals.

8. Central Nervous System

Symptoms range from mild drowsiness to acute psychoses, delirium, and coma. Preexisting psychotic tendencies appear to predispose to the pattern of psychotic manifestations. These can be controlled with paraldehyde. If barbiturates are to be used, the short-acting barbiturates (secobarbital, pentobarbital, and amobarbital) are preferred since they are largely inactivated in the liver and can be used in normal doses. Convulsions usually occur in a setting of hypertension, overhydration, and electrolyte disturbances. Fluid removal by ultrafiltration is the treatment of choice. Phenytoin in normal doses can be used to control convulsions.

9. Nutrition

Caloric intake must be maintained to minimize the hypercatabolic state and, therefore, the rate of rise of BUN. A high-caloric diet low in protein but high in essential amino acids should be used. All protein intake must be of high biological value. If the patient is being dialyzed, the daily protein intake should be 1 g/kg body weight or about 80 g. If the patient is not dialyzed, limit protein intake to 40 g/day. If the patient is capable of eating, oral nutrition is preferable; otherwise, use parenteral nutrition.

Although at present there is no conclusive evidence that in patients with acute renal failure mortality rate is influenced by hyperalimentation, this form of therapy should be strongly considered. Evidence that total parenteral nutrition (TPN) may affect the duration of renal failure and mortality has been advanced by some investigators but questioned by others. In rapidly deteriorating and seriously ill patients who usually succumb to their underlying disease and in patients with mild ARF who do not require dialysis, the course of the disease is most probably not influenced by hyperalimentation. It is in the relatively stable patients who require dialysis that TPN appears to be of benefit. As a rule, all patients with ARF requiring dialysis are best started on hyperalimentation.

The amount and type of essential amino acids to be administered in ATN are still unclear, but a high calorie-to-nitorgen ration (>450 : 1) is essential. Elevations in BUN during hyperalimentation may result from either insufficient carbohydrate calories per gram of nitrogen or excessive protein in the hydrolysate. In stable uncomplicated cases, 3000 kcal is required to prevent rises in BUN. In complicated cases (trauma, infection), 5000 to 6000 kcal is desirable. The following guidelines are useful to avoid unnecessary complications of TPN:

1. Monitor the blood glucose every 6 hr. Insulin, which has an anabolic effect of its own, must be given to maintain a reasonably normal blood glucose level.
2. Begin hyperalimentation slowly at a rate of 20 ml/hr. Increase infusion by 15 ml/hr daily until a rate of 125 ml/hr is attained.
3. If TPN is to be discontinued, taper the infusion over 48 hr. Hypoglycemia may occur if hyperalimentation is discontinued suddenly because of the continued hypersecretion of insulin by the pancreas. If infusion is discontinued, an intravenous infusion of 10% dextrose in water should be started to avoid the hypoglycemia.
4. With successful hyperalimentation, the increased anabolism will result in the intracellular translocatin of potassium, phosphate, and magnesium. These electrolytes must be monitored and carefully replaced to avoid the development of deficiencies.
5. Proper catheter care is an absolute must. Catheter sepsis is the most serious and potentially fatal complication of TPN but one that can be avoided with proper care.

10. Infection

Other than the underlying disease process, infection is frequently the most serious problem confronting the patient with ATN. Infections account for one-third of all deaths resulting from ATN. The primary sites of infection are the lung, peritoneum, and urinary tract. The latter is usually related to unnecessary catheterization. Following the initial in-and-out catheterization to exclude bladder outlet obstruction, the bladder should not be catheterized. Avoidance of unnecessary catheterizations and proper preventive care for catheter related sepsis in TPN are essential. Prophylactic antibiotics have no place in the prevention of infection and may prove harmful.

Early diagnosis and use of proper antibiotics are the cornerstone of management. In patients with renal failure, the usual finding of fever may be absent, and leukocytosis may not develop. Examination of the peripheral smear for toxic granulations of the leukocytes can be most useful. Unexplained tachycardia, hypotension, and dyspnea suggest an infection. A sudden increase in insulin requirements to control the blood glucose level in patients on TPN is also a useful sign to watch for infection.

11. Dialysis

Although most patients with ATN can be managed by conservative treatment, this is not possible for all, and many will eventually require dialysis. Definite indications for dialysis are (1) inability to control hyperkalemia in hypercatabolic patients; (2) fluid overload; (3) severe metabolic acidosis, particularly when volume overload curtails the administration of sodium bicarbonate; (4) severe uremia (BUN > 100 mg/dl or creatinine > 10 mg/dl) with uremic symptoms of pericarditis, gastrointestinal bleeding, and confusion. Early prophylactic and frequent daily dialysis has been advocated by some, and evidence presented that it might improve the course and reduce the mortality from ATN. Although this might be true in the hypercatabolic cases, no true generalizations can be made in this regard. The decision to institute early and frequent dialysis must be individualized.

A marked fall in urine output commonly occurs after the institution dialysis. This is because of the lowering of the blood urea nitrogen which acts as an osmotic agent and because of the correction of the volume expansion that might have been present.

12. Miscellaneous

Insulin is degraded by the kidneys. In diabetic patients who develop ARF, insulin requirements may, therefore, be decreased by as much as 40%. This is particularly true in otherwise uncomplicated cases of ARF such as those induced by contrast dye administration. Blood glucose levels should be carefully monitored, and the dose of insulin reduced to prevent hypoglycemic reactions.

Several of the drugs used in patients with ATN or their metabolites are excreted by the kidneys. The dosage of most need, therefore, to be adjusted to the level of renal function to avoid toxic blood levels. This is particularly true of patients who require antibiotic therapy for intercurrent infections. Dosages should be adjusted, and, where possible, blood levels monitored. Extensive lists of the appropriate dosages of drugs and their removal by dialysis have been published and should be consulted as the need arises (see Readings).

C. Diuretic Phase

The diuretic phase is heralded by a significant increase in the daily urine output over that established during the oliguric phase (<500 ml/day). Classically, the urine volume doubles on successive days until it attains a volume of 2000 to 3000 ml/day. This phase lasts from 7 to 14 days. Together with the onset of diuresis, the renal blood flow and glomerular filtration rate gradually increase. At first, the urine appears to be basically a pure plasma filtrate, for the total concentration of urine and that of each of its constituents are nearly identical to those in the plasma. As the tubules recover some ability to reabsorb sodium and concentrate urea, the urine will gradually contain less sodium and more urea than plasma. Consequently, the blood chemistries will not begin to correct with the onset of the diuretic phase, and it may be several days before the abnormal blood values begin to normalize. However, as diuresis continues, and renal function continues to improve, the azotemia gradually diminishes, and the blood chemistries begin returning to normal levels.

At present, more than 30% of deaths in ATN occur during the diuretic phase. Dialysis often has to be continued through the early stages of this phase, until the predialysis BUN levels begin dropping below 80 mg/dl and there are no problems associated with hyperkalemia from increased tissue injury. Sodium and potassium balance must continue to be followed closely by means of body weight and daily serum concentrations, applying the principles outlined above for the oliguric phase.

Factors contributing to the diuresis observed during this phase include the following:

1. Osmotic diuresis resulting from mobilization of the urea accumulated during the oliguric phase.
2. Functional inadequacy of the tubules to reabsorb the glomerular filtrate and concentrate the urine.
3. Mobilization of edema fluid accumulated during the oliguric phase.
4. "Pushing" of intravenous fluids. The overzealous replacement of urine output maintains the patient in a continuous state of volume expansion. Thus, one ends up "chasing" the urine output by infusing gradually larger volumes of fluid.

Although urine losses must be replaced, pushing fluids must be avoided. This can best be accomplished by replacing urine output no more frequently than every 8 to 12 hr. The volume should be two-thirds of the previous 8- to 12-hr output of urine in order to avoid the continued overexpansion of the extracellular fluid which the kidneys may be trying to correct in the first place. The type of fluid replacement may be estimated from the urine electrolytes. Changes in weight, blood pressure, pulse and skin turgor are useful clinical parameters of adequate replacement. In the alert patient, normal thirst and appetite may be the best guide to replacement therapy. Occasionally, the diuresis is marked, and the patient may require supplemental intravenous replacement therapy.

It is important to remember that many drugs are still poorly excreted during the diuretic phase, and continued dosage adjustments may be necessary if drug toxicity is to be avoided.

D. Recovery Phase

The blood urea nitrogen and creatinine values are usually normal within 5 to 60 days after the onset of the diuretic phase. Glomerular filtration rate, however, increases more slowly and is about 70–80% of normal within 1 to 2 years. The ability to concentrate the urine maximally will return but may take several months to do so. As a result, nocturia and polyuria may develop early during the recovery phase but will gradually disappear as the ability to concentrate the urine improves. As a rule, there is no evidence of progressive renal disease in patients who recover, although in some a mild loss of renal function because of fibrosis and atrophy may continue to develop over a period of several years.

Although urinary tract infection is common during the oliguric phase, usually because of the urethral catheterization, there is no evidence that persistent chronic urinary tract infection develops once urine flow and renal function return.

V. TREATMENT OF SPECIFIC TYPES OF ACUTE RENAL FAILURE

Specific therapy instituted during the initial phase of certain types of ARF may prevent the development of ATN or ameliorate its course.

A. Myoglobinuric Acute Renal Failure

Volume replacement is the cornerstone of therapy of myoglobinuric ARF. Mannitol may also provide a protective effect by overcoming intratubular obstruction, diluting the intratubular concentration of myoglobin, and decreasing renin production. In light of the pK of myoglobin, alkalinization of the urine may also provide protection. A protective effect of mannitol and sodium bicarbonate to reverse the azotemia and oliguria of myoglobinuric ARF has been reported. This can be accomplished by the intravenous infusion of 25 g mannitol and 100 mEq sodium bicarbonate in 1 liter of 5% dextrose in water at a rate of 200–500 ml/hr. If a diuretic response occurs, diuresis may be continued with saline. If no response is obtained, a trial dose of furosemide (240 mg IV over 15 min) may be tried. If there is a response, diuresis is continued with saline. If there is no response, the patient should be treated as outlined above for ATN.

Central venous pressures should be closely monitored during mannitol administration. Hypocalcemia, which is commonly present in these patients, may be aggravated following bicarbonate administration but need not be treated if no symptoms (tetany) develop.

B. Radiocontrast-Induced Acute Renal Failure

Radiopaque agents have emerged as a frequent cause of a relatively benign type of ARF, with deterioration of renal function peaking in 3 to 10 days and returning to near baseline levels shortly thereafter. Most common after intravenous pyelography, it may also occur after angiography or cholecystography in diabetic patients or patients with renal insufficiency. Volume depletion and large doses of radiocontrast agents are predisposing factors. Prior volume expansion may ameliorate the severity of the episode but fails to provide total protection. Mannitol has been reported to be useful in prevention. Diuresis should be instituted ½ hr prior to the procedure with 25 g mannitol and 100 mEq sodium bicarbonate in 1 liter of 5% dextrose in water to run at a rate of 150 ml/hr. Diuresis should be continued through the procedure with adequate replacement of fluid and electrolyte losses.

C. Acute Uric Acid Nephropathy

This classically reversible and potentially preventable type of ARF usually follows chemotherapy of lymphoproliferative disorders. Early diagnosis may be established from a spot of urine uric acid-to-creatinine ratio greater than one.

Reducing the urate load and maintaining a high urine flow is protective. This may be accomplished by adequate hydration prior to and through chemotherapy and the administration of allopurinol (300–800 mg daily). Alkalinization of the urine with sodium bicarbonate and osmotic diuresis with mannitol (same regimen as described above) are indicated both prophylactically or after the onset of renal dysfunction.

Hemodialysis is a very efficient method for removing uric acid. A 6-hr hemodialysis removes approximately 50% of the uric acid load. In oliguric patients who fail to respond to mannitol and bicarbonate diuresis, hemodialysis to remove urate is the treatment of choice.

D. Multiple Myeloma

Acute renal failure develops in a significant number of patients with multiple myeloma. Although this sometimes results from the coexistent hypercalcemia or hyperuricemia, Bence–Jones proteins are also nephrotoxic. Precipitation of B–J proteins is more likely to occur in a concentrated urine at a low pH. Adequate hydration with mannitol and alkalinization (same regimen as above) may prove helpful. Chemotherapy should be instituted to reduce the load of abnormal proteins. Peritoneal dialysis is also effective in removing light-chain proteins. Plasmapheresis, however, is the treatment of choice for the acute removal of abnormal light-chain protein.

SUGGESTED READINGS

General

Anderson RJ, Linas SL, Berns AS, et al: Non-oliguric acute renal failure. N Engl J Med 296:1134–1138, 1977.

Balslov JT, Jorgensen HE: A survey of 499 patients with acute anuric renal insufficiency: Causes, treatment, complications and mortality. Am J Med 34:754–764, 1963.

Bennett WM, Plamp C, Porter GA: Drug-related syndromes in clinical nephrology. Ann Intern Med 87:582–590, 1977.

Casali R, Simmons RL, Najarian JS, et al: Acute renal insufficiency complicating major cardiovascular surgery. Ann Surg 181:370–375, 1975.

Conger JD, Schrier RW: Renal hemodynamics in acute renal failure. Annu Rev Physiol 42:603–614, 1980.

Cronin RE: Aminoglycoside nephrotoxicity: Pathogenesis and prevention. Clin Nephrol 11:251–256, 1979.

Eknoyan G: The acute renal failure syndrome. Texas Med. 70:83–90, 1974.

Eknoyan G, Wacksman SJ, Glueck HI, et al: Platelet function in renal failure. N Engl J Med 280:677–681, 1969.

Espinel CH: The FE_{Na} test: Use in the differential diagnosis of acute renal failure. JAMA 236:579–581, 1976.

Flamenbaum W: Pathophysiology of acute renal failure. Arch Intern Med 131:911–928, 1973.

Hall JW, Johnson WJ, Maher FT, et al: Immediate and long-term prognosis in acute renal failure. Ann Intern Med 73:515–521, 1970.

Hollenberg NK, Epstein M, Rosen SM, et al: Acute oliguric renal failure in man: Evidence for preferential renal cortical ischemia. Medicine 47:455–474, 1968.

Koffler A, Friedler RM, Massry SM: Acute renal failure due to non-traumatic rhabdomyolysis. Ann Intern Med 85:23–28, 1976.

Levinsky NG: Pathophysiology of acute renal failure. N Engl J Med 296:1453–1458, 1977.

Lewers DT, Mathew TH, Maher JF, et al: Long-term follow-up of renal function and histology after acute tubular necrosis. Ann Intern Med 73:523–529, 1970.

Maher JR, Schreiner GE: Causes of death in acute renal failure. Arch Intern Med 110:493–504, 1962.

McLeish, KR, Luft FC, Kleit SA: Factors affecting prognosis in ARF following cardiac operations. Surg Gynecol Obstet 145:28–32, 1977.

McMurray SD, Luft FC, Maxwell DR, et al: Prevailing patterns and predictors in patients with acute tubular necrosis. Arch Intern Med 138:950–955, 1978.

Merrill JP: The Treatment of Renal Failure, ed 2. New York, Grune & Stratton, 1965.

Miller TR, Anderson RJ, Linas SL, et al: Urinary diagnostic indices in acute renal failure. A prospective study. Ann Intern Med 89:47–50, 1978.

Minuth AN, Terrell JB, Suki WN: Acute renal failure: A study of the course and prognosis of 104 patients and of the role of furosemide. Am J Med Sci 271:317–324, 1976.

O'Meara M, Eknoyan G: Acute renal failure associated with indomethacin administration. South Med J 73:587–589, 1980.

Skorecki KL, Brenner BM: Body fluid homeostasis in man: A contemporary overview. Am J Med 70:77–88, 1981.

Stein JH, Lifschitz MD, Barnes LD: Current concepts on the pathophysiology of acute renal failure. Am J Physiol 234:F171–F181, 1978.

Walshe JJ, Venuto RC: Acute oliguric renal failure induced by indomethacin: Possible mechanism. Ann Intern Med 91:47–49, 1979.

Wilson DM, Turner DR, Cameron JS, et al: Value of renal biopsy in acute intrinsic renal failure. Br Med J 2:459–463, 1976.

Management

Auger RG, Dayton DA, Harrison CE, et al: Use of ethacrynic acid in mannitol resistant oliguric renal failure. *JAMA* 206:891–893, 1968.

Aviram A, Pfau A, Czaczkes JW, et al: Hyperosmolality with hyponatremia caused by inappropriate administration of mannitol. *Am J Med* 42:648–650, 1967.

Bailey RR, Natale R, Turnbull DI, et al: Protective effect of furosemide in acute tubular necrosis and acute renal failure. *Clin Sci Mol Med* 45:1–17, 1973.

Barry KG, Malloy JP: Oliguric renal failure: Evaluation and therapy by the intravenous infusion of mannitol. *JAMA* 179:510–513, 1962.

Brown CB, Ogg CS, Cameron JS, et al: High-dose furosemide in acute reversible intrinsic renal failure. *Scot Med J* 19:S35–S39, 1974.

Doherty CC, O'Connor FA, Buchanan KD, et al: Cimetidine for duodenal ulceration in patients undergoing hemodialysis. *Brit Med J* 2:1506–1508, 1977.

Epstein M, Schneider NS, Befeler B: Effect of intrarenal furosemide on renal function and intrarenal hemodynamics in acute renal failure. *Am J Med* 58:510–516, 1975.

Jarnberg PO, Eklund J, Granberg PO: Acute effects of furosemide and mannitol on renal function in the early postoperative period. *Acta Anesthesiol Scan* 22:173–183, 1978.

Kjellstrand CM: Ethacrynic acid in acute tubular necrosis. Indications and effect on the natural course. *Nephron* 9:337–348, 1972.

Moreno M, Murphy C, Goldsmith C: Increase in serum potassium resulting from the administration of hypertonic mannitol and other solutions. *J Lab Clin Med* 73:291–298, 1969.

Ng RCK, Suki WN: Treatment of acute renal failure. *Contemp Issues Nephrol* 6:229–273, 1980.

Powers SR Jr, Boba A, Hostnik W, et al: Prevention of postoperative acute renal failure with mannitol in 100 cases. *Surgery* 55:15–23, 1964.

Stamm WE: Guideline for prevention of catheter-associated urinary infections. *Ann Intern Med* 82:386–390, 1975.

Tiller DJ, Mudge GH: Pharmacologic agents used in the management of acute renal failure. *Kidney Int* 18:700–711, 1980.

Dialysis

Chawla SK, Najafi H, Ing TS, et al: Acute renal failure complicating ruptured abdominal aortic aneurysm. *Arch Surg* 110:521–526, 1975.

Fischer RP, Griffen WO, Reiser M, et al: Early dialysis in the treatment of acute renal failure. *Surg Gynecol Obstet* 123:1019–1023, 1966.

Kleinknecht D, Jungers P, Chanard J, et al: Uremic and non-uremic complications in acute renal failure: Evaluation of early and frequent dialysis on prognosis. *Kidney Int* 1:190–196, 1972.

Teschan PE, Baxter CR, O'Brien TF, et al: Prophylactic hemodialysis in the treatment of acute renal failure. *Ann Intern Med* 53:992–1016, 1960.

Nutrition

Abel RM, Beck Ch, Abbott WM, et al: Improved survival from acute renal failure after treatment with intravenous essential L-amino acids and glucose: Results of a prospective, double-blind study. *N Engl J Med* 288:695–699, 1973.

Ausman RK, Hardy G: Metabolic complications of parenteral nutrition, in Johnson IDA (ed): *Advances in Parenteral Nutrition.* Baltimore, University Park Press, 1978, pp. 403–413.

Book SM, Makoheli CF, Brown Brown GW, et al: The influence of parenteral nutrition on the course of acute renal failure. *Surg Gynecol Obstet* 141:405–408, 1975.

Blumenkrantz MJ, Kopple JD, Koffler A, et al: Total parenteral nutrition in the management of acute renal failure. *Am J Clin Nutr* 31:1831–1838 1978.

Feinstein EI, Blumenkrantz MJ,, Healy M, et al: Clinical and metabolic responses to parenteral nutrition in acute renal failure. *Medicine* 60:124–137, 1981.

Kopple JD, Blumenkrantz MJ: Total parenteral nutrition and parenteral fluid therapy, in Maxwell MH, Kleeman CR (eds): *Clinical Disorders of Fluid and Electrolyte Metabolism*, New York, McGraw-Hill, 1980 pp. 413–458.

Maki DG, Goldmann DA, Rhame FS: Infection control in intravenous therapy. *Ann Intern Med* 79:867–887, 1973.

Toback FG: Amino acid enhancement of renal regeneration after acute tubular necrosis. *Kidney Int* 12:193–198, 1977.

Myoglobinuric Acute Renal Failure

Eneas JF, Schoenfeld PY, Humphreys MH: The effect of infusion of mannitol–sodium bicarbonate on the clinical course of myoglobinuria. *Arch Intern Med* 139:801–805, 1979.

Knochel JP: Renal injury in muscle disease, in: Suki WN, Eknoyan G (eds): *The Kidney in Systemic Disease*, ed 2. New York, John Wiley & Sons, 1981, p 263–284.

Koffler A, Friedler RM, Massry SG: Acute renal failure due to non-traumatic rhabdomyolysis. *Ann Intern Med* 85:23–28, 1976.

Radiocontrast-Induced Acute Renal Failure

Byrd L, Sherman RL: Radiocontrast-induced acute renal failure. *Medicine* 58:270279, 1979.

Gelman ML, Rowe JW, Coggins CH, et al: Effects of an angiographic contrast agent on renal function. *Cardiovasc Med* 4:313320, 1979.

Shafi J, Chou SY, Porush JG, et al: Infusion intravenous pyelography and renal function. *Arch Intern Med* 138:1218–1221, 1978.

Uric Acid-Induced Acute Renal Failure

Conger JD: Acute uric acid nephropathy. *Semin Nephrol* 1:69–74, 1981.

Kelton J, Kelley WN, Holmes EW: A rapid method for the diagnosis of acute urate nephropathy. *Arch Intern Med* 138:612–615, 1978.

Steinberg SM, Galen MA, Lazarus JM, et al: Hemodialysis for acute anuric acid nephropathy. *Am J Dis Child* 129:956–958, 1975.

Acute Renal Failure in Multiple Myeloma

Martinez-Maldonado M, Yium J, Suki WN, et al: Renal complications in multiple myeloma: Pathophysiology and some aspects of clinical management. *J Chron Dis* 24:221–227, 1971.

Misiani R, Remuzzi G, Bertani T, et al: Plasmapheresis in the treatment of acute renal failure in multiple myeloma. *Am J Med* 66:684–688, 1979.

Smithline N, Kassirer JP, Cohen JJ: Light-chain nephropathy: Renal tubular dysfunction associated with light-chain proteinuria. *N Engl J Med* 294:71–74, 1976.

Yium J, Martinez-Maldonado M, Eknoyan G, et al: Peritoneal dialysis in the treatment of renal failure in multiple myeloma. *South Med J* 64:1403–1405, 1971.

Drugs in Acute Renal Failure

Appel GB, Neu HC: The nephrotoxicity of antimicrobial agents. *N Engl J Med* 296:663–670, 722–728, 784–786, 1977.

Appel GB, Neu HC: The use of drugs in renal failure. *DM* 25:1–39, 1979.

Bennett WM, Muther RS, Parker RA, et al: Drug therapy in renal failure: Dosing guidelines for adults. *Ann Intern Med* 86:754–783, 1977.

20

Care of the Chronic Hemodialysis Patient

ALLAN J. COLLINS, CESAR E. PRU,
MANUEL MARTÍNEZ-MALDONADO, and
CARL M. KJELLSTRAND

I. INTRODUCTION

Hemodialysis has been available for the treatment of uremia for over 35 years. It was introduced into clinical use in the mid-1940s by Kolff, Alwall, and Murray and their co-workers. For the first 15 years, it was available only for patients with acute renal failure. Since the introduction of the arteriovenous shunt by Quinton and Schribner and their co-workers in the early 1960s, a phenomenal exponential growth of patients on chronic hemodialysis has occurred. Approximately 60,000 patients are presently on hemodialysis in the United States. The treatment is expensive. Assuming an approximate cost of $20,000 a year per patient, every individual in the United States pays $5.45 a year to the care of such patients.

Chronic hemodialysis is a very successful treatment and has undergone an astounding improvement during the 20 years it has been clinically available. In the mid-1960s, the first-year mortality rate on chronic hemodialysis

ALLAN J. COLLINS • Department of Medicine, University of Minnesota Medical School; and Renal Intensive Care Unit, Regional Kidney Disease Program, Hennepin County Medical Center, Minneapolis, Minnesota 55415.   CESAR E. PRU • Nephrology and Renal Transplant Unit, University Hospital, Caracas, Venezuela.   MANUEL MARTÍNEZ-MALDONADO • Medical Service, Veterans Administration Hospital, San Juan, Puerto Rico 00936; and Departments of Internal Medicine and Physiology, University of Puerto Rico School of Medicine, San Juan, Puerto Rico 00931.   CARL M. KJELLSTRAND • Departments of Medicine and Surgery, University of Minnesota Medical School; and Department of Medicine, Regional Kidney Disease Program, Hennepin County Medical Center, Minneapolis, Minnesota 55415.

was approximately 50%; in 1979, it had fallen to 14%. This remarkable improvement has occurred in spite of the fact that during the last decade, the mean age of a patient at the start of dialysis has gone from less than 40 to over 50 years of age. At the same time, much sicker patients are accepted for chronic hemodialysis. Thus, a decade ago, there were almost no patients with systemic disease such as diabetes, lupus, or malignancy being accepted for dialysis. Now these patients make up over 20% of all hemodialysis patients. Devastating complications such as severe neuropathy, bone disease, and anemia have decreased. However, symptoms will occur from all organ systems and account for the high morbidity of these patients with only moderately successful rehabilitation. Conservative management has an important part in preventing and treating these chronic long-term complications. Not only do chronic problems occur, but acute problems during each dialysis session are also common. Symptoms and morbidity occur as a mean every treatment.

The rest of this chapter will be devoted to the medical treatment of organ system complications and the treatment of problems occurring during the dialysis sessions in the patients on chronic hemodialysis.

II. ORGAN SYSTEM DISTURBANCES IN CHRONIC DIALYSIS PATIENTS

A. Cardiovascular Disturbances

1. General

Cardiovascular complications remain the leading cause of death in the patient on chronic hemodialysis. During the first 3 to 5 years of hemodialysis, approximately two-thirds of all deaths are the result of cardiovascular complications such as hypertension, myocardial infarcts, cerebrovascular accidents, and chronic heart failure. In the patient who survives these years of hemodialysis, the cardiovascular problems fall to second place as the cause of death. Infection, the second leading cause of death during the early dialysis years, then emerges as the number-1 killer of the dialysis patient.

For many years it was thought that hemodialysis invariably leads to vascular degeneration and accelerated atherosclerosis. It is now clear that this previously widely held observation was incorrect. The cardiovascular complications are not related to the duration of dialysis but are more closely correlated to preexisting hypertension and to hypertension during dialysis, to the age of the patient, and to a high calcium–phosphate product. To decrease such problems, it is therefore of extreme importance to aggressively treat hypertension long before dialysis is needed, to treat it vigorously in the patient on dialysis, and to carefully monitor calcium and phosphate levels.

2. Hypertension

Hypertension is generally regarded as the most important treatable factor of vascular degeneration. As in any hypertensive patient, the pathogenesis and pathophysiology are poorly understood. Although simplistic, it is clinically useful to divide hypertension into two main forms, one dependent on extracellular volume expansion as a result of salt and fluid overload and a form that is characterized by increased peripheral vasoconstriction.

a. Volume-Dependent Hypertension

Over 80% of all patients who begin hemodialysis have hypertension; 90–95% of these patients will become normotensive when fluid and water are removed by dialysis. Salt and water restriction is therefore of extreme importance and should be aggressively pursued. In almost all patients, the thirst center functions normally, and patients come to dialysis with normal serum sodium. Fluid restriction without salt restriction is essentially impossible to accomplish because salt ingestion, by raising tonicity, will elicit thirst and increased fluid intake. The patient who can avoid salt will not be thirsty, will gain very little fluid, is almost always normotensive, and has fewer problems during dialysis because the fluid removed will be small. One can derive an accurate estimation of salt intake between dialyses from the product of serum sodium and weight gain.

Although all hemodialysis personnel and most patients understand the importance of salt restriction, it is extremely difficult to impose. Eating is clearly one of the joys of a dialysis patient; salt is a basic spice, and as a result of its ingestion, weight gain and hypertension remain common in patients despite the most vigorous exhortation against its use. Excessive salt intake frequently leads to controversy between dialysis patients and personnel because patients tend to deny angrily that they have overeaten. Two grams of sodium or less (5 g sodium chloride) should be allowed per day. If this restriction can be kept, a patient gains only approximately 0.5 kg for every day he is without dialysis, since every 9 g of sodium chloride leads to a retention of approximately 1 kg of water.

b. Vasoconstriction

Five to ten percent of all patients on chronic hemodialysis have hypertension that cannot be controlled by sodium and fluid removal. In these cases, increased peripheral vasoconstriction exists. In two-thirds of these patients, the hypertension is associated with a high renin level. Excessive thirst, possibly secondary to angiotensin II stimulation of the thirst center, may also be present. Because of inappropriate thirst, hyponatremia sometimes occurs. Previously, such patients needed nephrectomy for control of blood pressure. The use of a combination of minoxidil and β blockers has obviated nephrectomy in many of these patients with vasoconstrictive hypertension. Preliminary clinical studies indicate that captopril will also be valuable in these patients. An occasional patient will be resistant to any combination of drugs or will have so many side effects from them that nephrectomy may be necessary. This occurs, however, in less than 1% of all dialysis patients. In most patients, the disadvantages of nephrectomy outweigh the advantages. Nephrectomy abolishes urinary output, and more rigid salt restriction will be required after removal of the kidneys. Nephrectomy uniformly decreases hematocrit and increases the need for transfusions. There is a 2–5% postoperative mortality following the procedure. Intestinal calcium absorption may decrease as a result of decreased $1,25(OH)_2D_3$.

On the other hand, nephrectomy may have a number of beneficial effects such as (1) easier control of hypertension, (2) decreased thirst drives, (3) diminished incidence of neuropathy, (4) elimination of dialysis-associated ascites, and (5) rare improvement of osteomalacia. Indications for nephrectomy in dialysis patients other than hypertension include (1) heavy urinary protein loss which is particularly common in pediatric patients with focal glomerulosclerosis, (2) renal infection, gross hematuria, or intrarenal bleeding in patients with polycystic kidney disease, or (3) patients with kidney tumors. These may occur many years after the start of chronic hemodialysis.

c. Therapy

The drug therapy of hypertension of patients on dialysis is similar to the treatment of hypertension in any patient (see Chapter 13). However, certain differences do exist. Diuretics are ineffective and should not be used. Certain antihypertensive drugs cause more problems during the dialysis sessions. Thus, a-methyldopa doubles the incidence of symptomatic hypotension during dialysis when compared to clonidine or β blockers. Theoretically, vasodilators such as prazosin, hydralazine, or minoxidil or drugs that decrease renin levels or activity such as β blockers or captopril should be preferable to those that interfere with the nervous regulation of vascular tone, as this mechanism is important in maintaining blood pressure during dialysis.

3. Arteriosclerosis

Hemodialysis in itself does not seem to lead to accelerated arteriosclerosis. Most vascular accidents occur in the early hemodialysis years, and there is no relationship between vascular accidents and arterial calcifications and the length of time a patient has been on hemodialysis.

a. Preexisting Vascular Disease

The vascular diseases that are found in many renal patients are not cured by hemodialysis. Patients with preexisting vascular disease, such as those who suffer from arteriosclerosis and nephrosclerosis secondary to hypertension and diabetic patients, are much more prone to vascular accidents. The death rate in these patients is two or three times that of patients without extensive vascular disease. The treatment of some of the conditions frequently found may be approached as in any other patient. For example, in the case of angina, it includes medications, angioplasty, and coronary bypass operations. Major intracardiac operations such as valve replacement have also been successfully performed on patients on chronic hemodialysis.

b. Calcium–Phosphate Product

Several studies have shown a relationship between vascular and extravascular calcifications and the calcium–phosphate product. It is clear that calcium and phosphate need to be carefully monitored. Phosphate concentration should be kept within normal levels between dialysis by the oral administration of aluminum hydroxide phosphate binders. The danger of calcification occurs when the product of serum calcium and serum phosphate concentration (in mg/dl) exceeds 60.

c. Serum Lipids

Fifty to 90% of all hemodialysis patients have hyperlipidemia, most commonly type IV with low high-density lipoprotein (HDL) as well as high levels of very-low-density lipoprotein (VLDL). The pathogenesis of the hyperlipidemia seems to be a decrease in removal rather than an increase in synthesis of triglycerides. Many believe that the hypertriglyceridemia and the high ratio of VLDL to HDL may contribute to arteriosclerosis in dialysis patients, although careful investigations have failed to establish such a correlation. The lipid abnormalities may be decreased by reducing carbohydrates in the diet from the usual 50% to 35% of calorie intake. Cloribrate effectively lowers triglycerides but has a high complication rate with painful myositis and neuritis even when minimal doses are used. Moreover, the effect of this drug on ischemic complications is uncertain. It should be used rarely if at all, and in dialysis patients the dosage must be reduced from the usual 2 g/day to 0.5 g/day.

Exercise appears to have a beneficial effect in dialysis patients, since it increases HDL and decreases triglycerides and VLDL. Anabolic steroids, D-thyroxin, and, experimentally, carnitine can also decrease triglyceride levels in such patients. Dietary control of plasma lipids in dialysis patients is difficult if not impossible. Thus, major dietary manipulation or drug treatment for moderate elevations of triglycerides and VLDL in patients on hemodialysis is not recommended.

d. Other Factors

The periodic infusion of glucose and acetate during dialysis has been thought to contribute to hypertriglyceridemia. Heparin infusion, by leading to lipoprotein lipase depletion, can also influence the development of athero-sclerosis.

Dialysis patients are under stress; furthermore, many of them smoke. Both of these could also be factors leading to vascular disease.

4. Pericarditis

In the renal patient, pericarditis may be divided into two groups: (1) uremic pericarditis, which can occur in any patient suffering from severe uremia, and (2) dialysis-associated pericarditis which may occur in the absence of severe uremia. The former group of pericarditis may be the result of the toxic effects of urea. At autopsy of patients who have died of uremia, urea crystals can be seen on the pericardial surface. The cause of dialysis pericarditis is not known. It usually occurs 6 to 12 months after the start of dialysis. Sometimes its development may coincide with surgical intervention or with episodes of localized or systemic bacterial or viral infections. Basically, however, the etiology remains unknown. Efforts to correlate it to levels of BUN, creatinine, uric acid, parathyroid hormone, or heparin administration have all failed.

The symptoms of pericarditis vary, and, actually, one-quarter (dialysis pericarditis) to two-thirds (uremic pericarditis) of the patients may be asymptomatic. The pericarditis is then discovered accidentally on a chest X-ray or a routine cardiac examination. Approximately 75% of all patients, however, have a combination of malaise, shortness of breath, and pain. The pain in half of these patients is so severe as to require narcotics. It is also common to encounter arrhythmias and a sudden onset or increase in hypotensive episodes during dialysis as the initial symptom.

The physical findings include fever, pericardial rub, or evidence of chronic heart failure with elevated CVP, the last being present in almost all patients. Of laboratory findings, an increase in heart size or change in the heart silhouette on chest X-ray is most common and present in almost all. Effusions are seen in over two-thirds of the cases on an ECHO examination and in almost all on a heart scan in symptomatic patients.

At least 90% of patients with uremic pericarditis show resolution when dialysis is started. Approximately 50% to 70% of all patients with dialysis-related pericarditis will show improvement simply by an increase in the frequency of dialysis or when resolution occurs of associated bacterial or viral infections. Patients with an asymptomatic effusion, estimated to be less than 100 ml on an ECHO examination of the heart, require no specific treatment. Those with an asymptomatic rub should be treated with low doses of heparin during dialysis until the rub disappears. The initial therapeutic approach in the other patients is to increase the frequency of dialysis. It is safer to use short, frequent dialyses than to prolong each dialysis session. This avoids problems with long heparinization. Some patients do not respond to this form of treatment, or the dialysis may become complicated by cardiac arrhythmia or hypotension. Such patients, and those with painful rub but without fluid, can be treated with oral prednisone, 1 mg/kg tapered over a 3- to 6-week period if the pain disappears and effusion decreases. If there is no response to this treatment within 3 or 5 days, it should be abruptly discontinued and invasive treatment as described below instituted. Systemic prednisone treatment carries a substantial risk of infectious complications.

Indomethacin has not been proven effective in controlled studies. Simple pericardiocentesis (except in acute cardiac tamponade) and creation of a small pericardial window should be avoided. These procedures are accompanied by a high rate of failure and recurrence. The major decision is whether to perform pericardiectomy or to do a pericardiocentesis with intrapericardial steroid instillation. The choice between these procedures depends on the availability of technically skilled operators, since they seem to be equally effective. Nevertheless, if the pericardial fluid is loculated or positioned posteriorly, it is probably best to do a pericardiectomy. In pericardiocentesis with steroid instillation, pericardiocentesis under ECG control is performed, and a tube is introduced through the needle, left in the pericardial sac, and used to drain the pericardial fluid. Triamcinolone (100 mg) is then injected into the pericardial sac. Every 6 hr fluid is drained, and another 100 mg triamcinolone injected. After 24 to 48 hr, there should be no or little fluid (<10 ml) to drain, and the catheter can be withdrawn after a further instillation of 50 mg triamcinolone. At all times, pericardial fluid should have been analyzed for bacteria, particularly acid-fast organisms, prior to the institution of this form of treatment. It should be pointed out that tuberculous pericarditis is not uncommon in renal patients whether on dialysis or not.

B. Immunologic Disturbances

1. General

Infections are the second leading cause of death during the first few years of hemodialysis, only to emerge as the most important cause of death 3 to 5 years after the beginning of treatment. Patients on chronic hemodialysis have subtle and overt immunologic defects. There are reduced counts of neutrophils and lymphocytes. In several patients, there is reduced bone marrow response to steroid stimulation. Chemotaxis, phagocytosis, and leukocyte adherence are also decreased in patients on chronic hemodialysis. Basal serum immunoglobulin levels and immunoglobulin production in response to a stimulus are also decreased. These patients show reduced delayed hypersensitivity, skin graft rejection, phytohemagglutinin, and mixed lymphocyte culture reactivity. Except for successful transplantation, there is no known treatment of these problems.

2. Infections

a. Viral Hepatitis

Patients on hemodialysis are susceptible to viral infections and should be vaccinated against influenza when epidemics threaten. But the overwhelming problem in these subjects is viral hepatitis. Although some of the cases of liver disease are caused by CMV, Epstein–Barr virus, hepatitis A, and a few isolated epidemics of non-A, non-B hepatitis, these are few when compared to hepatitis B. In addition to its distinction from other viruses, hepatitis B must be differentiated from iatrongenic hepatitis caused by the release of plasticizers from dialyzer tubing and from those produced by drugs such as methyldopa, anabolic steroids, azathioprine, or antibiotics. Up to 50% of patients and 33% of the hemodialysis unit staff develop hepatitis B. About 12% of the patients become carriers. A patient either reverts to negativity or becomes a carrier within 10 months. Hepatitis B infections are most often asymptomatic in patients on chronic hemodialysis. Only 15% will have clinical symptoms. These symptoms may range from only mild fatigue to fulminating liver necrosis with death. The fatality rate, however, is only 0.2% among patients. Most symptomatic patients have the usual gastrointestinal symptoms of anorexia, nausea, and vomiting. Itching and arthralgia are some symptoms seen in dialysis patients that one usually does not associate with hepatitis infections.

Patients on chronic hemodialysis need to be screened for hepatitis B. Because they are so commonly asymptomatic, they frequently become carriers and are a great risk as an infectious source. Radioimmunoassay, which is the most sensitive method, should be used. Patients should, every other month or monthly, have studies done for HBsAg antigen and HBs-antibody determinations with radioimmunoassay. Because HBs-antigenemia may only be very brief and transient, radioimmunoassay for anti-HBc is also recommended. With such tests, most cases of hepatitis B will be detected. It is also recommended that transaminase and alkaline phosphatase determinations be performed periodically to obtain a base line on the patient's liver function. It should be observed that transaminase levels sometimes are lower in patients on chronic dialysis who have normal livers. Any elevation, even if it is within the normal limit, should thus alert one to liver involvement.

If a patient develops clinical signs of hepatitis, or HBsAg is detected in blood, he should be treated with equipment designated (restricted) only for patients with hepatitis. The treatment should also occur in an area separate from other patients. Some patients develop persistent HBs-antigenemia. The risk of spreading hepatitis from any individual patient varies. It is believed that patients who continue to have circulating HBeAg are at high risk to infect other patients and staff.

Dialyzer, blood lines, and other equipment in contact with infected blood should be incinerated. Certain precautions (e.g., gloves, gown, and boots) should be employed as the virus has been detected on surfaces of dialysis equipment, and in rooms where such patients have been treated.

Personnel treating such patients should preferably be those who have already had hepatitis B. When hepatitis B vaccine is available, all personnel who lack hepatitis antibody should be vaccinated. At the present time, pregnant personnel should not work with HBeAg patients.

Hepatitis B immunoglobulin, 0.06 ml/kg body weight, should be administered immediately if personnel are exposed to blood from a HBeAg-positive patient.

b. Bacterial Infections

Bacterial infections are a leading cause of death in patients who have been on chronic hemodialysis for over 3 years. Fifty to 70% of all infections, particularly where bacteremia is present, originate from the blood access. Infections occur to a much higher frequency when silastic shunts are used compared to arteriovenous fistulae and are most common in prostheses and graft fistulae than in fistuale created from the patient's own vessels. The most common offending organism (over two-thirds of patients) is penicillinase-producing staphylococci. As many as one-fourth of blood access infections are caused by gram-negative bacteria. Infections originating in the blood access may spread to involve the lungs and the heart valves. Valve replacement has at times been necessary and successfully performed in dialysis patients with endocarditis. Arthritis and osteomyelitis may occur as secondary infections. Samples for culture of bacteria and determination of antibiotic sensitivity should be obtained from blood and the site of infection. These blood samples should be obtained from both sides of fistulae. Meanwhile, treatment may be initiated with those antibiotics known to be effective against the strains of staphylococci that predominate in the patient's hospital. The treatment is initiated with a parenteral penicillinase-resistant penicillin such as nafcillin, 2-g loading dose and then 1 g every 6 hr. In the presence of proven shunt infection, vancomycin, 1 g every 5 to 7 days, would be the agent of choice. It can be administered after every third dialysis for 6 weeks. If repeated episodes of bacteriemia occur, the blood access must be removed. If a new access is placed too soon after an infection, it frequently becomes infected from the old access site.

The second commonest infection is pneumonia which is responsible for 10% to 15% of all infections. In outpatients, S. pneumoniae is responsible for 50%, gram-negative organisms for 30%, and staphylococci for 20% of lung infections. When the infection is hospital acquired, gram-negative organisms are responsible for 85% of cases, whereas S. pneumoniae and S. aureus account for 5% and 10%, respectively. The remaining infections are genitourinary (6%), gastrointestinal (4%), meningitis, and skin infections.

c. Unusual Infections

Patients on chronic hemodialysis get infected with "usual organisms." Although there are case reports of infections with organisms that are unusual to see in the common population, such as Listeria monocytogenes, salmonella, or fungi, they are not a great problem in chronic hemodialysis, unlike in patients who are immunosuppressed after transplantation (see Chapter 22). Patients returning to chronic hemodialysis after rejection are at greater risk to develop intracellular infections. *Candida albicans* infection of a shunt should be treated with amphotericin B with the realization that the shunt probably will have to be removed.

Mycobacterium infections have been described to occur in an incidence ten times higher than in the general population. *Mycobacterium tuberculosis* has been seen in patients from populations in which tuberculosis is still prevelant. Tuberculosis has a nonspecific presentation with malaise and weight loss. Extrapulmonary disease is a common presenting pattern. Skin tests are unreliable, since at least one-third of the patients on hemodialysis are anergic, and biopsies have frequently been necessary to establish diagnosis. The most common drug program is rifampin, 600 mg once daily, and isoniazid, 300 mg daily. As dialysis removes significant amounts of isoniazid, it is best to give the drug immediately after dialysis has been performed. Treatment should continue for approximately 1 year. Frequent evaluation of hepatic function should be performed.

3. Cancer

The incidence of malignancies is three to ten times higher in patients on chronic hemodialysis than in the general population. Although there is an increase in the incidence of lymphoma, leukemia, and myeloma, most cancers are of "common type," unlike the malignancies occurring in patients after transplantation. Most common are cancer of the kidney and bladder followed by cancer of the gastrointestinal tract and skin. Patients with pyelonephritis and polycystic kidneys seem to be at particular risk.

The reason for the increased incidence of malignancies in hemodialysis patients is not known. It has been speculated that an impaired immune system or intestinal conversion of normal nitrogenous waste to carcinogenic compounds may contribute. Carcinogenic nitrogenous compounds may also be formed in deionizers used to purify water for hemodialysis. Such contaminants may be responsible for the periodic chromosome aberrations that have episodically been discovered in patients on chronic hemodialysis. Besides these general, speculated causes of malignancies, local changes occur in the kidneys of patients on chronic hemodialysis. These may contribute to the high incidence of cancer of the kidneys in such patients. These changes consist of cysts lined with abnormal epithelia that has been shown undergoing malignant metaplasia. The cysts appear after 3 or 4 years of chronic dialysis and may then affect up to 75% of all patients on chronic hemodialysis.

It is obvious that malignant transformations occurring in the kidneys of particular patients with pyelonephritis and polycystic kidney disease pose a difficult diagnostic dilemma. These patients often have both infections with local symptoms and hematuria. These may be symptoms of cancer of the kidney. The awareness of the problem and possibly periodic ultrasound examination of the kidneys, even when the patient is asymptomatic, may decrease the difficulty of the diagnosis. If a patient develops a malignancy, usual principles with operations and chemotherapy apply.

C. Nutrition

Many of the symptoms and signs of patients on chronic hemodialysis may result from depletion of various substances. One cause of depletion is that hemodialysis patients are frequently anorectic and suffer from nausea and vomiting. Infections are common and surgery frequent, so that metabolic stress is not rare. Approximately 1.25 g/kg body weight of protein and 30–50 calories/kg body weight must be given. Approximately 15% to 20% of the calories will be supplied as protein, 50% of the calories as carbohydrate, and the rest as fat. In patients with marked hypertriglyceridemia, the carbohydrate component should be decreased to 35%, and protein and fat intake, particularly of polyunsaturated fat, increased. Sodium should be restricted to approximately 2 g (90 mEq)/day; potassium to 3 g (75 mEq)/day. During episodes of stress, such as infections and operations, complications such as pericarditis, neuropathy, and dialysis encephalopathy may be increased. During such periods, nutritional support may be necessary and may include hyperalimentation. The usual care for the potential complications of this procedure prevail under these circumstances.

Several water-soluble vitamins are lost during dialysis. Folic acid (B_9), 1 mg/day, and pyridoxine (B_6), 10 mg/day, should always be given to patients. It may be necessary to increase pyridoxine to 20 mg/day during stress. An occasional patient with B_{12} deficiency has been reported. Only rarely has macrocytic or megaloblastic anemia been described. Vitamin C deficiencies have also been described, and 100 mg should also be given to patients. Excessive intake of vitamin C (over 100 mg/day) must be discouraged. Ascorbic acid is a major source of oxalate, and preliminary investigations suggest that blood oxalate levels are directly proportional to blood vitamin C levels. Tissue precipitation of oxalate may occur, and vascular damage ensue. Vitamin A should not be given. Blood levels of this vitamin are frequently high, and intoxication may result. This results in osteosclerosis, dermal hyperkeratosis, and hyperlipidemia. Tablets containing vitamin D should not be used. Use of vitamin D metabolites is discussed in detail in Chapters 3 and 18.

D. Hematological and Coagulation Disturbances

1. Anemia

Anemia is present in all patients with chronic renal failure whether or not they are treated by chronic hemodialysis. Anemia tends to be worse in interstitial renal diseases and least pronounced in patients with polycystic kidney disease. Similar to the anemia of chronic disease, it is normocytic and normochormic. The presence of micro- or macrocytic anemia suggests a deficiency syndrome. Burr and helmet cells may be present, which are a consequence of severe uremia or microangiopathy and hypertension. Iron utilization and incorporation are decreased in uremia but tend to slowly improve with dialysis. Despite the low hemoglobin and hematocrit values, acidosis through the Bohr effect and increased levels of diphosphoglycerate (2,3-DPG) improve oxygen delivery to tissues. The hyperphosphatemia of chronic renal disease is another factor that increases 2,3-DPG. The causes and treatment of anemia in dialyzed patients are summarized in Table I.

a. Decreased Production of Red Blood Cells

Erythropoietin deficiency and peripheral resistance to its action are present in chronic renal disease. It is secreted as one inactive form which is activated by an α-globulin from the liver. The origin of the 10% of erythro-poietin not made by the kidney is unknown. Anephric patients have very low levels of erythropoietin, whereas other patients with chronic renal failure may exhibit values within or slightly higher than normal but decidedly low for the degree of anemia present. The response to hypoxia, the most potent stimulus for erythropoietin production, is decreased in renal failure. The only treatment available for diminished erythropoietin is the use of androgen derivatives. Experimental and clinical investigation suggests that nan-drolone is the most effective and the least toxic of these agents. Nandrolone decanoate can be administered in a dose of 100–200 mg IM once a week or once every 2 weeks. Liver toxicity may result, but it is more pronounced with oral androgens. Cancer of the liver has been associated with androgen ther-apy. Masculinization and cancer and hypertrophy of the prostate are also possible complications. Other problems include nausea, acne, priapism, and cholestasis.

Cobalt salts can improve erythropoiesis; however, their clinical use is limited by severe gastrointestinal and cardiovascular toxicity. Erythropoietin preparations are not available for clinical use.

Some patients exhibit peripheral resistance to the action of erythropoie-tin. This may be the cause of anemia in patients with severe hyperparathy-roidism who also often have profound myelofibrosis. Parathyroidectomy, however, rarely improves anemia; anemia alone is never an indication for parathyroidectomy. A number of substances that accumulate in chronic renal disease, such as guanidinosuccinic acid, phenols, and so-called middle molecules, have been suggested as factors in the peripheral resistance to erythropoietin. Evidence for this has been adduced from the observations that prolonged hemodialysis, hemofiltration, or continuous ambulatory peri-toneal dialysis may improve anemia in certain patients.

When deficiencies of folate and pyridoxine lead to micro- or macrocytic anemia, replacement treatment becomes mandatory. Histidine and methio-nine have improved anemia in rare patients in whom the deficiency state did

Table I. Anemia in Patients on Hemodialysis

Cause	Characteristics	Treatment
Decreased production		
↓ Erythropoitin production and sensitivity	Normochromic, normocytic	Testosterone derivations (hemofiltration, CAPD), avoid nephrectomy
Myelofibrosis	Normochromic, normocytic	Suppress parathyroid (parathyroidectomy)
Deficiencies of: folate, pyridoxine, B_{12}, histamine, methionine, PO_4	Often micro- or macrocytic	Appropriate replacement
Iron deficiency	Microcytic, hypochromic	Oral (IV) iron
Hemolysis		
Endogenous "toxins"	Varied	Increase dialysis time, avoid oxidant drugs
Drug induced		Discontinue drugs
Exogenous toxins (nitrates, chloramines, zinc, copper, nickel, aluminum, formaldehyde)		Identify and remove toxin
Technical accidents (overheated or hypo-osmolar dialysate)		Recognize and correct
Hypersplenism	Pancytopenia	Splenectomy
Microangiopathic	Burr and helmet cells	(Remove native or transplanted kidneys)
External losses		
Excessive blood sampling	Normochromic, normocytic or microcytic, hypochromic	Identify, avoid
Poor technique for procedures of connecting/disconnecting of dialyzer, poor washback	Normochromic, normocytic or microcytic, hypochromic	Improve technique of personnel
Gastrointestinal losses	Normochromic, normocytic or microcytic hypochromic	Conservative or operative treatment of ulcers, diverticulae, or cancer

not respond to other treatment. Hypophosphatemia has also been associated with anemia.

Iron deficiency is a common and important factor in the anemia of the chronically dialyzed patient. Under these circumstances, serum iron and total binding capacity are not reliable indicators of iron stores. Ferritin levels and iron staining of bone marrow material are much more reliable. The response of patients on iron replacement therapy is best followed by these measurements.

Patients exhibiting ferritin levels below 50 ng/ml while on dialysis should be treated with iron. It is important to obtain ferritin levels before blood transfusions are given. Transfusions can cause an elevation of ferritin levels which may last for months in spite of iron deficiency. Oral iron is usually adequate replacement because intestinal absorption is normal in patients on dialysis; however, antacids may interfere with absorption. The usual replacement therapy (325 mg ferrous sulfate b.i.d. or 325 mg ferrous gluconate q.i.d.) suffices in almost all patients. Intramuscular or intravenous therapy should be used only if oral therapy fails to replete the iron stores. Hypersensitivity reactions and death have occurred with parenteral iron preparations. To reduce reactions to intravenous iron, 250–500 mg iron dextran can be diluted in 250–500 ml normal saline and given slowly into the venous return line during a dialysis once or twice every month. Only 25 mg should be given during the first hour of dialysis, with the hope of detecting hypersensitivity reactions before they become severe with the full dose.

b. Hemolysis

Hemolysis is always abnormal in patients on chronic hemodialysis who should have a normal red blood cell survival. Endogenous uremic toxins may cause hemolysis, but this responds to dialysis or an increase in dialysis time. One-third of dialysis patients are sensitive to oxidant drugs, and sulfa, antimalaria drugs, cephalosporin, penicillin, a-methyldopa, and others may cause hemolysis in such patients.

Microangiopathic hemolytic anemia can occur in patients with severely damaged microvasculature. It has responded to nephrectomy in patients with hemolytic uremic syndrome, malignant hypertension, and chronically rejected kidneys.

Hypersplenism is a rare cause of red cell destruction. It can be diagnosed by measuring the uptake of ^{51}Cr-tagged red cells over the spleen. It is associated with leukopenia and thrombocytopenia. Only when all of these factors exist should splenectomy be performed for anemia.

The commonest cause of exogenous hemolysis in dialysis patients is the presence in tap water of substances such as chloramines. Reverse osmosis procedures do not remove chloramines, and either charcoal filtration or deionizers are required for such purposes. Chloramines can also be neutralized by the addition of vitamin C to the dialysate. The addition of 2 to 4 g vitamin C per 120-liter dialysate usually suffices. Ascorbic acid can be dissolved directly in the concentrate, but its concentration in the dialysate as well as in the blood should be checked.

The use of well water containing nitrates and nitrites for hemodialysis has also caused hemolytic anemia. Hemolysis has also occurred as a result of the release of copper and zinc from dialysis machines. High dialysate aluminum has also been associated with anemia in patients on chronic dialysis. Persistence of formaldehyde after its use as a sterilizer of dialyzers is another cause of hemolysis. Hemolysis can also result from the use of dialysate that is either hypotonic or hypertonic to plasma. Over heating of the dialysate solutions has led to hemolysis which may last for weeks.

c. External Blood Loss

External blood loss during dialysis is a common cause of anemia. Meticulous care must be taken to minimize blood loss when connecting and disconnecting a patient to the dialyzer. Blood letting for laboratory tests must be kept to a minimum.

The decreased platelet count and diminished platelet adhesiveness as well as hypertrophy of mucosal folds are probably responsible for increased blood loss from the gastrointestinal tract. Unusual degrees of anemia (hematocrit below 25%) should lead to analysis of stool for occult blood.

d. Transfusion

In spite of extensive clinical investigation, some patients develop disabling anemia for which no cause can be found and consequently for which no etiologic treatment can be used. In these patients, transfusion becomes necessary.

Transfusion must never be given to maintain an arbitrary hematocrit or hemoglobin level but should be given only for symptoms that can be attributed to anemia. These include angina, shortness of breath, tiredness, or inability to perform reasonably normal physical activity. As many of these symptoms are nonspecific, their relationship to anemia and improvement by transfusion must be constantly evaluated. The general rule is to transfuse as little as possible to avoid hepatitis, iron overload, and hypersensitivity reactions. Overtransfusion, particularly if performed early during dialysis, may decrease erythropoietin production and thus initiate a vicious cycle of anemia, transfusions, more anemia, more transfusions.

For transfusions, a variety of blood cell products are available. Frozen packed red cells were at one time believed to decrease the risk of hepatitis. More recent investigations suggest that they are no safer than washed, white-cell-poor, packed red cells. This, therefore, remains the cheapest product equally safe to any other.

2. White Cell and Immunologic Alterations

Moderate decreases in total white blood cell count are common in patients on chronic hemodialysis. Severe granulocytopenia and simultaneous complement activation also develop within minutes after the start of each hemodialysis session. Hypoxemia commonly occurs at this time as well. It has been speculated that the dialysis membrane activates complement that in turn increases granulocyte adherence and makes granulocytes stick to lung capillaries, leading to the decreased diffusion of oxygen. This speculation has been challenged, as complement activation and granulocytopenia and hypoxemia can be disassociated with different dialysis membranes.

From a practical point it is important to know that white blood cell counts obtained during dialysis are unreliable.

Up to two-thirds of dialysis patients also fail to develop leukocytosis even when bacteremic and septicemic. However, even patients who do not increase their total granulocyte count usually show the expected increase in nonsegmented leucocyte count. Also, the temperature response to bacterial and viral infections may be blunted in patients on dialysis.

Between 25% and 30% of all dialysis patients develop transient or permanent eosinophilia (eosinophil counts over 700/mm^3). The cause is unknown in most, and most patients also remain asymptomatic. Severe hypersensitivity reaction to dialysis equipment has, however, been associated with eosinophilia. Preliminary information suggests that capillary hollow-fiber dialyzers may be more likely to lead to this complication. In a number of patients, eosinophilia and hypersensitivity reaction have disappeared when the patient switched to another dialyzer.

Finally, antibodies to extractable nuclear antigen and native deoxyribonucleic acid have been detected in up to 20% of dialysis patients. Free circulating deoxyribonucleic acid has also been found to increase during the hemodialysis procedure. There are no specific ill effects described with this.

3. Platelets

The platelet count exhibits an average fall of 20% to 30% during hemodialysis. In some patients, the drop can be as high as 90% of basal values. The pathogenetic mechanisms are unknown, but it is of interest that less thrombocytopenia is observed with the use of hollow-fiber dialyzers than with plate dialyzers. Patients with pronounced falls in platelet count should be treated on a different type of dialyzer. Recovery from dialysis-induced thrombocytopenia occurs within 12 to 48 hr after dialysis. The role of heparin, if any, in the thrombocytopenia of dialysis has not been clarified.

Platelet factor 3 is decreased in chronic renal failure. This defect is intimately linked to the blood concentration of guanidinosuccinic acid (GSA) which, in turn, is closely related to blood urea nitrogen levels. Increase in protein intake and catabolic stress raise the GSA value in plasma. It is decreased by approximately 50% during dialysis. An individual dialysis session immediately improves platelet function. Other substances such as so-called middle molecules may also affect platelet function. Some forms of platelet dysfunction in chronic renal failure have responded to infusion of cryoprecipitate; the mechanism of the effect of cryoprecipitate is unknown.

4. Coagulation

In addition to the platelet abnormalities, there are defects in other clotting factors, particularly factor VIII. Clotting factor deficiencies do not improve on dialysis but can be instantaneously corrected by infusion of fresh

frozen plasma. A prostaglandin-prostacyclinlike factor exists in high concentration in the blood vessels of patients with uremia and on chronic hemodialysis. The significance of this finding is as yet unknown.

E. Gastrointestinal Disturbances

1. Upper Tract

Anorexia, metallic taste, hiccups, nausea, and vomiting are common in
patients with severe uremia; all of these respond to dialysis therapy. Nausea
and vomiting, however, are also common complications during dialysis.
Peptic ulcer disease has been reported both to occur at the expected frequency or to be more common in patients on chronic hemodialysis. Increased mucosal folds seen in upper GI series may be mistaken for ulcer
disease. Gastrin levels are increased in patients on chronic dialysis. This is
probably because of a disturbed feedback loop, since it occurs most often in
patients with low gastric acidity, although diminished renal metabolism
because of parenchymal involvement may also be involved. Acid output
varies but does not correlate with the presence or absence of symptoms or
disease.

Short-term symptomatic treatment of nausea and vomiting or prophylaxis in patients with dialysis-related gastric upset can be accomplished by
trimethobenzamide HCl (Tigan®), 250 mg orally or 200 mg as a suppository
or 200 mg intramuscularly t.i.d. Another useful drug is diphenhydramine
HCl (Benadryl®), 50 mg three or four times daily. Phenothiazine derivatives
often cause extrapyramidal symptoms and profound hypotension during
dialysis and should be avoided.

2. Small and Large Bowel Problems

Constipation is common and is usually caused by the large amounts of
antacids and calcium medications dialysis patients require. Stool softeners
are usually sufficient to overcome constipation. Hematomas of the bowel
wall may result as a consequence of the bleeding defects and because of the
need for intermittent heparinization in the patients on chronic hemodialysis.
Bowel hematomas can be treated conservatively. Patients with polycystic
kidney disease have been reported to have higher incidence of diverticulosis,
diverticulitis, and colonic perforation than dialysis patients with other diag-
noses. Because of the increased incidence of gastrointestinal cancer, it is
important to determine blood in the stool and to do endoscopic examination
in patients with severe anemia.

3. Pancreas and Liver Problems

Patients on chronic hemodialysis frequently exhibit elevation of serum
amylase concentration without having symptoms of pancreatitis. On the

other hand, mild pancreatitis may be found at autopsy in patients who were clinically asymptomatic. Despite the frequency of hepatitis B in patients undergoing hemodialysis, SGOT and SGPT levels are frequently lower than normal.

4. Dialysis Ascites

A peculiar but rare problem for the patient on chronic dialysis is the occurrence of ascites. The ascites is of an exudative type with a high protein content. The etiology is obscure but may reflect a general defect in mesothelium function, as both pericarditis and pleuritis also occur with a greater frequency in patients on chronic hemodialysis. It is more common in those patients who have previously been treated by peritoneal dialysis and in patients who have had malignant hypertension as a primary cause of their renal disease. It is important to send samples of the ascites for bacterial cultures, as sometimes tuberculous peritonitis has presented as a "dialysis ascites."

The ascites may mainly be a nuisance to the patient because of a large amount of third-space fluid in the abdomen. In some patients, however, it is also associated with marked wasting.

The treatment consists of a series of more and more invasive procedures. Increased ultrafiltration during dialysis and simultaneous infusion of hyperoncotic albumin have been therapeutically successful in some rare patients. If this does not help, intraperitoneal installation of a nonabsorbable steroid such as triamcinolone has been successful. The dose is 0.5–1 g dissolved in 100–250 ml normal saline. It is introduced through a peritoneal catheter through which the ascites first has been drained. The steroids are then instilled, and a tight-fitting abdominal bandage applied. Sometimes the procedure needs to be repeated two or three times.

A more complicated maneuver is to introduce a catheter into the patient's abdomen and run the draining ascites fluid through a dialyzer with high ultrafiltration capacity and then infuse the concentrated protein solution into the patient's vein. Although this procedure has been performed with success by some, it has also been complicated by signs of fluid overload, with pulmonary edema, and severe intravascular coagulation. Recent anecdotal experience also suggests that some patients are cured of dialysis ascites when switched to CAPD. Although one would expect a large amount of protein losses, this has not been invariable in such patients. Three invasive procedures are available for patients who do not respond to conservative therapy. The Le Veen shunt has been implanted in such patients. This subcutaneous device shunts the ascites fluid into the jugular vein. A valve mechanism prevents fluid flowing to the venous system if the central venous pressure rises over a preset level. Although this can be successful, it has also been associated with a fluid overload and intravascular coagulation. In patients with much wasting and severe hypertension, bilateral nephrectomy has caused marked improvement with cure of hypertension, disappearance of ascites, and improvement in nutritional state. Finally, a renal transplant almost invariably cures the ascites.

What exact mode of treatment is used in the individual patient depends on the clinical circumstances. Nephrectomy and transplantation may be chosen quickly in the young, hypertensive patient. In the older patient who is not a transplant candidate, a long period of conservative management is necessary, and nephrectomy should be avoided because it will invariably make anemia worse.

F. Nervous System and Psychiatric Disturbances

1. Peripheral Neuropathy

Severe, crippling peripheral neuropathy seen during the early days when hemodialysis started as a form of chronic treatment is now rare. Hemodialysis is now started earlier, and the treatments are more frequent and intense. All of these factors are thought responsible for this improvement. Nevertheless, when dialysis is begun, over 50% of all patients have a marked decrease in nerve conduction velocity which usually improves as therapy progresses. The pathogenesis of the neuropathy is unknown. It is probably a mixed deficiency and toxicity syndrome, as both increasing and decreasing dialysis efficiency have been reported to improve it in different patients. The neuropathy is distal, symmetrical, and has mixed sensory and motor components. It is most common in males. The most prominent clinical symptoms are parethesias, burning feet, and a feeling of restlessness in the legs. The most accurate test predicting clinically overt neuropathy is a decrease in vibratory sense and a decrease or absence of ankle and knee jerks. Peripheral neuropathy is often precipitated or exacerabated by intercurrent infections, malnutritions, or surgical interventions.

An important aspect of treatment is to start dialysis as early as possible. If the patient does not respond, the dialysis should be intensified and its frequency increased in an attempt to improve dialysis efficiency. In patients who develop polyneuropathy in connection with intercurrent disease while on dialysis, the treatment should be the same. Hyperalimentation and vitamin supplementation should be used in patients with evidence of malnutrition and vitamin deficiencies who develop this complication. In the presence of severe hypertension, nephrectomy may result in improvement of the neuropathy. Parathyroidectomy in patients with severe hyperparathyroidism has also improved neuropathy. Carbamazepine, 100–300 mg twice daily, has been used to decrease severe pain caused by neuropathy in desperate situations in rare patients. When the neuropathy is progressive, transplantation should be planned for as soon as feasible, since neuropathy almost always improves after the procedure.

Other causes of peripheral neuropathy include amyloidosis and oxalosis. Vitamin B_6 deficiency has also been associated with neuropathy and should be always kept in mind. Drug-induced neuropathy has been caused by nitrofurantoin and clofibrate. Excess intake of vitamin A can also lead to neuropathy. The Guillain–Barre syndrome has been described in patients on dialysis, but it should be recognized that the syndrome may be mimicked by hypophosphatemia. Upper extremity neuropathy, particularly in the hands, should suggest the possibility of the carpal tunnel or ischemia secondary to the shunt or the fistula.

2. Autonomic Neuropathy

A whole series of subtle or overt symptoms of autonomic neuropathy exist in patients on dialysis. Approximately 50% of all patients have an abnormal Valsalva reaction. A similar percentage exhibit Raynaud's phenomenon. Patients with signs of autonomic dysfunction also tend to have more hypotension during dialysis. In uncontrolled studies, levodopa, in a dose of 100–250 mg q.i.d., appears to be useful in the treatment of patients with severe hypotensive episodes and evidence of autonomic dysfunction.

3. Dialysis Encephalopathy and Dementia

This disorder has been described with increasing frequency during the last few years. Initially patients develop speech difficulties. These are followed by dyspraxia and overt paranoia. Multifocal seizures, gait disturbances, and asterixis follow. Dementia completes the symptomatology of this horrible disorder. The presence of bursts of multifocal spikes on the EEG is diagnostic. Aluminum intoxication is generally thought to be a major factor in dialysis dementia, but tin intoxication and slow virus disease have also been suspected. The frequency of the disturbance is high when the dialysate aluminum concentration is over 50 mg/liter. Preliminary information suggests that when this aluminum concentration is exceeded, dialysis dementia is very common. Complications that lead to an increased bone dissolution and release of calcium, such as infections, immobilization, hypophosphatemia, and hyperparathyroidism, may trigger or aggravate dialysis dementia.
Treatment consists of stopping all aluminum-containing medications. The aluminum content of the dialysate should be reduced to less than 10 mg/liter. Parathyroidectomy, phosphate repletion, and mobilization of the patient whenever feasible have also improved the syndrome. Dialysis dementia is irreversible in its advanced stages unless a specific cause is found. If a clear-cut cause cannot be found, the patient should be transplanted as soon as possible. Symptomatic treatment with clonopin, initially 0.5 mg three times daily, has been associated with improvement. Chelation of aluminum by substances such as deferoxamine has been tried with little success. It is paradoxical that similar syndrome has been described with diazepam, one of the drugs initially used for its treatment. Intoxication with cephalosporin, penicillin, cyproheptadine, or analgesics can mimic the disorder.

4. Organic Encephalopathies

Subdural hematoma can occur in up to 4% of patients on dialysis. Pathogenetic mechanisms are believed to include intermittent brain edema which may result from dialysis. Heparinization no doubt also plays a role. Brain scintograms have a high incidence of both false-negative and false-positive findings. The usefulness of computerized axial tomography examination is not yet defined, and angiograms must be done on such patients. The hematomas are frequently bilateral and often associated with hypertension and headache that worsens during dialysis. Increased intracranial pressure may occur, and evacuation of the hematomas becomes necessary under these circumstances.

Intracerebral hemorrhage can also occur in these patients who suffer from hypertension and intermittent brain edema and who are anticoagulated. Granulomatous pachymeningitis, for which there is no known treatment, has rarely been reported. Wernicke's encephalopathy has also been described in patients on chronic hemodialysis. Treatment with thiamine should be started with 50 mg intravenously and 50 mg intramuscularly. The latter dose is repeated daily until the symptoms disappear.

5. Psychiatric Alterations

Suicide is between 5 and 20 times more common in dialyzed patients than in a nondialyzed population of comparable age and sex. It is responsible for approximately 1% of all dialysis deaths. Neurobehavioral deficiencies are present in all dialysis patients, but intellectual impairment as a result of the procedure does not occur. Most patients on dialysis show depression scores similar to psychiatric patients. Denial is used as the most common defense mechanism. The self-destructive behavior of many patients causes a great deal of stress for dialysis personnel. Hostile behavior by patients is also common.

G. Bone and Joint Involvement

Renal osteodystrophy is discussed in Chapter 18.

Patients on hemodialysis commonly use aluminum carbonate, calcium carbonate, and aluminum hydroxide antacids. Magnesium-containing antacids are contraindicated, as they may result in life-threatening magnesium intoxication. Overzealous patients may develop hypophosphatemic osteomalacia secondary to excessive intake of aluminum hydroxide. It is much more common, however, for patients not to tolerate phosphate binders. Although the normal dose is 1 g t.i.d., phosphate binder intake may vary from none at all to 20–30 g daily. If high doses are necessary, a dietary history should be obtained, as some patients develop peculiar dietary habits that may result in excessive phosphate intake. Soft drinks are common offenders.

Preparations of aluminum hydroxide and aluminum carbonate containing various sodium concentrations are available as tablets, capsules, and suspensions. Capsules are usually best tolerated. Frequently, many different brands and formulations must be tried on individual patients before satisfactory therapy and acceptance by the individual is achieved. Aluminum phosphate gel can be used in the rare patient who needs an antacid but has hypophosphatemia.

All phosphate binders can produce constipation. This may be prevented or treated by the use of a bulk-producing laxative or a stool softener such as psyllium, 3–5 g daily (use low-sodium preparation). Sodium- or potassium-containing laxatives should be avoided.

Diseases of joints in dialysis patients include acute attacks of gout. The treatment is intensified dialysis and allopurinol (50 to 100 mg once or twice daily) with observation of serum uric acid levels. Colchicine is also effective for the acute attack. Pseudogout also responds to short courses of colchicine or nonsteroidal antiinflammatory agents. Tight control of serum phosphorus levels helps to prevent pseudogout. Aspiration of joint fluid is necessary to make a diagnosis of pseudogout (pyrophosphate) and distinguish it from gout (uric acid).

H. Other Endocrine and Metabolic Disturbances

Most women on dialysis remain amenorrhic. Less than a dozen pregnancies have been reported to the European Transplant Registry which covers a 10-year period with well over 20,000 dialyzed women of childbearing age. There is no known treatment for this disturbance.

Thyroid function tests are not easily interpretable in patients on hemodialysis. Almost all tests have been described to be either increased, unchanged, or decreased in chronic hemodialysis patients who are seemingly clinically euthyroid. Serial determinations of various functions and much reliance on clinical observation are necessary.

Hyperinsulinemia and hyperglucagonemia exist in patients on chronic dialysis. Resistance to the peripheral actions of insulin occurs, and moderate elevations of blood glucose are not unusual. As a consequence, patients are prone to develop hyperglycemia and hyperosmolality. Careful monitoring of blood glucose must be undertaken when large amounts of glucose are given (e.g., during hyperalimentation), and supplemental insulin is then often required, particularly in septic patients.

I. Dermatological Complications

Although a variety of dermatological disturbances have been described in patients on chronic hemodialysis, a specific relationship to the procedure is not clear in all of the conditions. Some of the commonest skin manifestations include necrotizing dermatitis associated with secondary hyperparathyroidism and possibly plasticizer release, porphyria cutanea tarda, bullous dermatosis, and prurigo nodularis.

Pruritis is a very common problem in the patient on chronic hemodialysis. It may be a manifestation of severe hyperparathyroidism, since it is frequently associated with high calcium–phosphorus product and very high PTH levels. Moreover, it may be controlled by lowering the calcium and phosphorus product through the use of phosphate-binding antacids, a lower dialysate calcium concentration, or by parathyroidectomy. Pruritus, particularly when it appears suddenly, may also be the initial manifestation of hepatitis. A role for urea in the genesis of pruritus has been considered, since some patients note its disappearance if they can decrease protein intake and if a lower level of BUN is achieved by either diet or dialysis. Nevertheless, a specific cause is not always identified in many patients.

Symptomatic treatment consists of hydroxyzine HCl (Atarax®) in a dose of 25 to 50 mg q.i.d. or trimeprazine (Temaril®), 2.5 mg t.i.d. However, as with other phenothiazine derivatives, the latter drug may make dialysis hypotension worse and cause extrapyramidal symptoms. Cholestyramine (5–10 g twice daily) and oral charcoal (6 g daily) have been tried with occasional success. These two drugs are thought to bind uremic toxins in the intestinal tract. Ultraviolet B light (UVB, sunburn-spectrum UV light) has been used successfully in some patients. Lidocaine (200 mg infusion over an hour during dialysis), lowering the magnesium content of the dialysate, simple skin emollients, and sauna baths may also improve pruritus.

J. Special Problems

1. Operations

Postoperative mortality after elective surgery on patients with end-stage renal disease is only one-tenth of that after emergency surgery. Thus, whenever possible, surgery should be carefully planned. The treatment falls into three phases: preparation, intraoperative, and postoperative management.

The patient should be well dialyzed before he goes to major surgery. If possible, dialysis should be done in two consecutive days to normalize serum potassium, magnesium, bicarbonate, and urea levels. The serum albumin should be brought to a level of between 3 and 4 g/dl, and the hematocrit should be above 30%. Both of these procedures will decrease postoperative complications. It is best to give the blood with sufficient time before surgery so that potassium release may be controlled by the last dialysis prior to the surgery. Careful adjustment of heparin requirements should be made, since anticoagulation of the patient must be avoided. The patient's clotting state needs to be carefully checked. Platelet dysfunction is usually reversed by two consecutive dialyses. Some also need cryoprecipitate for normalization of bleeding time. The platelet count should be checked after both dialyses, since, for unexplainable reasons, some patients develop thrombocytopenia during dialysis. Hollow-fiber dialyzers seem to cause less thrombcytopenia than plate dialyzers. Meticulous control of fluid and blood pressure should also be attempted during the last few days before the operation.

Short-acting barbiturates are commonly used and well tolerated for induction of anesthesia. Gallamine and pancuronium should be avoided as muscle relaxants because they are excreted by the kidneys. Succinylcholine and tubocurarine can be used instead. The former may cause sudden hyperkalemia, and both are sometimes followed by prolonged muscle paralysis which may require prolonged respirator treatment. The exact mechanism for these changes is unknown, but the hypermagnesemia present in these patients may contribute to muscle paralysis. The use of inhalation anesthetics, particularly nitrous oxide and halothane, has been extensive and without much complication.

Hyperkalemia is a common postoperative complication, and potassium should be checked at least every 6 hr for the first 2 to 3 days after an operation. It may necessitate emergency dialysis. To try to avoid it, a 20% glucose solution can be infused at 20 ml/hr. Dialyses for 1 week to 10 days after the operation should all be done with low-dose heparin infusion. Protamine, calculated to neutralize half of the heparin given during the dialysis, should be given intravenously at the end of the dialysis run. The dialysis should be shortened because prolonged dialysis with large amounts of heparin increase the risk of bleeding. Hyperalimentation should be considered in patients who are unable to eat normally. This procedure is of great value since it decreases postoperative complications including infections.

2. Diabetic Patients and Chronic Hemodialysis

These patients have many more problems than nondiabetic dialysis patients. The mortality is much higher because of preexisting vascular disease. Both chronic and acute dialysis complications are greatly increased in these patients. Nutrition needs to be particularly closely supervised. Malnutrition is common because the gastroenteropathy of diabetes aggravates the gastrointestinal tract disturbances common in all dialysis patients.

The requirement for insulin usually doubles when dialysis is started. The insulin almost always needs to be given at least twice daily and should include both a long- and a short-acting insulin in a ratio of 1 : 3 to 1 : 5. In spite of this, the glucose of these patients has a tendency to vary widely, and the new methods of constant infusion may be particularly beneficial to these patients.

3. Children

Children need to be dialyzed with special miniaturized equipment. The volume of the dialyzers and the efficiency of the dialysis procedure must be gauged by their body weight. If these principles are observed, there are no more long- or short-term complications of hemodialysis in children than in adults. Growth, however, is almost never normal in dialyzed children.

III. ACUTE COMPLICATIONS OF HEMODIALYSIS

A. General

Hemodialysis is an uncomfortable procedure. In general, one of the following symptoms occurs during every dialysis: hypotension, hypertension, nausea, vomiting, headache, and cramps. The symptoms are always much more severe and common during the first weeks of hemodialysis and stabilize to one per dialysis after 1 full month of hemodialysis (after 13–15 dialyses). The symptoms are also related to dialysis efficiency. Short, vigorous dialyses with a high small-molecule clearance have more symptoms than long, gentle, and slow dialyses.

The pathogenesis and pathophysiology of these symptoms are complex and controversial. It has been difficult to separate the various factors involved in these disturbances. Figure 1 represents an attempt to categorize various factors involved in the hypotension of dialysis.

Because of the increased susceptibility to side effects during the early period of dialysis, dialysis should be initiated gently in these patients. One method is to treat the patient for 1 to 2 weeks with peritoneal dialysis. Another is to use short, slow, and frequent hemodialysis for the first few treatments. Stabilized hemodialysis patients tolerate dialysis with a BUN clearance of 150–200 ml/min or a BUN clearance of approximately 3 ml/min per kg body weight. One should adjust the blood flow during dialysis to the patient's body weight. Thus, very heavy patients should have a higher blood flow to achieve the desired BUN clearance. Smaller patients, particularly children, need much less blood flow. Allowance should be made for body fat, since it contains no body water and thus no urea. During the first two dialyses, the blood flow should be much slower, giving dialyzer BUN clearance of only between 1 and 2 ml/min per kg body weight. In the next two dialyses, it is increased to between 2 and 3 ml/min per kg, and during the fifth to sixth dialyses, full BUN clearance efficiency may be used. In the patient who does not tolerate hemodialysis, the new method of continuous ambulatory peritoneal dialysis may be particularly suitable, although the

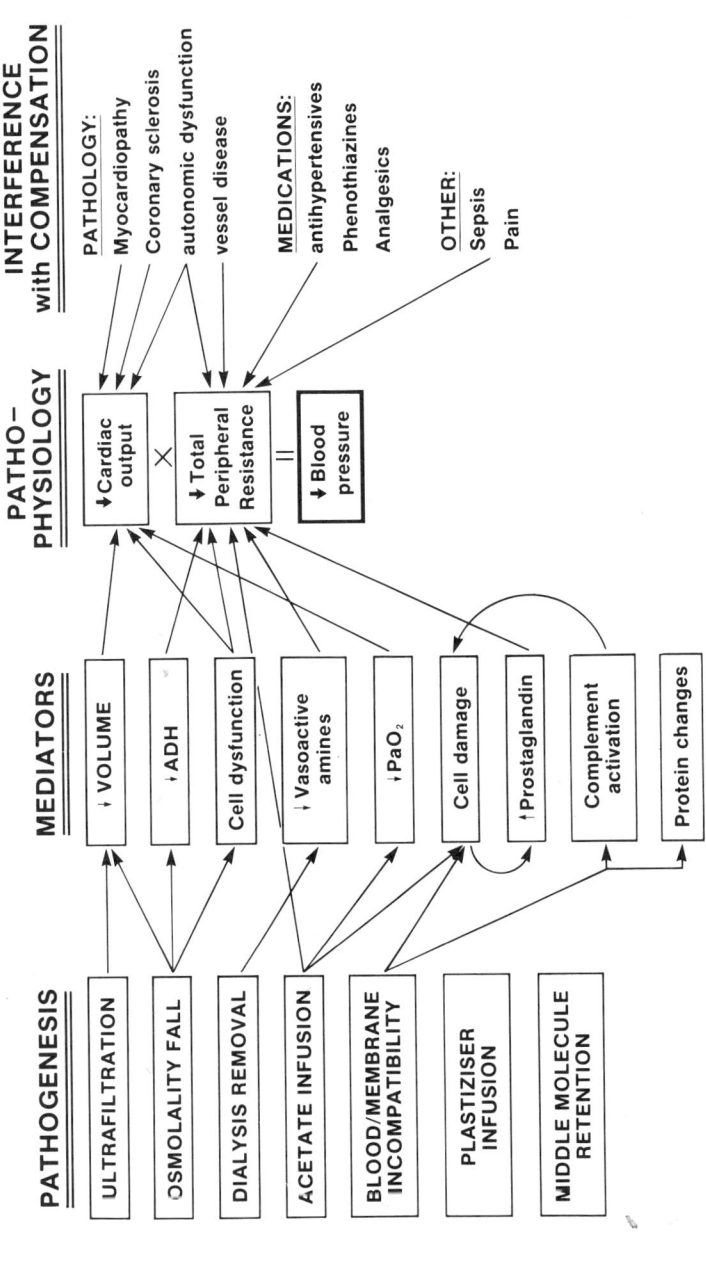

Figure 1. Schedule of events leading to dialysis hypotension. Many factors remain speculative. Most factors seem to decrease total peripheral resistance. (Reproduced with the permission of the editors of *Replacement of Renal Function by Diclysis*, Martinus Nijhoff, The Hague, 1982.)

final role of this treatment is not yet defined (see Chapter 21). In the rest of this section, we first go through the mechanisms of acute problems and later deal with specific symptoms during dialysis.

B. Mechanisms of Acute Complications during Hemodialysis

1. Pathogenetic Factors

a. Ultrafiltration and Sequence Dialysis–Ultrafiltration

Volume removal alone, unless excessive, is rarely a cause of hypotension, but hypotension is common when simultaneous ultrafiltration and dialysis are performed. Hypotension is the most common of all acute dialysis symptoms, occurring in 15–50% of all dialyses. One method of avoiding hypotension is therefore to separate dialysis from ultrafiltration (sequence dialysis–ultrafiltration). Some patients will respond to this treatment, but it is also very common to see hypotension occur when the ultrafiltration phase is over and dialysis begun. In these patients, it may be better to separate the dialysis and ultrafiltration by 1 day. Thus, one day the patient is ultrafiltered, the other day he is dialyzed. Unfortunately, this requires a large increase in the time the patient spends on the artificial kidney, which patients almost uniformly resist.

b. Osmolality Fall

The fall in osmolality that occurs during dialysis causes a number of symptoms such as hypotension, nausea, vomiting, headache, and cramps. The osmolality fall is almost entirely caused by a decline in blood urea nitrogen, with additional changes in the serum sodium and serum glucose. Any factor that decreases the osmolality fall also tends to alleviate many of the symptoms. Thus, an increase in dialysate sodium reduces hypotension, muscle cramps, and postdialysis fatigue, but this may lead to more thirst and fluid gain between dialyses. Sodium chloride can also be infused slowly during dialysis (3–5 mEq/kg body weight). The present trend is to use approximately 140 mEq/liter dialysate. Mannitol in a dose of 1 g/kg can be slowly infused during the dialysis and will also decrease many symptoms. Also, this causes thirst and more fluid retention between dialyses. It cannot be used more than every third dialysis on a long-term basis because of toxicity resulting from accumulation. As the symptoms of dialysis are much more common during the first few dialyses, one can use 1 g mannitol/kg slowly infused during the first two dialyses, 0.5 g/kg slowly infused during the next two dialyses, and then use it only once weekly for patients who are particularly symptomatic.

If no glucose is used in the dialysate there are more catabolism, hypotension, muscle cramps, and postdialysis fatigue. These can be alleviated without increased thirst or weight gain by adding some glucose to the dialysate. The ideal concentration is not known. Levels over 1 g/dl are almost never used, since postdialysis hypoglycemia and convulsions may occur. Glycerol has also been used experimentally in dialysis. Controversy regarding its efficiency still exists, and it is not used routinely.

c. Acetate Infusion

Acetate is commonly used instead of bicarbonate in the dialysate because it is cheaper and technically easier to deal with. Some patients develop symptoms such as hypotension and postdialysis fatigue more readily when acetate is used. Such patients can be treated by switching to bicarbonate dialysis. The exact benefits in long-term dialysis are not known, and an empirical approach should therefore be used because of the expense and technical difficulties of bicarbonate dialysate.

d. Dialysis Removal

Small vasoactive amines such as epinephrine and norepinephrine are readily removed by the dialysis procedure. Although most patients do not exhibit a decreased serum concentration of either, when large volumes of fluid are to be removed, it is helpful to infuse vasoactive amines such as norepinephrine, dopamine, or metaramine.

e. Blood–Membrane Incompatibility—Hemofiltration

Presently, commonly available dialysis membranes are very blood incompatible. Leukopenia, thrombocytopenia, and complement activation occur when blood comes into contact with these membranes. Effective treatment is not available at present. High-dose steroids and antihistaminics have failed to influence these phenomena. The membranes used for hemofiltration may be more blood compatible, and this may explain why hemofiltration seems to be much better tolerated by patients. Particularly, hypotension and postdialysis fatigue seem less with this procedure. Other factors that contribute to this may be that the hemofiltration procedure is usually somewhat slower than hemodialysis and that more sodium seems to be infused into the patient. Reuse of dialyzers may also increase blood compatibility and lessen discomfort.

f. Plasticizer Infusion, Middle-Molecule Retention

Plasticizers, plastics, rubber particles, etc. are inevitably infused into patients during dialysis. Episodes of hepatitis and exfoliative dermatitis in patients and cardiotoxicity in animal experiments have been blamed on these contaminants, but direct evidence is nonexistent. Middle-molecule retention may also contribute to dialysis symptoms. This may partly explain the superiority of hemofiltration over hemodialysis.

2. Mediators

a. Volume Removal

See the section on ultrafiltration above. In some patients, it is useful to infuse 25% or 5% albumin solution in a trial to compensate the volume reduction of ultrafiltration. This is particularly useful in the hypoalbuminemic patient.

b. Decreased ADH Secretion; Removal of Vasoactive Amines

The importance of these factors is unknown.

c. Cell Dysfunction/Damage; Prostaglandin Release

Prostaglandins and prostaglandin metabolites are known to increase during dialysis and may be the cause of hypotension. Preliminary trials with prostaglandin inhibitors have not been of help in ameliorating dialysis hypotension.

d. Hypoxemia

A fall in PaO_2 regularly occurs after 15–20 min of hemodialysis. The cause of this is not known. Complement activation increases leukocyte adherence, and this may result in leukocytes sticking to lung capillaries with a decrease in oxygen diffusion. Other mechanisms involve a decrease in respiratory drive secondary to a fall in PCO_2. Carbon dioxide is removed through the hemodialysis membrane. The increase of pH during hemodialysis, independent of whether bicarbonate or acetate dialysate is used, may also decrease respiratory drive. Oxygen consumption also increases during acetate metabolism. The only therapy available is to give the patient supplemental oxygen.

3. Factors That Interfere with a Compensatory Increase of Cardiac Output or Total Peripheral Resistance

a. Underlying Pathology

Several pathological changes are present in patients on chronic dialysis that prevent an increase in cardiac output in response to a decrease in total peripheral resistance and vice versa. Many of those, such as myocardiopathy, coronary artery sclerosis, and peripheral vessel dysfunction, may be untreatable. Another factor may be autonomic nervous dysfunction. This factor can be treated by infusing vasoactive amines during dialysis. Levodopa, as discussed above, has also decreased dialysis hypotension in some rare patients with severe autonomic dysfunction.

b. Medications

Many medications used for patients on chronic hemodialysis aggravate some symptoms of acute hemodialysis. Commonly used antihypertensives frequently increase dialysis hypotension. Changes in antihypertensive medications may therefore make dialysis more comfortable.

Phenothiazines are also notorious for causing hypotension during dialysis. They should therefore not be used for nausea and vomiting in this setting.

c. Other Factors

Infected and septic patients have many more problems with hypotension during dialysis, and therefore, if unexpected hypotension occurs, infection should be suspected. Pain occurring, for example, in patients shortly after operations is frequently associated with hypotension during dialysis. Vaso-vagal blockers such as atropine could possibly be tried.

C. Specific Symptoms

1. Hypotension

The treatment of hypotension as mentioned above consists of sequencing dialysis–ultrafiltration and increasing the osmolality in the dialysate by adding more sodium, glucose, or glycerol or by infusing mannitol or sodium intravenously. Some patients benefit from switching from acetate to bicarbonate dialysate. An infusion of vasoactive amines, hemofiltration, and supplemental oxygen may also help.

2. Hypertension

Some patients develop hypertension during dialysis. Symptomatically, it is best dealt with by giving hydralazine, 10–15 mg intravenously, repeated as necessary. It almost always suggests that the patient is fluid overloaded and that the patient's ideal weight should be adjusted downward. Some patients, particularly children on rare occasions, paradoxically respond with a decrease in blood pressure to a sudden infusion of 5% albumin in bolus doses. These patients seem to have vasoactive amine secretions that are greater in response to volume removal.

3. Disequilibrium

The dialysis disequilibrium syndrome is one of the first recognized and best studied of the acute side effects of dialysis. The pathophysiology of the syndrome is brain edema secondary to hyperosmolality in brain cells relative to extracellular fluid. Although the clinical presentation of the problem is not precise, the following have been described: headache, restlessness, nausea, vomiting, confusion, seizures, stupor, coma, and death. Sometimes, hypo- and hypertension as well as muscle cramps may be present. The symptom usually occurs late in dialysis or after a dialysis session is over. It is always worse during the first few dialyses and whenever dialysis is performed for extreme uremia. Dialysis in patients with marked acidosis, hypernatremia, or hyperglycemia also leads to more disequilibrium. It is also much more pronounced with rapid dialysis but has been described even after peritoneal dialysis. Children are particularly susceptible, as are patients with preexisting brain disease. These patients often have seizures. Older patients are also susceptible but tend to develop confusion or psychosis.

Although the exact pathogenesis is not known, idiogenic osmol generation is the most likely explanation. Idiogenic osmol generation may result from the interconversion of glutamine to glutamic acid with ammonium ions displacing protein-bound sodium or potassium. Another possibility is the accumulation of intracellular small-acid radicals. Older theories such as reverse urea effect, paradoxical acidosis, changes in sodium, glucose, or oncotic pressure are presently not thought to be important.

Autopsy and brain biopsies show increased brain water because of intracellular edema; CSF pressure is also increased. On EEG, there is an increase of the background abnormality of uremia, such as slow waves and a burst of abnormal waves. The differential diagnosis includes erroneous, particularly hypoosmolar but also hyperosmolar, dialysate, cerebrovascular accidents, subdural hematoma, hyper- and hypoglycemia, and hypotension or cardiac arrhythmias with seizures.

The treatment consists of etiologic and symptomatic treatment. Intracellular brain edema is proportional to the degree of uremia and rapidity of dialysis as well as being worse during the first few dialyses. These dialyses should be done particularly slowly as mentioned above. Osmotically active substances can also be added to blood during dialysis as mentioned under hypotension.

Symptomatic treatment of dialysis seizures consists of phenytoin or short-acting barbiturates. However, intravenous diazepam is the recommended drug in a dose from 5 to 10 mg slowly IV. If seizures occur during dialysis, diazepam should be given, dialysis immediately terminated, and approximately 50 g mannitol rapidly infused. Seizures caused by disequilibrium are one of the few absolute indications for discontinuing dialysis. Life-threatening brain edema might otherwise ensue.

4. Nausea–Vomiting

These symptoms also respond to a decrease of the osmolality fall that occurs during dialysis. Symptomatic treatment consists of using trimethobenzamide, diphenhydramine, or metoclopramide as mentioned above. Sometimes patients may conveniently be treated prophylactically with a 200-mg trimethobenzamide suppository shortly before dialysis is started. Phenothiazines should not be used because of hypotension.

5. Headache

This symptom is often decreased by preventing too fast an osmolality fall. Symptomatic treatment with a mild analgesic such as acetominophen or propoxyphene can be used. Some patients benefit from being switched from acetate to bicarbonate dialysate or being given nasal oxygen.

6. Leg Cramps

This is a common, very uncomfortable, and frightening symptom for the patient. It can be avoided by preventing a rapid fall in osmolality. Other maneuvers that give almost instantaneous relief are the infusion of 50–100 ml 3% or 20 ml 14.5% sodium chloride given over a few seconds as an intravenous bolus. Glucose, 50 ml of a 50% solution given over 1 to 2 min, also instantaneously relieves the symptoms, as does a dose of 50 ml 20% mannitol. It is probably better to use glucose later during dialysis, as otherwise sodium or mannitol will remain in the patient and give rise to more thirst and weight gain.

Some patients respond well to 200–300 mg quinine sulfate (with or without aminophylline 200 mg) given immediately before dialysis. Diazepam, 5 mg before dialysis, may also help.

7. Arrhythmia and Angina Pectoris during Dialysis

Continuous Holter monitoring has shown that cardiac rhythm disturbances are common in patients on chronic hemodialysis, particularly when they are being hemodialyzed. Patients with preexisting arrhythmias develop worse and more frequent arrhythmias during dialysis. A rapid fall in potassium and increase in calcium and pH during dialysis are thought to be responsible. The hypoxemia and hypotension of dialysis also contribute. In patients with preexisting arrhythmias, this should therefore be treated as appropriate, utilizing digoxin, quinidine, procainamide, disopyramide, lidocaine, phenytoin, propranolol, or bretylium as indicated. Appropriate adjustment of the dose as described in Chapter 11 must be performed.

The arrhythmias can sometimes be prevented by avoiding a rapid fall in serum potassium, by using more potassium in the dialysate, or by lowering the calcium content. Prophylactic oxygen and gentle ultrafiltration should also be used in patients with arrhythmias. If a patient has many clinical problems with arrhythmias, it is probably best, at least temporarily, to transfer him to peritoneal dialysis. Unexplained arrhythmias during dialysis may be a sign of pericarditis.

Angina frequently gets worse during dialysis. Usual symptomatic treatment with oxygen, nitroglycerin, and analgesics should be used. If severe, patients should be switched to peritoneal dialysis, or coronary artery bypass or angioplasty of the coronary arteries performed.

If cardiac arrest occurs during dialysis, the usual resuscitation measures should be initiated. It is probably best to leave the patients on hemodialysis but to reduce the blood flow. The dialysis can be useful in removing the sodium accompanying large amounts of bicarbonate infusions. If resuscitation is successful but has led to the infusion of large amounts of fluids, this may be removed by resuming ultrafiltration.

8. Postdialysis Fatigue

This is also decreased by preventing too rapid an osmolality fall. Some patients have a marked improvement of this symptom when dialyzed on bicarbonate rather than acetate dialysate. Hemofiltration patients are said to have less of this complication.

D. Accidents during Dialysis

1. Hypotonic–Hypertonic Dialysate

The extreme of hypotonic dialysis is dialysis against water to which electrolytes have not been added. The symptoms are those of severe disequilibrium syndrome with headache, severe muscle cramps, abdominal pain, seizures, and death. The hemolyzed blood appears dark in the return blood line, and pain in the vein into which the blood is returned is a specific complaint. Treatment consists of a rapid infusion of 100 to 300 ml of 5% sodium chloride solution. Potassium should not be given because hemolysis has often led to hyperkalemia. Dialysis should then be resumed with a correct dialysate and dialysis continued until all blood electrolytes are normal. Seizures can be treated symptomatically with intravenous diazepam, 5 to 10 mg. Transfusions or exchange transfusions may be necessary in cases with extreme hemolysis.

The symptoms of hypertonic dialysis are varied. If extremely hypertonic dialysate is used, such as dialyzing against an undiluted concentrate, hyperkalemia with cardiac arrest ensues. The hyperkalemia is treated with intravenous 10% calcium gluconate under ECG observation until P waves have returned. They may require 50 to 100 ml 10% calcium gluconate. If a less erroneous dialysate is used, the patient often complains of hot feeling, thirst, blurred and yellow vision, paresthesia and pruritus, nausea and vomiting, and develops confusion. The diagnosis is made on a blood electrolyte battery showing hypernatremia. Treatment with a correct dialysate should be immediately instituted. It is dangerous to wait, as idiogenic osmol generation in the brain then occurs. This may then lead to brain edema during dialysis if this is delayed.

2. Erroneous Temperature of Dialysate

Cold dialysate results in chills and a feeling of being cold, and it is easily diagnosed by checking the temperature of the dialysate. Overheated dialysate may result in long-term hemolysis that continues for several weeks after the episode is over.

3. Specific Toxins

a. Nitrates–Nitrites; Chloramines

Nitrates and nitrites may contaminate dialysate preparation, particularly during home dialysis and particularly if animal urine contamination of well water has occurred. Methemoglobin formation and hemolysis occur which sometimes lead to marked darkening of the blood as it passes through the dialyzer. Diagnosis is through identification of the substances in the water, and therapy consists of removal of the offending substances. Chloramines are a common additive to city drinking water. The chloramines readily pass reverse osmosis membranes. As with nitrates and nitrites, they induce methemoglobin formation and hemolysis. They can be removed by boiling, by charcoal filtration, and by deionization. They can be neutralized by adding vitamin C to the dialysate.

b. Zinc, Copper, Nickel, Fluoride, and the Hard-Water Syndrome

Zinc, copper, and nickel may be released from dialysis machines to contaminate the dialysate. Zinc and copper in low concentration induce hemolysis. Copper has been released from heating elements in dialysis machines secondary to acid dialysate and from deionizers that have not been regenerated at the appropriate time. Severe acute copper intoxication has caused nausea, vomiting, headache, and weakness. One accident with a very high concentration of fluoride resulted in the death of several dialysis patients. The fluoride spilled into the central city water supply. Calcium may vary considerably in tap water, and if deionizer or reverse osmosis water purification are not used, the patient may be dialyzed against a very high calcium concentration. A feeling of warmth, nausea, vomiting, hypertension, and rarely pancreatitis may result. Treatment consists of dialysis against a normal-calcium dialysate or, if the patient is acutely ill, against a dialysate containing no calcium.

c. Miscellaneous Endotoxins, Formaldehyde, and Plasticizers

Contrary to previous opinion, endotoxin probably can not pass the dialysis membrane from the dialysate into the patient, but contamination of dialyzers with endotoxin has been described. Fever, chills, and, in severe cases, shock occurring after a few hours of dialysis ensue. The Limulus test is used to diagnose this complication.

Formaldehyde, particularly if reuse is employed, has also caused patient problems. Pain in the vein to which the blood is returned from the dialyzer results; hemolysis partially caused by an anti-N-like antibody has also been reported. The antibody is detected by screening patients' sera at 20°C by saline agglutination technique against a panel of group O, MM, MN, and NN red cells. The anti-N-like antibody can cause hemolysis, particularly of cooled blood. Isolating the blood lines to the dialyzer from a patient with such an antibody has decreased hemolysis. Formaldehyde can be detected by the clinitest.

Plasticizers and plastic hardeners are released from dialyzers and blood tubing sets and are believed to be the cause of dialysis eosinophilia; when they are released in high concentrations, hepatitis and a necrotizing dermatitis occur.

4. Bacterial Contamination of Dialyzers

Fever, chills, vomiting, and shock 15–60 min after the start of dialysis is the usual presentation. However, this rarely occurs with present-day dialysis technology.

5. Air Emboli

This is also a rare complication of dialyzers with present-day air detectors. However, all air detectors can malfunction. Those that utilize a light beam through blood tubing may not detect air if the blood tubing is coated with a clot. If the light beam passes through the clot trap, air foam may also be missed. Those detectors that measure conductance in clot traps will detect air foaming, but a big central clot may allow air to run along its side without triggering the air leak detector. The symptoms of air emboli consist of substernal pain, dyspnea, headache, shock, confusion, seizures, often with focal neurological signs, coma, and death. The patient often complains of a swishing noise and blindness, thought to be caused by air emboli going through the lungs and lodging in the capillaries of the brain. Treatment consists of immediately clamping the venous return line and stopping the dialysis procedure and putting the patient on his left side with the head down and feet up. The purpose of this is to prevent the air from entering the heart and allow it to float out into the inferior vena cava. It has also been suggested that a central venous catheter or an intracardial needle should be introduced and used to remove the air. Although this can probably be tried, few would have the dexterity to perform such a maneuver in an unstable patient, and under no circumstances must this interfere with the proper positioning of the patient. Oxygen supplementation, intravenous dextran and heparin to improve microcirculation, and dexamethasone to decrease brain edema are conventional measures with uncertain effect. Hyperbaric oxygenation with rapid compression to 6 atm has been reported to be highly successful. The air will be absorbed out of the blood within several hours. Periodic X-rays including the inferior caval vein can be used to check this.

SUGGESTED READINGS

Alfrey AC, LeGendre GR, Kaehny WD: The dialysis encephalopathy syndrome. *N Engl J Med* 294:184–188, 1976.

Brynger H, Brunner FP, Chantler C, et al: Combined report on regular dialysis and transplantation in Europe, X, 1979. *Proc Eur Dialysis Transplant Assoc* 17:2–86, 1980.

Higgins MR, Grace M, Ulan R, et al: Anemia in hemodialysis patients. *Arch Intern Med* 137:172–178, 1977.

Johnson WJ, Goldsmith RS, Beabout JW, et al: Prevention and reversal of progressive secondary hyperparathyroidism in patients maintained by hemodialysis. *Am J Med* 56:827–830, 1974.

Kjellstrand CM, Pru C, Jahnke W, et al: Acute renal failure, in Drukker W, Parson FM, Maher JF (eds): *Replacement of Renal Function by Dialysis*, The Hague, Martinus Nijhoff, 1983, in press.

Lazarus, JM, Kjellstrand CM: Dialysis: Medical Aspects. in Brenner BM, Rector FC (eds): *The Kidney*, Philadelphia, WB Saunders, 1981, p 2490–2543.

Linder A, Charra B, Sherrard DJ, et al: Accelerated atherosclerosis in prolonged maintenance hemodialysis. *N Engl J Med* 290:697–701, 1974.

Prince AM, Szmuness W, Mann MK, et al: Hepatitis B "immune" globulin: Effectiveness in prevention of dialysis-associated hepatitis. *N Engl J Med* 4:557–559, 1974.

Ramirez G, O'Neill WM, Jubiz W, et al: Thyroid dysfunction in uremia: Evidence with thyroid and hypophyseal abnormalities. *Ann Intern Med* 84:672–681, 1973.

Rostand SG, Gretes JC, Kirk KA, et al: Ischemic heart disease in patients with uremia undergoing maintenance hemodialysis. *Kidney Int* 16:600–611, 1979.

21

Care of the Patient on Acute and Chronic Peritoneal Dialysis

HANS J. GLOOR and KARL D. NOLPH

I. INTRODUCTION

Peritoneal dialysis has been utilized clinically for blood purification since 1923. It was used sparingly until the 1960s when stylet catheters and commercial dialysis solutions became available. In the 1960s, it was used primarily for the treatment of acute renal failure or for temporary maintenance dialysis in chronic dialysis patients awaiting the availability of blood access.

Two important advances made chronic peritoneal dialysis practical. First, Tenckhoff introduced the chronic indwelling silastic catheter in 1968. Secondly, automated dialysate delivery systems became available. Only a small portion, less than 2%, of the total chronic dialysis population has ever been maintained on chronic intermittent peritoneal dialysis (IPD). This is because chronic intermittent peritoneal dialysis requires 30 to 40 hr of treatment per week as compared to less than 12 hr of therapy per week with efficient modern hemodialysis equipment.

In 1976, continuous ambulatory peritoneal dialysis (CAPD) was introduced by Popovich, Moncrief, and colleagues. Patients undergoing CAPD perform long-dwell (4 to 8 hr) exchanges; CAPD represents a portable internal dialysis system and has been used with increasing frequency over the past 4 years. As of the beginning of 1981, there were nearly 3000 patients in the United States on CAPD and probably fewer than 500 patients on IPD. Both of these numbers continue to represent small portions of the total

HANS J. GLOOR and KARL D. NOLPH • Division of Nephrology, Department of Medicine, University of Missouri Health Sciences Center; and Harry S. Truman Memorial Veterans Hospital, Columbia, Missouri 65211. Present address for Dr. Gloor: Kantonsspital Schaffhausen, Geissberg, Switzerland.

chronic dialysis population which now approaches 60,000. Peritoneal dialysis continues to be used frequently for acute renal failure and temporary maintenance therapy.

II. PERITONEAL MEMBRANE

A. Anatomy

The abdominal cavity is lined by a thin serous membrane called the peritoneum (derived from the Greek word *peritonaion*, meaning stretched around). It is composed of a mesothelial cell surface and an underlying interstitium. Capillaries and lymphatics course through this interstitium. The visceral portion of the peritoneum covers the bowels and other abdominal organs and forms connecting mesentery between loops of bowel. This visceral peritoneum includes the major portion of the peritoneal surface area. The peritoneum covering the inner surface of the abdominal wall is referred to as the parietal peritoneum.

Mesothelial cells project microvilli into the peritoneal cavity. Between adjacent mesothelial cells, there are intercellular gaps which probably serve as the major pathways of solute movement through the peritoneum. In some areas of the peritoneum, these gaps may be more than 50 nm in width.

The interstitium of the peritoneum is predominantly formed of connective tissue. There appears to be a network of aqueous channels penetrating mucopolysacchride and collagenous materials. Interstitial pathways from capillaries to mesothelium may be 100 μm or more in length.

Peritoneal arterioles usually branch into five or more capillaries. The number perfused at any time may vary with the state of vasodilation. Endothelial cell intercellular gaps may represent the predominant pathways for solute movement across the endothelium. In venules, these gaps may be greater than 4 nm in width; in proximal capillaries, many may be much smaller. It has been estimated that endothelial intercellular gaps represent no more than 0.2% of the total capillary luminal surface. Since capillaries are not plentiful in many areas of the peritoneum, the effective pore area of the peritoneum is thus far less than total gross peritoneal surface area. This "low pore density" of the peritoneum contrasts with the "high pore density" in synthetic cellulosic membranes. On the other hand, pore width in cellulosic membranes is usually less than 2 nm. Thus, the peritoneum would appear to have a much smaller total pore area but a much larger mean pore size. This explains why molecules the size of albumin can cross the peritoneal membrane but not the cellulosic membranes.

A summary of the peritoneal membrane characteristics in comparison to the synthetic fibers in a hollow fiber dialyzer is shown in Table I. A most important difference between the living and synthetic fibers is the dynamic

Table I. Peritoneal Membrane versus Synthetic Fiber Characteristics

	Hollow fiber kidney	Peritoneum
Anatomy of capillaries		
Number	7000–20,000	Unknown
Diameter (μm)	200–215	5–10
Wall thickness (μm)	26–30	1–2
Distance lumen to dialysate (μm)	16–30	30–100
Mean pore diameter (nm)	<2	>4
Pore density	High	<0.2% of endothelial surface
Interconnections	None	Many
Length	Fixed	Variable
Channels around capillaries	Narrow	Variable, wide
Perfusion		
Blood flow (ml/min)	200	60–70
Perfused capillaries (%)	100	20–80
Interactions between blood and membrane	Clotting and complement activation	None, except when vascular damage
Dialysate flow	Countercurrent	Stagnant
Ultrafiltration and clearance		
Transmembrane pressure (mm Hg)	100–600	40
Oncotic pressure (mm Hg)	25	25
Dialysate osmolality (mOsm/kg)	280–300	340–490
Maximum ultrafiltration (ml/min)	20–30	12
Sodium in the ultrafiltrate	$\cong$Plasma sodium	<Plasma sodium
Small solutes (urea)	High clearance	Low clearance
Large solutes (inulin)	Low clearance	Low, but same as HFK
Protein loss in dialysate (g)	None	~5–10/24 hr in CAPD

behavior of the peritoneal capillaries which can vary in terms of lumen diameter, permeability, and in the number of capillaries perfused, depending on physiological and pharmacological stimuli.

B. Transport

1. Resistances to the Solute Movement

In order to move from the capillary lumen into the peritoneal cavity or *vice versa*, solutes must cross various histological structures and fluid films. These resistances are shown diagrammatically in Fig. 1. They include (1) stagnant fluid films in the capillary blood, (2) capillary endothelium, (3) capillary basement membranes, (4) interstitium, (5) mesothelium, and (6) stagnant fluid films within the peritoneal cavity. The sum of these resistances for a large molecule (greater than 5000 daltons) is less than the sum of resistances in hemodialyzers, since synthetic membranes are less permeable

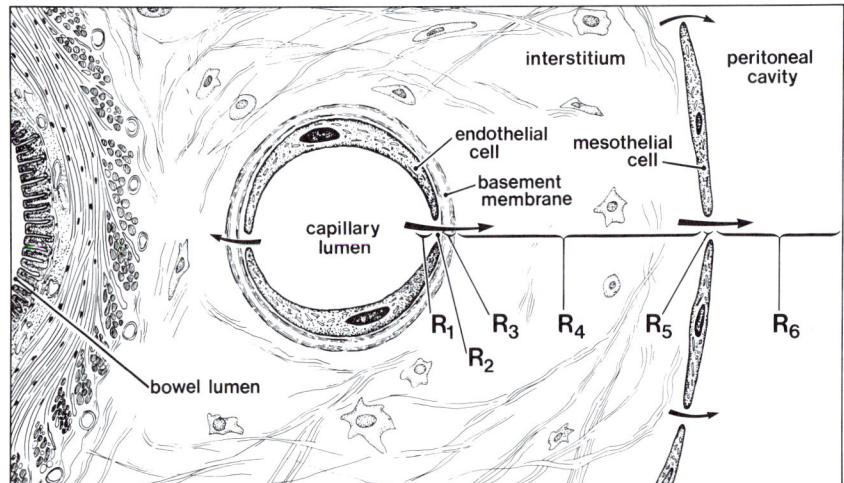

Figure 1. Resistances (R_1–R_6, see text) to solute movement during peritoneal dialysis. (Published with permission of *Kidney International*, Nolph et al., 1980.)

to such molecules. On the other hand, the sum of resistances for very small molecules (such as urea, 60 daltons) is much higher in the peritoneal membrane, since the fluid films become significant. Fluid films are minimized in hemodialyzers. The combination of low total pore area and high fluid film resistances may explain why peritoneal urea clearances usually cannot exceed 40 ml/min even with very rapid dialysate cycling techniques. For solutes with molecular weights near 5000 such as inulin, peritoneal and hemodialysis clearances are similar (near 5 ml/min). For very large solutes such as albumin, some losses occur during peritoneal dialysis; albumin losses are not seen with hemodialysis.

2. Diffusion and Ultrafiltration

Solutes cross the peritoneal membrane from capillary blood into dialysis solution or in the opposite direction, depending on concentration differences between blood and the dialysate. Such movements represent passive diffusion.

The osmolality of dialysis solution is increased above that in blood by the addition of glucose. Water movement as a result of the osmotic pressure can sweep solutes along by the process of convection.

The net removal of solute during an exchange by diffusion and/or convection can be calculated as (drainage volume × drainage concentration) minus (inflow volume × inflow concentration). For solutes such as urea, the inflow concentration is 0, and the second part of the equation can be deleted. For electrolytes present in the instilled solution, the entire equation must be used. If solutes such as glucose are absorbed from the dialysis solution, a negative mass transfer may be generated, representing the amount of substance absorbed during an exchange.

3. Peritoneal Clearance

If net removal is divided by plasma concentration, the resulting value represents the volume of plasma "cleared" of the substance during an exchange. If this value is in turn divided by the total duration of the exchange, an average clearance rate is determined and usually expressed in ml/min. This is the average clearance rate during the exchange; at the beginning of an exchange, clearances are maximum at a time when concentration gradients and ultrafiltration rates are maximum. As concentration differences and ultrafiltration rates are diminished, clearances decrease and approach 0 at equilibrium. For some solutes, such as urea, equilibrium is approached in several hours. For larger molecules, such as inulin, peritoneal dialysis solution may be less than 50% equilibrated even after 8 hr of dwell.

During peritoneal dialysis with 2-liter 1-hr exchanges, urea clearances are about 20 ml/min in most patients. They can be increased to 25 ml/min with 30-min cycles. Maximum clearances reported are near 30 to 40 ml/min with very rapid cycling.

Clearances of small molecules are modestly affected by dialysis solution flow rate and can be increased somewhat by rapid cycling or larger dialysis solution volumes if tolerated. Clearances of the larger solutes are more dependent on the permeability of the membrane and can be increased by agents that alter capillary permeability. Intraperitoneal vasodilators such as nitroprusside may double inulin clearances and protein losses. This is thought to reflect primary increases in venular permeability. Small-solute clearances may increase slightly, but usually less than 20%. Typical clearances at various cycle times for different solutes are summarized in Table II.

Table II. Clearances of Different Solutes at Various Dialysate Flow Rates[a]

Solute	Dialysate flow (liter/hr)	Clearance (ml/min)
Urea	1	15
	2	21
	3.5	28.5
	10	41
Creatinine	1	5
	2	13
	3	17
Uric acid	1	7
	2	12
	3	15
Inulin	2	5

[a] According to Boen ST: *Peritoneal Dialysis in Clinical Medicine.* Springfield, Illinois, Charles C Thomas, 1964.

III. ACCESS TO THE PERITONEAL CAVITY

A. Catheter for Acute Dialysis

In 1959, Maxwell introduced the first catheter made of plastic material designed for insertion through a trocar. In 1965, the Weston stylet catheter was introduced. A stylet inside the catheter is used to perforate the abdominal wall. The stylet is then withdrawn as the catheter is introduced into the peritoneal cavity. Most nephrologists prefer not to permit acute catheters to remain in place for more than 48 to 72 hr. Repeated treatments require repeated punctures. For patients who will probably need more than one peritoneal dialysis, many prefer to place a chronic indwelling catheter to avoid the need for repeated punctures.

Insertion of the stylet catheter involves the following steps:

1. Insure that the bladder is empty.
2. After appropriate preparation of a sterile field and local anesthesia, make a small incision about 2 cm below the umbilicus in the midline.
3. Insert the stylet with the catheter perpendicular to the abdominal wall until resistance at the peritoneum is felt.
4. With the patient tightening the abdominal muscles, increase the pressure of the stylet handle and puncture the peritoneum.
5. Advance the catheter and remove the stylet. Advance the catheter until all the catheter holes are felt to be within the peritoneal cavity.
6. Connect the catheter to tubing and instill 2 liters of peritoneal dialysis solution.
7. With the abdominal cavity filled with fluid, advance the catheter into one of the posterior lower quandrants of the abdominal cavity.
8. Drain the peritoneal cavity and instill fresh solution.
9. Run several in-and-out cycles with no dwell until the acceptable mechanics are assured and drainage flows freely.
10. If drainage is not complete over 15 to 20 min, replace the catheter.
11. If the initial drainage is bloody or contains fibrin particles, add heparin, 1000 units/2 liters, until the solution is clear.
12. Failure to achieve adequate outflow may indicate malplacement, early obstruction of the catheter with clots, or aspiration of omentum into the catheter holes.
13. In some patients, the entire procedure must be repeated several times to achieve an adequate functioning catheter.

B. Chronic Indwelling Catheters

The most commonly used chronic catheter is the Tenckhoff double-cuff catheter (see Fig. 2). Some nephrologists place this catheter through a trocar. Tunnel design and cuff placement are carried out at the bedside.

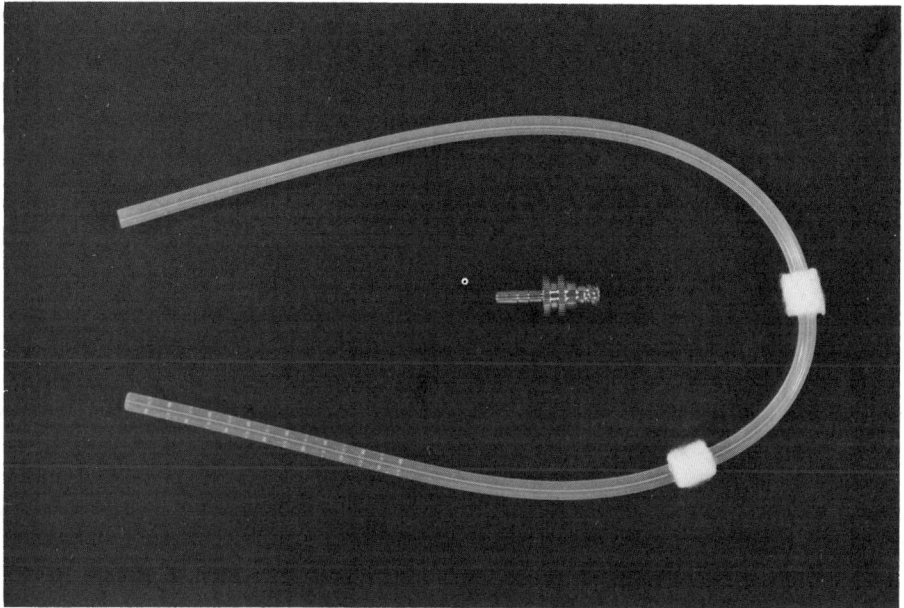

Figure 2. A double-cuff (Dacron® felt) Tenckhoff catheter. A screw-type titanium connector is also shown (see text).

We prefer to have the catheter placed in the operating room by surgeons. Local anesthesia can be used. Tunnel and cuff placement can take place in a cleaner environment. The inner cuff is placed outside the peritoneum below or above the fascia. A subcutaneous tunnel (4 to 5 cm) is created. The exit cuff is placed deep in the subcutaneous space approximately 2 to 3 cm below the skin.

Some centers use a catheter with a single cuff placed in the same position below the skin exit site. There is a short subcutaneous tunnel and no deep cuff. The latter may be particularly advantageous for acute renal failure in which it is anticipated that the catheter will soon be removed. Cuffs are made of dacron felt, and fibroblasts grow into the dacron and allow firm fixation between tissue and catheter. The cuffs thereby form a bacterial seal.

There are other chronic indwelling catheters available such as the Toronto Western catheter with soft disk protrusions at the distal part of the catheter which help to prevent catheter migration into upper parts of the abdominal cavity. The Column Disk Catheter is fixed to the parietal wall of the peritoneum and thus cannot migrate.

C. Complications of Catheter Insertions

Acute insertion of a stylet catheter at the bedside risks puncture of organs or blood vessels. Perforations of intestines, bladder, and aorta have all been reported. Fortunately, these are all unusual. Puncture of the abdominal wall by such a stylet should be avoided in patients with an extended abdomen. Also, patients who have undergone previous abdominal surgery may have adhesion of loops of bowel to the anterior abdominal wall. The bowel will not float away during catheter puncture and is more easily perforated. If the incision for catheter insertion is too large, leaking of dialysis solution around the catheter is common. This may be corrected with a suture around the catheter.

Chronic indwelling catheters require time for healing around the dacron cuffs. Peritoneal dialysis immediately after placement frequently results in leaking. This can be prevented by not dialyzing the patient peritoneally the first 3 days after operation. Heparinized saline may be instilled from an attached bag in 50-cc amounts three times per day to prevent catheter obstruction without opening the tubing system. This irrigation technique can be followed by 3 days of 1-liter exchanges. When the patient needs immediate postoperative dialysis treatment, automated equipment may be operated with 1-liter, 30-min cycles rather than 2-liter, 1-hr cycles. It is important to avoid leaking, since this often will interfere with healing, and the leak may become chronic. In the immediate postplacement period, catheters are particularly susceptible to kinking or migration.

During episodes of peritonitis, catheters may be obstructed with clots. Catheter exit sites and catheter tunnels may become infected; if the internal cuff is inadequate, this may result in peritonitis. Chronic leaks can be a problem if acute leaks do not resolve. A low-grade cellulitis around the exit site is not uncommon. Incisional hernias can be seen. Migration of the catheter or kinking can occur as late complications.

IV. PERITONEAL DIALYSATE SOLUTIONS, ACCESSORIES, AND MACHINES

A. Composition of Solutions

Table III summarizes the characteristic composition of available dialysis solutions. The commercial solutions differ mainly in whether lactate or acetate is used as the buffer anion. Glucose concentrations are typically 1.5%, 2.5%, or 4.25% and range in osmolality from 347 to 486 mOsm/kg. Sodium, chloride, calcium, and magnesium concentrations approach diffusible concentrations in normal serum. Potassium is usually not present, allowing the option of adjusting potassium concentrations depending on the need to remove potassium in the patient. Even with no potassium in dialysis solution, potassium removal rates during peritoneal dialysis are relatively low. For example, a 2-liter, 1-hr exchange in a patient with a serum potassium of 6 mEq/liter will usually not remove more than 4 to 5 mEq/liter or 8 to 10

Table III. Commercial Peritoneal Dialysis Solutions

	Low (1.5%)	Medium (2.5%)	High (4.25%)
Dextrose (g/liter)	15	25	42.5
Osmolality (mOsm/liter)	347	398	486
Acidity (pH)	5.5	5.5	5.5
Ions (mEq/liter)			
Sodium	132	132	132
Potassium	0	0	0
Chloride	102	102	102
Calcium	3.5	3.5	3.5
Magnesium	1.5	1.5	1.5
Lactate or acetate	35	35	35

mEq/exchange. On contrast, a 30-g Kayexelate® enema can remove 30 mEq of potassium per hour. Hemodialysis can remove potassium at even higher rates. Peritoneal dialysis can be helpful in shifting potassium into cells subsequent to absorption of buffer anion and glucose. In acute hyperkalemia, potassium shifts may be as effective as potassium removal in reducing elevated serum potassium levels.

Even though potassium removal rates are low, it may be undesirable to remove any potassium in patients who have low-normal or low serum potassium concentrations. This is particularly true if patients are taking digitalis preparations. Under these circumstances, it is reasonable to add potassium to the dialysis solution prior to instillation to prevent potassium removal.

Bicarbonate would theoretically be the ideal anion for peritoneal dialysis solution; however, calcium does not readily remain in solution with bicarbonate present. Also, glucose carmelization during heat sterilization is a problem at physiological pH. With acetate or lactate as the buffer anions, hydrochloric acid can be added to solutions prior to heat sterilization. For this reason, solutions have pH values near 5.5. Acetate and lactate are readily absorbed, however, and metabolism of these anions results in the production of bicarbonate. Bicarbonate generation from this process exceeds bicarbonate removal rates during peritoneal dialysis. Thus, serum bicarbonate concentrations increase during peritoneal dialysis.

B. Manual Drainage Systems

There are a number of closed drainage systems available for manual peritoneal dialysis. For CAPD, an extension tube is connected to the catheter. Currently, a titanium screw-type adaptor is popular (Fig. 2). The other end is a spike connecting system for entry into solution in plastic bags. In CAPD patients, this tubing is changed every 6 to 8 weeks by the CAPD nurses to avoid tube kinks and excessive wear of the spike connector.

C. Automated Peritoneal Dialysis Delivery Systems

With the exception of CAPD, it is difficult to carry out safe peritoneal dialysis with manual methods without a very high nurse–patient staffing ratio. Overworked personnel can easily contaminate the system. There are several types of automated systems available that are closed and require less personnel time.

1. Peritoneal Dialysis Cyclers

In 1969, Lasker introduced an automated cycling device consisting of a simple timer that automatically regulates instillation and drainage cycles. Eight 2-liter containers filled with dialysis solution are connected to the system which can then operate unattended for 8 hr utilizing 2-liter, 1-hr cycles (Fig. 3). Dialysis solution first runs through a heating box and into the peritoneal cavity. Inflow times, dwell times, and outflow times can be adjusted on clocks on the instrument panel. The machine is relatively inexpensive, requires little space, and is easy to operate. Personnel time is reduced, and the system remains closed over the 8-hr period.

2. Reverse Osmosis Machines

The disadvantage of the cycler is that prepared commercial solution is required as in manual dialysis. This increases expense. Reverse osmosis machines (Fig. 4) prepare dialysis solutions from tap water. Tap water is first deionized and then pumped under high pressure through a filter membrane which removes solutes and microorganisms. Glucose and electrolyte concentrate are added to sterilized water. The machine automatically cycles peritoneal dialysis solution into and from the peritoneal cavity. Series of alarms and devices automatically monitor temperature, conductivity, and flow alterations. The handling of the machine requires specifically trained technicians.

V. ACUTE PERITONEAL DIALYSIS

A. Indications

Acute peritoneal dialysis can be considered for the treatment of acute renal failure or of chronic renal failure when hemodialysis is not readily available (Table V). In the patient with an unstable cardiovascular system or in shock, peritoneal dialysis may be of less risk. Hemodialysis requires blood volume shifts into the dialyzer and frequently results in rapid ultrafiltration and rapid changes in body fluid chemistries. Peritoneal dialysis is less efficient and takes place over longer periods of time. Acute symptomatic hypo-

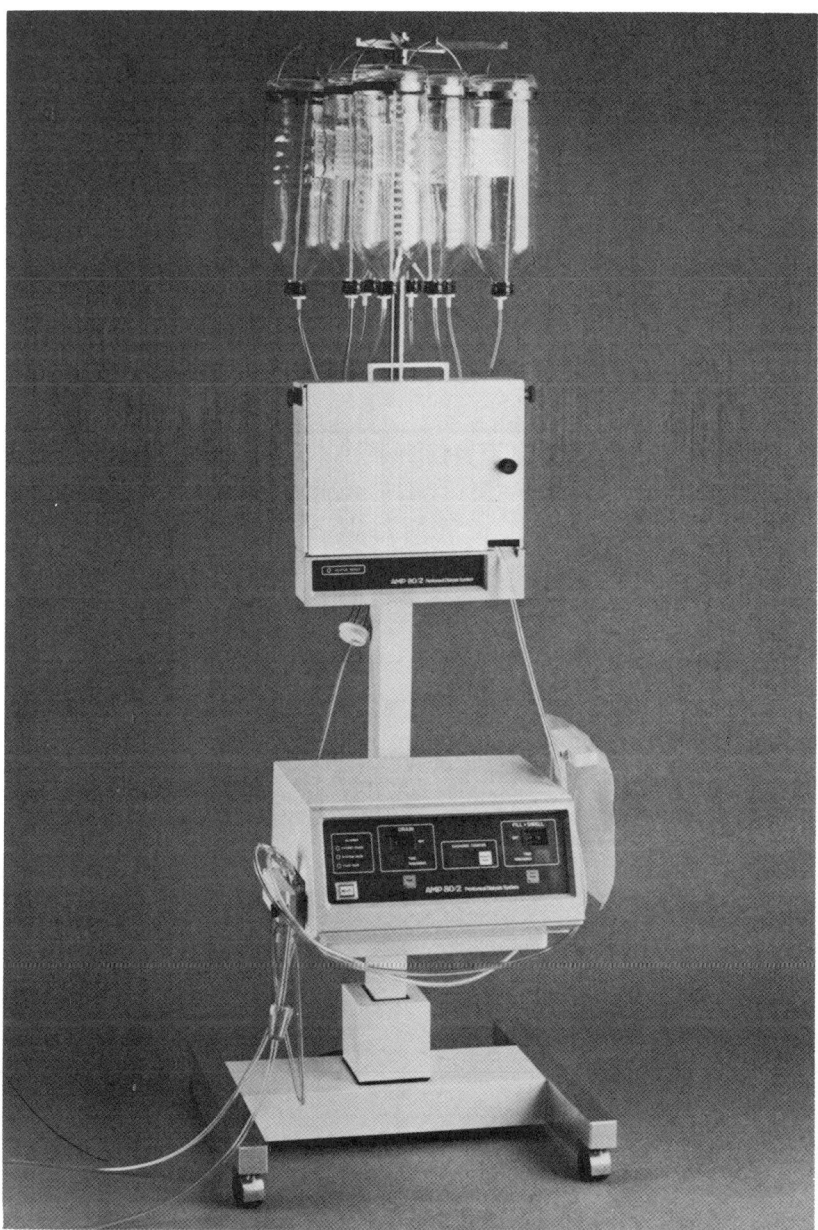

Figure 3. A peritoneal dialysis cycler (American Medical Products).

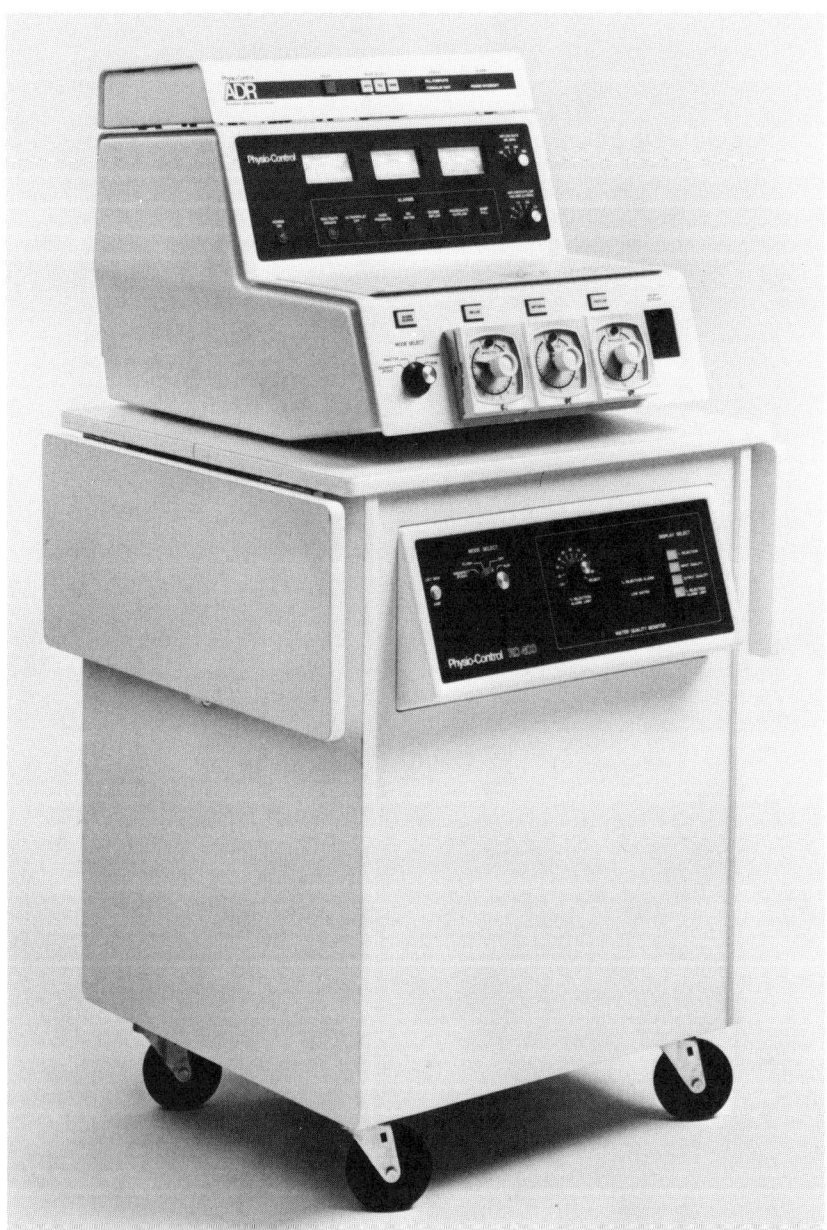

Figure 4. A reverse osmosis peritoneal dialysis machine (Physio-Control).

Table IV. Indications for Acute Peritoneal Dialysis

	Rationale for PD	Potential hazard of PD
Acute renal failure	Less hypotension than with hemodialysis	Low efficiency in cleansing toxins
Hyperuricemia	Rapid urate removal (7 g per 24-hr PD); indicated in oliguric patients.	Too "invasive" compared to drug management; alkalinized dialysate preferable
Hypercalcemia	Indicated when adequate diuresis is not achievable	Ca-free dialysate required Drug management usually effective
Lactic acidosis	Bicarbonate absorption and lactate removal; avoids hypervolemia and metabolic alkalosis	Bicarbonate-buffered dialysate required
Poisoning	Numerous reports about many different poisonings	Extracorporeal dialysis usually more effective; no controlled studies
Pulmonary edema	May be utilized in refractory congestive heart failure	May induce arrhythmias
Pancreatitis	Consider when pancreatitis severe or hemorrhagic; removal of proteolytic enzymes	May in itself lead to infection No controls
Hypothermia	"Central" heat; big surface area	Experimental

tension is less likely. Adequate delivery of blood flow to a hemodialyzer may be difficult in shock. Although splanchnic blood flow may be reduced in peritoneal dialysis, it would appear adequate under most circumstances to yield acceptable clearances.

Acute peritoneal dialysis has also been used for the treatment of hyperuricemia. The addition of adequate amounts of sodium bicarbonate or sodium hydroxide to dialysis solution may favor higher urate clearances.

Calcium-free solutions can be prepared for use in the treatment of refractory hypercalcemia. Effective diuresis and hemodialysis are capable of removing much larger amounts of calcium than is peritoneal dialysis. Peritoneal dialysis with calcium-free solutions, however, can result in a slow, steady calcium removal. Commercially available solutions have calcium concentrations above normal diffusible concentrations in human serum. This is because they are designed for use in patients with renal failure in whom calcium absorption is thought to be beneficial. They are not effective for removing calcium in the presence of hypercalcemia.

Peritoneal dialysis may be helpful in the treatment of severe lactic acidosis. Recent studies suggest that bicarbonate solutions are preferable. In lactic acidosis, there may be less efficient metabolism of lactate and acetate, resulting in small generation of bicarbonate. With hypertonic exchanges, net sodium chloride removal can occur while bicarbonate is being absorbed along concentration gradients for diffusion. Therefore, extracellular volume expansion is less likely to occur with peritoneal dialysis than with intravenous sodium bicarbonate administration.

Peritoneal dialysis has been used in the treatment of exogenous poisoning of many types. Because peritoneal dialysis has relatively low clearances of small solutes compared to hemodialysis, it is not nearly as effective for the treatment of acute poisoning with low-molecular-weight poisons.

Acute peritoneal dialysis has been used for the treatment of refractory pulmonary edema. Hypertonic exchanges can remove as much as 1 liter/hr of edema fluid.

Peritoneal dialysis is frequently used for the treatment of acute hemorragic pancreatitis. Removal of pancreatic enzymes may diminish the extent of local tissue necrosis. Animal and clinical studies suggest lower morbidities and improved survivals with peritoneal dialysis.

Severe hypothermia treated by peritoneal dialysis allows central core warming and has other advantages over peripheral rewarming.

Acute peritoneal dialysis is technically simple and can be performed eventually as a bedside treatment without surgical assistance and without the availability of sophisticated equipment. Trained personnel are essential, however, and minimize the risk of infection.

B. Contraindications

Acute peritoneal dialysis is not the treatment of choice in the severely catabolic patient. Relatively low clearances as compared to hemodialysis may result in inadequate control of blood concentrations of small-molecular-weight toxins (Table V).

Peritoneal dialysis cannot be performed in the postoperative abdomen. Technical difficulties become a major problem. Bloody drainage may clot the catheter. Leaks through drains and wounds may be nonaesthetic and make the monitoring of fluid balance difficult.

Table V. Relative Contraindications for Peritoneal Dialysis

Hypercatabolism	PD insufficient
Postoperative abdomen (first 2 weeks)	Clotting, leakage, perforation
Aortic graft surgery	Peritonitis risk too high
Hernia (inguinal, umbilical, incisional)	Progression, leakage, scrotal edema
Hydrothorax	Acute dyspnea
Other abdominal abnormalities	Colostomy, malignancy, abdominal adhesions, skin infections, chronic bowel disease
Vascular disease	PD occasionally insufficient
	Progression?

Many surgeons are reluctant to use peritoneal dialysis in the presence of a fresh aortic graft. Peritonitis, as a complication, could involve the graft and anastomoses which are exposed to the peritoneal cavity and peritoneal dialysis solution until the peritoneum recovers the aorta.

The presence of an inguinal hernia may result in aggravation of the hernia or dissecting leak into the scrotum.

A large diaphragmatic defect resulting in a major hydrothorax with peritoneal dialysis is an absolute contraindication. Patients with severe respiratory disease may have their respirations further compromised by elevation of the diaphragms with intraperitoneal solution. This is usually of minor significance in the absence of pulmonary disease.

Patients with colostomies, skin infections of abdominal wall, intestinal adhesions, abdominal malignancy, or other intraabdominal disease are more prone to risks of infection, perforation, bleeding, and other obvious related complications.

Patients with severe vascular diseases may have very low peritoneal clearances. Such findings have been observed in diabetes mellitus, scleroderma, malignant hypertension, and systemic lupus erythematosis.

C. Patient Management during Acute Peritoneal Dialysis

The choice of manual peritoneal dialysis or automated equipment must be made. Manual peritoneal dialysis and cyclers involve the use of preprepared solutions. On the other hand, if reverse osmosis is utilized, concentrates are used. In most instances, 2 liters of concentrate make 40 liters of peritoneal dialysis solution and are thus diluted 1 to 20. A 30% dextrose concentrate results in a 1.5% dextrose solution. Most concentrates will dilute to yield an electroyte concentration similar to those of commercial solutions.

Other decisions must be made (Table VI). First, the desirable rate of ultrafiltration must be determined. With manual peritoneal dialysis, this can be altered from exchange to exchange. Two-liter 1.5% dextrose exchanges usually yield 100 to 200 ml of ultrafiltration. Two liters of 4.25% exchanges usually yield 500 ml or more of ultrafiltrate over a 60-min exchange. We recommend using the more hypertonic solutions intermittently with hourly cycling and avoid using more than three consecutive 4.25% dextrose exchanges. With automated peritoneal dialysis equipment, one is committed to 40 liters of dialysis solution with the 2 liters of concentrate. The concentrate can be changed, but it is reasonable to attempt to continue serial exchanges, since each concentrate bottle will last for 20 hours. The 1.5% exchanges will result in 100- to 200-ml/hr ultrafiltration rates which are adequate for many patients. For the grossly edematous patient, 2.5% exchanges will result in approximately 300 ml/hour ultrafiltration rates.

One must decide whether to add potassium. For the hyperkalemic patient, potassium need not be added until serum potassium concentrations approach lower values. For patients without hyperkalemia, we would sug-

Table VI. Management during Acute Peritoneal Dialysis

	Problem	Approach
Dialysate osmolality	ECV normal or decreased	30% concentrate = 1.5% Glucose/exchange
	ECV expanded	50% concentrate = 2.5% Glucose/exchange
Potassium supplement	Digitalized hypoxic and acidotic patients	3–4 mE K/liter exchange
Heparin supplement	Peritonitis, bleeding, and other increased clotting tendencies	500–1000 units/liter exchange
Inflow volume	New catheter inserted	1-liter exchanges for 6 hr 1.5-liter exchanges for 6 hr, then 2 liters if no leak
Dwell time	First three exchanges Routine	0 min 20–30 min (45- to 60-min cycles)
Duration of acute PD	Depending on patient's status	24–48 hr
Some complications	Constipation	Preventive stool softeners Laxatives
	Pain (often initially)	Lidocaine 1% 10 cc IP
	Leak	Interruption of PD for 24–48 hr If reoccurrence, removal and replacement of catheter
	Bleeding (often initially)	Continue PD, add heparin to prevent clotting
	Incomplete drainage	Check position of catheter (X-ray) Eventually replacement
Antibiotics	Routine Peritonitis	None See Table X

gest adding 2–3 mEq of potassium chloride per liter of dialysis solution or 40 to 60 mEq per liter of concentrate. For patients on digitalis preparations, slightly higher amounts of potassium might be added if serum potassium concentrations approach low normal levels.

We suggest the use of heparin, 1000 units per 2 liters of dialysis solution, if drainage contains fibrin clots or if bleeding or peritonitis occurs.

We do not suggest the routine addition of antibiotics to peritoneal dialysis solution.

The choice of volumes and cycle times depends on a number of circumstances. With the fresh stylet catheter, 2-liter volumes can be immediately used. For the new chronic catheter, we suggest 1 liter, 30-min cycles to operate at lower intraabdominal pressures and avoid leakage. Some small patients may require smaller volumes on instillation. In normal-sized adults with acute catheters or the well-established chronic catheter, we usually utilize 2-liter exchanges every hour. If the patient is catabolic, and it is imperative to increase small solute clearances, 2 liters per 30 min is reasonable.

All connections of chronic catheters to automated equipment or to special tubing should be done by well-trained personnel. If the system is contaminated, peritonitis is almost certain to follow. Personnel trained to make connections with the lowest risk of peritonitis should be available.

It must be remembered that aggressive ultrafiltration can lead to hypernatremia and hyperglycemia. Only about 70 mEq of sodium accompany each liter of ultrafiltrate removed from the body. Most of the ultrafiltrate would appear to come from the extracellular fluid space. Thus, the membrane exerts what is called a sodium-sieving effect. The sodium left behind increases the serum sodium concentration as the extracellular fluid compartment decreases in volume. Glucose absorption can result in hyperglycemia, particularly in diabetic patients. Serum sodium concentrations and serum glucose concentrations should be monitored closely. Increases in sodium must be combated by increased water intake or reduced ultrafiltration rates. Increases in serum glucose can be minimized by using less hypertonic solutions or administering subcutaneous or intraperitoneal insulin.

Several common problems may occur during acute peritoneal dialysis. Inadequate drainage may reflect an obstructed catheter. The catheter may also be malpositioned. For acute catheters, it is often easier to simply remove them and place a new one. For chronic catheters, an X-ray can be obtained to see if the catheter is in an appropriate position. The use of radioopaque catheters prevents the necessity of injecting catheters with contrast materials. Acute catheters may cause pain if the tip of the catheter touches the bladder or rectum. Pain on inflow can often be relieved by simply pulling the catheter out very slightly. Some patients seem sensitive to the low pH of dialysis solutions. This discomfort can be relieved with addition of small amounts of sodium hydroxide or sodium bicarbonate. Two milliliters of 1% lidocaine added to 2 liters of solution can alleviate this discomfort. It is not unusual to see air in the peritoneal cavity. This causes no serious problem but seems to cause diaphragmatic irritation with pain radiating to the shoulder in some patients. Peritonitis does occur in acute peritoneal dialysis. The diagnosis and treatment of peritonitis are discussed in Section VIII.

VI. CHRONIC INTERMITTENT PERITONEAL DIALYSIS

Prior to the development of continuous ambulatory peritoneal dialysis (CAPD) in 1976, chronic peritoneal dialysis was predominantly carried out with intermittent techniques using automated equipment. Most patients were trained to operate the equipment in their homes. Thirty to 40 hr of therapy were considered necessary per week. This was frequently accomplished in four 10-hr sessions.

The number of patients on chronic intermittent peritoneal dialysis probably never exceeded 2% of the total chronic dialysis population. This related primarily to the time requirements as compared to chronic hemodialysis which requires three 4- to 5-hr sessions per week.

Chronic intermittent peritoneal dialysis is still a viable alternative for home dialysis. Not all patient can be trained to perform CAPD. It is more reasonable to utilize a partner to help with chronic IPD than with CAPD. With rare exceptions, CAPD should be entirely self-care.

Essential training for chronic IPD includes catheter care, maintenance and utilization of automated equipment, and monitoring vital signs during and between treatments. The patients must be familiar with complications of a technical nature that could occur during treatment. They must be aware of problems associated with excessive dehydration or the development of peritonitis. An understanding of their diet and medications is also essential.

VII. CONTINUOUS AMBULATORY PERITONEAL DIALYSIS

A. Definition

In 1976, Popvich and Moncrief described a new approach to chronic peritoneal dialysis: CAPD involves continuous peritoneal dialysis, 24 hr a day, 7 days a week. The patients drain the peritoneal cavity and instill fresh solution three to five times a day depending on their size and clearance requirements. Daytime cycles usually last 4–6 hr, and nighttime cycles 8 hr. This provides low efficiency but continuous dialysis. On a weekly basis, it provides almost as much clearance of urea as intermittent hemodialysis therapy and exceeds the clearances provided by intermittent peritoneal dialysis. For large molecules, for example, in the 5000-dalton range, CAPD clearances per week may be five times those provided by intermittent hemodialysis (Table VII).

Initially, in the United States, the technique involved the use of peritoneal dialysis solutions in bottles. Each exchange required connection and disconnection of tubing. In 1977, Oreopoulos described a form of CAPD using peritoneal dialysis solutions in plastic bags. The plastic bags can be left in place during cycles and used for drainage. Fresh bags can be easily attached to the connecting tubing with a spike connection. Connecting tubing can be joined to the catheter by a screw-lock system that prevents disconnections and is water safe. This connecting tube can be replaced every 4–8 weeks in clinic by trained nurses. Thus, patients need to be trained only to make bag changes. The latter does require very careful technique in order to avoid contamination of the spike. Details of the technique are beyond the scope of this chapter.

Table VII. Clearances of Different Solutes with Different Dialysis Techniques over Different Lengths of Time

	IPD	CAPD	Standard HD	IPD	CAPD	Standard HD
Rate/frequency	2 liters/hr	4 × 2 liters/day	200 ml blood flow/min	4 × 10 hr per week	4 × 2 liters/day, 7 days a week	3 × 5 hr per week
Urea (60 daltons)	20 ml/min	8 ml/min	159 ml/min	50 liters/week	81 liters/week	143 liters/week
Creatinine (113 daltons)	13 ml/min	6 ml/min	130 ml/min	31 liters/week	60 liters/week	117 liters/week
Vitamin B_{12} (1355 daltons)	8 ml/min	5 ml/min	17 ml/min	19 liters/week	50 liters/week	15 liters/week
Inulin (5200 daltons)	5 ml/min	3 ml/min	5 ml/min	12 liters/week	30 liters/week	5 liters/week

The term "ambulatory" refers to the fact that the CAPD patient is totally independent of any kind of machine. After hospitalization for catheter placement and break-in, he can be trained to perform CAPD as an outpatient. Patients can vary the use of 1.5%, 2.5%, or 4.25% exchanges depending on the need to remove edema fluid to maintain their weight. Chemistries remain essentially steady state. Ultrafiltration is slow and steady. This represents an internal portable wearable continuous dialysis system.

B. Patient Selection

Conditions favoring consideration of CAPD would include blood access failure, an unstable cardiovascular system, small children with difficulties in achieving blood access, problems in being inactive during intermittent therapy, the patient who lives alone and desires home dialysis, and patients prone to hypotension during hemodialysis. There are those who feel that diabetic retinopathy may be aggravated by fluctuating blood pressure and anticoagulation during hemodialysis. This remains to be proven, but many now prefer CAPD for diabetics.

Unfavorable conditions for CAPD would include blindness, poor motor coordination, severe weakness in assuring the ability to carry out the technique, poor hygiene, and a lack of motivation to self-care.

C. Training and Follow-up

Training can actually begin during the catheter break-in period. It can be continued on an outpatient basis. The CAPD training typically takes 5–10 days and includes items summarized in Table VIII. This training must be carried out by a well-qualified, experienced CAPD nurse. The duration of training must be adjusted to individual patients.

The patient/nurse contact must be frequent following completion of training. This is established by telephone communications at regular scheduled intervals as well as additional times when necessary.

The patient must be scheduled to be examined in clinic, initially at 4-week intervals. Clinic visits may be at 6- to 8-week intervals later if patients are doing well. During clinic visits, patients are also subjected to numerous laboratory evaluations (Table IX); tube changes should be made by the CAPD nurses during clinic visits.

D. Some Aspects of Medical Management on CAPD

Most patients on CAPD gain weight. This is attributed to a return of excellent appetite coupled with absorption of glucose from the dialysis solu-

Table VIII. CAPD Patient Education Outline

1. Normal kidney function
2. Kidney disease
3. Uremic complications
4. Principles of dialysis therapy
    A. Hemodialysis
    B. Peritoneal dialysis
    C. CAPD
5. Peritoneal anatomy
6. Indwelling peritoneal catheter
7. Kinetics of CAPD
8. Catheter and exit site care
9. CAPD
    A. CAPD system
    B. Solution concentration
    C. Exchange cycles
    D. Exchange schedules
10. Principles of asepsis
11. Procedures
    A. CAPD exchange
    B. Tubing change
    C. Addition of IP medication
    D. Collection of sterile dialysate samples
12. Fluid balance
13. Diet
14. Medications
15. Monitoring of vital signs, blood pressure, weight
16. Maintenance of home dialysis records
17. Routine laboratory interpretations
18. Diagnostic procedures
19. Procedures for contamination of the CAPD system
20. Technical problems
21. Complications
22. Activities and exercise program
23. Social, psychological, and sexual implications
24. Patient responsibilities
25. Home dialysis supplies
26. Unit, staff directory
27. Emergency call system

tion. From each 2-liter 1.5% dextrose exchange, approximately 25 g of glucose is absorbed. Approximately 70 g of glucose is absorbed from 4.25% dextrose exchanges. Each exchange can add 100–280 calories to the daily oral caloric intake. Glucose absorption may aggravate hypertriglyceridemia which is frequently found in chronic renal failure and in all chronic dialysis populations. Long-term effects of hypertriglyceridemia are uncertain. It is not known whether it contributes to or aggravates arteriosclerotic cardiovascular disease.

Blood pressure can usually be readily controlled in CAPD patients by adequate ultrafiltration. Interesting studies suggest that blood pressure control may be more readily accomplished in CAPD patients than in other dialysis populations.

Patients on CAPD lose about 5–10 g of protein per day in their dialysate. Nitrogen balance studies suggest that this can easily be replaced with adequate oral intake and that malnutrition should not be encountered in most patients who eat well. During episodes of peritonitis, protein losses regularly increase. Patients with inadequate diets such as alcoholics may develop signs of malnutrition on CAPD.

It is interesting that hematocrits usually increase to above 30% in CAPD patients. The reason for the better control of anemia on CAPD is unknown.

Patients do receive oral supplementation of water-soluble vitamins to replace peritoneal losses.

Potassium is usually controlled in the normal range. This is of interest, since four exchanges per day yield about 10 liters of drainage. Equilibrated dialysate with serum values of 4 mEq/liter should thus result in the removal of nearly 40 mEq of potassium in dialysate at most. Patients are frequently eating more than this (60 mEq/day). Differences between dialysate losses and oral intake may be explained for the most part by stool losses. Mechanisms responsible for the adjustment of stool losses in these patients are unknown.

Control of serum inorganic phosphate often requires some phosphate binders.

Table IX. Clinical and Laboratory Parameters for Patient Follow-up

Every clinic visit (4–6 weeks)	Check-up (½–1 year)
Clinical	Clinical
Weight	Complete physical exam
Blood pressure (supine, upright)	Fundoscopic eye exam
Fluid status (edema)	Neurological exam, including nerve
Catheter status (exit site, cuff palpation)	conduction velocity
Dialysate drainage (volume, appearance)	
Brief physical exam (heart, lungs,	
abdomen, pulses)	
Laboratory	Laboratory
Hemoglobin, hematocrit	Complete blood count
White blood cells	Complete serum chemistry
Electrolytes	Dialysate cell count and differential
BUN, creatinine	Dialysate cultures
Calcium, phosphate	Peritoneal clearances for urea and
Alkaline phosphatase	creatinine
Total protein	Residual renal function (urine volume,
Albumin	clearances)
Uric acid	Electrocardiogram
Cholesterol, triglycerides	Chest X-ray
	Bone X-rays
	PTH, magnesium

VIII. PERITONITIS AND CATHETER TUNNEL INFECTIONS

A. Incidence

The major complication of CAPD in the early years was peritonitis. This was particularly the case in the United States during the period 1977–1978 when CAPD was performed with dialysis solutions in bottles. Subsequent to the development of the technique with solutions in bags in Canada and the approval of dialysis solutions in bags in the United States in September of 1978, the incidence of peritonitis has decreased. In our own center, the incidence of peritonitis in the first year with bottles was six episodes per patient year. In 1980, using the solutions in plastic bags the incidence has decreased to one episode per patient year. This trend also reflects increasing staff experience, increasing numbers of patients with long-term experience, and improvements in connectors and techniques. The screw-type connection between the catheter and the connecting tube eliminates loose connections at this site. This was a frequent problem with prior tubing.

In other forms of peritoneal dialysis, in which the connections are made primarily by experts and are much less frequent, there is a very low incidence of peritonitis. In some IPD programs, the incidence of peritonitis is less than one episode per hundred connect/disconnect procedures. Actually, CAPD patients do very well in terms of numbers of connect/disconnnect procedures, since the openings of the system reoccur so frequently. Episodes of peritonitis per unit time are higher than in IPD.

B. Diagnosis

Peritonitis usually begins with turbid drainage. The turbidity is caused by increased leukocyte counts in the dialysis solution. There are several causes of turbidity other than peritonitis. These include lymphatics leaking into dialysate. Also, increased amounts of fibrin particles when dispersed can cause slight turbidity. In both instances, dialysate leukocyte counts will be well below 100 cells per cubic millimeter in the absence of peritonitis. More than 100 leukocytes per cubic millimeter in dialysate drainage strongly suggests peritoneal inflammation. In the absence of peritonitis, the mean leukocyte count in our center has been 23 leukocytes per cubic millimeter. In the latter situation, lymphocytes, monocytes, and mesothelial cells predominate, and neutrophils are in the minority.

In contrast, neutrophils tend to predominate in bacterial peritonitis and with fungal peritonitis. Elevated leukocyte counts with predominantly mononuclear cells over a prolonged period of time might raise a suspicion of tuberculous peritonitis.

One type of peritonitis that can occur but does not appear to be infectious is eosinophilic peritonitis. Here, leukocyte counts are elevated, and eosinophils predominate. This could represent some type of allergic reaction or chemical irritation of the peritoneum and may be transient and disappear without therapy.

Most patients with peritonitis develop abdominal symptoms . Abdominal tenderness to palpation may be mild to severe. Rebound tenderness is often present. Other findings include fever, nausea and vomiting, chills, and other nonspecific symptoms. In our experience, chills and fever occur in the minority of patients.

It is important to examine the exit site and tunnel to see if they may be primarily or secondarily infected. Tunnel involvement may develop from an exit site infection and actually lead to peritonitis. On the other hand, if the internal cuff does not prevent back leak into the tunnel, infested fluid can enter the tunnel and cause a secondary tunnel infection in association with peritonitis that results from tubing contamination. Tunnel involvement is indicated by erythema, tunnel tenderness, and purulent discharge from the catheter exit site. Leaking of infected fluid into the subcutaneous tissue from the tunnel can result in cellulitis. In our experience, tunnel involvement of any kind is an indication for catheter removal.

C. Cultures and Gram Stains

If dialysate cell counts are elevated, the sediment of centrifuged dialysate should be examined by gram stain. In about 50% of cases of peritonitis, an organism can be seen on gram stain.

Specific culture techniques should be used to identify very low numbers of bacteria in dialysate (as low as one bacterium per 100 ml). Centrifugation or filter culture techniques are recommended. We do not routinely obtain fungal or anerobic cultures. Fungal cultures are obtained when patients are not responding after 48 hr of therapy, in patients exposed to multiple antibiotics previously, or in patients who are immunosuppressed. Anaerobic cultures are obtained in patients who do not respond to initial therapy or if a perforated viscus is suspected. The latter is highly suspect if multiple organisms (mixed gram-positive/gram-negative) are seen on gram stain or more than one organism is identified on culture. In our experience, multiple organisms have been almost invariably indicative of a perforated bowel with poor prognosis despite catheter removal.

D. Treatment

We do not delay the initiation of therapy once elevated neutrophil counts have been identified in dialysate drainage and gram stains and cultures have been obtained. Usually, 60–75% of episodes of peritonitis are caused by gram-positive organisms. Unless gram-negative organisms are seen on gram stains, we would start therapy with a cephalosporin. This is

usually given intraperitoneally for 10–14 days. If gram-negative organisms
are seen on gram stain, we are more likely to start initial therapy with an
intramuscular loading dose of an aminoglycoside followed by intraperitoneal therapy. Once cultures and sensitivities are obtained, antibiotic therapy is changed if necessary. Table X summarizes typical doses of numerous
antibiotics for intraperitoneal administration during long-dwell CAPD exchanges or during rapid-cycling intermittent peritoneal dialysis. In the latter
cases, the doses are somewhat lower, since so many more exchanges are
being instilled per day, and total antibiotic absorption would most likely be
greater. Although peritoneal dialysis does not remove antibiotics from the
blood stream rapidly enough to require significant adjustment of antibiotic
systemic doses, it presumably provides enough absorption at intraperitoneal
concentrations listed to maintain adequate blood levels (see Table X).

Table X. Intraperitoneal Administration of Antibiotics

	IPD (mg/liter)	CAPD (mg/liter)	Comments

Cephalosporins
  Cephalothin
  Cephazolin
  Cephaloridin
	100	125	Readily absorbed
			First drug of choice in gram-
			  positive peritonitis

Aminoglycosides
  Gentamycin
  Tobramycin
  Amikacin
	5	5–8	Slow absorption
			Parenteral priming dose required:
			  1–1.5 mg/kg B.W.
			First drug of choice in gram-
			  negative peritonitis
			Follow serum levels: 4–8 μg/ml

Penicillins
  Penicillin G
  Ampicillin
  Cloxacillin
	
	50,000 u/liter
	50
	100
		
		50,000 u/liter
		50
		100
			
			Not used routinely

Chloramphenicol	—	—	Inactive intraperitoneally
Tetracycline	—	—	Not recommended
Erythromycin	—	—	Not recommended

Vancomycin	15	15–30	Indicated in peritonitis with
			  tunnel infections
			Parenteral priming dose required:
			  1 g IV drip (30–60 min)

Sulfa drugs	5 TMP 25 SMZ	5 TMP 25 SMZ	Indicated for *Nocardia* peritonitis
Amphotericin B	1–2	2–4	Indicated in fungal peritonitis Consider catheter removal Painful Additional parenteral treatment required

In CAPD patients, we prefer to treat peritonitis with CAPD-type exchanges. This can be done on an outpatient basis initially, but patients must be hospitalized if they do not promptly clear within 12–24 hr. In the hospital, they may continue their own CAPD if able or be maintained on CAPD by trained CAPD nurses. Since this becomes impractical over long periods of time, CAPD patients may be switched to automated cycling equipment.

There are preliminary studies to suggest that fresh instilled dialysis solutions may paralyze leukocyte phagocytosis for 30 min. Mechanisms to explain this inhibition of leukocyte function may relate to the low pH of the solution and the relatively high osmolality. In the long-dwell exchanges, leukocyte-killing properties may return for most of the latter portions of exchanges. Washing out leukocytes and inhibiting their phagocytic properties may not be advantageous during rapid cycling.

On the other hand, rapid cycling often does result in more dramatic relief in symptoms. Rapid cycling may wash out fibrin debris and help to prevent catheter clotting. In patients who continue CAPD during peritonitis, it is reasonable to flush out fibrin particles with several shorter exchanges early in therapy. In peritonitis with slow or rapid cycling, we recommend the addition of heparin to the dialysis solution (1000 units/2 liters).

The decision to use long-dwell exchanges or hourly exchanges with automated equipment has to be individualized in each patient.

If patients do not promptly improve within 24–48 hr on an antibiotic to which the organism is supposedly sensitive, then fungal peritonitis, a tunnel infection, a leaky perforated viscus, or a resistant organism becomes highly suspect. We find that improvement often follows quickly with catheter removal in the case of a fungal infection (where fungus may grow in silastic) or in the presence of a tunnel infection. A perforated viscus may obviously require surgical intervention. Numerous cultures for fungus, anaerobes, and tuberculosis are also necessary to determine therapy in the refractory case.

If a fungus is identified on gram stain or in a culture, we promptly remove the catheter and initiate 10–14 days of intravenous amphotericin B therapy. After a test dose of 1 mg of amphotericin B, we increase at increments of 5 mg/day until an intravenous dose of 25 mg/day is reached. This is then continued 10–14 days. With catheter removal, patients may clear without amphotericin B therapy. However, we prefer to administer the latter and not simply rely on catheter removal. Some fungal organisms may require longer periods of therapy. In our experience, most are *Candida* organisms and seem to do well with very brief courses. Patients can be discharged to outpatient hemodialysis, and the drug can be given on hemodialysis days until a total of 200–300 mg of amphotericin B has been given.

In patients who have catheter removal as part of the treatment of peritonitis, we usually wait 2 weeks for replacement of a new catheter and the reinstitution of chronic peritoneal dialysis. If hemodialysis cannot be carried out by femoral or subclavian routes, acute peritoneal dialysis can be performed with an acute catheter.

Table XI. Complications of Peritoneal Dialysis

Catheter-related complications	
Abdominal pain	Often postsurgically
	Altered dialysate temperature
	Catheter touches organs
Fullness	Increased ultrafiltration
	Small abdominal cavity
	Incomplete drainage
Bleeding	Postsurgical
	Ovulation, retrograde menstruation
	Trauma
Leakage	Around catheter exit
	Through incision
	Into abdominal wall
	Scrotal edema
Perforation	Postsurgical
	Peritonitis with multiple organisms on culture
Obstruction	Kinked catheter
	Fibrin clots
	Omentum in lumen
Cuff and tunnel infections	Exit site irritation
	Cuff extrusion
	Too short tunnel
	Chronic leakage
Peritonitis	See Section VIII
Complications of organ systems	
Pulmonary	Aspiration
	Pneumonia
	Atelectasis
	Hydrothorax
Cardiovascular	Pulmonary edema
	Hypotension
	Arrhythmia
Gastrointestinal	Constipation
	Hemorrhoids
	Hernias
	Peptic ulcers
Neurological	Convulsions
	Disequilibrium
Metabolic complications	Hyper- and hypoglycemia
	Hypernatremia
	Metabolic alkalosis
	Protein depletion
	Hypertriglyceridemia
	Weight gain

IX. COMPLICATIONS OF PERITONEAL DIALYSIS

Table XI lists numerous other complications of peritoneal dialysis that have been reported. Detailed discussion of the diagnosis and management of these complications can be found in the suggested readings.

X. SUMMARY

Peritoneal dialysis represents low-efficiency dialysis for the removal of small solutes, and, for such, hemodialysis is five to six times more efficient. For the dialysis of large solutes, peritoneal dialysis is comparable to hemodialysis. Peritoneal dialysis can be used when rapid removal of small solutes is not the major goal of the dialysis therapy. It is not the dialysis therapy of choice for the treatment of the hypercatabolic patient or in the treatment of poisoning.

It is adequate for the treatment of most cases of acute renal failure. It can be used for temporary maintenance therapy in patients awaiting blood access.

Chronic intermittent peritoneal dialysis required much longer treatment times than hemodialysis. For patients with cardiovascular problems or situations aggravated by rapid hemodialysis, it may be a better choice. This is especially true for those patients who are not capable of learning and carrying out self-care in the form of CAPD.

Continuous ambulatory peritoneal dialysis represents a form of self-care dialysis that will probably increase in the years to come. It may be especially advantageous for patients with cardiovascular problems or intolerance to hemodialysis treatments for medical or other reasons. It represents a very good treatment modality for the diabetic patient with retinopathy, who would then have less risk for bleeding than he would on hemodialysis. It can also permit home dialysis for patients who live alone. It should be avoided in patients who are not highly motivated towards self-care.

Most recently, another form of maintanence peritoneal dialysis has been proposed: continuous cycling peritoneal dialysis (CCPD). Thereby, the patient is connected overnight to a peritoneal dialysis cycler with 2- to 3-hr dwells while he is asleep. During the daytime, the patient fullfills his duties uninterrupted by exchange procedures, carrying 2 liters of dialysate solution in his abdomen. The potential benefit of CCPD is fewer connect/disconnect procedures and, thus, less risk of introducing infection. Further comparative studies are needed to validate this hypothesis.

SUGGESTED READINGS

Boen ST (ed): *Peritoneal Dialysis in Clinical Medicine*. Springfield, Illinois, Charles C Thomas, 1964.

Cairus KB, Porter GA, Kloster IE, et al: Clinical and hemodynamic results of peritoneal dialysis for severe cardiac failure. *Am Heart J* 76:227, 1968.

Dege GE, Wagoner RO: Peritoneal dialysis in acute uric acid nephropathy. *Mayo Clin Proc* 47:189, 1972.

Diamond LH (ed): *Renal Physicians Association. Northeastern Meeting Proceedings, Symposium: Peritoneal Dialysis*, New York, 1979.

Gjessing J: Peritoneal dialysis in severe acute hemorrhagic pancreatitis. *Acta Clin Scand* 133:645, 1967.

Grossheim RL: Hypothermia and frostbite treated with peritoneal dialysis. *Alaska Med* 15:23, 1973.

Henderson LW: Peritoneal dialysis, in Massry SG, Sellers AL (eds): *Clinical Aspects of Uremia and Dialysis*, Springfield, Illinois, Charles C Thomas, 1976, pp 555–582.

Legrain M (ed): *Continuous Ambulatory Peritoneal Dialysis: Proceedings of an International Symposium in Paris*. Amsterdam, Excerpta Medica, 1980.

Maher JF (ed): *An Introduction to Continuous Ambulatory Peritoneal Dialysis*. Deerfield, Illinois, Travenol Laboratories, 1980.

Nolph KD: Peritoneal dialysis, in Drukker W, Parsons FM, Maher JF (eds): *Replacement of Renal Function by Dialysis*. The Hague, Martinus Nijhoff, 1978, pp 277–321.

Nolph KD: CAPD—a logical approach to peritoneal dialysis limitations (a comparison of the peritoneal dialysis system and hollow fiber kidneys), *Nua* 1:5–8, 1980.

Nolph KD: *Peritoneal Dialysis*. The Hague, Martinus Nijhoff, 1981.

Nolph KD, Miller F, Rubin J, et al: New directions in peritoneal dialysis concepts and applications. *Kidney Int* 18(Suppl 10):S111–S116, 1980.

Sorkin MI: Peritoneal dialysis, in Jones NF, Peters DK (eds): *Recent Advances in Renal Medicine—2*. Edinburgh, Churchill Livingstone, 1982.

Tenckhoff H: Home peritoneal dialysis, in Massry SG, Sellers AL (eds): *Clinical Aspects of Uremia and Dialysis*, Springfield, Illinois, Charles C Thomas, 1976, pp 583–615.

Vaziri ND, Ness R, Wellikson L, et al: Bicarbonate buffered peritoneal dialysis. An effective adjunct in the treatment of lactic acidosis. *Am J Med* 67:392–396, 1979.

Williams P, Khahna R. Vas S. et al: The treatment of peritonitis in patients on CAPD: To lavage or not? *Peritoneal Dial Bull* 1:14–17, 1980.

Winchester JS, Gelfond MC, Knepshield JH, et al: Dialysis and hemoperfusion of poisons and drugs—update. *Trans Am Soc Artif Intern Organs* XXIII:762–842, 1977.

22

Care of the Transplant Recipient

K. VENKATESWARA RAO, CESAR E. PRU, and
CARL M. KJELLSTRAND

I. INTRODUCTION

In this chapter, the management of a renal transplant recipient is discussed under three distinct headings: (1) preparation of recipient, (2) evaluation of the donor (live related versus cadaver), and (3) management of complications in the immediate posttransplant period, the intermediate period, and the late posttransplant period.

The first question that arises is how would one select a patient for transplantation from the large number of people undergoing chronic dialysis. If an HLA-identical sibling is available, few would dispute that renal transportation is the best treatment for anyone with end-stage renal failure. Considerable controversy exists, however, of the relative merits of transplantation using poorly matched living related donors versus cadaver donors and chronic dialysis. Some groups actively push for any form of living related donor transplantation, as this can be done quickly. Other groups find no significant difference in the success rate between mismatched related donor transplants and cadaver kidneys. Therefore, they exclude all related donors except HLA-identical siblings. There is no convincing study which suggests that cadaveric transplant recipients have better survival than a rigorously matched group of dialysis patients. Most of the large-scale

K. VENKATESWARA RAO • Department of Medicine, University of Minnesota Medical School; and Department of Nephrology, Regional Kidney Disease Program, Hennepin County Medical Center, Minneapolis, Minnesota 55415.   CARL M. KJELLSTRAND • Departments of Medicine and Surgery, University of Minnesota Medical School; and Department of Medicine, Regional Kidney Disease Program, Hennepin County Medical Center, Minneapolis, Minnesota 55415.   CESAR E. PRU • Nephrology and Renal Transplant Unit, University Hospital, Caracas, Venezuela.

statistical studies indicate that age-matched patients have better survival on chronic hemodialysis than after cadaveric transplantation. However, the freedom and quality of life with a functioning allograft will convince many patients and physicians that cadaveric transplantation is preferable to being tied up to a chronic hemodialysis machine.

The relative indications for chronic dialysis or transplantation are unclear. Cardiovascular deaths are by far the most common cause of death in dialysis patients. Those with cardiac problems who tolerate chronic hemodialysis poorly may do well after transplantation. The patients in whom the infectious foci cannot be eradicated and those with chronic pulmonary problems are better after receiving chronic hemodialysis. Infections are the most common cause of death even after several years following transplantation, and the lungs are the common portal of entry. After a few years of chronic hemodialysis or transplantation, the mode of death changes. Vascular disease now becomes the leading cause of death in the transplanted patients. In contrast, infection is the most common cause of death in the long-term dialysis patients.

Once the decision is made that the patient is a candidate for transplantation, a search should be made for a potential live related donor, or else the patient should be placed on a waiting list for cadaveric transplantation. At the same time, the recipient should undergo a series of preparatory steps. These consist of immunologic preparation (HLA-A and -B typing, DR typing, mixed lymphocyte culture), cytotoxic antibody screening, blood transfusions, and cross-match studies. Other considerations are splenectomy, thoracic duct drainage, and total lymphoid irradiation. Prophylactic measures against infections and gastrointestinal complications should also be taken. Finally, some patients require bilateral nephrectomy. Before the transplant operation takes place, it has to be carefully timed with dialysis.

Immediately after transplantation, 10% to 30% of the patients develop acute renal failure which necessitates appropriate diagnostic and therapeutic intervention. Intermediate problems include the selection of a suitable immunosuppression protocol, diagnosis and management of acute rejection episodes, and close monitoring of the patient for infectious complications, years after transplantation, long-term problems arise. These are yet only partially known. They include hypertension, vascular catastrophes, liver failure, cancer, and suicide.

II. PREPARATION OF THE TRANSPLANT RECIPIENT

Table I outlines the general work-up of the renal transplant recipient, and Table II, the evaluation of the living related kidney donor.

Table I. Renal Transplant Recipient Work-up Protocol

History and physical examination	
Biochemical profile	Na, K, Cl, HCO_3, PO_4, Ca, BUN, creatinine, uric acid, triglycerides, cholesterol, serum protein and lipoprotein electrophoresis, blood glucose
Hematology	CBC, platelets (before and after dialysis)[a]
Coagulation	Ivy bleeding time, protime, PTT, serum fibrinogen, thrombin time, (factor VIII)
Immunology	Immunoelectrophoresis, serum complement, antinuclear antibodies, VDRL, AB–O typing, HLA-A, -B, and -C and DR typing, MLC, cytotoxic antibody screening
Infection	Hepatitis-B antigen and antibody determination, base serum sample for antibody titers (i.e., herpes group), pneumococcal and influenza vaccination, (CMV and hepatitis vaccination)[b] (hydrocortisone test), X-ray of sinuses, lungs, teeth (dental, ENT consult), cultures of urine, throat, sputum; any additional work-up as per local practice
Liver	Serum bilirubin, alkaline phosphatase, SGOT, SGPT, 5'-nucleotidase
Lungs	Chest X-ray, PA and lateral views, arterial blood gases, (lung function tests)
Heart	ECG (Stress ECG, thallium imaging)
Kidneys	24-hr urine protein, urinalysis, voiding cystourethrogram, ultrasound examination, X-ray of the abdomen, KUB scout film
Gastrointestinal	Esophagogram and upper GI series, oral cholecystogram, barium enema (endoscopy)
Neurological	Motor nerve conduction velocities, (EEG, EMG, audiometry)
Endocrine–gynecological	Pap smear, (glucose-tolerance test), serum PTH level, X-ray of hands, clavicles, and skull for evidence of hyperparathyroidism

[a] Tests in parentheses are desirable but not necessary.
[b] May be available in near future.

A. Immunologic Preparation

1. Tissue Typing, Mixed Lymphocyte Culture, Cytotoxicity, Cross Match

The value of HLA-A and -B typing in living related donor transplantation is undisputed. The four-antigen-matched sibling-donor kidney transplant provides the best survival for any patient with end-stage renal disease. The value of this typing in cadaver transplantation is disputed. The benefits

Table II. Living Related Donor Work-up Protocol

History and physical examination	
Biochemical profile	Na, K, HCO$_3$, Cl, Ca, PO$_4$, BUN, creatinine, blood sugar, uric acid, triglycerides, cholesterol, serum protein electrophoresis, and oral glucose-tolerance test in patients with family history of diabetes
Heart	Chest X-ray, ECG
Lungs	Arterial blood gases (lung function tests)[a]
Liver	Serum bilirubin, SGOT, alkaline phosphatase
Hematology	Complete blood count, platelets
Coagulation	Bleeding time, protime, PTT, thrombin time, serum fibrinogen
Renal	Urinanalysis × 2, urine culture × 2, 24-hr creatinine clearance × 2, (24-hr calcium and uric acid excretion) (renogram), intravenous pyelogram, renal arteriogram
Psychosocial evaluation	

[a] Tests in parentheses desired but not necessary.

vary from program to program but seem relatively modest. Currently, DR typing is undergoing clinical evaluation and is strongly prompted by some groups. The mixed lymphocyte culture (MLC) reaction is of undoubted value in living related donor transplantation. A low stimulation index in the MLC predicts a good long-term survival of the transplanted kidney even in non-HLA-identical sibling donor transplants. However, it is too time consuming to be of use in cadaver transplantation. Attempts at using primed cells in MLC that would allow earlier interpretation within hours have been done, but still there is no practical method of using MLC typing in cadaver transplantation at the present time.

Monthly serum samples for cytotoxic antibody screening should be obtained on all dialysis patients waiting for cadaver transplantation. A cross-match test utilizing both the latest and the earlier serum sample with the highest cytotoxic antibody titer should be done before scheduling the transplant surgery. A positive warm T-cell antibody cross match predicts hyperacute rejection. If possible, all serum samples collected should be used for the cross match. From a review of the monthly serum samples, a cytotoxicity profile can be obtained on all patients. If there is a high percentage of positive reaction against a panel of random lymphocytes, the patient in a practical sense is untransplantable. Transplantation should be avoided if the antibody titer is on the rise. However, even in the presence of a high percentage of cytotoxic antibodies, successful transplantation can be performed, if the level remains stable over several months.

2. Blood Transfusions

Blood transfusions improve the survival of cadaver kidney transplants. Some controversy still exists on what type of blood has to be used, how many transfusions are required, and what the optimal timing is. Present data indicate that between five and 20 transfusions given within a few months before transplantation are optimal. A reasonable clinical approach is to give the recipient fractions of approximately 5 to 10 units of packed red blood cells a few weeks before transplantation. The transfusions can be spaced over a period of time and should not be given in one single day.

3. Splenectomy, Total Lymphoid Irradiation, Thoracic Duct Drainage, and Thymectomy

These procedures are not used universally. Recent large-scale comparative studies indicate an improvement in kidney survival of 10–15% in splenectomized patients with cadaver as well as related-donor transplants. The benefit does not appear to be present in patients with HLA-identical sibling-donor transplants.

Total-body lymphoid irradiation as used in Hodgkin's disease has been tried experimentally by some transplant groups. Preliminary data in humans suggest that it is of some value in patients who have quickly rejected their first transplant and wish to receive a second. If the rejection took place within 1 year, the success rate with a second transplant without some form of special treatment is very limited. The undesirable effects of lymphoid irradiation include severe gastrointestinal dysfunction, malnutrition, and posttransplant lymphoma. The procedure still remains experimental. Thoracic duct drainage has recently been revived and used by a few transplant groups. It also appears to improve kidney survival in patients with cadaver transplants. Thymectomy is not performed at the present time.

B. Prophylactic Measures against Infectious Complications

Even after several years following successful transplantation, infections are still the most frequent causes of death. All infectious foci must therefore be eradicated before transplantation. The only incurable infection that does not contraindicate transplantation is inactive hepatitis B with stable liver enzymes.

X-ray of the teeth is mandatory, and radical treatment, frequently with extraction, should be done for root canal infections. The sinuses must also be X-rayed and cleaned if necessary. The shunt site must be free of infection for at least 6 weeks before transplantation. If this is not possible, the shunts should be removed, and subclavian catheterization or preferably intermittent femoral vein catheterization employed for several weeks while the shunt infection is being cured. Lungs must also be X-rayed, and the patient should not smoke for 6 months before transplantation. A urine culture should be obtained, and if positive, systemic antibiotics or repeated instillation of the antibiotic solution into the bladder should be done. If there is past or present evidence of active infection within the native kidneys, they have to be removed.

Patients who have undergone splenectomy should receive polyvalent pneumococcal vaccine before transplantation. This can be done with a satisfactory antibody response in well-dialyzed patients. The antibody response is less in the severely uremic undialyzed patient or in the patient who is heavily immunosuppressed immediately after transplantation. The splenectomized patients, especially children, should receive 250 mg of penicillin orally each morning as a prophylactic measure against pneumococcal septicemia. Tri methoprim and sulfa combinations are not as effective prophylactically against pneumococcal infections.

C. Prophylaxis against Gastrointestinal Complications

Gastrointestinal perforation or bleeding in the early posttransplant period is a dangerous complication with a high mortality rate. All transplant recipients should therefore undergo X-ray studies of the upper gastrointestinal tract. If there is a history of peptic ulcer disease or X-ray evidence of scarring or craters, vagotomy and pyloroplasty or, in severe cases, a vagotomy and antrectomy should be performed. This decreases the risk of bleeding and perforation during the immediate posttransplant period. Although some claim that a combination of cimetidine and antacids makes the operation unnecessary, there are no large-scale controlled studies addressing this problem. Until such studies become available, these prophylactic surgical procedures should be performed.

The patient with a history of cholecystitis or gallstones should undergo an elective cholecystectomy. Some transplant surgeons perform cholecystectomy even for asymptomatic gallstones. In most transplant centers, routine barium enemas are obtained in patients over the age of 45 years. In those with diverticulosis of the colon or other abnormal X-ray findings, a colonscopy and biopsy should be performed. Some transplant groups advocate colectomy for patients with asymptomatic diverticular disease. Diverticulosis is particularly common in patients with polycystic kidney disease.

D. Bilateral Nephrectomy, Ileal Bladder

Originally, many transplant groups performed bilateral nephrectomy on all potential renal transplant recipients, but nowadays, nephrectomy is performed only on strict indications. The most important indication is infected kidneys. If ureterovesical reflux is present, the kidneys should be removed along with the refluxing ureters. For patients with severe bladder dysfunction, an ilial bladder may need to be constructed many weeks before transplantation.

Intractable hypertension also necessitates the removal of the kidneys whether the patient is a candidate for transplantation or not. With the advent of more effective antihypertensive drugs such as minoxidil, β blockers, and captopril, this indication is becoming less common. There is presently no clinical agreement on what levels of hypertension are acceptable prior to subjecting the patient to bilateral nephrectomy. High renin levels are thought to weigh the decision in favor of nephrectomy. A well-dialyzed patient with optimal body weight who continues to require antihypertensive drugs may need to undergo bilateral nephrectomy prior to transplantation.

Large amounts of protein in the urine may also necessitate nephrectomy even if the patient is not going to have a transplant. This indication is present almost exclusively in small children with focal glomerulosclerosis. Such patients may be impossible to treat successfully with dialysis because of heavy protein loss resulting in malnutrition. Conservative management of such patients includes embolization of the kidneys or medical nephrectomy with high-dose mercurial diuretics.

Other indications for nephrectomy include measures to prevent recurrence of the original kidney disease in the renal allografts. This has been done in Goodpasture's syndrome, focal glomerulosclerosis, and rapidly progressive glomerulonephritis. Consensus that nephrectomy is necessary in these conditions exists only for Goodpasture's syndrome. In these patients, the kidneys should be removed, and periodic measurements of circulating antiglomerular basement membrane antibodies performed. A transplant should not be done until this test is negative.

E. Pretransplant Hemo- and Peritoneal Dialysis

Dialysis patients must be meticulously prepared for surgery. This preparation is discussed in detail in Chapter 20 of this manual. In cadaver transplantation, such meticulous preparation may not be feasible. However, preoperative dialysis is advisable in these patients while waiting for the results of the final cross match. Transplantation has been safely performed even in patients undergoing continuous ambulatory peritoneal dialysis (CAPD).

III. EVALUATION OF THE DONOR

A. The Living Related Donor

The work-up of the donor is outlined in Table II. What minor abnormalities one is willing to accept is a matter of difference among transplant teams, as is their conviction of how important related donor transplantation is. When in doubt, live donors should be excluded. Minor abnormalities of one kidney such as smaller size, cyst, or a scar are acceptable if that kidney is transplanted. Stone disease and hypertension are absolute contraindications.

B. The Cadaver Donor

Cadaver donors are always in short supply, even to the most successful donor-recruiting teams. One should therefore not exclude a potential donor. The only absolute contraindications are disseminated cancer and septicemia. Localized infections in the lung with negative blood cultures or malignancies confined to the CNS are not contraindications for transplantation, nor is hyperthermia *per se* in the brain-damaged patient. Transient hypotension in the donor or mild renal insufficiency does not rule out the use of the cadaver kidneys. Decisions regarding this can be made on the perfusion machine when flow characteristics of the kidneys are evaluated.

A whole series of pharmaceutical agents have been used in the potential cadaver donor. They include anticoagulation with heparin and platelet inhibitors; drugs presumed to improve the renal blood flow such as mannitol, rheomacrodex, furosemide, ethacrynic acid, and dopamine; drugs that would inhibit the noxious influence of the autonomic nervous system such as α and β blockers; phenothiazines; and peripheral vasodilators such as hydralazine and minoxidil. Other drugs are used in an attempt to induce better immunologic acceptance of the transplanted kidney. Such pretreatment includes very high doses of cyclophosphamide, corticosteroids, and azathioprine. Most of these protocols are used in a complicated routine that is unique for each transplant team. Almost none have been vigorously tested in large controlled trials. Most of them seem to be relatively innocuous to the function of the kidney.

IV. MANAGEMENT OF IMMEDIATE POSTTRANSPLANT COMPLICATIONS

These fall into two groups, which may partially overlap: posttransplant acute renal failure and surgical complications.

A. Acute Renal Failure

This is not a catastrophic complication if a simple noninvasive clinical approach is used. Approximately 90% of patients with posttransplant acute renal failure have acute tubular necrosis. Acute tubular necrosis occurs in 15 to 30% of patients receiving cadaver kidney transplants and in 5 to 10% of those receiving related-donor kidney transplants. It is not uncommon for the patient who develops acute tubular necrosis to have good urinary output for several hours and then develop oliguria and acute renal failure.

Diagnostically, it is important to first check the indwelling catheter, which may be plugged by blood clots, and make sure that the patient is adequately hydrated. A [131I]hippuran renogram should then be performed. Approximately 80% of patients with acute tubular necrosis have good uptake and delayed excretion on the renogram. In contrast, patients with hyperacute rejection or renal artery or vein thrombosis usually have no uptake on the renogram.

This approach may not establish the diagnosis in an occasional patient with a urological cause of acute renal failure. However, in these patients, the diagnosis becomes clinically evident by graft swelling or by leakage of urine through the transplant incision. On [131I]hippuran renogram with late-γ camera pictures, the extravasated urine can often be seen. An ultrasound of the transplanted kidney may also aid in the diagnosis by revealing the dilated urinary pelvis or extravasated urine. A patient with acute tubular necrosis often has a collapsed urinary pelvis. Methylene blue exuding through the transplant incision after intravenous injection or a high urea or creatinine content of this fluid can also be used to diagnose urinary leak. A renal biopsy is rarely indicated before the end of the second or third week. However, it becomes increasingly necessary and useful to delineate the cause of renal failure and to formulate long-range treatment plans.

In patients with acute tubular necrosis, the usual prednisone schedule can be used, but the dose of azathioprine has to be reduced. Although azathioprine is not metabolized in the kidneys, the association of uremia, dialysis, and full-dose azathioprine leads to a high incidence of infections. The renogram should be repeated once or twice a week. Routine antirejection therapy should not be used unless the renogram shows deterioration or the renal function had not improved within 2 to 3 weeks. An arteriogram should be done only in the rare patient whose renogram shows a poor uptake. If the vessels are relatively normal, the patient is then presumed to have acute tubular necrosis with decreased uptake on the renogram. These patients may have prolonged periods of oliguria but will eventually regain their renal function as do those who show better uptake on the renograms.

If renal artery thrombosis or severe pruning of small blood vessels suggesting hyperacute rejection is present, transplant nephrectomy should be done. Radioisotopic renal blood flow studies are noninvasive and are presently used in the place of renal arteriogram at many transplant centers. Digital subtraction angiography is a recent diagnostic tool that can be employed without subjecting the patient to the risk of high-dose contrast media and the inherent technical complications of renal arteriography. Short and frequent dialysis with low-dose heparin should be used in the postoperative period for patients who have acute renal failure (see Chapter 20 of this volume for postoperative dialysis).

B. Surgical Complications

Thrombosis of the transplant renal artery may present as acute renal failure. The treatment invariably is nephrectomy. Severe renal artery kinking may also present as ischemic acute tubular necrosis and be amenable to surgical correction once the diagnosis is made by arteriography. Renal vein thrombosis frequently leads to heavy proteinuria, hematuria, and acute renal failure. Rupture of the kidney occurs particularly in connection with hyperacute or accelerated acute rejection. The clinical manifestations are severe abdominal pain and shock. This necessitates emergency surgery. Urinary tract obstruction has been discussed under acute posttransplant renal failure. Lymphocele can also cause acute renal dysfunction but tends to occur in the later weeks. Associated clinical signs are unilateral leg edema or drainage of fluid through the transplant incision.

V. IMMUNOSUPPRESSION AND REJECTION

A. Prophylactic Immunosuppression

Routine immunosuppression consisting of azathioprine and prednisone is used universally by all transplant groups. Antilymphocyte serum preparations are also often used. Azathioprine and prednisone must be continued indefinitely. Extensive clinical experience suggests that rejection occurs if immunosuppression is discontinued, even after several years of successful transplantation. Presently, a new immunosuppressive drug, cyclosporin-A, is undergoing clinical trials. It may change the immunosuppressive regimen if early enthusiastic reports are confirmed by large-scale and long-term clinical investigations.

1. Azathioprine

Azathioprine has for 20 years remained the mainstay of immunosuppressive therapy for renal allograft recipients. The therapeutic spectrum is narrow. The principal side effect is bone marrow suppression with leukopenia, thrombocytopenia, and anemia. Seventy percent of all patients receiving azathioprine develop macrocytosis. Cholestasis with a hepatitislike picture is an idiosyncratic reaction that necessitiates discontinuation of the drug. The usual starting dose is 4 to 5 mg/kg body weight. The usual maintenance dose is 2 to 3 mg/kg. Some patients have an increased sensitivity to the drug and may need only small doses such as 25 to 50 mg (0.3 to 0.5 mg/kg). The dose should be decreased in patients with poor renal function. In patients who are receiving allopurinol, the dose of azathioprine must be decreased to one-half or one-third of normal. Otherwise, the combined effect of both drugs leads to severe leukopenia.

2. Prednisone

Prednisone is used by almost all groups after transplantation. Every transplant team seems to use a different dose schedule. The most commonly used protocol is 2 mg/kg per day of oral prednisone initially for cadaver transplantation and 1 mg/kg per day for related-donor transplantation. This dose is slowly tapered to approximately 0.25 mg/kg per day after 4 to 6 months.

Recent clinical investigations indicate that it is not necessary to use such large doses of prednisone for prophylactic immunosuppression. Very impressive results have been obtained by starting with a much lower dose of only 0.5 mg/kg per day and reaching a dose of 0.25 mg/kg every other day at 12 to 14 months after transplantation. Table III outlines a number of side effects caused by corticosteroids. Most common of these are infections. Posterior, subcapsular cataracts occur in one-third of the patients but rarely interfere with vision. In contrast to this, hip necrosis, which occurs in 15% of patients, is a serious clinical problem and often requires prosthetic replacement.

Some transplant groups use high-dose intravenous steroid pulses such as 1.0 g/day of methylprednisolone which is quickly tapered down during the first week following transplantation. This is replaced by oral prednisone at a dose of 60 mg/day during the second week and gradually reduced to 20 mg/day by 3 months and 15 mg/day by 6 months after transplantation. The advantages and drawbacks of using prophylactic steroid pulses remain controversial.

There is no agreement on the minimum dose of maintenance steroids. An enormous individual patient tolerance for prednisone exists. Clinical impressions are that when the dose is lowered below 0.25 mg/kg per day, rejection tends to occur. Therefore, more frequent monitoring of renal function should be done when the dose is lowered below this level. A temporary increase in prednisone dosage may be necessary after mild infections which may trigger an acute rejection. Almost all patients develop rejection if they discontinue even minute amounts of prednisone.

There is considerable controversy with regard to the use of every-other-day steroids in renal transplantation. When one uses low-dose prednisone, there is no convincing proof either that Cushingoid appearance or hypertension is decreased or that there is any increase in the incidence of rejection episodes. Some transplant centers have adopted the protocol of slowly switching from every-day to every-other-day prednisone in patients with stable graft function a year following successful transplantation. The main benefit appears to be that of restoration of the hypothalamic–hypophyseal–adrenal hormonal axis. Transplant groups with excellent cadaver

Table III. Side Effects of Corticosteroids[a]

Metabolic	Carbohydrates	Steroid diabetes
	Fat	Lipemia
		Accelerated atherogenesis
	Protein	Increased catabolism
	Electrolytes	Na$^+$–fluid retention (hypertension)
		K$^+$ loss
Immunosuppressive, antiinflammatory	Infections	Viruses
		Bacteria
		Fungi
		Protozoan
	Decreased wound healing	
	Intestinal perforation and bleeding	
CNS	Psychosis	
	Extrapyramidal symptoms	
	Pseudotumor cerebri	
	Dependency	
Locomotor	Myopathy	
	Osteopororis	
	Aseptic necrosis of bone	
Gastrointestinal	Ulcers	Esophageal
		Gastroduodenal (peptic)
		Jejunal–ileal
		Colon
	Pancreatitis	
	Decreased Ca^{2+} absorption	
Eye	Cataracts	
	Glaucoma	
	Exophthalmos	
Vascular	Vascular occlusions	(Hypercoagulability)
	Vasculitis	
	Ecchymosis	
Other	Cushingoid appearance	Moonface
		Hump
		Acne
		Hirsutism
	Growth failure, pregnancy-related complications	Increased congenital abnormalities
		Increased incidence of stillbirths
	Disturbed hypothalamus–hypophyseal–adrenal gland axis	Sudden collapse
		Severe malaise
	Allergic reactions	Includes anaphylaxis

[a] From Kjellstrand CM: Side effects of steroids and their treatment, *Transplant Proc* 7:123, 1975, with permission from Grune and Stratton, Inc.

patient and kidney survival have reduced the dose of prednisone to 0.25 mg/kg every other day or approximately 15 mg orally every other day.

3. Antilymphocyte and Antithymocyte Globulin

Large prospective controlled studies show that these preparations delay the onset and the incidence of acute rejections. Thus, at 3 to 6 months, there is a 10 to 15% better kidney survival in patients treated with these drugs than in those who have not received them. The survival advantage then persists for many years. The optimal dose seems to be between 10 to 20 mg/kg per day given intravenously for 2 to 4 weeks after transplantation. There seems to be great difficulty in standardizing the product and evaluating its potency. This may explain some of the earlier controversy regarding the efficacy of these drugs. Side effects include anaphylactic reactions, an early increase in virus infections, fever, joint pain, thrombocytopenia, glomerulonephritis, and an increase in the incidence of neoplasms.

4. Cyclosporin-A

At the time of this writing, this promising drug is undergoing clinical trials. The early trials were complicated by a relatively high incidence of lymphoma, nephrotoxicity, and hepatic dysfunction. By reducing the dosage from approximately 25 mg/kg body weight to between 10 and 15 mg/kg, many of these problems seem to have been decreased, with immunosuppression still maintained. The drug is said to be particularly effective when given with an antigen load and thus appears to be a more specific immunosuppressive drug than azathioprine and steroids.

5. Other Immunosuppressive Medications

Cyclophosphamide has been used in the place of azathioprine in patients who have had sensitivity or idiosyncracy to this drug. The dosage is 2 to 3 mg/kg per day. Clinical impressions from its use in transplantation are that it is more toxic. Toxicity consists of bone marrow suppression, macrocytosis, alopecia, leukemia, urinary tract tumors, and hemorrhagic cystitis. The latter problem can be decreased by encouraging a large fluid intake. Imidazole compounds such as bredinin and niridazole have been tried in Europe and Japan with satisfactory results. However these trials were made on such a limited number of patients that we cannot comment on their routine use at the present time.

Extracorporeal blood irradiation and anticoagulation with heparin, dicumarol, and antiplatelet agents have been abandoned as ineffective in controlled clinical trials. Thymectomy and maternal g-globulin are experimental methods without any practical clinical use at this time.

B. Antirejection Therapy

1. Hyperacute and Accelerated Acute Rejection

Hyperacute rejection occurs within minutes or hours after completion of the renal transplant vascular anastomosis. It is caused by preexisting antibodies against donor cells resulting in diffuse microvascular thrombosis and cortical necrosis. It can be avoided with appropriate cross-matching technique. The treatment consists of removal of the renal allograft; otherwise, life-threatening events such as disseminated intravascular coagulation and microangiopathic hemolytic anemia may ensue.

Accelerated acute rejection occurs from 1 day to 1 week after transplantation. It may be caused by an anamnestic antibody response. A definitive diagnosis is made only after evaluating the renal histology. The response to conventional antirejection therapy has been poor, and invariably, this type of rejection leads to loss of the transplanted kidney.

2. Acute Rejection

HLA-identical recipients of related-donor transplants may not ordinarily experience rejection. Most other related-donor kidney recipients and almost all recipients of cadaver kidneys undergo acute rejections. The onset of first rejection occurs between 1 and 3 weeks in patients who have not received ALG. Rejection is less common and occurs later in the course in ALG-treated patients. The incidence of acute rejections decreases with time. It may be triggered at any time by such unrelated factors as trauma, surgery, intravascular contrast media, infections, or when the prednisone dose is decreased below 0.25 mg/kg per day. The rejection phenonemon leads to decreased renal blood flow with sodium and fluid retention and decreased glomerular filtration. Uremia ensues thereafter.

a. Diagnosis—Classical

Early rejections are often heralded by fever, malaise, abdominal pain in the area of the graft, decreased urine flow, and edema especially occurring in the leg below the graft. Weight gain and hypertension then ensue. These classic features are often modified because of the immunosuppressive therapy and the individual host response. Rejections occurring in the late posttransplant period are often asymptomatic, the patient presenting only with abnormal renal function. Biochemical studies reveal increased levels of creatinine and urea in the blood, decreased urinary creatinine and sodium, and a low Fe_{Na}. The diagnosis is further suggested by $[^{131}I]$hippuran renogram. Renal biopsy is the only confirmatory test and should always be done when diagnostic uncertainties exist. A biopsy is also useful to predict response to therapy. The presence of interstitial edema and inflammatory cellular infiltration in the biopsy specimen indicates good prognosis; vascular involvement, a poor prognosis.

b. Diagnosis—Nonclassical

Many other tests have been suggested in the diagnosis of rejection. To be helpful, they need either to be more specific or should aid in the detection of rejection early. Immunologic monitoring has been found useful under experimental conditions. These tests are expensive and time consuming and therefore have not gained large-scale acceptance. Sophisticated urine tests for fibrin degradation products or various enzyme levels have been tried. Most of them appear to be nonspecific and have not gained widespread clinical acceptance. Urinary cytopathology has been found useful by some investigators. It also has not gained widespread use. Fine-needle aspiration biopsies have been successfully employed by some.

c. Differential Diagnosis

The differential diagnosis of immediate posttransplant renal failure has been discussed above.

After renal function has been restored in a transplanted kidney, different diagnostic problems arise. In an analysis of approximately 600 episodes of presumed acute rejection, 16% were caused by factors other than rejection ("pseudorejection"). Two-thirds of these were the result of renal insufficiency associated with infections. Although infections can trigger a rejection, they can also lead to prerenal failure or even acute tubular necrosis. Some of the viral infections, particularly CMV, may induce a special form of glomerulopathy tht can lead to renal dysfunction. Such difficult dilemmas require a biopsy for diagnosis. In diabetic patients, hyperglycemia is often associated with an increase in serum creatinine. When insulin is given, and the hyperglycemia is controlled, serum creatinine normalizes.

Factors such as ureteral obstruction caused by calculi, scarring, or lymphocele, renal arterial stenosis, recurrence of the original disease, and invasive lymphoma of the kidneys may lead to renal insufficiency in 1–2% of the patients. Other rare causes include acute tubular necrosis secondary to intravascular dye and drug nephrotoxicity. Hypercalcemia, fungus balls in the urinary bladder, and lymphocele with pressure on the transplanted kidney or ureter are other conditions to consider. Special studies such as allograft biopsy, ultrasound examination, renogram, intravenous pyelogram, arteriogram, or cystoscopy may be necessary to establish the correct diagnosis.

d. Treatment of Acute Rejection

The mainstay of acute rejection treatment is to increase the dose of corticosteroids for a limited time. The most common practice is to increase oral prednisone to 2 mg/kg per day and taper the dose to the prerejection level in approximately 2 to 3 weeks. Another approach is to use daily intravenous steroid (methylprednisolone) pulses for a brief period. There are recent encouraging reports that 10 to 20 mg/kg per day of ALG given intravenously for 1 to 2 weeks is effective in the treatment of acute rejection episodes.

Graft irradiation, often in a dose of 150 R given on days 1, 3, and 5, is also commonly employed, although controlled trials indicate that it is ineffective. The total dose should not exceed 1500 R because of the risk of radiation nephritis. It may be particularly useful in infected patients who also have a rejection and in whom one does not dare to use high-dose corticosteroids. Intravenous heparin or other forms of anticoagulation have not been proved useful when added to the conventional antirejection therapy. Intense plasmapheresis seems effective in some cases of intractable rejection, although the trials to date are small and uncontrolled.

If severe renal failure occurs (creatinine over 3 mg/dl) secondary to rejection, the dose of azathioprine should be reduced.

e. Danger of Treatment and the Number of Rejections That Can Be Treated

The main danger of rejection treatment is a fatal infection. In one series, over 90% of the patients who never rejected survived. In contrast, almost a third of the patients who had one or more rejections died.

There is no unanimity as to how many rejection episodes one should treat. All groups will treat one rejection unless it is associated with a serious infection. Most will treat two rejection episodes. Improved patient survival has been reported when no more rejections were treated. Many groups also treat a third rejection, taking into account the severity, histological lesion, and time interval between the rejection episodes.

3. Chronic Rejection

There is no known treatment for chronic vascular rejection. Unfortunately, many patients lose their kidneys years after transplantation. Although most have been said to represent "chronic rejection," some are caused by recurrence of the original disease in the renal allografts. Some of them represent *de novo* glomerulonephritis, as circulating immune complexes have been found commonly in such patients. The classical clinical triad of chronic rejection is proteinuria, sometimes in the nephrotic range, hypertension, and progressive renal insufficiency. It is important to rule out other treatable disorders mimicking chronic rejection such as renal artery stenosis, nephrotoxic drugs, and obstruction. If uncertainty exists, a biopsy should be performed.

VI. INFECTIOUS COMPLICATIONS

A. General Causes and Timing of Infections

Infections account for 60 to 75% of all early posttransplant deaths. Even many years after transplantation, infections can occur and lead to fatality, but at this point their incidence is lower than that of vascular deaths.

Patients who are treated for multiple rejections and those who develop leukopenia or suffer from posttransplant technical problems are all at an increased risk for infections. Unexplained fever, graft swelling, chest pain, or cough requires thorough evaluation, and frequently these patients need to be hospitalized. Infections are often caused by uncommon organisms and patients can present with unusual and confusing symptoms. Extensive and often invasive diagnostic procedures are required. After appropriate cultures are obtained, antibiotics should be given while one awaits definite diagnosis. Antibiotics do little harm in 2 to 3 days, but an infection can easily escalate out of control during this brief period. Usual clinical diagnostic clues are unreliable. Temperature may be decreased by steroids and raised by rejections. Similarly, white blood cell counts are raised by steroid treatment and lowered by cytostatic drugs.

Although the various infections will be discussed under appropriate subheadings such as viral, bacterial, fungal, protozoal, and parasitic, it must be understood that they are often mixed. The time and clinical circumstances when infections occur are very important to arrive at a preliminary diagnosis. Common bacterial infections occur immediately after transplantation and following antirejection treatment. They also occur following surgical procedures. One to 2 months after transplantation, infection with the herpes group of viruses, particularly cytomegalovirus and herpes simplex, becomes a common entity.

Opportunistic infections can occur without any discernable predisposing causes. These include herpes zoster, primary or recurrent infection with cytomegalovirus, fungal infections, tuberculosis, and salmonella infections. The transplant patient is never home safe from these infectious complications.

B. Viral Infections

1. Herpes Group of Viruses

a. Cytomegalovirus Infection

This is the most common infection in renal allograft recipients. Laboratory evidence such as presence of the virus in the urine or a fourfold or greater rise in the serum antibody titers occurs in up to 90% of all posttransplant patients. They may represent either a primary infection or reactivation of a latent infection. Transmission may occur with the graft, or following blood transfusions. Clinical problems are common in those who don't have preexisting antibodies, particularly if they receive the renal allograft or transfusions from donors with a CMV infection. The virus by itself can be immunodepressive and thus invite opportunistic infections even after cessation of all immunosuppressive therapy. It can occasionally stimulate an immune response and trigger a rejection episode. The virus can also damage the kidney by a direct glomerulopathic effect. This diagnosis can be made only after evaluating the renal histology.

The clinical expression of CMV infection is extremely varied. Many patients have no symptoms, although the serum antibody titers increase and viral inclusion bodies are detected in the urine. Other patients die of viremia. Common manifestations of CMV infection are leukopenia, fever, and malaise. Pneumonia with interstitial pattern on chest X-ray and hepatic dysfunction is also common. In some instances, gastrointestinal bleeding and bowel perforation have been blamed on the virus. Conjunctivitis, retinitis, episcleritis, pancreatitis, and nonspecific skin rashes and arthritis are some of the other manifestations of this disease. Nervous system involvement including encephalitis, polyneuritis, and autonomic dysfunction with orthostatic hypotension has also been reported.

In the majority of instances, the diagnosis of CMV infection is made retrospectively by demonstrating fourfold or greater rise in serum antibody titer. The virus can be cultured from the blood, or the inclusion bodies can be found in the biopsy specimens obtained from the liver, kidney, or lungs. Bronchial washing or brushing can be done even in very ill patients, and thus, the need for a lung biopsy may be obviated.

There is no good treatment for the CMV infections. In patients who are severely ill, immunosuppression should be decreased or discontinued. Adenine arabinoside (Vidarabine®) has been used but is probably ineffective. Other treatments that are experimental include transfer factor, leukocyte interferon, immunoglobulin infusions, and the recent antiviral drug acyclovir.

b. Herpes Simplex

Lip infections with this virus (canker sores) are common during maximal immunosuppressive treatment. These infections are treated with local iodoxyuridine or adenine arabinoside. The virus may spread and cause stomatitis, esophagitis, gastritis, proctitis, as well as involvement of the perigenital area. Sometimes it is associated with urinary retention. Widespread skin lesions simulating chicken pox may also occur. Mononucleosislike illness has also been reported with this virus. The most feared complications are hepatitis and encephalitis. The encephalitis should be treated early with intravenous adenine arabinoside (Vidarabine®) in a dose of 15 mg/kg per day for 10 days. The exact role of brain biopsy is controversial. Other diagnostic studies include a rise in serum and spinal fluid antibody levels. Acyclovir is presently undergoing clinical testing for the treatment of disseminated herpes simplex infection.

c. Herpes Zoster

This infection usually occurs during the late posttransplant period. It runs a benign course, but sometimes it can be prolonged. It is recommended that immunosuppression be decreased somewhat during these infections. Carbamepazine (Tegretol®) may be beneficial in controlling the postherpetic neuralgia. Zoster immune globulin is ineffective. Treatment with acyclovir appears promising.

d. Varicella

This disease is extremely malignant in posttransplant patients and often is lethal. Children who have not had chicken pox should therefore be allowed to get this infection while on dialysis before they receive the immunosuppressive drugs. In patients who have not had this disease earlier and are exposed after transplantation, prophylactic immune serum (10 mg/kg IV) should be given as a single dose immediately.

e. Epstein–Barr

This virus disorder is recognized with increased frequency in renal transplant recipients. It may run a benign course, but in an occasional young patient, it may be the responsible agent for a rapidly growing malignant lymphoma. Anecdotal evidence suggests that acyclovir is helpful in treating this sort of lymphoma.

2. Hepatitis

Hepatitis B infection in dialysis patients is not a contraindication for renal transplantation if the infection is chronic. Long-term ill effects are unknown, but some patients, particularly those with chronic active hepatitis, may die with liver failure in the late posttransplant period. There is little clinical experience with hepatits A or non-A, non-B after transplantation.

3. Other Viral Infections

Infection with influenza virus has been described in immunosuppressed patients. When epidemics threaten, vaccination should be given, utilizing the dead or attenuated virus. Live-virus vaccines should not be used. Sometimes viral infections can trigger an acute rejection which is difficult to diagnose.

Papovavirus infections, particularly warts, are common after transplantation. Although not lethal, they cause endless problems. Local treatment is the only one that can be offered to these unfortunate patients. A progressive multifocal leukoencephalopathy caused by a papovavirus has been described in immunosuppressed patients. There is no known therapy.

4. Summary of Therapy for Viral Diseases

The treatment for viral diseases is presently disappointing. In most instances, all one can do is to decrease the immunosuppression and hope that the patient can eradicate the virus infection without rejecting his kidney. Adenine arabinoside (Vidarabine®) seems to be effective against herpes simplex and possibly zoster and hepatitis. Fatal CNS complications have occurred in patients treated with adenine arabinoside. Acyclovir is presently undergoing clinical trial and may be ideal for the treatment of the herpes group of viruses. The recommended dose is 5 mg/kg three times a day for 5 days. Side effects include uremia. At the time of this writing, it was not commercially available but may soon be released into the market.

Vaccination against cytomegalovirus and other herpes viruses is undergoing clinical testing. Interferon and transfer factors are presently used only under experimental conditions.

C. Bacterial Infections

1. Common Bacterial Infections

Infections with staphylococci, streptococci, and gram-negative rods occur in renal transplant patients after technical procedures and following antirejection therapy, when the patients are maximally immunosuppressed. They complicate fistulae and shunts, hematomas, wound dehesions, and late operations. They may also be the cause of death in patients who are hospitalized for prolonged periods with other disorders such as virus infection or liver failure.

Patients should therefore undergo transplantation only after all infectious foci have been cleaned out, as suggested earlier in this chapter (Section II.B).

2. Urinary Tract Infections

These infections are extremely common. Those occurring within the first 3 to 4 months are serious and need vigorous treatment. Many groups use the combination drug trimethoprim–sulfamethoxazole prophylactically while the patients are receiving high-dose corticosteroids. In those with recurrent urinary tract infections, anatomic abnormalities should be ruled

out. Urinary tract infections late in the posttransplant period are not uncommon. Routine urine culture may show a positive growth, but patients generally do not experience clinical symptoms. There is no convincing evidence
that these need treatment.

3. Unusual Bacterial Infections

a. *Diplococcus Pneumonia*

Pneumococcal pneumonia occurs with increased frequency in splenectomized patients. Such patients, particularly if children, should be given
prophylactic oral penicillin, 250 mg daily indefinitely. For adults, pretrans-
plant vaccination with a polyvalent pneumococcal vaccine is recommended.

b. *Salmonella Infections*

These infections often involve the blood vessels leading to mycotic
aneurysms. Rupture of these may have a fatal consequence. Osteomyelitis
involving the extremities is not uncommon in diabetic patients with renal
allografts. Sepsis, icterus, and prolonged gastrointestinal shedding are sometimes encountered.

c. *Mycobacteria*

Mycobacteria, particularly tuberculosis, are seen with increased incidence after transplantation. Patients known to have tuberculosis before may
be safely transplanted if INH prophylaxis is used indefinitely after transplantation. Tuberculosis occurring after transplantation is usually from reactivation of a latent infection. Monoarthritis, pneumonia, and meningitis have
also been described. The diagnosis is made by demonstrating the organism
in the acid-fast stain or by culturing the specimens obtained by broncho-
scopic brushing or lavage. Usual drug therapy should be employed for a
period of 18 to 24 months. Atypical mycobacteria may be extremely difficult
or impossible to eradicate or may need years of treatment.

d. *Nocardiosis*

This usually presents as a cavitating lung nodule or a cerebral abscess.
Disseminated nocardiosis involving multiple sites including the skin, joints,
muscles, lymph nodes, and liver has been described in immunosuppressed
patients. Diagnosis is easily made by the characteristic morphology in gram-
stained specimens and cultures. Invasive procedures such as bronchial
washings or lung biopsy may be necessary at times to establish the correct
diagnosis. Treatment consists of 8–10 g sulfisoxazole (Gantrisin®) for 2–3
months or the combination drug trimethoprim–sulfamethoxazole (Septra),

two tablets b.i.d. for 2–3 months. Other drugs that have been used to treat nocardiosis include cycloserine and minocycline.

e. Listeriosis

This infection is being increasingly recognized as a complication of renal transplantation. Most often it presents as sepsis. Meningitis, cerebritis, and endophthalmitis have also been described. The bacterium, a gram-negative rod, is easily grown in blood cultures but may be mistaken for diphtheroids. The infection tends to recur, and therefore, treatment with high-dose ampicillin for at least 6 weeks is recommended.

f. Legionnaires' Disease

This has been described as a virulent epidemic in some transplantation units. The clinical presentation is that of a rapidly changing nodular or lobar consolidation seen on chest X-ray. Diagnosis is made by culture or by direct fluorescent antibody staining of the tissue sections or by the increase in antibody titers in the serum. The treatment consists of a prolonged course of erythromycin given in high doses.

g. Other

A growing family of bacteria, either newly encountered or previously thought to be saprophytes, are discovered to cause disease in immunosuppressed patients. They include Legionella-like bacteria, WIGA, Pittsburgh agent, RBC-assoicated bacteria, rhodochros, and Chlamydia.

4. Summary of Treatment for Bacterial Infections

In treating the bacterial infections one would follow the usual guidelines. Antibiotics, however, must be started as soon as possible after appropriate cultures have been obtained. The usual criteria followed in medical wards, such as delaying treatment while awaiting culture results, are not appropriate in these patients. The immunosuppressive drugs should be decreased or discontinued in patients with severe infection. These clinical situations are often difficult to deal with, and all factors have to be carefully considered in arriving at the right decision. Sudden withdrawal of steroids should be avoided in a septic patient, as it may precipitate an addisonian crisis. High caloric intake either by intravenous or oral route is essential to minimize tissue catabolism and to improve the body defense. Uremia resulting from graft failure following discontinuation of immunosuppression has to be managed with frequent dialysis using low-dose heparin.

Granulocyte transfusions should be considered in patients who are granulocytopenic. Infusion of broad-spectrum γ-globulin may be beneficial in an occasional patient.

D. Fungal Infections

Fungal infections are common in the late posttransplant period. Most run a slow indolent course, presenting with general malaise or as incidental findings. The lungs are a common portal of entry. Discrete, slowly changing pulmonary nodules are often seen on chest X-ray.

1. *Candida*

Localized *Candida* infections are common in immunosuppressed patients. Nystatin prophylaxis 250,000 units swish and swallow four times a day or clotrimazole troches slowly dissolved in the mouth four times a day should therefore be used for several weeks after transplantation. In recalcitrant cases of oral candidiasis, local application of gentian violet is recommended. *Candida* is frequently found in the urine, particularly in diabetic patients. In the absence of clinical symptoms, no treatment is needed. In patients who are symptomatic, local lavage with amphotericin B in a concentration of 0.05–0.2 mg/ml or bladder irrigation with 0.25% acetic acid is recommended.

Severe localized candidiasis or candidemia most often complicates other bacterial and viral infections. Pneumonia with lobar infiltrates is the most common presentation. The diagnosis is made by culturing the specimens obtained by bronchial lavage; sometimes endophthalmitis, meningitis, and endocarditis are also seen. A peculiar sign is muscle tenderness, and *Candida* can be demonstrated on biopsy of the muscle or the skin rashes. Another complication of this infection is that of arterial thromboembolism. The exact status of the precipitin and agglutinin tests is not known. Countercurrent immunoelectrophoresis is a promising new test.

It is often difficult to know when to treat *Candida* infection. Involvement of two or three sites in a sick patient is generally considered an indication for therapy. The mainstay of treatment is amphotericin B. 5-Fluorocytosine can be used as an adjuvant but should not be used alone because of the development of resistance. Rifampin and miconazole have also been used. In patients with peritonitis, amphotericin B added to the peritoneal dialysate in a concentration of 2–4 mg/liter has been effective. Clotrimazole orally is also worth a trial.

2. *Aspergillus*

The most common presentation of *Aspergillus* infection is an upper lobe nodule in the lungs. Sputum cultures are often negative. Invasive studies such as transbronchial lung biopsy may be required for establishing the correct diagnosis. An immunoassay has recently been described. The mainstay of treatment is amphotericin B and 5-fluorocytosine. Surgery is often necessary to complement the antibiotic treatment in order to eradicate this infection.

3. *Cryptococcus*

Central nervous system involvement is the most common clinical presentation. Both meningitis and cerebral abscess can occur. During the process of evaluation, one may detect pulmonary infections which are often asyptomatic. India ink preparation from the cerebrospinal fluid is frequently positive, although sometimes cisternal puncture may be necessary. Staining for the polysaccharide antigen should also be done, and in some cases bone marrow stains may be necessary. Treatment consists of amphotericin B and 5-fluorocytosine or intravenous miconazole. Sometimes intraventricular infusions are necessary.

4. Other Fungal Infections

Histoplasmosis presenting with high fever and diagnosed by lung biopsy or bone marrow culture has been described in posttransplant patients. Coccidiomycosis with pulmonary symptoms is another late infection. Mucormycosis (phycomycosis) occurs with pulmonary and rhinocerebral symptoms. *Torulopsis glabrata* often mimics *Candida*. Other rare types of fungal infections are chromoblastomycosis, dessiminated trichosporon capitatum, sporotrichosis, and *Allescheria boydii* (maduromycosis).

5. Summary of Treatment for Fungal Infections

The mainstay of systemic fungal infections is amphotericin B. The common way of using this drug is to give a test dose of approximately 0.1 mg/kg diluted in 500 cc of 5% dextrose in water infused slowly over 4 to 6 hr. If the patient has no serious reactions to the drug, then the dose can slowly be escalated up to 1 mg/kg per day over the next several days. It is necessary to continue the treatment for several weeks to reach a cumulative total dose of 1.0 to 1.5 g. Every-other-day treatment has been successful in patients who could not tolerate the drug on a daily basis.

The main problem with amphotercin B is its nephrotoxicity. Although mannitol has been thought to decrease the nephrotoxicity of amphotericin, controlled trials have not shown it to be effective. High-dose intravenous potassium and bicarbonate are necessary, as hypokalemia and acidosis often ensue. Hypokalemia perhaps also increases the nephrotoxicity of amphotericin. Many patients develop fever, chills, muscle pains, and hypertension while the drug is being administered. These reactions can be controlled with diphenhydramine (Benadryl®), 25–50 mg given intravenously or intramuscularly shortly before administering the amphotericin. Intravenous meperidine (Demerol®) in a dose of 25–50 mg and intravenous hydrocortisone, 50–100 mg, are also beneficial in avoiding these reactions. Sometimes a combination of these drugs may be advantageous.

5-Flurocytosine often enhances the effect of amphotericin B but should not be used alone because resistance develops rapidly. The dosage of 5-fluorocytosine is 10–20 mg/kg four times daily in patients with normal renal function.

E. Protozoan and Parasitic Infections

1. *Pneumocystis carinii*

Pneumocystis carinii is a common infectious agent in immunosuppressed patients. The infection almost always is limited to the lungs and frequently occurs in combination with other viral or fungal infections. The clinical manifestations include nonproductive cough, tachypnea, cyanosis, and severe hypoxia. There are often no diagnostic signs on physical examination. Peripheral alveolar infiltrate with pronounced air brochogram is a frequent finding on chest X-ray. Localized nodular appearance is rare. The diagnosis can be made by staining the specimens obtained by bronchial lavage or brushing. Often, an open lung biopsy with touch imprints is necessary. The organism appears as a folded cyst with a double outer membrane on silver methenamine staining. Treatment consists of the trimethoprim–sulfamethoxazole combination. Pentamidine is no longer used because of its many toxic side effects.

2. Toxoplasmosis

Toxoplasmosis can also occur in transplanted patients. It presents with meningitis, encephalitis, or endophthalmitis. Diagnosis is made by lymph node biopsy or the Sabin–Feldman dye test. Recent diagnostic studies include immunofluorescence, complement fixation, and hemagglutination tests. Treatment consists of sulfadiazine and pyrimethamine combination.

3. Strongyloidosis

Strongyloidosis is recognized as an infection characterized by cavitating pneumonia and sepsis. It is diagnosed by finding the larvae in the sputum or bronchial washings or from a lung biopsy specimen showing the larvae within the alveoli.

4. Other

Other protozoan and parasitic infections include malaria, sparagonimus, and protatacosis. Leprosy has been reported after transplantation in Brazil.

VII. INFECTIONS—ORGAN SYSTEM INVOLVEMENT

A. Pulmonary Infection

All types of infectious agents, viruses, bacteria, fungi, protozoa, and parasites, can involve the lung. Bacterial and viral infections tend to occur during the early posttransplant period. They may complicate other diseases or antirejection treatment. Pneumocystis and fungi tend to occur late without any precipitating causes.

Along with timing of infections and clinical examinations, frequent chest X-rays are invaluable. They allow the clinician to formulate a preliminary diagnosis long before results of cultures and biopsies become available. Thus, they offer the advantage of allowing the selection of an early and life-saving therapy. Table IV summarizes the different patterns of lung involvement in bacterial, fungal, viral, and Pneumocystis infections.

It is useful to describe the findings of the chest X-ray in six different patterns, although these are not absolutely diagnostic. The first pattern is that of bacterial infection. The infiltrates tend to be segmental or lobar and change rapidly. The second pattern is an interstitial pneumonia, often occurring in association with viral infections. It is most pronounced in the hilar area. The third pattern seen in infections with Pneumocystis carinii also tends to start in the hilar area, but rapidly spreads to the peripheral parts of the lung, resulting in air bronchograms. Fungal infections cause the fourth pattern, that of soft, slowly changing nodules. The fifth pattern is that of pulmonary edema. It is often difficult to differentiate this pattern from that seen during viral and Pneumocystis carinii infections. However, it usually occurs with cardiomegaly and is more patchy than the pattern of virus or Pneumocystis infections. It is particularly common in older patients and in very young patients. Pulmonary edema is frequently associated with rejection when a rapid increase in body weight occurs secondary to fluid retention. The sixth pattern, that of wedge-shaped infiltrates, occurs in pulmonary embolism and infarctions. This pattern may also be seen in Candida lung infections.

If the diagnosis is not established by history, physical examination, or chest X-ray or after microscopic examination and culture of the sputum, bronchoscopy and lavage should be performed immediately. Transbronchial lung biopsy should also be done liberally. Specimens have to be sent for culture of all organisms. Special stains such as acid-fast stain, Giemsa, and silver–methenamine stains should also be performed. If the diagnosis is still in doubt, an open lung biopsy which should include touch imprints should be performed. Although it is technically more complicated than percutaneous needle biopsy, the diagnostic yield is considerably better.

B. Central Nervous System Involvement

Organisms often found in patients with CNS infections include cytomegalovirus, herpes simplex, pneumococcus, listeriosis, crytococcus, toxoplasmosis, Nocardia, and Aspergillus. Lumbar puncture must be performed immediately, and India ink stain and tests for fungal antigens performed routinely. Cisternal puncture may be necessary in some patients. Radioisotopic scans and computerized tomography cannot be trusted, as these studies can be normal in patients with even serious CNS infections. Cerebral angio-

Table IV. Summary of the Six Clinical Patterns of Lung Involvement after Transplantation

Disease	Chest X-ray appearance	Timing after transplantation	Precipitating event	Clinical presentation
Bacterial infection	Segmental or lobar pattern; changes rapidly	Any time, but most common early	Operations, antirejection therapy, other viral and fungal infections	Fulminant course, very ill patients
Virus infection	Interstitial pattern	Most common at 1–4 months	None	Fever, dyspnea
Pneumocystis carinii	Alveolar pattern, air bronchogram	6–12 months	None	Marked dyspnea, cyanosis, and hypoxia; few physical findings
Fungal infections	Soft, often nodular infiltrates; slowly changing	Late, 1–5 years	None	Indolent course
Pulmonary edema	Hilar, spreading to periphery; cardio-megaly	Most often early, 1–6 months	Acute tubular necrosis, rejection, renal failure	Very young and very old patients are susceptible
Pulmonary embolism	Wedge shaped	Early, 1–6 months	Congestive heart failure, iliofemoral thrombosis, none (candidiasis)	Sudden onset of pleuritic chest pain and hemoptysis or circulatory collapse

grams may be necessary at times. In patients with encephalitis, brain biopsy may be useful.

C. Oropharynx and the Gastrointestinal Tract

These are frequently infested with *Candida* and sometimes with herpes simplex virus. Endoscopy, computerized tomography, and gallium scan may be necessary to diagnose these infections.

D. Bacteremia

Bacteremia is not unusual during the early months following renal transplantation. A urinary tract infection precedes bacteremia in 65 to 70% of patients. Other sources of entry include lungs, open wounds, skin and subcutaneous tissue, oropharynx, and the gastrointestinal tract. In some instances, no source for bacteremia can be found. The bacteria most often discovered in blood cultures are gram-negative rods such as *E. coli, Klebsiella,* and *Proteus.* Other bacteria detected less commonly include *Clostridia, Pseudomonas, Salmonella,* staphylococci, streptococci, *Hemophilus, Bacteroides, Listeria, Herella,* and enterococci. The factors predisposing to bacteremia include ureteral complications such as leakage or necrosis of the ureter, leukopenia, overimmunosuppression during rejection episodes, and diabetes mellitus with circulatory impairment. Despite adequate antibiotic therapy, the death rate continues to be high in these patients, ranging from 20 to 40% in different series.

E. Hepatitis

Hepatitis may be caused by cytomegalovirus or herpes simplex virus. Hepatitis with A and B and non-A, non-B viruses is also common. Other causes include *Salmonella* and *Candida.* Differential diagnosis from azathioprine toxicity is obviously important. Biopsy, computerized tomography, and sometimes retrograde cannulation of the common hepatic duct with injection of contrast media may be necessary to distinguish the various etiologic factors in a jaundiced patient.

F. Urinary Tract Infections

Urinary tract infections are extremely common. During the first 4 months after transplantation, they should be vigorously treated because of the risk of bacteremia in a highly immunosuppressed patient. These infections seem to do less harm in the late posttransplant period. In a patient with repeated urinary tract infections, a voiding cystourethrogram should be obtained. Although reflux may not have been present in the patients' own ureters, it may occur after ureteroneocystostomy, especially following repeated urinary tract infections. Ultrasound examination to detect perinephric fluid collection is an important diagnostic study.

G. Skin

Skin infections are common after transplantation. Warts are most common. Disseminated herpes simplex with a varicellalike picture can occur and may necessitate a skin biopsy. *Pseudomonas aeruginosa*, bacteroides, erysipilothrix, histoplasmosis, *Candida*, mucorymcosis, *Cryptococcus*, and *Aspergillus* have also been found in skin rashes. When there is doubt, a skin biopsy should be performed immediately.

VIII. INTERMEDIATE SURGICAL PROBLEMS

A. Vascular

Renal artery stenosis is not an uncommon problem during the late post-transplant period. This can be due to an atherosclerotic plaque or it could be idiopathic. Whatever the cause, the symptomatology is the same, that is, increasing severity of hypertension sometimes associated with erythrocytosis. A peculiar feature is that of a rise in serum creatinine which responds temporarily to an increase in the prednisone dose (pseudorejection). The treatment is either surgical or by intravascular balloon dilatation. Surgical repair is difficult, and the operation carries a high risk of graft loss. There are now several reports of successful balloon dilatations. Spontaneous resolution has occurred in rare instances.

Thrombosis of the renal vein can occur in the transplanted kidney. This is usually associated with nephrosis, hematuria, and decreased renal function. A conservative approach with anticoagulation is recommended in most instances.

B. Renal

1. Rupture

Rupture of the transplanted kidney usually occurs in association with rejection but can also occur spontaneously. The symptoms consist of pain and tenderness over the transplanted kidney and shock. Nephrectomy is necessary in almost all instances, although a few reports of successful surgical repair have appeared.

2. Obstruction

Obstruction of the urinary tract can result from renal stones, particularly common in previous stone formers and in those with urinary infection. *Candida* and fungus balls have also caused obstruction of the transplanted renal pelvis. Fibrosis of the transplanted ureter, perirenal abscess, and lymphocele are other causes of obstruction. The diagnosis is usually made by ultrasound examination during investigation of the causes of transplant malfunction. Obstruction is also a cause of pseudorejection that may temporarily respond to an increase in prednisone dose. The treatment is surgical, with drainage of abscesses and lymphoceles or reimplantation of the ureter. Sometimes the patient's own ureter may be used to bypass a hopelessly obstructed ureter from the transplanted kidney.

3. Lymphocele

Lymphocele may cause obstruction of the ureter, vascular occlusion, ascites, or unilateral leg edema. Frequently, there is a functional deterioration of the transplanted kidney. The diagnosis is made on ultrasound examination. The therapy consists of surgical drainage into the peritoneal cavity. Prior to the internal drainage, it is important to make sure that the fluid is not infected.

4. Reflux

Reflux may occur along the transplanted ureter and give rise to dilatation of the collecting system and repeated urinary tract infections. It may also occur free of any symptoms. The treatment consists of reimplantation or long-term antibacterial prophylaxis. Reflux may also occur into the patient's own ureters. Although the ureters may have been normal during the voiding cystourethrogram that was done before transplantation, reflux into the native ureters can occur during the posttransplant period. If recurrent urinary tract infections occur, the refluxing ureters may have to be removed.

C. Gastrointestinal

A whole series of gastrointestinal complications occur in these patients. Gastroduodenal ulcers may be complicated by bleeding or perforation. Mesenteric artery or vein thrombosis with bowel necrosis has also been reported. Colonic perforation, particularly in patients with preexisting diverticulosis, is not an uncommon finding. Ulceration of any part of the gastrointestinal tract can occur even in patients without predisposing factors. Cytomegalovirus infection has been thought to cause some of these problems. Ileus secondary to adhesions, particularly in patients who have had many previous abdominal operations, can also occur. The symptoms of the gastrointestinal disease may be obscured by high-dose steroids during rejection treatment when they seem to occur most commonly. A high index of suspicion is necessary, and early operative intervention is mandatory. Despite adequate management, these complications continue to carry a formidable mortality rate.

Pancreatitis also occurs with increased frequency in the transplanted patient. Steroid treatment, particularly high-dose prednisone during rejection, is one of the causes. Hypercalcemia and hyperparathyroidism are others. Usual treatment principles apply.

IX. LONG-TERM COMPLICATIONS

Long-term complications occurring after transplantation are now becoming known and are being publicized in the transplant literature.

A. Vascular Complications and Hypertension

1. Arteriosclerotic Vascular Disease

Patients with preexisting vascular disease, such as diabetes, coronary artery disease, and arteriolar nephrosclerosis, have increased incidence of vascular deaths. It is presently unclear whether these factors are operating many years after transplantation or if other factors have come into existence. Preexisting hypertension, obesity, and old age probably contribute to the vascular deaths. Renal insufficiency caused by chronic rejection, hyperlipidemia, and high-dose prednisone therapy may also be contributory.

2. Thromboembolic Disease and Pulmonary Embolism

These problems occur with high frequency during the first 6 months following transplantation. Sudden deaths from massive pulmonary embolism have been reported in graft recipients. Older patients and those receiving high-dose prednisone are particularly prone to this complication.

Aggressive treatment of hypertension, hyperlipidemia, and the institution of alternate-day steroid therapy may be beneficial. Prophylactic antiplatelet drugs may reduce the risk of thromboembolism. In those patients who have severe hypertension and transplant malfunction, it is probably best to remove the allograft and return them to dialysis.

B. Infections

Infectious complications have been discussed in detail (Sections VI and VII).

C. Liver Disorders

Hepatic failure is an important late cause of death after transplantation. Only a few deaths are caused by known infectious agents. Liver disease may result from multiple factors including alcoholism, infections, gall bladder disease, and drug toxicity. Hemosiderosis and hemochromatosis due to iron overload has recently been described.

Since the etiology is not known in the majority of cases, the treatment remains unsatisfactory. It may be worthwhile to decrease the dose of azathioprine or even substitute with cyclophosphamide to prevent azathioprine toxicity in patients with severe liver disease. Intermittent phlebotomies are beneficial in patients with iron overload.

D. Neoplasms

There is a seven- to tenfold increase in the incidence of neoplasms in these patients compared to the age-matched, nontransplant population. Between 2 and 5% of posttransplant deaths are caused by malignancy. There is no evidence that the relative number of deaths from malignancy increases with time, during the posttransplant period.

Skin tumors are particularly common, and are responsible for approximately 40% of the neoplasms. The ratio of squamous cell carcinoma to basal cell carcinoma is much increased. All skin tumors are much more common in areas exposed to light. They are particularly common in places such as Australia where the exposure to ultraviolet light is higher. Usual treatment principles apply.

Lymphomas are the second most common tumors occurring in these patients, constituting approximately 20% of all neoplasms. Half of them occur in the brain. There are two types of lymphomas: a slow-growing lymphoma occurring late after transplantation, usually seen in older patients, and an aggressive and rapidly growing tumor which is more common in younger patients and occurs during the early months after transplantation. Preliminary information suggests tht many of the latter types of lymphomas may be caused by Epstein–Barr viruses.

The third most common tumors involve the female reproductive system. Brain tumors other than lymphomas occur in approximately 10% of all patients. The remaining 30% of tumors are a mixture. Kaposi's sarcoma is not uncommon.

E. Suicide

Suicides are the fourth most common cause of death after transplantation. It is obviously stressful for these patients to live on borrowed time. No thorough investigation seems to exist with reference to this problem. Awareness of the problem and psychiatric consultation when appropriate is necessary.

F. Other Medical Problems

Other medical complications that occur late after transplantation are frequently induced by prednisone. Musculoskeletal problems include steroid myopathy, hypophosphatemia, and aseptic necrosis. Some of these complications may be decreased by a reduction in the dose of prednisone or conversion to every-other-day therapy. The most common site of aseptic necrosis is the femoral head. It has also been described in the tibia, calcaneus, and humerus. Prosthetic replacement or arthroplasty is the preferred treatment for patients with pronounced clinical symptoms such as pain or difficulty in locomotion. The initial success rate with surgery has been quite good.

Eye problems include infections as mentioned previously in this chapter. Cataracts occur in 30% of patients. They usually occur many months after transplantation and are centrally located. They usually interfere with vision only in bright light such as in the sun or when meeting cars with headlights on during the night. Removal of the lens is necessary in patients with significant visual impairment.

Many endocrine disorders occur in these patients. Addisonian crisis is a constant threat but has rarely been described, probably because of awareness of this problem. The patient needs to be protected with parenteral cortisone during operations or other catastrophic illnesses. Secondary diabetes develops in approximately 15% of patients. It is more common in patients over 40 years of age and in obese females. Nonketotic hyperosmolar coma has been the presenting symptom in several such patients. Hyperparathyroidism is not a common problem in renal transplant patients. Although mild hypercalcemia may be present in many patients, symptomatic hyperparathyroidism requiring surgery is quite rare. Other renal complications such as hyperchloremic acidosis may occur but tends to disappear spontaneously after months or years and rarely causes any clinical problems.

G. Late Loss of the Transplanted Kidney

Late loss of the transplanted kidney occurs with an unknown frequency. It may be caused by chronic rejection, recurrence of the original disease, or de novo glomerulonephritis. If transplant malfunction occurs in the late posttransplant period, appropriate investigations including [^{131}I]hippuran renogram and ultrasound examination of the kidney must be performed. Computerized tomography and renal allograft biopsy are sometimes necessary. Some patients suffer from chronic vascular rejection. There is no known treatment for this. When the diagnosis of chronic rejection is established, high-dose prednisone must not be used.

The exact incidence of recurrence is not known, but most of the common kidney diseases do not seem to recur. Included in this category are most forms of glomerulonephritis, pyelonephritis, nephrosclerosis, and polycystic disease. Only certain diseases seem to recur with increased frequency in the renal allografts. Thus, microvascular disease is seen commonly in the renal allografts of diabetic patients. However, renal malfunction does not occur for at least 8 to 10 years. Focal glomerulosclerosis, if associated with mesangial proliferation, is frequently associated with rapid recurrence and renal transplant malfunction. By contrast, if there is no mesangial proliferation, such recurrence seems to be uncommon, and the patient can be safely transplanted. Membranoproliferative glomerulonephritis with dense deposits also recurs and ultimately leads to transplant loss. Immunoglobulin A nephritis is seen frequently in allograft biopsies but rarely associated with renal malfunction.

Anti-GBM nephritis (Goodpasture's syndrome) also recurs in the transplanted kidney. However, if the patient's own kidneys have been removed, and the transplant surgery is delayed until the anti-GBM antibodies have disappeared, the risk of recurrence is considerably decreased. Oxalosis recurs in approximately two-thirds of the patients, in one-third of these rather fast. Rapidly progressive cresenteric glomerulonephritis, hemolytic uremic syndrome, scleroderma, membranous glomerulonephritis, amyloidosis, and anaphylactoid purpura nephritis have been reported to occur in the transplanted kidney. The incidence, however, is quite low in these disorders. Only isolated case reports exist in the literature. Recurrence in the renal allografts has not been reported in patients with Wegener's granulomatosis, Fabry's disease, cystinosis, myeloma, and lupus erythematosus.

The problem of recurrence is particularly confusing, as chronic rejection may take a varied form and mimic many primary glomerular diseases. A variety of circulating immune complexes are commonly found in transplant recipients, but the association with these and *de novo* glomerulonephritis remains to be delineated. There is no treatment known for these disorders except to return the patient to chronic dialysis when the transplant function deteriorates.

H. Return to Dialysis

Whatever is the cause of death in the late posttransplant period, it is often associated with malfunction of the transplanted kidney. The association of renal dysfunction and immunosuppression is a lethal one. Patients should therefore be returned to dialysis at a lower serum creatinine level than in patients who have chronic renal failure but are not receiving immunosuppressive drugs. It is advantageous to plot the serum creatinine level of patients developing renal insufficiency on a hyperbolic scale rather than simply estimating the progression without such an accurate measurement. It is probably best to return the patient when the serum creatinine remains persistently high at 5 or 6 mg/dl. If severe hypertension is present, an even earlier return to dialysis is indicated. Vascular access surgery should be performed many months before the patients are actually returned to dialysis.

Table V. Causes of Death in 61 of 526
Patients (11.6%) Surviving 3–14 Years
after Transplantation

Infection	16	(25%)
Cardiovascular accidents	20	(32%)
Liver failure	7	(11%)
Suicide	5	(9%)
Malignancy	4	(7%)
Gastrointestinal problems	4	(7%)
Other	5	(9%)
Total	61	(100%)
Renal failure present	23	(38%)

I. Causes of Death

Table V summarizes the causes of death occurring after 3 to 5 years and up to 15 years following transplantation. Infections, which have been the most common cause of death during the first few years after transplantation, have dropped to second place, and vascular complications have become the leading causes of death in the late posttransplant period. Diseases of the liver are the third most common, followed by suicide. Uremia, hyperparathyroidism, and other rare causes make up the remaining percentages.

SUGGESTED READINGS

Guttmann RD: Renal transplantation. N Engl J Med 301:975–982, 1038–1048, 1979.

Kjellstrand CM, Simmons RL: Long-term survivors after renal transplantation, in Avram AA (ed): Prevention of Kidney Disease and Survival on Dialysis. New York, Plenum Press, 1981, pp 281–290.

Kjellstrand CM, Casali RE, Simmons RL, et al: Etiology and prognosis in acute post-transplant renal failure. Am J Med 61:190–199, 1976.

McGeown MG, Douglas JF, Brown WA, et al: Advantages of low dose steroid from the day after renal transplantation. Transplantation. 29:287–289, 1980.

Nephritogenic immunopathologic mechanisms and human renal transplants: The problem of recurrent glomerulonephritis, editorial. Kidney Int 10:135–138, 1976.

Opelz G, Graver B, Terasaki PI: Induction of high kidney graft survival rate by multiple transfusions. Lancet 1:1223–1225, 1981.

Peterson PK, Balfour HH, Fryd DS, et al: Fever in renal transplant recipients: Causes, prognostic significance and changing patterns at the University of Minnesota Hospital. Am J Med 71:345–351, 1981.

Rao KV, Smith EJ, Alexander JW, et al: Thromboembolic disease in renal allograft recipients. Arch Surg 111:1086–1092, 1976.

Standards Committee of the American Society of Transplant Surgeons: Current results and expectations of renal transplantation. JAMA 246:1330–1331, 1981.

Zoller KM, Cho SI, Cohen JJ: Cessation of immunosuppressive therapy after successful transplantation: A national survey. Kidney Int 18:110–114, 1980.

Index